THIRD EDITION

BASIC BIOMECHANICS
of the
MUSCULOSKELETAL
SYSTEM

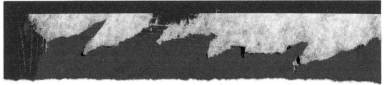

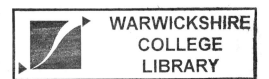

BASIC BIOMECHANICS
of the
MUSCULOSKELETAL SYSTEM

Margareta Nordin, P.T., Dr. Sci.
Director, Occupational and Industrial Orthopaedic Center (OIOC)
Hospital for Joint Diseases Orthopaedic Institute
Mt. Sinai NYU Health
Program of Ergonomics and Biomechanics, New York University
Research Professor
Department of Orthopaedics and Environmental Health Science
School of Medicine, New York University
New York, New York

Victor H. Frankel, M.D., Ph.D., KNO
President Emeritus
Hospital for Joint Diseases Orthopaedic Institute
Professor of Orthopaedic Surgery
New York University School of Medicine
New York, New York

Dawn Leger, Ph.D., Developmental Editor
Kajsa Forssen, Illustrator
Angela Lis, P.T., M.A., Editorial Assistant

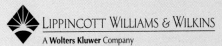
LIPPINCOTT WILLIAMS & WILKINS
A **Wolters Kluwer** Company
Philadelphia · Baltimore · New York · London
Buenos Aires · Hong Kong · Sydney · Tokyo

Editor: John Butler
Managing Editor: Ulita Lushnycky
Marketing Manager: Debby Hartman
Production Editor: Paula C. Williams
Compositor: Graphic World, Inc.
Printer: Courier

Library of Congress Cataloging-in-Publication Data

Basic biomechanics of the musculoskeletal system / [edited by] Margareta Nordin,
Victor H. Frankel.—3rd ed.
  p. ; cm.
Includes bibliographical references.
ISBN 0-683-30247-7
 1. Human mechanics. I. Nordin, Margareta. II. Frankel, Victor H. (Victor Hirsch),
1925-
 [DNLM: 1. Biomechanics. WE 103 B311 2001]
QP303 .N57 2001
612.7'6—dc21   00-065519

To purchase additional copies of this book call our customer service department at **(800) 638-3030** or fax orders to **(301) 824-7390**. International cus-
tomers should call **(301) 714-2324.**

02 03 04 05
2 3 4 5 6 7 8 9 10

This book, and all our work, is dedicated to students of biomechanics, past, present, and future.

Foreword

Mechanics and biology have always fascinated humankind. The importance of understanding the biomechanics of the musculoskeletal system cannot be underestimated. Much attention has been paid in recent years to genetic and biomolecular research, but the study of the mechanics of structure and of the whole body system is still of immense importance. Musculoskeletal ailments are among the most prevalent disorders in the world and will continue to grow as the population ages.

Since the days when I first studied biomechanics in Sweden with Carl Hirsch, through my years as an orthopaedic surgeon, teacher, and researcher, I have always emphasized combining basic and applied research with clinical experience. This text represents my fifth effort to integrate biomechanical knowledge into clinical training for patient care. It is not a simple task but by relating the basic concepts of biomechanics to everyday life, rehabilitation, orthopaedics, traumatology, and patient care are greatly enhanced. Biomechanics is a multidisciplinary specialty, and so we have made a special effort to invite contributors from many disciplines so that individuals from different fields may feel comfortable reading this book.

Together with an invaluable team, Margareta Nordin and I have produced this third edition of *Basic Biomechanics of the Musculoskeletal System.* The new edition is sharpened and improved thanks to the input from the students and residents in orthopaedics that during the past 10 years have used the text. This book is written for students and with a major input from students and will hopefully be used to educate students and residents for many years to come. Although the basic information contained in the book remains largely unchanged, a considerable amount of extra information has been provided throughout. We have also made a special point to document with the key references any significant changes in the field of biomechanics and rehabilitation.

It has always been my interest to bridge the gap between engineering knowledge and clinical care and practice. This book is written primarily for clinicians such as orthopaedists, physical and occupational therapists, clinical ergonomists, chiropractors, and other health professionals who are acquiring a working knowledge of biomechanical principles for use in the evaluation and treatment of musculoskeletal dysfunction. We only hope that if you find this book interesting, you will seek more in-depth study in the field of biomechanics. Enjoy it, discuss it, and become a better clinician and/or researcher.

We are extremely proud that *Basic Biomechanics of the Musculoskeletal System* has been designated "A Classic" by the publishers, Lippincott Williams & Wilkins. We thank the readers, students, professors, and all who acquire the text and use it.

Victor H. Frankel, M.D., Ph.D., KNO

Preface

Biomechanics uses physics and engineering concepts to describe the motion undergone by the various body segments and forces acting on these body parts during normal activities. The inter-relationship of force and motion is important and must be understood if rational treatment programs are to be applied to musculoskeletal disorders. Deleterious effects may be produced if the forces acting on the areas with disorders rise to high levels during exercise or other activities of daily living.

The purpose of this text is to acquaint the readers with the force-motion relationship within the musculoskeletal system and the various techniques used to understand these relationships. The third edition of *Basic Biomechanics of the Musculoskeletal System* is intended for use as a textbook either in conjunction with an introductory biomechanics course or for independent study. The third edition has been changed in many ways, but it is still a book that is designed for use by students who are interested in and want to learn about biomechanics. It is primarily written for students who do not have an engineering background but who want to understand the most basic concepts in biomechanics and physics and how these apply to the human body.

Input from students has greatly improved this third edition. We have used the book for 10 years in the Program of Ergonomics and Biomechanics at New York University, and it is the students and residents who have suggested the changes and who have continuously shown an interest in developing and improving this book. This edition has been further strengthened by the contribution of the students over the past year. We formed focus groups to understand better what the students wanted and applied their suggestions wherever possible. We retained the selected examples to illustrate the concepts needed for basic knowledge of the musculoskeletal biomechanics; we also have kept the important engineering concepts throughout the volume. We have added four chapters on applied biomechanics topics. Patient case studies and calculation boxes have been added to each chapter. We incorporated flowcharts throughout the book as teaching tools.

The text will serve as guide to a deeper understanding of musculoskeletal biomechanics gained through further reading and independent research. The information presented should also guide the reader in assessing the literature on biomechanics. We have attempted to provide therapeutic examples but it was not our purpose to cover this area; instead, we have described the underlying basis for rational therapeutic or exercise programs.

An introductory chapter describes the importance of the study of biomechanics, and an appendix on the international system of measurements serves as an introduction to the physical measurements used throughout the book. The reader needs no more than basic knowledge of mathematics to fully comprehend the material in the book, but it is important to review the appendix on the SI System and its application to biomechanics.

The body of the third edition is then divided into three sections. The first section is the Biomechanics of Tissues and Structures of the Musculoskeletal System and covers the basic biomechanics of bone, ligaments, cartilage, tendons, muscles, and nerves. The second section covers the Biomechanics of Joints, including every joint system in the human body. Chapters range from the foot and ankle through the cervical spine, and cover every joint in between. The third section covers some topics in Applied Biomechanics, including chapters on fracture fixation; arthroplasty; sitting, standing and lying; and gait. These are basic chapters that serve to introduce topics in applied biomechanics; they are not in-depth explorations of the subject.

Finally, we hope that the revision and expansion of this third edition of *Basic Biomechanics* *of the Musculoskeletal System* will bring about an increased awareness of the importance of biomechanics. It has never been our intention to completely cover the subject, but instead provide a basic introduction to the field that will lead to further study of this important topic.

Margareta Nordin and Victor H. Frankel

Acknowledgments

This book was made possible through the outstanding contributions of many individuals. The chapter authors' knowledge and understanding of the basic concepts of biomechanics and their wealth of experience have brought both breadth and depth to this work. Over the past 10 years, questions raised by students and residents have made this book a better teaching tool. The Third Edition could not have been done without the students who have shared their comments and really scrutinized the Second Edition. There are too many names to list here, but we thank each student who asked a question or made a suggestion during the course of his or her studies. Special thanks to the students who participated in several focus groups, whose input was invaluable in finalizing the contents and design of the text.

We are honored and grateful for the contributions of everyone who has worked to prepare this new edition. We can honestly say that this third edition is written for the student and by students and residents who leave the classroom with the knowledge to enhance our life and existence.

A book of this size with its large number of figures, legends, and references cannot be produced without a strong editorial team. As project editor, Dawn Leger's continuous effort and perseverance and thoughtfulness shines through the entire book. She has contributed not just to the editing but also to logistics, and as a stylist, as an innovator, and a friend. Our editorial assistant, Angela Lis, is a physical therapist and recent recipient of the MA degree in Ergonomics and Biomechanics from NYU. As a recent graduate, Angela was also a recent user of the book, and she devoted several months to help finalize this edition. She created the flowcharts and scrutinized all the figures, patient cases, and calculation boxes. Angela took this book to her heart, and we are all the better for her passion and attention to detail.

The illustrator, Kajsa Forssen, has now worked on all three editions of this text. Her never-failing grasp of biomechanical illustrations, her simplicity and exactness of figures, is always appreciated. In drawing all the figures and graphs, she considers how they would translate into a slide or into a computer-generated presentation. Kajsa Forssen is one of the top illustrators that we have ever worked with, and she has been an important member of the publication team.

This book was also made when publication companies merged and merged again, and in the end we are deeply grateful to Ulita Lushnycky, who has with her team at Lippincott Williams & Wilkins been responsible for the production. She has worked with tremendous energy and positive thinking, put the book together in record speed, and we forward our sincerest gratitude to her. We are also thankful for a development grant provided by Lippincott Williams & Wilkins to finance this effort.

Our colleagues at the Occupational and Industrial Orthopaedic Center and the Department of Orthopaedics of the Hospital for Joint Diseases Orthopaedic Institute functioned as critical reviewers and contributors to the chapters. Special thanks is extended to David Goldsheyder for assistance in reviewing the biomechanical calculation boxes, to Marco Campello as a contributor and reviewer, and to Shira Schecter-Weiner for contributing to the spine chapter. Much thanks to Dr. Mark Pitman for supplying vital x-rays for the new edition. We are particularly grateful to Dr. Markus Pietrek for contributing with the latest on intra-abdominal pressure, to Dr. Ali Sheikhzadeh for reviewing chapters and contributing new references, to Dr. Tobias Lorenz for his work on the first section, and to all other staff at the Occupational and Industrial Orthopaedic Center who have been managing the center while we are absorbed with the book.

We are most grateful to Drs. Bejjani, Lindh, Pitman, Peterson, and Stuchin for their contributions to the second edition which served as a framework for the updated third edition.

The third edition of *Basic Biomechanics of the Musculoskeletal System* was supported throughout its production by the Research and Development Foundation of the Hospital for Joint Diseases Orthopaedic Institute and the hospital administration, to whom we forward our sincere gratitude.

To all who helped, we say again, thank you and TACK SA MYCKET.

Margareta Nordin and Victor H. Frankel

Contributors

Gunnar B. J. Andersson, M.D., Ph.D.
Professor and Chairman
Department of Orthopaedic Surgery
Rush-Presbyterian-St. Luke's Medical Center
Chicago, IL

Thomas P. Andriacchi, Ph.D.
Biomechanical Engineering Division
Stanford University
Stanford, CA

Sherry I. Backus, M.D., P.T.
Senior Research Physical Therapist and Research Associate
Motion Analysis Laboratory
Hospital for Special Surgery
New York, NY

Ann E. Barr, Ph.D., P.T.
Assistant Professor
Physical Therapy Department
College of Allied Health Professionals
Temple University
Philadelphia, PA

Fadi Joseph Bejjani, M.D., Ph.D.
Director of Occupational Musculoskeletal Diseases
Department
University Rehabilitation Association
Newark, NJ

Maureen Gallagher Birdzell, Ph.D.
Department of Orthopaedic Surgery
Hospital for Joint Diseases/Mt. Sinai NYU Health
New York, NY

Marco Campello, P.T., M.A.
Associate Clinical Director
Occupational and Industrial Orthopaedic Center
Hospital for Joint Diseases/Mt. Sinai NYU Health
New York, NY

Dennis R. Carter, Ph.D.
Professor
Biomechanical Engineering Program
Stanford University
Stanford, CA

Craig J. Della Valle, M.D.
NYU-HJD Department of Orthopaedic Surgery
Hospital for Joint Diseases
School of Medicine
New York University
New York, NY

Victor H. Frankel, M.D., Ph.D., KNO
President Emeritus
Hospital for Joint Diseases Orthopaedic Institute
Professor of Orthopaedic Surgery
New York University School of Medicine
New York, NY

Ross Todd Hockenbury, M.D.
River City Orthopaedic Surgeons
Louisville, KY

Clark T. Hung, Ph.D.
Assistant Professor
Department of Mechanical Engineering and Center for
Biomedical Engineering
Columbia University
New York, NY

Debra E. Hurwitz, Ph.D.
Assistant Professor
Department of Orthopaedics
Rush-Presbyterian-St. Luke's Medical Center
Chicago, IL

Laith M. Jazrawi, M.D.
NYU-HJD Department of Orthopaedic Surgery
Hospital for Joint Diseases
School of Medicine
New York University
New York, NY

Frederick J. Kummer, Ph.D.
Associate Director, Musculoskeletal Research Center
Hospital for Joint Diseases/Mt. Sinai NYU Health
Research Professor, NYU-HJD Department of Orthopaedic
Surgery
School of Medicine
New York University
New York, NY

Dawn Leger, Ph.D.
Adjunct Assistant Professor
NYU-HJD Department of Orthopaedics
School of Medicine
New York University
New York, NY

Jane Bear-Lehman, Ph.D., OTR, FAOTA
Assistant Professor of Clinical Occupational Therapy
Department of Occupational Therapy
Columbia University College of Physicians and Surgeons
New York, NY

Margareta Lindh, M.D., Ph.D.
Associate Professor
Department of Physical Medicine and Rehabilitation
Sahlgren Hospital
Gothenburg University
Gothenburg, Sweden

Angela Lis, M.A., P.T.
Research Physical Therapist
Occupational and Industrial Orthopaedic Center
Hospital for Joint Diseases/Mt. Sinai NYU Health
New York, NY
Associate Professor
Physical Therapy Program
Corporación Universitaria Iberoamericana
Bogotá, COLOMBIA

Tobias Lorenz, M.D.
Fellow
Occupational and Industrial Orthopaedic Center
Hospital for Joint Diseases/Mt. Sinai NYU Health
New York, NY

Goran Lundborg, M.D.
Professor
Department of Hand Surgery
Lunds University
Malmo Allmanna Sjukhus
Malmo, Sweden

Ronald Moskovich, M.D.
Associate Chief
Spine Surgery
NYU-HJD Department of Orthopaedic Surgery
Hospital for Joint Diseases
School of Medicine
New York University
New York, NY

Van C. Mow, Ph.D.
Director
Orthopaedic Research Laboratory
Department of Orthopaedic Surgery
Columbia University
New York, NY

Robert R. Myers, Ph.D.
Associate Professor
Department of Anesthesiology
University of California San Diego
La Jolla, CA

Margareta Nordin, P.T., Dr. Sci.
Director, Occupational and Industrial Orthopaedic Center (OIOC)
Hospital for Joint Diseases Orthopaedic Institute
Mt. Sinai NYU Health
Program of Ergonomics and Biomechanics
New York University
Research Professor
Department of Orthopaedics and Environmental Health Science
School of Medicine, New York University
New York, NY

Kjell Olmarker, M.D., Ph.D.
Associate Professor
Department of Orthopaedics
Sahlgren Hospital
Gothenburg University
Gothenburg, Sweden

Nihat Özkaya (deceased)
Associate Professor
Occupational and Industrial Orthopaedic Center
Hospital for Joint Diseases
Research Associate Professor
Department of Environmental Medicine
New York University
New York, NY

Lars Peterson, M.D., Ph.D.
Gruvgat 6
Vastra Frolunda
Sweden

Mark I. Pitman, M.D.
Clinical Associate Professor
NYU-HJD Department of Orthopaedic Surgery
School of Medicine
New York University
New York, NY

Andrew S. Rokito, M.D.
Associate Chief, Sports Medicine Service
Assistant Professor
NYU-HJD Department of Orthopaedic Surgery
School of Medicine
New York University
New York, NY

Bjorn Rydevik, M.D., Ph.D.
Professor and Chairman
Department of Orthopaedics
Sahlgren Hospital
Gothenburg University
Gothenburg, Sweden

G. James Sammarco, M.D.
Program Director
Fellowship in Adult Reconstructive Surgery
Foot and Ankle Orthopaedic Surgery Program
The Center for Orthopaedic Care, Inc.
Volunteer Professor of Orthopaedic Surgery
Department of Orthopaedics
University of Cincinnati Medical Center
Cincinnati, OH

Chris J. Snijders, Ph.D.
Professor
Biomedical Physics and Technology
Faculty of Medicine
Erasmus University
Rotterdam, The Netherlands

Steven Stuchin, M.D.
Director Clinical Orthopaedic Services
Director Arthritis Service
Associate Professor
NYU-HJD Department of Orthopaedics
School of Medicine
New York University
New York, NY

Shira Schecter Weiner, M.A., P.T.
Research Physical Therapist
Occupational and Industrial Orthopaedic Center
Hospital for Joint Diseases/Mt. Sinai NYU Health
New York, NY

Joseph D. Zuckerman, M.D.
Professor and Chairman
NYU-HJD Department of Orthopaedic Surgery
Hospital for Joint Diseases
School of Medicine
New York University
New York, NY

Contents

BASIC BIOMECHANICS
of the
MUSCULOSKELETAL SYSTEM

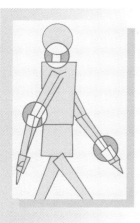

CHAPTER 1

Introduction to Biomechanics: Basic Terminology and Concepts

Nihat Özkaya, Dawn Leger

Introduction

Biomechanics is considered a branch of bioengineering and biomedical engineering. Bioengineering is an interdisciplinary field in which the principles and methods from engineering, basic sciences, and technology are applied to design, test, and manufacture equipment for use in medicine and to understand, define, and solve problems in physiology and biology. Bioengineering is one of several specialty areas that come under the general field of biomedical engineering.

Biomechanics considers the applications of classical mechanics to the analysis of biological and physiological systems. Different aspects of biomechanics utilize different parts of applied mechanics. For example, the principles of statics have been applied to analyze the magnitude and nature of forces involved in various joints and muscles of the musculoskeletal system. The principles of dynamics have been utilized for motion description, gait analysis, and segmental motion analysis and have many applications in sports mechanics. The mechanics of solids provides the necessary tools for developing the field constitutive equations for biological systems that are used to evaluate their functional behavior under different load conditions. The principles of fluid mechanics have been used to investigate blood flow in the circulatory system, air flow in the lung, and joint lubrication.

Research in biomechanics is aimed at improving our knowledge of a very complex structure—the human body. Research activities in biomechanics can be divided into three areas: experimental studies, model analyses, and applied research. Experimental studies in biomechanics are done to determine the mechanical properties of biological materials, including the bone, cartilage, muscle, tendon, ligament, skin, and blood as a whole or as parts constituting them. Theoretical studies involving mathematical model analyses have also been an important component of research in biomechanics. In general, a model that is based on experimental findings can be used to predict the effect of environmental and operational factors without resorting to laboratory experiments.

Applied research in biomechanics is the application of scientific knowledge to benefit human beings. We know that musculoskeletal injury and illness is one of the primary occupational hazards in industrialized countries. By learning how the musculoskeletal system adjusts to common work conditions and by developing guidelines to assure that manual work conforms more closely to the physical limitations of the human body and to natural body movements, these injuries may be combatted.

Basic Concepts

Biomechanics of the musculoskeletal system requires a good understanding of basic mechanics. The basic terminology and concepts from mechanics and physics are utilized to describe internal forces of the human body. The objective of studying these forces is to understand the loading condition of soft tissues and their mechanical responses. The purpose of this section is to review the basic concepts of applied mechanics that are used in biomechanical literature and throughout this book.

SCALARS, VECTORS, AND TENSORS

Most of the concepts in mechanics are either scalar or vector. A scalar quantity has a magnitude only. Concepts such as mass, energy, power, mechanical work, and temperature are scalar quantities. For example, it is sufficient to say that an object has 80 kilograms (kg) of mass. A vector quantity, conversely, has both a magnitude and a direction associated with it. Force, moment, velocity, and acceleration are examples of vector quantities. To describe a force fully, one must state how much force is applied and in which direction it is applied. The magnitude of a vector is also a scalar quantity. The magnitude of any quantity (scalar or vector) is always a positive number corresponding to the numerical measure of that quantity.

Graphically, a vector is represented by an arrow. The orientation of the arrow indicates the line of action and the arrowhead denotes the direction and sense of the vector. If more than one vector must be shown in a single drawing, the length of each arrow must be proportional to the magnitude of the vector it represents. Both scalars and vectors are special forms of a more general category of all quantities in mechanics called tensors. Scalars are also known as "zero-order tensors," whereas vectors are "first-order tensors." Concepts such as stress and strain, conversely, are "second-order tensors."

FORCE VECTOR

Force can be defined as mechanical disturbance or load. When an object is pushed or pulled, a force is applied on it. A force is also applied when a ball is thrown or kicked. A force acting on an object may deform the object, change its state of motion, or both. Forces may be classified in various ways according to their effects on the objects to which they are applied or according to their orientation as compared with one another. For example, a force may be internal or external, normal (perpendicular) or tangential; tensile, compressive, or shear; gravitational (weight); or frictional. Any two or more forces acting on a single body may be coplanar (acting on a two-dimensional plane surface); collinear (have a common line of action); concurrent (lines of action intersecting at a single point); or parallel. Note that weight is a special form of force. The weight of an object on Earth is the gravitational force exerted by Earth on the mass of that object. The magnitude of the weight of an object on Earth is equal to the mass of the object times the magnitude of the gravitational acceleration, which is approximately 9.8 meters per second squared (m/s^2). For example, a 10-kg object weighs approximately 98 newtons (N) on Earth. The direction of weight is always vertically downward.

TORQUE AND MOMENT VECTORS

The effect of a force on the object it is applied upon depends on how the force is applied and how the object is supported. For example, when pulled, an open door will swing about the edge along which it is hinged to the wall. What causes the door to swing is the torque generated by the applied force about an axis that passes through the hinges of the door. If one stands on the free-end of a diving board, the board will bend. What bends the board is the moment of the body weight about the fixed end of the board. In general, torque is associated with the rotational and twisting action of applied forces, while moment is related to the bending action. However, the mathematical definition of moment and torque is the same.

Torque and moment are vector quantities. The magnitude of the torque or moment of a force about a point is equal to the magnitude of the force times the length of the shortest distance between the point and the line of action of the force, which is known as the lever or moment arm. Con-

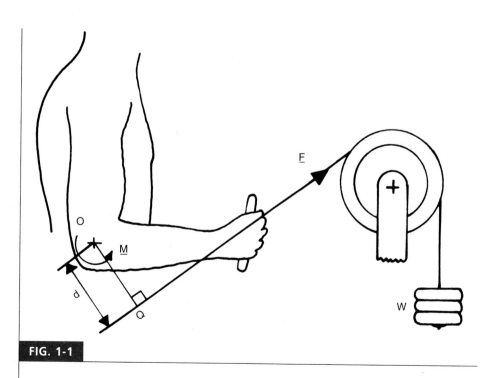

FIG. 1-1

Definition of torque. *Reprinted with permission from Özkaya, N. (1998). Biomechanics. In W.N. Rom,* Environmental and Occupational Medicine *(3rd ed., pp. 1437–1454). New York: Lippincott-Raven.*

sider a person on an exercise apparatus who is holding a handle that is attached to a cable (Fig. 1-1). The cable is wrapped around a pulley and attached to a weight pan. The weight in the weight ̥ stretches the cable such that the magnitude F the tensile force in the cable is equal to the ̥ght of the weight pan. This force is transmitted ̥he person's hand through the handle. At this in- ̥nt, if the cable attached to the handle makes an angle θ with the horizontal, then the force $\underline{F}$ exerted by the cable on the person's hand also makes an angle θ with the horizontal. Let O be a point on the axis of rotation of the elbow joint. To determine the magnitude of the moment due to force $\underline{F}$ about O, extend the line of action of force $\underline{F}$ and drop a line from O that cuts the line of action of F at right angles. If the point of intersection of the two lines is Q, then the distance d between O and Q is the lever arm, and the magnitude of the moment $\underline{M}$ of force $\underline{F}$ about the elbow joint is M = dF. The direction of the moment vector is perpendicular to the plane defined by the line of action of $\underline{F}$ and line OQ, or for this two-dimensional case, it is counterclockwise.

NEWTON'S LAWS

Relatively few basic laws govern the relationship between applied forces and corresponding motions. Among these, the laws of mechanics introduced by Sir Isaac Newton (1642–1727) are the most important. Newton's first law states that an object at rest will remain at rest or an object in motion will move in a straight line with constant velocity if the net force acting on the object is zero. Newton's second law states that an object with a nonzero net force acting on it will accelerate in the direction of the net force and that the magnitude of the acceleration will be proportional to the magnitude of the net force. Newton's second law can be formulated as $\underline{F} = m \underline{a}$. Here, $\underline{F}$ is the applied force, m is the mass of the object, and $\underline{a}$ is the linear (translational) acceleration of the object on which the force is applied. If more than one force is acting on the object, then $\underline{F}$ represents the net or the resultant force (the vector sum of all forces). Another way of stating Newton's second law of motion is $\underline{M} = I \underline{\alpha}$, where $\underline{M}$ is the net or resultant moment of all forces acting on the object, I is the mass moment of inertia of the object, and $\underline{\alpha}$ is the angular (rotational) acceleration of the object. The mass m and mass moment of inertia I in these equations of motion are measures of resistance to changes in mo-

tion. The larger the inertia of an object, the more difficult it is to set in motion or to stop if it is already in motion.

Newton's third law states that to every action there is a reaction and that the forces of action and reaction between interacting objects are equal in magnitude, opposite in direction, and have the same line of action. This law has important applications in constructing free-body diagrams.

FREE-BODY DIAGRAMS

Free-body diagrams are constructed to help identify the forces and moments acting on individual parts of a system and to ensure the correct use of the equations of mechanics to analyze the system. For this purpose, the parts constituting a system are isolated from their surroundings and the effects of surroundings are replaced by proper forces and moments.

The human musculoskeletal system consists of many parts that are connected to one another through a complex tendon, ligament, muscle, and joint structure. In some analyses, the objective may be to investigate the forces involved at and around various joints of the human body for different postural and load conditions. Such analyses can be carried out by separating the body into two parts at the joint of interest and drawing the free-body diagram of one of the parts. For example, consider the arm illustrated in Figure 1-2. Assume that the forces involved at the elbow joint are to be analyzed. As illustrated in Figure 1-2, the entire body is separated into two at the elbow joint and the free-body diagram of the forearm is drawn (Fig. 1-2B). Here,

$\underline{F}$ is the force applied to the hand by the handle of the cable attached to the weight in the weight pan,

$\underline{W}$ is the total weight of the lower arm acting at the center of gravity of the lower arm,

$\underline{F}_{M1}$ is the force exerted by the biceps on the radius,

$\underline{F}_{M3}$ is the force exerted by the brachioradialis muscles on the radius,

$\underline{F}_{M2}$ is the force exerted by the brachialis muscles on the ulna, and

$\underline{F}_J$ is the resultant reaction force at the humero-ulnar and humeroradial joints of the elbow. Note that the muscle and joint reaction forces represent the mechanical effects of the upper arm on the lower arm. Also note that as illustrated in Figure 1-2A (which is not a complete free-body diagram), equal magnitude but opposite muscle and joint reaction forces act on the upper arm as well.

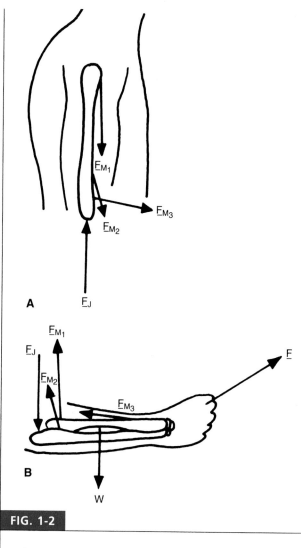

FIG. 1-2

Forces involved at and around the elbow joint and the free-body diagram of the lower arm. *Reprinted with permission from Özkaya, N. (1998). Biomechanics. In W.N. Rom,* Environmental and Occupational Medicine *(3rd ed., pp. 1437–1454). New York: Lippincott-Raven.*

CONDITIONS FOR EQUILIBRIUM

Statics is an area within applied mechanics that is concerned with the analysis of forces on rigid bodies in equilibrium. A rigid body is one that is assumed to undergo no deformations. In reality, every object or material may undergo deformation to an extent when acted on by forces. In some cases, the amount of deformation may be so small that it may not affect the desired analysis and the object is assumed to be rigid. In mechanics, the term equilib-

rium implies that the body of concern is either at rest or moving with constant velocity. For a body to be in a state of equilibrium, it has to be both in translational and rotational equilibrium. A body is in translational equilibrium if the net force (vector sum of all forces) acting on it is zero. If the net force is zero, then the linear acceleration (time rate of change of linear velocity) of the body is zero, or the linear velocity of the body is either constant or zero. A body is in rotational equilibrium if the net moment (vector sum of the moments of all forces) acting on it is zero. If the net moment is zero, then the angular acceleration (time rate of change of angular velocity) of the body is zero, or the angular velocity of the body is either constant or zero. Therefore, for a body in a state of equilibrium, the equations of motion (Newton's second law) take the following special forms:

$$\Sigma \underline{F} = 0 \text{ and } \Sigma \underline{M} = 0$$

It is important to remember that force and moment are vector quantities. For example, with respect to a rectangular (Cartesian) coordinate system, force and moment vectors may have components in the x, y, and z directions. Therefore, if the net force acting on an object is zero, then the sum of forces acting in each direction must be equal to zero ($\Sigma F_x = 0, \Sigma F_y = 0, \Sigma F_z = 0$). Similarly, if the net moment on an object is zero, then the sum of moments in each direction must also be equal to zero ($\Sigma M_x = 0, \Sigma M_y = 0, \Sigma M_z = 0$). Therefore, for three-dimension force systems there are six conditions of equilibrium. For two-dimensional force systems in the xy-plane, only three of these conditions ($\Sigma F_x = 0, \Sigma F_y = 0,$ and $\Sigma M_z = 0$) need to be checked.

STATICS

The principles of statics (equations of equilibrium) can be applied to investigate the muscle and joint forces involved at and around the joints for various postural positions of the human body and its segments. The immediate purpose of static analysis is to provide answers to questions such as: What tension must the neck extensor muscles exert on the head to support the head in a specified position? When a person bends, what would be the force exerted by the erector spinae on the fifth lumbar vertebra? How does the compression at the elbow, knee, and ankle joints vary with externally applied forces and with different segmental arrangements? How does the force on the femoral head vary with loads carried in the hand? What are the forces involved in various muscle groups and joints during different exercise conditions?

In general, the unknowns in static problems involving the musculoskeletal system are the magnitudes of joint reaction forces and muscle tensions. The mechanical analysis of a skeletal joint requires that we know the vector characteristics of tensions in the muscles, the proper locations of muscle attachments, the weights of body segments, and the locations of the centers of gravity of the body segments. Mechanical models are obviously simple representations of complex systems. Many models are limited by the assumptions that must be made to reduce the system under consideration to a statically determinate one. Any model can be improved by considering the contributions of other muscles, but that will increase the number of unknowns and make the model a statically indeterminate one. To analyze the improved model, the researcher would need additional information related to the muscle forces. This information can be gathered through electromyography measurements of muscle signals or by applying certain optimization techniques. A similar analysis can be made to investigate forces involved at and around other major joints of the musculoskeletal system.

MODES OF DEFORMATION

When acted on by externally applied forces, objects may translate in the direction of the net force and rotate in the direction of the net torque acting on them. If an object is subjected to externally applied forces but is in static equilibrium, then it is most likely that there is some local shape change within the object. Local shape change under the effect of applied forces is known as deformation. The extent of deformation an object may undergo depends on many factors, including the material properties, size, and shape of the object; environmental factors such as heat and humidity; and the magnitude, direction, and duration of applied forces.

One way of distinguishing forces is by observing their tendency to deform the object they are applied upon. For example, the object is said to be in tension if the body tends to elongate and in compression if it tends to shrink in the direction of the applied forces. Shear loading differs from tension and compression in that it is caused by forces acting in directions tangent to the area resisting the forces causing shear, whereas both tension and compression are caused by collinear forces applied perpendicular to the areas on which they act. It is common to call tensile and compressive forces normal or axial forces; shearing forces are tangential forces. Objects also deform when they are subjected to forces that cause bending and torsion, which are related to the moment and torque actions of applied forces.

A material may respond differently to different loading configurations. For a given material, there may be different physical properties that must be considered while analyzing the response of that material to tensile loading as compared with compressive or shear loading. The mechanical properties of materials are established through stress analysis by subjecting them to various experiments such as uniaxial tension and compression, torsion, and bending tests.

NORMAL AND SHEAR STRESSES

Consider the whole bone in Figure 1-3A that is subjected to a pair of tensile forces of magnitude F. The bone is in static equilibrium. To analyze the forces induced within the bone, the method of sections can be applied by hypothetically cutting the bone into two pieces through a plane perpendicular to the long axis of the bone. Because the bone as a whole is in equilibrium, the two pieces must individually be in equilibrium as well. This requires that at the cut section of each piece there is an internal force that is equal in magnitude but opposite in direction to the externally applied force (Fig. 1-3B). The internal force is distributed over the entire cross-sectional area of the cut section, and $\underline{F}$ represents the resultant of the distributed force (Fig. 1-3C). The intensity of this distributed force (force per unit area) is known as stress. For the case shown in Figure 1-3, because the force resultant at the cut section is perpendicular to the plane of the cut, the corresponding stress is called a normal or axial stress. It is customary to use the symbol σ (sigma) to refer to normal stresses. Assuming that the intensity of the distributed force at the cut section is uniform over the cross-sectional area A of the bone, then $\sigma = F/A$. Normal stresses that are caused by forces that tend to stretch (elongate) materials are more specifically known as tensile stresses; those that tend to shrink them are known as compressive stresses. According to the Standard International (SI) unit system (see Appendix), stresses are measured in newton per square meter (N/m^2), which is also known as pascal (Pa).

There is another form of stress, shear stress, which is a measure of the intensity of internal forces acting tangent (parallel) to a plane of cut. For

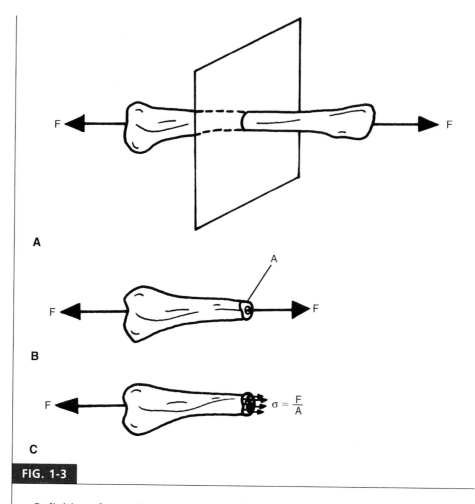

FIG. 1-3

Definition of normal stress. *Reprinted with permission from Özkaya, N. (1998). Biomechanics. In W.N. Rom, Environmental and Occupational Medicine (3rd ed., pp. 1437–1454). New York: Lippincott-Raven.*

example, consider the whole bone in Figure 1-4*A*. The bone is subject to a number of parallel forces that act in planes perpendicular to the long axis of the bone. Assume that the bone is cut into two parts through a plane perpendicular to the long axis of the bone (Fig. 1-4*B*). If the bone as a whole is in equilibrium, its individual parts must be in equilibrium as well. This requires that there must be an internal force at the cut section that acts in a direction tangent to the cut surface. If the magnitudes of the external forces are known, then the magnitude F of the internal force can be calculated by considering the translational and rotational equilibrium of one of the parts constituting the bone. The intensity of the internal force tangent to the cut section is known as the shear stress. It is customary to use the symbol τ (tau) to refer to shear stresses (Fig. 1-4*C*).

Assuming that the intensity of the force tangent to the cut section is uniform over the cross-sectional area A of the bone, then $\tau = F/A$.

NORMAL AND SHEAR STRAINS

Strain is a measure of the degree of deformation. As in the case of stress, two types of strains can be distinguished. A normal strain is defined as the ratio of the change (increase or decrease) in length to the original (undeformed) length, and is commonly denoted with the symbol ϵ (epsilon). Consider the whole bone in Figure 1-5. The total length of the bone is l. If the bone is subjected to a pair of tensile forces, the length of the bone may increase to l' or by an amount $\Delta\lambda = l' - l$. The normal strain is the ratio of the amount of elongation to the original

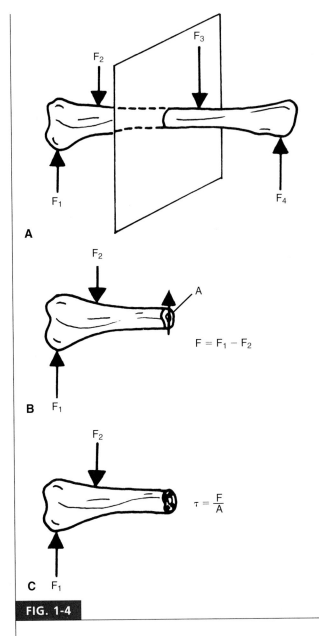

FIG. 1-4

Definition of shear stress. *Reprinted with permission from Özkaya, N. (1998). Biomechanics. In W.N. Rom, Environmental and Occupational Medicine (3rd ed., pp. 1437–1454). New York: Lippincott-Raven.*

length, or $\epsilon = \Delta l / l$. If the length of the bone increases in the direction in which the strain is calculated, then the strain is tensile and positive. If the length of the bone decreases in the direction in which the strain is calculated, then the strain is compressive and negative.

Shear strains are related to distortions caused by shear stresses and are commonly denoted with the symbol γ (gamma). Consider the rectangle (ABCD) shown in Figure 1-6 that is acted on by a pair of tangential forces that deform the rectangle into a parallelogram (AB'C'D). If the relative horizontal displacement of the top and the bottom of the rectangle is d and the height of the rectangle is h, then the average shear strain is the ratio of d and h, which is equal to the tangent of angle γ. The angle γ is usually very small. For small angles, the tangent of the angle is approximately equal to the angle itself measured in radians. Therefore, the average shear strain is $\gamma = d/h$.

Strains are calculated by dividing two quantities measured in units of length. For most applications, the deformations and consequently the strains involved may be very small (e.g., 0.001). Strains can also be given in percentages (e.g., 0.1%).

STRESS-STRAIN DIAGRAMS

Different materials may demonstrate different stress-strain relationships. Consider the stress-strain diagram shown in Figure 1-7. There are six distinct points on the curve, which are labeled as O, P, E, Y, U, and R. Point O is the origin of the stress-strain diagram, which corresponds to the initial (no load, no deformation) state. Point P represents the proportionality limit. Between O and P, stress and strain are linearly proportional and the stress-strain diagram is a straight line. Point E represents the elastic limit. Point Y is the yield point, and the stress σ_y corresponding to the yield point is called the yield strength of the material. At this stress level, considerable elongation (yielding) can occur without a corresponding increase of load. U is the highest stress point on the stress-strain diagram. The stress σ_u is the ultimate strength of the material. The last point on the stress-strain diagram is R, which represents the rupture or failure point. The stress at which the failure occurs is called the rupture strength of the material. For some materials, it may not be easy to distinguish the elastic limit and the yield point. The yield strength of such materials is determined by the offset method, which is applied by drawing a line parallel to the linear section of the stress-strain diagram that passes through a strain level of approximately 0.2%. The intersection of this line with the stress-strain curve is taken to be the yield point, and the stress corresponding to this point is called the apparent yield strength of the material.

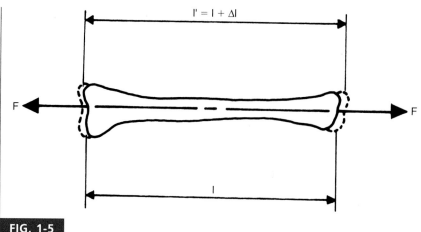

FIG. 1-5

Definition of normal strain. *Reprinted with permission from Özkaya, N. (1998). Biomechanics. In W.N. Rom, Environmental and Occupational Medicine (3rd ed., pp. 1437–1454). New York: Lippincott-Raven.*

Note that a given material may behave differently under different load and environmental conditions. If the curve shown in Figure 1-7 represents the stress-strain relationship for a material under tensile loading, there may be a similar but different curve representing the stress-strain relationship for the same material under compressive or shear loading. Also, temperature is known to alter the relationship between stress and strain. For some materials, the stress-strain relationship may also depend on the rate at which the load is applied on the material.

ELASTIC AND PLASTIC DEFORMATIONS

Elasticity is defined as the ability of a material to resume its original (stress-free) size and shape on removal of applied loads. In other words, if a load

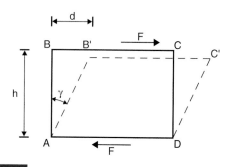

FIG. 1-6

Definition of shear strain. *Reprinted with permission from Özkaya, N. (1998). Biomechanics. In W.N. Rom, Environmental and Occupational Medicine (3rd ed., pp. 1437–1454). New York: Lippincott-Raven.*

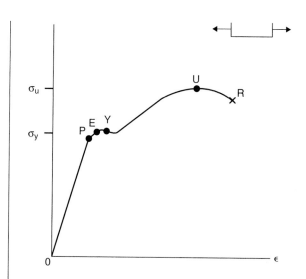

FIG. 1-7

Stress-strain diagrams. *Reprinted with permission from Özkaya, N. (1998). Biomechanics. In W.N. Rom, Environmental and Occupational Medicine (3rd ed., pp. 1437–1454). New York: Lippincott-Raven.*

is applied on a material such that the stress generated in the material is equal to or less than the elastic limit, the deformations that took place in the material will be completely recovered once the applied loads are removed. An elastic material whose stress-strain diagram is a straight line is called a linearly elastic material. For such a material, the stress is linearly proportional to strain. The slope of the stress-strain diagram in the elastic region is called the elastic or Young's modulus of the material, which is commonly denoted by E. Therefore, the relationship between stress and strain for linearly elastic materials is $\sigma = E\epsilon$. This equation that relates normal stress and strain is called a material function. For a given material, different material functions may exist for different modes of deformation. For example, some materials may exhibit linearly elastic behavior under shear loading. For such materials, the shear stress τ is linearly proportional to the shear strain γ, and the constant of proportionality is called the shear modulus, or the modulus of rigidity. If G represents the modulus of rigidity, then $\tau = G\gamma$. Combinations of all possible material functions for a given material form the constitutive equations for that material.

Plasticity implies permanent deformations. Materials may undergo plastic deformations following elastic deformations when they are loaded beyond their elastic limits. Consider the stress-strain diagram of a material under tensile loading (Fig.1-7). Assume that the stresses in the specimen are brought to a level greater than the yield strength of the material. On removal of the applied load, the material will recover the elastic deformation that had taken place by following an unloading path parallel to the initial linearly elastic region. The point where this path cuts the strain axis is called the plastic strain, which signifies the extent of permanent (unrecoverable) shape change that has taken place in the material.

Viscoelasticity is the characteristic of a material that has both fluid and solid properties. Most materials are classified as either fluid or solid. A solid material will deform to a certain extent when an external force is applied. A continuously applied force on a fluid body will cause a continuous deformation (also known as flow). Viscosity is a fluid property that is a quantitative measure of resistance to flow. Viscoelasticity is an example of how areas in applied mechanics can overlap, because it utilizes the principles of both fluid and solid mechanics.

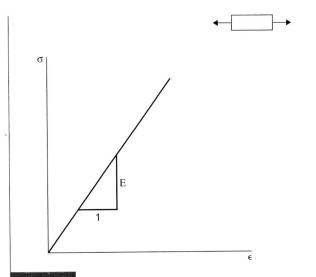

FIG. 1-8

Linearly elastic material behavior. *Reprinted with permission from Özkaya, N. (1998). Biomechanics. In W.N. Rom,* Environmental and Occupational Medicine *(3rd ed., pp. 1437–1454). New York: Lippincott-Raven.*

VISCOELASTICITY

When they are subjected to relatively low stress levels, many materials such as metals exhibit elastic material behavior. They undergo plastic deformations at high stress levels. Elastic materials deform instantaneously when they are subjected to externally applied loads and resume their original shapes almost instantly when the applied loads are removed. For an elastic material, stress is a function of strain only, and the stress-strain relationship is unique (Fig. 1-8). Elastic materials do not exhibit time-dependent behavior. A different group of materials, such as polymer plastics, metals at high temperatures, and almost all biological materials, exhibits gradual deformation and recovery when subjected to loading and unloading. Such materials are called viscoelastic. The response of viscoelastic materials is dependent on how quickly the load is applied or removed. The extent of deformation that viscoelastic materials undergo is dependent on the rate at which the deformation-causing loads are applied. The stress-strain relationship for a viscoelastic material is not unique but is a function of time or the rate at which the stresses and strains are developed in the material (Fig. 1-9). The word "viscoelastic" is made of two words. Viscosity is a fluid property and

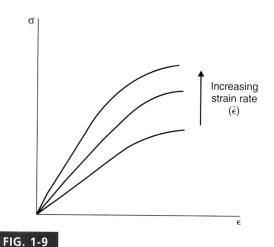

FIG. 1-9

Strain rate-dependent viscoelastic material behavior. *Reprinted with permission from Özkaya, N. (1998). Biomechanics. In W.N. Rom,* Environmental and Occupational Medicine *(3rd ed., pp. 1437–1454). New York: Lippincott-Raven.*

with an instantaneous strain that would remain at a constant level until the load is removed (Fig. 1-10*B*). At the instant when the load is removed, the deformation will instantly and completely recover. To the same constant loading condition, a viscoelastic material will respond with a strain increasing and decreasing gradually. If the material is viscoelastic solid, the recovery will eventually be complete (Fig. 1-10*C*). If the material is viscoelastic fluid, complete recovery will never be achieved and there will be a residue of deformation left in the material (Fig. 1-10*D*). As illustrated in Figure 1-11*A*, a stress-relaxation experiment is conducted

is a measure of resistance to flow. Elasticity is a solid material property. Therefore, viscoelastic materials possess both fluid- and solid-like properties.

For an elastic material, the energy supplied to deform the material (strain energy) is stored in the material as potential energy. This energy is available to return the material to its original (unstressed) size and shape once the applied load is removed. The loading and unloading paths for an elastic material coincide, indicating no loss of energy. Most elastic materials exhibit plastic behavior at high stress levels. For elasto-plastic materials, some of the strain energy is dissipated as heat during plastic deformations. For viscoelastic materials, some of the strain energy is stored in the material as potential energy and some of it is dissipated as heat regardless of whether the stress levels are small or large. Because viscoelastic materials exhibit time-dependent material behavior, the differences between elastic and viscoelastic material responses are most evident under time-dependent loading conditions.

Several experimental techniques have been designed to analyze the time-dependent aspects of material behavior. As illustrated in Figure 1-10*A*, a creep and recovery test is conducted by applying a load on the material, maintaining the load at a constant level for a while, suddenly removing the load, and observing the material response. Under a creep and recovery test, an elastic material will respond

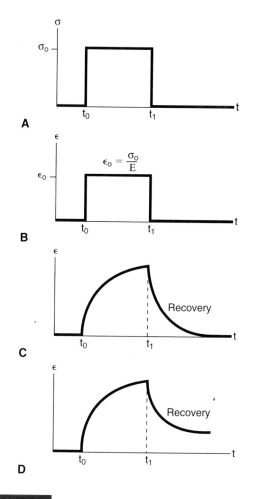

FIG. 1-10

Creep and recovery test. *Reprinted with permission from Özkaya, N. (1998). Biomechanics. In W.N. Rom,* Environmental and Occupational Medicine *(3rd ed., pp. 1437–1454). New York: Lippincott-Raven.*

by straining the material to a level and maintaining the constant strain while observing the stress response of the material. Under a stress-relaxation test, an elastic material will respond with a stress developed instantly and maintained at a constant level (Fig. 1-11*B*). That is, an elastic material will not exhibit a stress-relaxation behavior. A viscoelastic material, conversely, will respond with an initial high stress level that will decrease over time. If the material is a viscoelastic solid, the stress level will never reduce to zero (Fig. 1-11*C*). As illustrated in Figure 1-11*D*, the stress will eventually reduce to zero for a viscoelastic fluid.

MATERIAL PROPERTIES BASED ON STRESS-STRAIN DIAGRAMS

The stress-strain diagrams of two or more materials can be compared to determine which material is relatively stiffer, harder, tougher, more ductile, or more brittle. For example, the slope of the stress-strain diagram in the elastic region represents the elastic modulus that is a measure of the relative stiffness of materials. The higher the elastic modulus, the stiffer the material and the higher its resistance to deformation. A ductile material is one that exhibits a large plastic deformation prior to failure. A brittle material, such as glass, shows a sudden failure (rupture) without undergoing a considerable plastic deformation. Toughness is a measure of the capacity of a material to sustain permanent deformation. The toughness of a material is measured by considering the total area under its stress-strain diagram. The larger this area, the tougher the material. The ability of a material to store or absorb energy without permanent deformation is called the resilience of the material. The resilience of a material is measured by its modulus of resilience, which is equal to the area under the stress-strain curve in the elastic region.

Although they are not directly related to the stress-strain diagrams, other important concepts are used to describe material properties. For example, a material is called homogeneous if its properties do not vary from location to location within the material. A material is called isotropic if its properties are independent of direction. A material is called incompressible if it has a constant density.

PRINCIPAL STRESSES

There are infinitely many possibilities of constructing elements around a given point within a structure. Among these possibilities, there may be

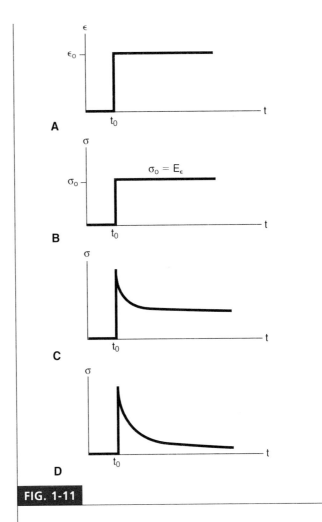

FIG. 1-11

Stress-relaxation experiment. *Reprinted with permission from Özkaya, N. (1998). Biomechanics. In W.N. Rom, Environmental and Occupational Medicine (3rd ed., pp. 1437–1454). New York: Lippincott-Raven.*

one element for which the normal stresses are maximum and minimum. These maximum and minimum normal stresses are called the principal stresses, and the planes whose normals are in the directions of the maximum and minimum stresses are called the principal planes. On a principal plane, the normal stress is either maximum or minimum, and the shear stress is zero. It is known that fracture or material failure occurs along the planes of maximum stresses, and structures must be designed by taking into consideration the maximum stresses involved. Failure by yielding (excessive deformation) may occur whenever the largest principal stress is equal to the yield strength of the material or failure by rupture may occur whenever the largest principal stress is equal to the ultimate strength of the material. For a given structure and loading condition, the principal stresses may be within the limits of operational safety. However, the structure must also be checked for critical shearing stress, called the maximum shear stress. The maximum shear stress occurs on a material element for which the normal stresses are equal.

FATIGUE AND ENDURANCE

Principal and maximum shear stresses are useful in predicting the response of materials to static loading configurations. Loads that may not cause the failure of a structure in a single application may cause fracture when applied repeatedly. Failure may occur after a few or many cycles of loading and unloading, depending on factors such as the amplitude of the applied load, mechanical properties of the material, size of the structure, and operational conditions. Fracture resulting from repeated loading is called fatigue.

Several experimental techniques have been developed to understand the fatigue behavior of materials. Consider the bar shown in Figure 1-12A. Assume that the bar is made of a material whose ultimate strength is σ_u. This bar is first stressed to a mean stress level σ_m and then subjected to a stress fluctuating over time, sometimes tensile and other times compressive (Fig. 1-12B). The amplitude σ_a of the stress is such that the bar is subjected to a maximum tensile stress less than the ultimate strength of the material. This reversible and periodic stress is applied until the bar fractures and the number of cycles N to fracture is recorded. This experiment is repeated on specimens having the same material properties by applying stresses of varying amplitude. A typical result of a fatigue test is plotted in Figure 1-12C on a diagram showing stress amplitude versus number of cycles to failure. For a given N, the corresponding stress value is called the fatigue strength of the material at that number of cycles. For a given stress level, N represents the fatigue life of the material. For some materials, the stress amplitude versus number of cycles curve levels off. The stress σ_e at which the fatigue curve levels off is called the endurance limit of the material. Below the endurance limit, the material has a high probability of not failing in fatigue, regardless of how many cycles of stress are imposed on the material.

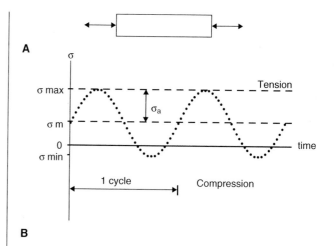

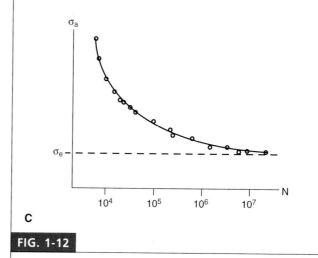

FIG. 1-12

Fatigue and endurance. *Reprinted with permission from Özkaya, N. (1998). Biomechanics. In W.N. Rom, Environmental and Occupational Medicine (3rd ed., pp. 1437–1454). New York: Lippincott-Raven.*

The fatigue behavior of a material depends on several factors. The higher the temperature in which the material is used, the lower the fatigue strength. The fatigue behavior is sensitive to surface imperfections and the presence of discontinuities within the material that can cause stress concentrations. The fatigue failure starts with the creation of a small crack on the surface of the material, which can propagate under the effect of repeated loads, resulting in the rupture of the material.

Orthopaedic devices undergo repeated loading and unloading as a result of the activities of the patients and the actions of their muscles. Over a period of years, a weight-bearing prosthetic device or a fixation device can be subjected to a considerable number of cycles of stress reversals as a result of normal daily activity. This cyclic loading and unloading can cause fatigue failure of the device.

Basic Biomechanics of the Musculoskeletal System

Understanding even a simple task executed by the musculoskeletal system requires a broad, in-depth knowledge of various fields that may include motor control, neurophysiology, physiology, physics, and biomechanics. For example, based on the purpose and intention of a task and the sensory information gathered from the physical environment and orientation of the body and joints, the central nervous system plans a strategy for a task execution. According to the strategy adopted, muscles will be recruited to provide the forces and moments required for the movement and balance of the system. Consequently, the internal forces will be changed and soft tissues will experience different load conditions.

The purpose of this book is to present a well-balanced synthesis of information gathered from various disciplines, providing a basic understanding of biomechanics of the musculoskeletal system. The material presented here is organized to cover three areas of musculoskeletal biomechanics.

PART I: BIOMECHANICS OF TISSUES AND STRUCTURES

The material presented throughout this textbook provides an introduction to basic biomechanics of the musculoskeletal system. Part I includes chapters on the biomechanics of bone, articular cartilage, tendons and ligaments, peripheral nerves, and skeletal muscle. These are augmented with case studies to illustrate the important concepts for understanding the biomechanics of biological tissues.

PART II: BIOMECHANICS OF JOINTS

Part II of this textbook covers the major joints of the human body, from the spine to the ankle. Each chapter contains information about the structure and functioning of the joint, along with case studies illuminating the clinical diagnosis and management of joint injury and illness. The chapters are written by clinicians to provide an introductory level of knowledge about each joint system.

PART III: APPLIED BIOMECHANICS

A new section in the third edition of this book introduces important issues in applied biomechanics. These include the biomechanics of fracture fixation; arthroplasty; sitting, standing, and lying; and gait. It is important for the beginning student to understand the application of biomechanical principles in different clinical areas.

Summary

1 Biomechanics is a young and dynamic field of study based on the recognition that conventional engineering theories and methods can be useful for understanding and solving problems in physiology and medicine. Biomechanics considers the applications of classical mechanics to biological problems. The field of biomechanics flourishes from the cooperation among life scientists, physicians, engineers, and basic scientists. Such cooperation requires a certain amount of common vocabulary: an engineer must learn some anatomy and physiology, and medical personnel need to understand some basic concepts of physics and mathematics.

2 The information presented throughout this textbook is drawn from a large scholarship. The authors aim to introduce some of the basic concepts of biomechanics related to biological tissues and joints. The book does not intend to provide a comprehensive review of the literature, and readers are encouraged to consult the list of suggested reading below to supplement their knowledge. Some basic textbooks are listed here, and students should consult peer-reviewed journals for in-depth presentations of the latest research in specialty areas.

SUGGESTED READING
Black, J. (1988). Orthopaedic Biomaterials in Research and Practice. New York: Churchill Livingstone.

Bronzino, J.D. (Ed.) (1995). The Biomedical Engineering Handbook. Boca Raton, FL: CRC Press.

Burstein, A.H., & Wright, T.M.(1995). Fundamentals of Orthopaedic Biomechanics. Baltimore: Williams & Wilkins.

Chaffin, D.B., & Andersson, G.B.J. (1991). Occupational Biomechanics (2nd ed.). New York: John Wiley & Sons.

Fung, Y.C. (1981). Biomechanics: Mechanical Properties of Living Tissues. New York: Springer-Verlag.

Fung, Y.C. (1990). Biomechanics: Motion, Flow, Stress, and Growth. New York: Springer-Verlag.

Hay, J.G., & Reid, J.G. (1988). Anatomy, Mechanics and Human Motion (2nd ed.). Englewood Cliffs, NJ: Prentice-Hall.

Kelly, D.L. (1971). Kinesiology: Fundamentals of Motion Description. Englewood Cliffs, NJ: Prentice-Hall.

Mow, V.C., & Hayes, W.C. (1997). Basic Orthopaedic Biomechanics (2nd ed.). New York: Raven Press.

Mow, V.C., Ratcliff, A., & Woo, S.L.-Y. (Eds.). (1990). Biomechanics of Diarthrodial Joints. New York: Springer-Verlag.

Nahum, A.M., & Melvin, J. (Eds.). (1985). The Biomechanics of Trauma. Norwalk, CT: Appleton-Century-Crofts.

Nordin, M., Andersson, G.B.J., & Pope, M.H. (Eds.). (1997). Musculoskeletal Disorders in the Workplace. Philadelphia: Mosby-Year Book.

Nordin, M., & Frankel, V.H. (Eds.). (1989). Basic Biomechanics of the Musculoskeletal System (2nd ed.). Philadelphia: Lea & Febiger.

Özkaya, N. (1998). Biomechanics. In W.N. Rom, Environmental and Occupational Medicine (3rd ed., pp. 1437–1454). New York: Lippincott-Raven.

Özkaya, N., & Nordin, M. (1999). Fundamentals of Biomechanics: Equilibrium, Motion, and Deformation (2nd ed.). New York: Springer-Verlag.

Schmid-Schonbein, G.W., Woo, S.L.-Y., & Zweifach, B.W. (Eds.). (1985). Frontiers in Biomechanics. New York: Springer-Verlag.

Skalak, R., & Chien, S. (Eds.). (1987). Handbook of Bioengineering. New York: McGraw-Hill.

Thompson, C.W. (1989). Manual of Structural Kinesiology (11th ed.). St. Louis, MO: Times Mirror/Mosby.

Williams, M., & Lissner, H.R. (1992). Biomechanics of Human Motion (3rd ed.). Philadelphia: Saunders.

Winter, D.A. (1990). Biomechanics and Motor Control of Human Behavior (2nd ed.). New York: John Wiley & Sons.

Winters, J.M., & Woo, S.L.-Y. (Eds.). (1990). Multiple Muscle Systems. New York: Springer-Verlag.

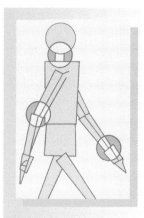

The System International d'Unites (SI)

Dennis R. Carter

The SI Metric System

The System International d'Unites (SI), the metric system, has evolved into the most exacting system of measures devised. In this section, the SI units of measurement used in the science of mechanics are described. SI units used in electrical and light sciences have been omitted for the sake of simplicity.

BASE UNITS

The SI units can be considered in three groups: 1, the base units; 2, the supplementary units; and 3, the derived units (Fig. App-1). The base units are a small group of standard measurements that have been arbitrarily defined. The base unit for length is the meter (m), and the base unit for mass is the kilogram (kg). The base units for time and temperature are the second (s) and the kelvin (K), respectively. Definitions of the base units have become increasingly sophisticated in response to the expanding needs and capabilities of the scientific community (Table App-1). For example, the meter is now defined in terms of the wavelength of radiation emitted from the krypton-86 atom.

SUPPLEMENTARY UNITS

The radian (rad) is a supplementary unit to measure plane angles. This unit, like the base units, is arbitrarily defined (Table App-1). Although the radian is the SI unit for plane angle, the unit of the degree has been retained for general use because it is firmly established and is widely used around the world. A degree is equivalent to $\pi/180$ rad.

DERIVED UNITS

Most units of the SI system are derived units, meaning that they are established from the base units in accordance with fundamental physical principles. Some of these units are expressed in terms of the base units from which they are derived. Examples are area, speed, and acceleration, which are expressed in the SI units of square meters (m^2), meters per second (m/s), and meters per second squared (m/s^2), respectively.

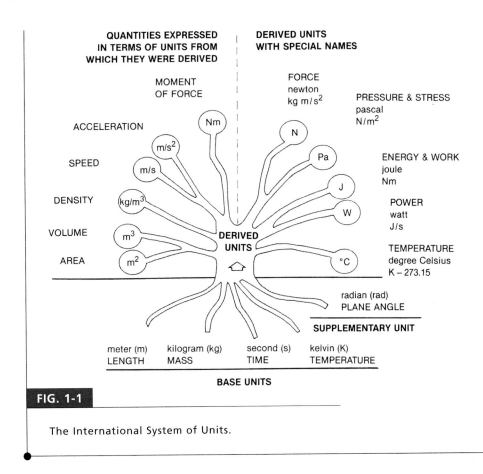

FIG. 1-1

The International System of Units.

Specially Named Units

Other derived units are similarly established from the base units but have been given special names (Fig App-1 and Table App-1). These units are defined through the use of fundamental equations of physical laws in conjunction with the arbitrarily defined SI base units. For example, Newton's second law of motion states that when a body that is free to move is subjected to a force, it will experience an acceleration proportional to that force and inversely proportional to its own mass. Mathematically, this principle can be expressed as:

$$\text{force} = \text{mass} \times \text{acceleration}$$

The SI unit of force, the newton (N), is therefore defined in terms of the base SI units as:

$$1 \text{ N} = 1 \text{ kg} \times 1 \text{ m/s}^2$$

The SI unit of pressure and stress is the pascal (Pa). Pressure is defined in hydrostatics as the force divided by the area of force application. Mathematically, this can be expressed as:

$$\text{pressure} = \text{force/area}$$

The SI unit of pressure, the pascal, is therefore defined in terms of the base SI units as:

$$1 \text{ Pa} = 1 \text{N} / 1 \text{ m}^2$$

Although the SI base unit of temperature is the kelvin, the derived unit of degree Celsius (°C or c) is much more commonly used. The degree Celsius is equivalent to the kelvin in magnitude, but the absolute value of the Celsius scale differs from that of the Kelvin scale such that °C = K − 273.15.

When the SI system is used in a wide variety of measurements, the quantities expressed in terms of the base, supplemental, or derived units may be either very large or very small. For example, the area on the head of a pin is an extremely small number when expressed in terms of square meters. Conversely, the weight of a whale is an extremely large number when expressed in terms of newtons. To accommodate the convenient representation of small or large quantities, a system of prefixes has been incorporated into the SI system (Table App-2). Each prefix has a fixed meaning and can be used with all SI units. When used with the name of the unit, the prefix indicates that the quantity described is being expressed in some multiple of

TABLE 1

Definitions of SI Units

Base SI Units

meter (m)	The meter is the length equal to 1,650,763.73 wavelengths in vacuum of the radiation corresponding to the transition between the levels $2p_{10}$ and $5d_5$ of the krypton-86 atom.
kilogram (kg)	The kilogram is the unit of mass and is equal to the mass of the international prototype of the kilogram.
second (s)	The second is the duration of 9,192,631,770 periods of the radiation corresponding to the transition between the two hyperfine levels of the ground state of the cesium-133 atom.
kelvin (k)	The kelvin, a unit of thermodynamic temperature, is the fraction 1/273.16 of the thermodynamic temperature of the triple point of water.

Supplementary SI Unit

radian (rad)	The radian is the plane angle between two radii of a circle that subtend on the circumference of an arc equal in length to the radius.

Derived SI Units With Special Names

newton (N)	The newton is that force which, when applied to a mass of 1 kilogram, gives it an acceleration of 1 meter per second squared. $1 \text{ N} = 1 \text{ kg m/s}^2$.
pascal (Pa)	The pascal is the pressure produced by a force of 1 newton applied, with uniform distribution, over an area of 1 square meter. $1 \text{ Pa} = 1 \text{ N/m}^2$.
joule (J)	The joule is the work done when the point of application of a force of 1 newton is displaced through a distance of 1 meter in the direction of the force. $1 \text{ J} = 1 \text{ Nm}$.
watt (W)	The watt is the power that in 1 second gives rise to the energy of 1 joule. $1 \text{ W} = 1 \text{ J/s}$.
degree Celsius ((C)	The degree Celsius is a unit of thermodynamic temperature and is equivalent to K − 273.15.

TABLE 2

SI Multiplication Factors and Prefixes

Multiplication Factor	SI Prefix	SI Symbol
1 000 000 000 = 10^9	giga	G
1 000 000 = 10^6	mega	M
1 000 = 10^3	kilo	k
100 = 10^2	hecto	h
10 = 10^1	deka	da
.1 = 10^{-1}	deci	d
.01 = 10^{-2}	centi	c
.001 = 10^{-3}	milli	m
.000 001 = 10^{-6}	micro	μ
.000 000 001 = 10^{-9}	nano	n
.000 000 000 001 = 10^{-12}	pico	p

Reprinted with permission from Özkaya, N., & Nordin, M. (1999). Fundamentals of Biomechanics: Equilibrium, Motion, and Deformation (2nd ed.) New York: Springer-Verlag, p. 10.

ten times the unit used. For example, the millimeter (mm) is used to represent one thousandth (10^{-3}) of a meter and a gigapascal (Gpa) is used to denote one billion (10^9) pascals.

Standard Units Named for Scientists

One of the more interesting aspects of the SI system is its use of the names of famous scientists as standard units. In each case, the unit was named after a scientist in recognition of his contribution to the field in which that unit plays a major role. Table App-3 lists a number of SI units and the scientist for which each was named.

For example, the unit of force, the newton, was named in honor of the English scientist Sir Isaac Newton (1624–1727). He was educated at Trinity College at Cambridge and later returned to Trinity College as a professor of mathematics. Early in his career, Newton made fundamental contributions to mathematics that formed the basis of differential and integral calculus. His other major discoveries were in the fields of optics, astronomy, gravitation, and mechanics. His work in gravitation was purportedly spurred by being hit on the head by an apple falling from a tree. It is perhaps poetic justice that the SI unit of one newton is approximately equivalent to the weight of a medium-sized apple. Newton was knighted in 1705 by Queen Mary for his monumental contributions to science.

TABLE 3

SI Units Named After Scientists

Symbol	Unit	Quantity	Scientist	Country of Birth	Dates
A	ampere	electric current	Amphere, Andre-Marie	France	1775–1836
C	coulomb	electric charge	Coulomb, Charles Augustin de	France	1736–1806
°C	degree celsius	temperature	Celsius, Anders	Sweden	1701–1744
F	farad	electric capacity	Faraday, Michael	England	1791–1867
H	henry	inductive resistance	Henry, Joseph	United States	1797–1867
Hz	hertz	frequency	Hertz, Heinrich Rudolph	Germany	1857–1894
J	joule	energy	Joule, James Prescott	England	1818–1889
K	kelvin	temperature	Thomson, William (Lord Kelvin)	England	1824–1907
N	newton	force	Newton, Sir Isaac	England	1642–1727
Ω	ohm	electric resistance	Ohm, Georg Simon	Germany	1787–1854
Pa	pascal	pressure/stress	Pascal, Blaise	France	1623–1662
S	siemens	electric conductance	Siemens, Karl Wilhelm (Sir William)	Germany (England)	1823–1883
T	testa	magnetic flux density	Testa, Nikola	Croatia (US)	1856–1943
V	volt	electrical potential	Volta, Count Alessandro	Italy	1745–1827
W	watt	power	Watt, James	Scotland	1736–1819
Wb	weber	magnetic flux	Weber, Wilhelm Eduard	Germany	1804–1891

BOX APP-1 *Conversion of Units*

Length

1 centimeter (cm) = 0.01 meter (m)

1 inch (in) = 0.0254 m

1 foot (ft) = 0.3048 m

1 yard (yd) = 0.9144 m

1 mile = 1609 m

1 angstrom (Å) = 10^{-10} m

Time

1 minute (min) = 60 second (s)

1 hour (h) = 3600 s

1 day (d) = 86400 s

Mass

1 pound mass (1bm) = 0.4536 kilogram (kg)

1 slug = 14.59 kg

Force

1 kilogram force (kgf) = 9.807 Newton (N)

1 pound force (lbf) = 4.448 N

1 dyne (dyn) = 10^{-5} N

Pressure and Stress

1 kg/ m-s^2 = 1 N/m^2 = 1 Pascal (Pa)

1 lbf / in^2 (psi) = 6896 Pa

1 lbf / ft^2 (psf) = 92966 Pa

1 dyn / cm^2 = 0.1 Pa

Moment (Torque)

1 dyn-cm = 10^{-7} N-m

1 lbf-ft = 1.356 N-m

Work and Energy

1 kg-m^2 / s^2 = 1 N-m = 1 Joule (J)

1 dyn-cm = 1 erg = 10^{-7} J

1 lbf-ft = 1.356 J

Power

1 kg- m^2 / s^3 = 1 J/s = 1 Watt (W)

1 horsepower (hp) = 550 lbf-ft/s = 746 W

Plane Angle

1 degree (°) = π / 180 radian (rad)

1 revolution (rev) = 360°

1 rev = 2π rad = 6.283 rad

Temperature

°C = °K − 273.2

°C = 5 (°F − 32)/9

Reprinted with permission from Özkaya, N., & Nordin, M. (1999). Fundamentals of Biomechanics: Equilibrium, Motion, and Deformation (2nd ed.) New York: Springer-Verlag, p. 11.

The unit of pressure and stress, the pascal, was named after the French physicist, mathematician, and philosopher Blaise Pascal (1623–1662). Pascal conducted important investigations on the characteristics of vacuums and barometers and also invented a machine that would make mathematical calculations. His work in the area of hydrostatics helped lay the foundation for the later development of these scientific fields. In addition to his scientific pursuits, Pascal was passionately interested in religion and philosophy and thus wrote extensively on a wide range of subjects.

The base unit of temperature, the kelvin, was named in honor of Lord William Thomson Kelvin (1824–1907). Named William Thomson, he was ed-ucated at the University of Glasgow and at Cambridge University. Early in his career, Thomson investigated the thermal properties of steam at a scientific laboratory in Paris. At the age of 32, he returned to Glasgow to accept the chair of Natural Philosophy. His meeting with James Joule in 1847 stimulated interesting discussions on the nature of heat, which eventually led to the establishment of Thomson's absolute scale of temperature, the Kelvin scale. In recognition of Thomson's contributions to the field of thermodynamics, King Edward VII conferred on him the title of Lord Kelvin.

The commonly used unit of temperature, the degree Celsius, was named after the Swedish astronomer and inventor Anders Celsius (1701–1744).

Celsius was appointed professor of astronomy at the University of Uppsala at the age of 29 and remained at the university until his death 14 years later. In 1742, he described the centigrade thermometer in a paper prepared for the Swedish Academy of Sciences. The name of the centigrade temperature scale was officially changed to Celsius in 1948.

Converting to SI From Other Units of Measurement

Box App-1 contains the formulae for the conversion of measurements expressed in English and non-SI metric units into SI units. One fundamental source of confusion in converting from one system to another is that two basic types of measurement systems exist. In the "physical" system (such as SI), the units of length, time, and *mass* are arbitrarily defined, and other units (including force) are derived from these base units. In "technical" or "gravitational" systems (such as the English system), the units of length, time, and *force* are arbitrarily defined, and other units (including mass) are derived from these base units. Because the units of force in gravitational systems are in fact the *weights* of standard masses, conversion to SI is dependent on the acceleration of mass due to the Earth's gravity. By international agreement, the acceleration due to gravity is 9.806650 m/s^2. This value has been used in establishing some of the conversion factors in Box App-1.

REFERENCES

Feirer, J.L. (1977). *SI Metric Handbook.* New York: Charles Scribner's Sons.

Özkaya, N., & Nordin, M. (1999). *Fundamentals of Biomechanics: Equilibrium, Motion, and Deformation* (2nd ed.) New York: Springer-Verlag.

Pennychuick, C.J. (1974). *Handy Matrices of Unit Conversion Factors for Biology and Mechanics.* New York: John Wiley & Sons.

World Health Organization. (1977). *The SI for the Health Professions.* Geneva: WHO.

PART I

Biomechanics of Tissue and Structures of the Musculoskeletal System

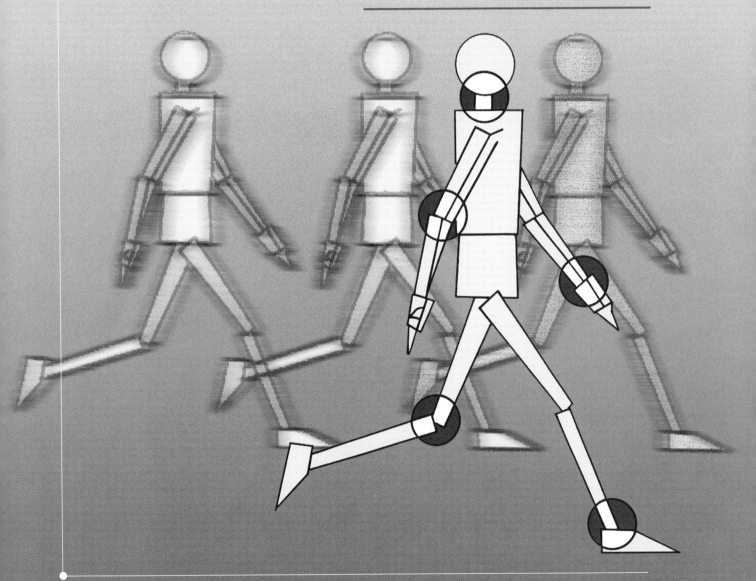

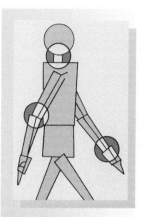

CHAPTER 2

Biomechanics of Bone

Victor H. Frankel, Margareta Nordin

Introduction

The purpose of the skeletal system is to protect internal organs, provide rigid kinematic links and muscle attachment sites, and facilitate muscle action and body movement. Bone has unique structural and mechanical properties that allow it to carry out these roles. Bone is among the body's hardest structures; only dentin and enamel in the teeth are harder. It is one of the most dynamic and metabolically active tissues in the body and remains active throughout life. A highly vascular tissue, it has an excellent capacity for self-repair and can alter its properties and configuration in response to changes in mechanical demand. For example, changes in bone density are commonly observed after periods of disuse and of greatly increased use; changes in bone shape are noted during fracture healing and after certain operations. Thus, bone adapts to the mechanical demands placed on it.

This chapter describes the composition and structure of bone tissue, the mechanical properties of bone, and the behavior of bone under different loading conditions. Various factors that affect the mechanical behavior of bone in vitro and in vivo also are discussed.

Bone Composition and Structure

Bone tissue is a specialized connective tissue whose solid composition suits it for its supportive and protective roles. Like other connective tissues, it consists of cells and an organic extracellular matrix of fibers and ground substance produced by the cells. The distinguishing feature of bone is its high content of inorganic materials, in the form of mineral salts, that combine intimately with the organic matrix (Buckwalter et al., 1995). The inorganic component of bone makes the tissue hard and rigid, while the organic component gives bone its flexibility and resilience. The composition of bone differs depending on site, animal age, dietary history, and the presence of disease (Kaplan et al., 1993).

In normal human bone, the mineral or inorganic portion of bone consists primarily of calcium and phosphate, mainly in the form of small crystals resembling synthetic hydroxyapatite crystals with the composition $Ca_{10}(PO_4)_6(OH)_2$. These minerals, which account for 60 to 70% of its dry weight, give bone its solid consistency. Water accounts for 5 to 8% and the organic matrix makes up the remainder

of the tissue. Bone serves as a reservoir for essential minerals in the body, particularly calcium.

Bone mineral is embedded in variously oriented fibers of the protein collagen, the fibrous portion of the extracellular matrix—the inorganic matrix. Collagen fibers (type I) are tough and pliable, yet they resist stretching and have little extensibility. Collagen composes approximately 90% of the extracellular matrix and accounts for approximately 25 to 30% of the dry weight of bone. A universal building block of the body, collagen also is the chief fibrous component of other skeletal structures. (A detailed description of the microstructure and mechanical behavior of collagen is provided in Chapters 3 and 4.)

The gelatinous ground substance surrounding the mineralized collagen fibers consists mainly of protein polysaccharides, or glycosaminoglycans (GAGs), primarily in the form of complex macromolecules called proteoglycans (PGs). The GAGs serve as a cementing substance between layers of mineralized collagen fibers. These GAGs, along with various noncollagenous glycoproteins, constitute approximately 5% of the extracellular matrix. (The structure of PGs, which are vital components of articular cartilage, is described in detail in Chapter 3.)

Water is fairly abundant in live bone, accounting for up to 25% of its total weight. Approximately 85% of the water is found in the organic matrix, around the collagen fibers and ground substance, and in the hydration shells surrounding the bone crystals. The other 15% is located in the canals and cavities that house bone cells and carry nutrients to the bone tissue.

At the microscopic level, the fundamental structural unit of bone is the osteon, or haversian system (Fig. 2-1). At the center of each osteon is a small channel, called a haversian canal, that contains blood vessels and nerve fibers. The osteon itself consists of a concentric series of layers (lamellae) of mineralized matrix surrounding the central canal, a configuration similar to growth rings in a tree trunk.

Along the boundaries of each layer, or lamella, are small cavities known as lacunae, each containing one bone cell, or osteocyte (Fig. 2-1C). Numerous small channels, called canaliculi, radiate from each lacuna, connecting the lacunae of adjacent lamellae and ultimately reaching the haversian canal. Cell processes extend from the osteocytes into the canaliculi, allowing nutrients from the blood vessels in the haversian canal to reach the osteocytes.

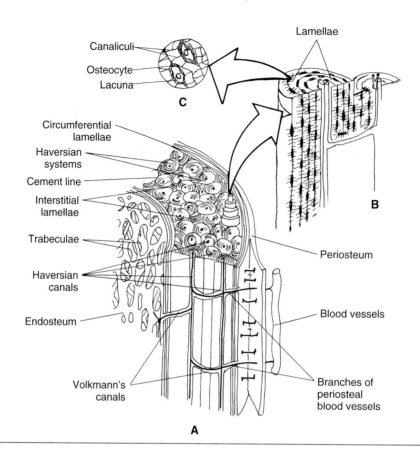

FIG. 2-1

A, The fine structure of bone is illustrated schematically in a section of the shaft of a long bone depicted without inner marrow. The osteons, or haversian systems, are apparent as the structural units of bone. The haversian canals are in the center of the osteons, which form the main branches of the circulatory network in bone. Each osteon is bounded by a cement line. One osteon is shown extending from the bone (20×). *Adapted from Bassett, C.A.L. (1965). Electrical effects in bone.* Sci Am, 213,18. **B,** Each osteon consists of lamellae, concentric rings composed of a mineral matrix surrounding the haversian canal. *Adapted from Tortora G.J., & Anagnostakos, N.P. (1984). Principles of Anatomy and Physiology (4th ed.). New York: Harper & Row.* **C,** Along the boundaries of the lamellae are small cavities known as lacunae, each of which contains a single bone cell, or osteocyte. Radiating from the lacunae are tiny canals, or canaliculi, into which the cytoplasmic processes of the osteocytes extend. *Adapted from Tortora G.J., & Anagnostakos, N.P. (1984). Principles of Anatomy and Physiology (4th ed.). New York: Harper & Row.*

At the periphery of each osteon is a cement line, a narrow area of cement-like ground substance composed primarily of GAGs. The canaliculi of the osteon do not pass this cement line. Like the canaliculi, the collagen fibers in the bone matrix interconnect from one lamella to another within an osteon but do not cross the cement line. This intertwining of collagen fibers within the osteon undoubtedly increases the bone's resistance to mechanical stress and probably explains why the cement line is the weakest portion of the bone's microstructure.

A typical osteon is approximately 200 micrometers (μ) in diameter. Hence, every point in the osteon is no more than 100 μm from the centrally located blood supply. In the long bones, the osteons usually run longitudinally, but they branch frequently and anastomose extensively with each other.

Interstitial lamellae span the regions between complete osteons (Fig. 2-1*A*). They are continuous with the osteons and consist of the same material in a different geometric configuration. As in the os-

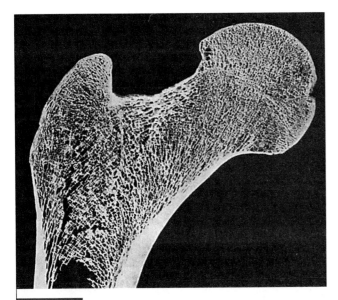

FIG. 2-2

Frontal longitudinal section through the head, neck, greater trochanter, and proximal shaft of an adult femur. Cancellous bone, with its trabeculae oriented in a lattice, lies within the shell of cortical bone. *Reprinted with permission from Gray, H. (1985).* Anatomy of the Human Body. *(13th American ed.). Philadelphia: Lea & Febiger.*

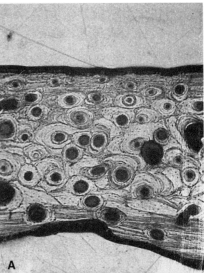

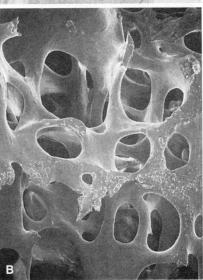

FIG. 2-3

A, Reflected-light photomicrograph of cortical bone from a human tibia (40×). **B,** Scanning electron photomicrograph of cancellous bone from a human tibia (30×). *Reprinted with permission from Carter, D.R., & Hayes, W.C. (1977). Compact bone fatigue damage. A microscopic examination. Clin Orthop, 127, 265.*

teons, no point in the interstitial lamellae is farther than 100 μm from its blood supply. The interfaces between these lamellae contain an array of lacunae in which osteocytes lie and from which canaliculi extend.

At the macroscopic level, all bones are composed of two types of osseous tissue: cortical, or compact, bone and cancellous, or trabecular, bone (Fig. 2-2). Cortical bone forms the outer shell, or cortex, of the bone and has a dense structure similar to that of ivory. Cancellous bone within this shell is composed of thin plates, or trabeculae, in a loose mesh structure; the interstices between the trabeculae are filled with red marrow (Fig. 2-3). Cancellous bone tissue is arranged in concentric lacunae-containing lamellae but does not contain haversian canals. The osteocytes receive nutrients through canaliculi from blood vessels passing through the red marrow. Cortical bone always surrounds cancellous bone, but the relative quantity of each type varies among bones and within individual bones according to functional requirements.

On a microscopic level, bone consists of woven and lamellar bone (Fig. 2-4). Woven bone is considered immature bone. This type of bone is found in the embryo, in the newborn, in the fracture callus, and in the metaphysial region of growing bone as well as in tumors, osteogenesis imperfecta, and pagetic bone. Lamellar bone begins to form 1 month after birth and actively replaces woven bone. Lamellar bone is therefore a more mature bone.

All bones are surrounded by a dense fibrous membrane called the periosteum (Fig. 2-1A). Its outer layer is permeated by blood vessels (Fig. 2-5) and nerve fibers that pass into the cortex via Volkmann's canals, connecting with the haversian canals and extending to the cancellous bone. An inner, osteogenic layer contains bone cells responsible for generating new bone during growth and repair (osteoblasts). The periosteum covers the entire bone except for the joint surfaces, which are covered with articular cartilage. In the long bones, a thinner membrane, the endosteum, lines the central (medullary) cavity, which is filled with yellow fatty marrow. The endosteum contains osteoblasts and also giant multinucleated bone cells called osteoclasts, both of which play important roles in the remodeling and resorption of bone.

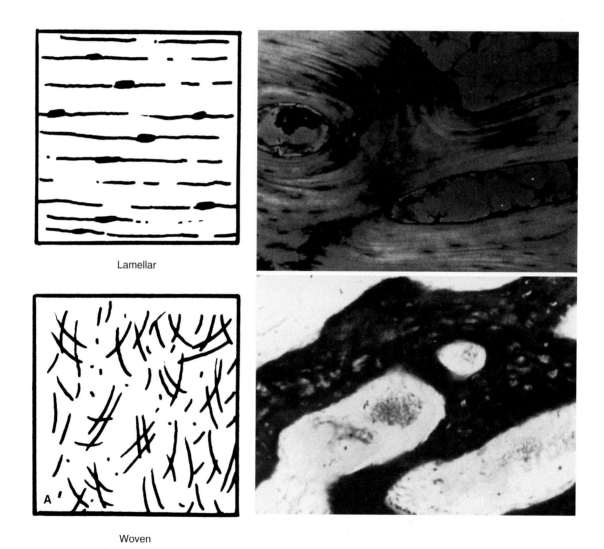

Lamellar

Woven

FIG. 2-4

Schematic drawing and photomicrographs of lamellar and woven bone. *Adapted from Kaplan, F.S., Hayes, W.C., Keaveny, T.M., et al. (1994). Form and function of bone. In S.R. Simon (Ed.). Orthopaedic Basic Science (pp. 129, 130). Rosemont, IL: AAOS.*

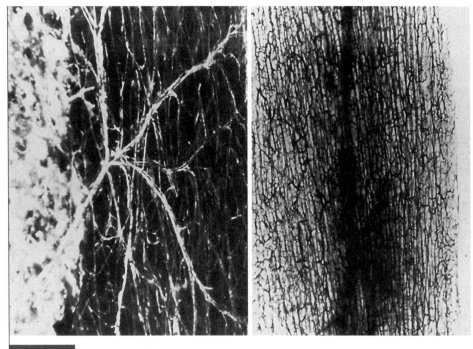

FIG. 2-5

Photomicrograph showing the vasculature of cortical bone. *Adapted from Kaplan, F.S., Hayes, W.C., Keaveny, T.M., et al. (1994). Form and function of bone. In S.R. Simon (Ed.).* Orthopaedic Basic Science *(p. 131). Rosemont, IL: AAOS.*

Biomechanical Properties of Bone

Biomechanically, bone tissue may be regarded as a two-phase (biphasic) composite material, with the mineral as one phase and the collagen and ground substance as the other. In such materials (a nonbiological example is fiberglass) in which a strong, brittle material is embedded in a weaker, more flexible one, the combined substances are stronger for their weight than is either substance alone (Bassett, 1965).

Functionally, the most important mechanical properties of bone are its strength and stiffness. These and other characteristics can best be understood for bone, or any other structure, by examining its behavior under loading, that is, under the influence of externally applied forces. Loading causes a deformation, or a change in the dimensions, of the structure. When a load in a known direction is imposed on a structure, the deformation of that structure can be measured and plotted on a load-deformation curve. Much information about the

strength, stiffness, and other mechanical properties of the structure can be gained by examining this curve.

A hypothetical load-deformation curve for a somewhat pliable fibrous structure, such as a long bone, is shown in Figure 2-6. The initial (straight line) portion of the curve, the elastic region, reveals the elasticity of the structure, that is, its capacity for returning to its original shape after the load is removed. As the load is applied, deformation occurs but is not permanent; the structure recovers its original shape when unloaded. As loading continues, the outermost fibers of the structure begin to yield at some point. This yield point signals the elastic limit of the structure. As the load exceeds this limit, the structure exhibits plastic behavior, reflected in the second (curved) portion of the curve, the plastic region. The structure will no longer return to its original dimensions when the load has been released; some residual deformation will be permanent. If loading is progressively increased, the structure will fail at some point (bone will fracture). This point is indicated by the ultimate failure point on the curve.

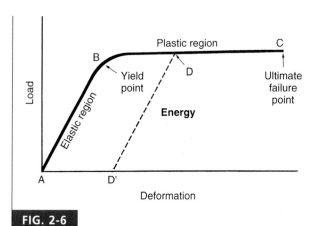

FIG. 2-6

Load-deformation curve for a structure composed of a somewhat pliable material. If a load is applied within the elastic range of the structure (A to B on the curve) and is then released, no permanent deformation occurs. If loading is continued past the yield point (B) and into the structure's plastic range (B to C on the curve) and the load is then released, permanent deformation results. The amount of permanent deformation that occurs if the structure is loaded to point D in the plastic region and then unloaded is represented by the distance between A and D. If loading continues within the plastic range, an ultimate failure point (C) is reached.

Three parameters for determining the strength of a structure are reflected on the load-deformation curve: 1, the load that the structure can sustain before failing; 2, the deformation that it can sustain before failing; and 3, the energy that it can store before failing. The strength in terms of load and deformation, or ultimate strength, is indicated on the curve by the ultimate failure point. The strength in terms of energy storage is indicated by the size of the area under the entire curve. The larger the area, the greater the energy that builds up in the structure as the load is applied. The stiffness of the structure is indicated by the slope of the curve in the elastic region. The steeper the slope, the stiffer the material.

The load-deformation curve is useful for determining the mechanical properties of whole structures such as a whole bone, an entire ligament or tendon, or a metal implant. This knowledge is helpful in the study of fracture behavior and repair, the response of a structure to physical stress, or the effect of various treatment programs. However, char-

acterizing a bone or other structure in terms of the material of which it is composed, independent of its geometry, requires standardization of the testing conditions and the size and shape of the test specimens. Such standardized testing is useful for comparing the mechanical properties of two or more materials, such as the relative strength of bone and tendon tissue or the relative stiffness of various materials used in prosthetic implants. More precise units of measurement can be used when standardized samples are tested—that is, the load per unit of area of the sample (stress) and the amount of deformation in terms of the percentage of change in the sample's dimensions (strain). The curve generated is a stress-strain curve.

Stress is the load, or force, per unit area that develops on a plane surface within a structure in response to externally applied loads. The three units most commonly used for measuring stress in standardized samples of bone are newtons per centimeter squared (N/cm^2); newtons per meter squared, or pascals (N/m^2, Pa); and meganewtons per meter squared, or megapascals (MN/m^2, MPa).

Strain is the deformation (change in dimension) that develops within a structure in response to externally applied loads. The two basic types of strain are linear strain, which causes a change in the length of the specimen, and shear strain, which causes a change in the angular relationships within the structure. Linear strain is measured as the amount of linear deformation (lengthening or shortening) of the sample divided by the sample's original length. It is a nondimensional parameter expressed as a percentage (e.g., centimeter per centimeter). Shear strain is measured as the amount of angular change (γ) in a right angle lying in the plane of interest in the sample. It is expressed in radians (one radian equals approximately 57.3°) (International, Society of Biomechanics, 1987).

Stress and strain values can be obtained for bone by placing a standardized specimen of bone tissue in a testing jig and loading it to failure (Fig. 2-7). These values can then be plotted on a stress-strain curve (Fig. 2-8). The regions of this curve are similar to those of the load-deformation curve. Loads in the elastic region do not cause permanent deformation, but once the yield point is exceeded, some deformation is permanent. The strength of the material in terms of energy storage is represented by the area under the entire curve. The stiffness is represented by the slope of the curve in the elastic region. A value for stiffness is obtained by dividing the stress at a point in the elastic (straight line) portion of the curve by the strain at that point. This value is called the modulus of elasticity (Young's modulus). Young's modulus (E) is derived from the relationship between stress (σ) and strain (ϵ):

$$E = \sigma / \epsilon$$

The elasticity of a material or the Young's modulus E is equal to the slope of the stress (σ) and strain (ϵ) diagram in the elastic linear region. E represents the stiffness of the material, such that the higher the elastic modulus or Young's modulus, the stiffer the material (Özkaya & Nordin, 1999).

Mechanical properties differ in the two bone types. Cortical bone is stiffer than cancellous bone, withstanding greater stress but less strain before failure. Cancellous bone in vitro may sustain up to 50% of strains before yielding, while cortical bone yields and fractures when the strain exceeds 1.5 to 2.0%. Because of its porous structure, cancellous bone has a large capacity for energy storage (Keaveny & Hayes, 1993). The physical difference between the two bone tissues is quantified in terms of the apparent density of bone, which is defined as the mass of bone tissue present in a unit of bone volume (gram per cubic centimeter [g/cc]). Figure 2-9 depicts typical stress-strain qualities of cortical and trabecular bone with different bone densities tested under similar conditions. In general, it is not enough to describe bone strength with a single number. A better way is to examine the stress-strain curve for the bone tissue under the circumstances tested.

To better understand the relationship of bone to other materials, schematic stress-strain curves for bone, metal, and glass illustrate the differences in mechanical behavior among these materials (Fig. 2-10). The variations in stiffness are reflected in the different slopes of the curves in the elastic region. Metal has the steepest slope and is thus the stiffest material.

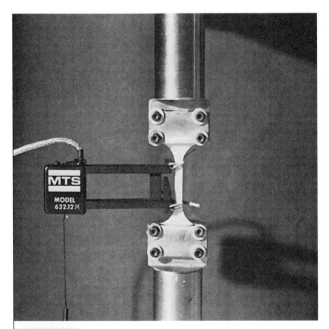

FIG. 2-7

Standardized bone specimen in a testing machine. The strain in the segment of bone between the two gauge arms is measured with a strain gauge. The stress is calculated from the total load measured.
Courtesy of Dennis R. Carter, Ph.D.

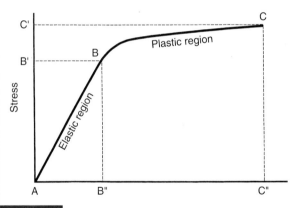

FIG. 2-8

Stress-strain curve for a cortical bone sample tested in tension (pulled). Yield point (B): point past which some permanent deformation of the bone sample occurred. Yield stress (B'): load per unit area sustained by the bone sample before plastic deformation took place. Yield strain (B"): amount of deformation withstood by the sample before plastic deformation occurred. The strain at any point in the elastic region of the curve is proportional to the stress at that point. Ultimate failure point (C): the point past which failure of the sample occurred. Ultimate stress (C'): load per unit area sustained by the sample before failure. Ultimate strain (C"): amount of deformation sustained by the sample before failure.

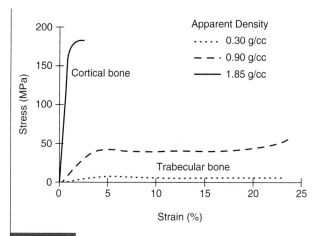

FIG. 2-9

Example of stress-strain curves of cortical and trabecular bone with different apparent densities. Testing was performed in compression. The figure depicts the difference in mechanical behavior for the two bone structures. *Reprinted with permission from Keaveny, T.M., & Hayes, W.C. (1993). Mechanical properties of cortical and trabecular bone. Bone, 7, 285-344.*

The elastic portion of the curve for glass and metal is a straight line, indicating linearly elastic behavior; virtually no yielding takes place before the yield point is reached. By comparison, precise testing of cortical bone has shown that the elastic portion of the curve is not straight but instead slightly curved, indicating that bone is not linearly elastic in its behavior but yields somewhat during loading in the elastic region (Bonefield & Li, 1967). Table 2-1 depicts the mechanical properties of selected biomaterials for comparison. Materials are classified as brittle or ductile depending on the extent of deformation before failure. Glass is a typical brittle material, and soft metal is a typical ductile material. The difference in the amount of deformation is reflected in the fracture surfaces of the two materials (Fig. 2-11). When pieced together after fracture, the ductile material will not conform to its original shape whereas the brittle material will. Bone exhibits more brittle or more ductile behavior depending on its age (younger bone being more ductile) and the rate at which it is loaded (bone being more brittle at higher loading speeds).

After the yield point is reached, glass deforms very little before failing, as indicated by the ab-

sence of a plastic region on the stress-strain curve. By contrast, metal exhibits extensive deformation before failing, as indicated by a long plastic region on the curve. Bone also deforms before failing but to a much lesser extent than metal. The difference in the plastic behavior of metal and bone is the result of differences in micromechanical events at yield. Yielding in metal (tested in tension, or pulled) is caused by plastic flow and the formation of plastic slip lines; slip lines are formed when the molecules of the lattice structure of metal dislocate. Yielding in bone (tested in tension) is caused

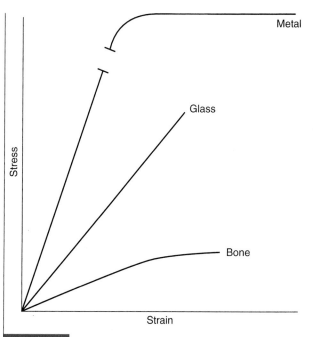

FIG. 2-10

Schematic stress-strain curves for three materials. Metal has the steepest slope in the elastic region and is thus the stiffest material. The elastic portion of the curve for metal is a straight line, indicating linearly elastic behavior. The fact that metal has a long plastic region indicates that this typical ductile material deforms extensively before failure. Glass, a brittle material, exhibits linearly elastic behavior but fails abruptly with little deformation, as indicated by the lack of a plastic region on the stress-strain curve. Bone possesses both ductile and brittle qualities demonstrated by a slight curve in the elastic region, which indicates some yielding during loading within this region.

TABLE 2-1

Mechanical Properties of Selected Biomaterials

	Ultimate Strength (MPa)	Modulus (GPa)	Elongation (%)
Metals			
Co-Cr alloy			
Cast	600	220	8
Forged	950	220	15
Stainless steel	850	210	10
Titanium	900	110	15
Polymers			
Bone cement	20	2.0	2–4
Ceramic			
Alumina	300	350	<2
Biological			
Cortical bone	100–150	10–15	1–3
Trabecular bone	8–50		2–4
Tendon, ligament	20–35	2.0–4.0	10–25

Adapted from Kummer, J.K. (1999). Implant biomaterials. In J.M. Spivak, P.E. DiCesare, D.S. Feldman, K.J. Koval, A.S. Rokito, & J.D. Zuckerman (Eds.). *Orthopaedics: A Study Guide* (pp. 45–48). New York: McGraw-Hill.

by debonding of the osteons at the cement lines and microfracture (Fig. 2-12), while yielding in bone as a result of compression is indicated by cracking of the osteons (Fig. 2-13).

Because the structure of bone is dissimilar in the transverse and longitudinal directions, it exhibits different mechanical properties when loaded along different axes, a characteristic known as anisotropy.

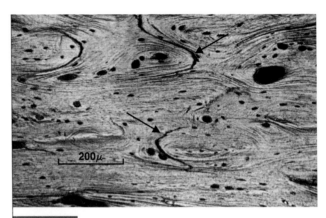

FIG. 2-12

Reflected-light photomicrograph of a human cortical bone specimen tested in tension (30×). *Arrows* indicate debonding at the cement lines and pulling out of the osteons. *Courtesy of Dennis R. Carter, Ph.D.*

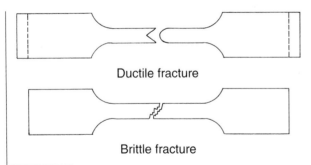

FIG. 2-11

Fracture surfaces of samples of a ductile and a brittle material. The *broken lines* on the ductile material indicate the original length of the sample, before it deformed. The brittle material deformed very little before fracture.

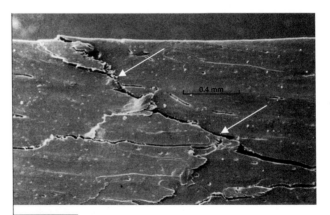

FIG. 2-13

Scanning electron photomicrograph of a human cortical bone specimen tested in compression (30×). *Arrows* indicate oblique cracking of the osteons. *Courtesy of Dennis R. Carter, Ph.D.*

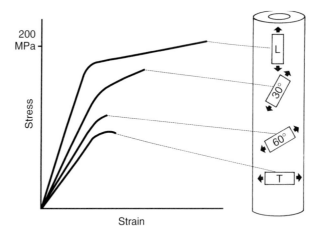

FIG. 2-14

Anisotropic behavior of cortical bone specimens from a human femoral shaft tested in tension (pulled) in four directions: longitudinal (L), tilted 30° with respect to the neutral axis of the bone, tilted 60°, and transverse (T). Data from Frankel, V.H., & Burstein, A.H. (1970). Orthopaedic Biomechanics. **Philadelphia: Lea & Febiger.**

Figure 2-14 shows the variations in strength and stiffness for cortical bone samples from a human femoral shaft, tested in tension in four directions (Frankel & Burstein, 1970; Carter, 1978). The values for both parameters are highest for the samples loaded in the longitudinal direction. Figures 2-9 and 2-15 show trabecular bone strength and stiffness tested in two directions: compression and tension. Trabecular or cancellous bone is approximately 25% as dense, 5 to 10% as stiff, and five times as ductile as cortical bone.

Although the relationship between loading patterns and the mechanical properties of bone throughout the skeleton is extremely complex, it generally can be said that bone strength and stiffness are greatest in the direction in which daily loads are most commonly imposed.

Biomechanical Behavior of Bone

The mechanical behavior of bone—its behavior under the influence of forces and moments—is affected by its mechanical properties, its geometric characteristics, the loading mode applied, direction of loading, rate of loading, and frequency of loading.

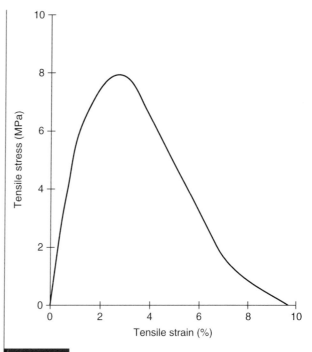

FIG. 2-15

Example of tensile stress-strain behavior of trabecular bone tested in the longitudinal axial direction of the bone. Adapted from Gibson, L.J., & Ashby, M.F. (1988). Cellular Solids: Structure and Properties. New York: Pergamon, Press.

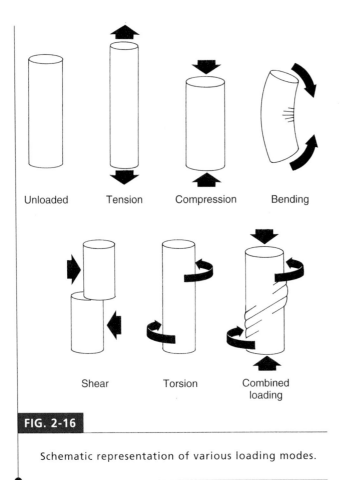

Unloaded   Tension   Compression   Bending

Shear   Torsion   Combined loading

FIG. 2-16

Schematic representation of various loading modes.

pendicular to the applied load (Fig. 2-17). Under tensile loading, the structure lengthens and narrows.

Clinically, fractures produced by tensile loading are usually seen in bones with a large proportion of cancellous bone. Examples are fractures of the base of the fifth metatarsal adjacent to the attachment of the peroneus brevis tendon and fractures of the calcaneus adjacent to the attachment of the Achilles tendon. Figure 2-18 shows a tensile fracture through the calcaneus; intense contraction of the triceps surae muscle produces abnormally high tensile loads on the bone.

Compression

During compressive loading, equal and opposite loads are applied toward the surface of the structure and compressive stress and strain result inside the structure. Compressive stress can be thought of as many small forces directed into the surface of the structure. Maximal compressive stress occurs on a plane perpendicular to the applied load (Fig. 2-19). Under compressive loading, the structure shortens and widens.

Clinically, compression fractures are commonly found in the vertebrae, which are subjected to high compressive loads. These fractures are most often seen in the elderly with osteoporotic bone tissue. Figure 2-20 shows the shortening and widening

BONE BEHAVIOR UNDER VARIOUS LOADING MODES

Forces and moments can be applied to a structure in various directions, producing tension, compression, bending, shear, torsion, and combined loading (Fig. 2-16). Bone in vivo is subjected to all of these loading modes. The following descriptions of these modes apply to structures in equilibrium (at rest or moving at a constant speed); loading produces an internal, deforming effect on the structure.

Tension

During tensile loading, equal and opposite loads are applied outward from the surface of the structure, and tensile stress and strain result inside the structure. Tensile stress can be thought of as many small forces directed away from the surface of the structure. Maximal tensile stress occurs on a plane per-

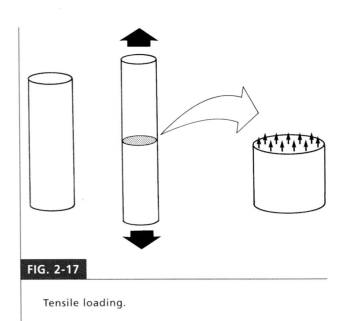

FIG. 2-17

Tensile loading.

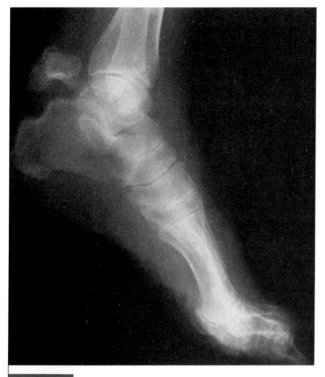

FIG. 2-18

Tensile fracture through the calcaneus produced by strong contraction of the triceps surae muscle during a tennis match. *Courtesy of Robert A. Winquist, M.D.*

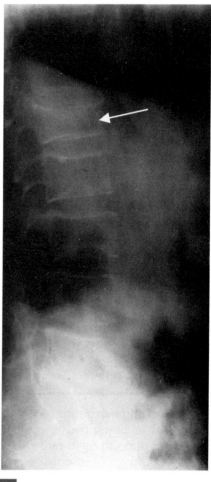

FIG. 2-20

Compression fracture of a human first lumbar vertebra. The vertebra has shortened and widened.

that takes place in a human vertebra subjected to a high compressive load. In a joint, compressive loading to failure can be produced by abnormally strong contraction of the surrounding muscles. An example of this effect is presented in Figure 2-21; bilateral subcapital fractures of the femoral neck

were sustained by a patient undergoing electroconvulsive therapy; strong contractions of the muscles around the hip joint compressed the femoral head against the acetabulum.

Shear

During shear loading, a load is applied parallel to the surface of the structure, and shear stress and strain result inside the structure. Shear stress can be thought of as many small forces acting on the surface of the structure on a plane parallel to the applied load (Fig. 2-22). A structure subjected to a shear load deforms internally in an angular manner; right angles on a plane surface within the structure

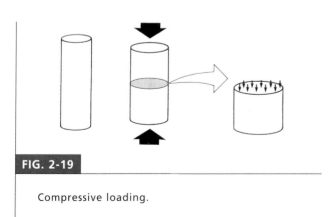

FIG. 2-19

Compressive loading.

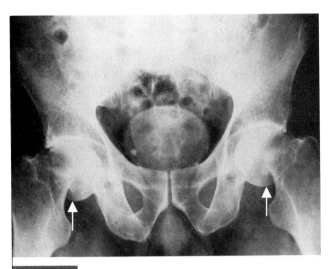

FIG. 2-21

Bilateral subcapital compression fractures of the femoral neck in a patient who underwent electroconvulsive therapy.

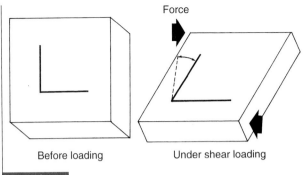

Force

Before loading   Under shear loading

FIG. 2-23

When a structure is loaded in shear, lines originally at right angles on a plane surface within the structure change their orientation, and the angle becomes obtuse or acute. This angular deformation indicates shear strain.

become obtuse or acute (Fig. 2-23). Whenever a structure is subjected to tensile or compressive loading, shear stress is produced. Figure 2-24 illustrates angular deformation in structures subjected to these loading modes. Clinically, shear fractures are most often seen in cancellous bone.

Human adult cortical bone exhibits different values for ultimate stress under compressive, tensile, and shear loading. Cortical bone can withstand greater stress in compression (approximately 190 Mpa) than in tension (approximately 130 Mpa) and greater stress in tension than in shear (70 Mpa). The elasticity (Young's modulus) is approximately 17 GPa in longitudinal or axial loading and approximately 11 GPa in transverse loading. Human trabecular bone values for testing in compression are approximately 50 Mpa and are reduced to approxi-

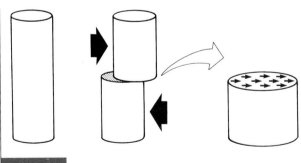

FIG. 2-22

Shear loading.

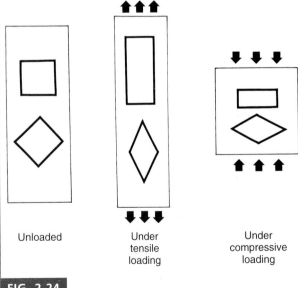

Unloaded   Under tensile loading   Under compressive loading

FIG. 2-24

The presence of shear strain in a structure loaded in tension and in compression is indicated by angular deformation.

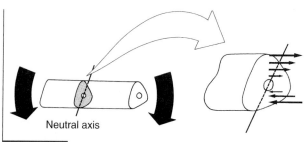

FIG. 2-25

Cross-section of a bone subjected to bending, showing distribution of stresses around the neutral axis. Tensile stresses act on the superior side, and compressive stresses act on the inferior side. The stresses are highest at the periphery of the bone and lowest near the neutral axis. The tensile and compressive stresses are unequal because the bone is asymmetrical.

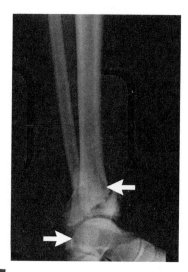

FIG. 2-27

Lateral roentgenogram of a "boot top" fracture produced by three-point bending. *Courtesy of Robert A. Winquist, M.D.*

mately 8 Mpa if loaded in tension. The modulus of elasticity is low (0.0–0.4 GPa) and dependent on the apparent density of the trabecular bone and direction of loading. The clinical biomechanical consequence is that the direction of compression failure results in general in a stable fracture, while a fracture initiated by tension or shear may have catastrophic consequences.

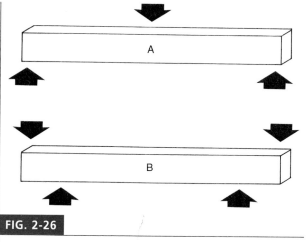

FIG. 2-26

Two types of bending. **A,** Three-point bending. **B,** Four-point bending.

Bending

In bending, loads are applied to a structure in a manner that causes it to bend about an axis. When a bone is loaded in bending, it is subjected to a combination of tension and compression. Tensile stresses and strains act on one side of the neutral axis, and compressive stresses and strains act on the other side (Fig. 2-25); there are no stresses and strains along the neutral axis. The magnitude of the stresses is proportional to their distance from the neutral axis of the bone. The farther the stresses are from the neutral axis, the higher their magnitude. Because a bone structure is asymmetrical, the stresses may not be equally distributed.

Bending may be produced by three forces (three-point bending) or four forces (four-point bending) (Fig. 2-26). Fractures produced by both types of bending are commonly observed clinically, particularly in the long bones.

Three-point bending takes place when three forces acting on a structure produce two equal moments, each being the product of one of the two peripheral forces and its perpendicular distance from the axis of rotation (the point at which the middle force is applied) (Fig. 2-26*A*). If loading continues to the yield point, the structure, if homogeneous, symmetrical, and with no structural or tissue de-

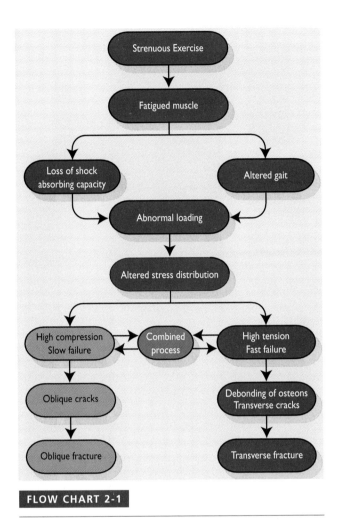

FLOW CHART 2-1

Four-point bending takes place when two force couples acting on a structure produce two equal moments. A force couple is formed when two parallel forces of equal magnitude but opposite direction are applied to a structure (Fig. 2-28A). Because the magnitude of the bending moment is the same throughout the area between the two force couples, the structure breaks at its weakest point. An example of a four-point bending fracture is shown in Figure 2-28B. A stiff knee joint was manipulated incorrectly during rehabilitation of a patient with a postsurgical infected femoral fracture. During the

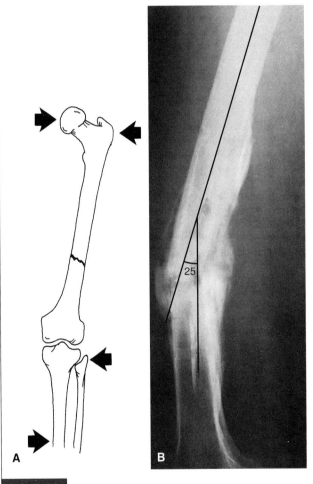

FIG. 2-28

A, During manipulation of a stiff knee joint during fracture rehabilitation, four-point bending caused the femur to refracture at its weakest point, the original fracture site. B, Lateral radiograph of the fractured femur. *Courtesy of Kaj Lundborg, M.D.*

fect, will break at the point of application of the middle force.

A typical three-point bending fracture is the "boot top" fracture sustained by skiers. In the "boot top" fracture shown in Figure 2-27, one bending moment acted on the proximal tibia as the skier fell forward over the top of the ski boot. An equal moment, produced by the fixed foot and ski, acted on the distal tibia. As the proximal tibia was bent forward, tensile stresses and strains acted on the posterior side of the bone and compressive stresses and strains acted on the anterior side. The tibia and fibula fractured at the top of the boot. Because adult bone is weaker in tension than in compression, failure begins on the side subjected to tension. Because immature bone is more ductile, it may fail first in compression, and a buckle fracture may result on the compressive side (Flowchart 2-1).

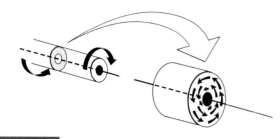

FIG. 2-29

Cross-section of a cylinder loaded in torsion, showing the distribution of shear stresses around the neutral axis. The magnitude of the stresses is highest at the periphery of the cylinder and lowest near the neutral axis.

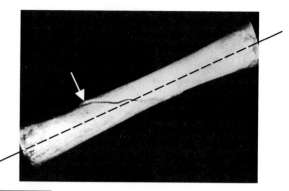

FIG. 2-31

Experimentally produced torsional fracture of a canine femur. The short crack *(arrow)* parallel to the neutral axis represents shear failure; the fracture line at a 30° angle to the neutral axis represents the plane of maximal tensile stress.

manipulation, the posterior knee joint capsule and tibia formed one force couple and the femoral head and hip joint capsule formed the other. As a bending moment was applied to the femur, the bone failed at its weakest point, the original fracture site.

Torsion

In torsion, a load is applied to a structure in a manner that causes it to twist about an axis, and a torque (or moment) is produced within the structure. When a structure is loaded in torsion, shear

stresses are distributed over the entire structure. As in bending, the magnitude of these stresses is proportional to their distance from the neutral axis (Fig. 2-29). The farther the stresses are from the neutral axis, the higher their magnitude.

Under torsional loading, maximal shear stresses act on planes parallel and perpendicular to the neutral axis of the structure. In addition, maximal tensile and compressive stresses act on a plane diagonal to the neutral axis of the structure. Figure 2-30 illustrates these planes in a small segment of bone loaded in torsion.

The fracture pattern for bone loaded in torsion suggests that the bone fails first in shear, with the formation of an initial crack parallel to the neutral axis of the bone. A second crack usually forms along the plane of maximal tensile stress. Such a pattern can be seen in the experimentally produced torsional fracture of a canine femur shown in Figure 2-31.

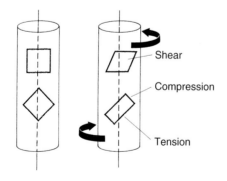

— Shear

— Compression

— Tension

FIG. 2-30

Schematic representation of a small segment of bone loaded in torsion. Maximal shear stresses act on planes parallel and perpendicular to the neutral axis. Maximal tensile and compressive stresses act on planes diagonal to this axis.

Combined Loading

Although each loading mode has been considered separately, living bone is seldom loaded in one mode only. Loading of bone in vivo is complex for two principal reasons: bones are constantly subjected to multiple indeterminate loads and their geometric structure is irregular. In vivo measurement of the strains on the anteromedial surface of a human adult tibia during walking and jogging demonstrates the complexity of the loading patterns during these common physiological activities (Lanyon et al., 1975). Stress values calculated from these strain measurements by Carter (1978) showed that during normal walking, the stresses were compressive during heel strike, tensile during the stance phase, and again compressive during push-off (Fig. 2-32A). Values for shear stress were relatively high in the later portion of the gait cycle, denoting significant torsional loading. This torsional loading was associated with external rotation of the tibia during stance and push-off.

During jogging, the stress pattern was quite different (Fig. 2-32B). The compressive stress predominating at toe strike was followed by high tensile stress during push-off. The shear stress was low throughout the stride, denoting minimal torsional loading produced by slight external and internal rotation of the tibia in an alternating pattern. The increase in speed from slow walking to jogging in-

creased both the stress and the strain on the tibia (Lanyon et al., 1975). This increase in strain with greater speed was confirmed in studies of locomotion in sheep, which demonstrated a fivefold increase in strain values from slow walking to fast trotting (Lanyon & Bourn, 1979).

INFLUENCE OF MUSCLE ACTIVITY ON STRESS DISTRIBUTION IN BONE

When bone is loaded in vivo, the contraction of the muscles attached to the bone alters the stress distribution in the bone. This muscle contraction decreases or eliminates tensile stress on the bone by producing compressive stress that neutralizes it either partially or totally.

The effect of muscle contraction can be illustrated in a tibia subjected to three-point bending. Figure 2-33A represents the leg of a skier who is falling forward, subjecting the tibia to a bending

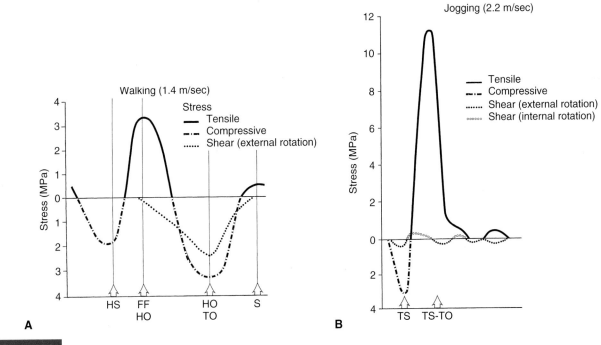

FIG. 2-32

A, Calculated stresses on the anterolateral cortex of a human tibia during walking. HS, heel strike; FF, foot flat; HO, heel-off; TO, toe off; S, swing. *Calculated from Lanyon, L.E., Hampson, W.G.J., Goodship, A.E., et al. (1975). Bone deformation recorded in vivo from strain gauges attached to the human tibial shaft. Acta Orthop Scand, 46, 256. Figure courtesy of Dennis R. Carter, Ph.D.*

B, Calculated stresses on the anterolateral cortex of a human tibia during jogging. TS, toe strike; TO, toe off. *Calculated from Lanyon, L.E., Hampson, W.G.J., Goodship, A.E., et al. (1975). Bone deformation recorded in vivo from strain gauges attached to the human tibial shaft. Acta Orthop Scand, 46, 256. Figure courtesy of Dennis R. Carter, Ph.D.*

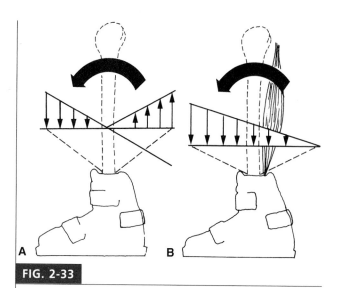

FIG. 2-33

A, Distribution of compressive and tensile stresses in a tibia subjected to three-point bending. **B,** Contraction of the triceps surae muscle produces high compressive stress on the posterior aspect, neutralizing the high tensile stress.

moment. High tensile stress is produced on the posterior aspect of the tibia, and high compressive stress acts on the anterior aspect. Contraction of the triceps surae muscle produces great compressive stress on the posterior aspect (Fig. 2-33*B*), neutralizing the great tensile stress and thereby protecting the tibia from failure in tension. This muscle contraction may result in higher compressive stress on the anterior surface of the tibia and thus protect the bone from failure. Adult bone can usually withstand this stress, but immature bone, which is weaker, may fail in compression.

Muscle contraction produces a similar effect in the hip joint (Fig. 2-34). During locomotion, bending moments are applied to the femoral neck and tensile stress is produced on the superior cortex. Contraction of the gluteus medius muscle produces compressive stress that neutralizes this tensile stress, with the net result that neither compressive nor tensile stress acts on the superior cortex. Thus, the muscle contraction allows the femoral neck to sustain higher loads than would otherwise be possible.

STRAIN RATE DEPENDENCY IN BONE

Because bone is a viscoelastic material, its biomechanical behavior varies with the rate at which the bone is loaded (i.e., the rate at which the load is applied and removed). Bone is stiffer and sustains a higher load to failure when loads are applied at higher rates. Bone also stores more energy before failure at higher loading rates, provided that these rates are within the physiological range.

The in vivo daily strain can vary considerably. The calculated strain rate for slow walking is 0.001 per second, while slow running displays a strain rate of 0.03 per second.

In general, when activities become more strenuous, the strain rate increases (Keaveny & Hayes, 1993). Figure 2-35 shows cortical bone behavior in tensile testing at different physiological strain rates. As can be seen from the figure, the same change in strain rate produces a larger change in ultimate stress (strength) than in elasticity (Young's modulus). The data indicates that the bone is approximately 30% stronger for brisk walking than for slow

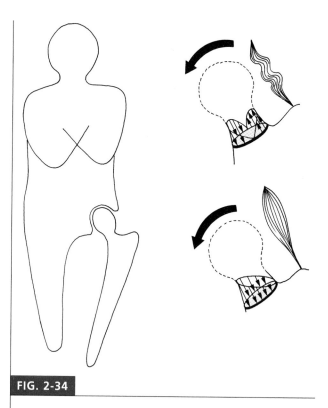

FIG. 2-34

Stress distribution in a femoral neck subjected to bending. When the gluteus medius muscle is relaxed *(top),* tensile stress acts on the superior cortex and compressive stress acts on the inferior cortex. Contraction of this muscle *(bottom)* neutralizes the tensile stress.

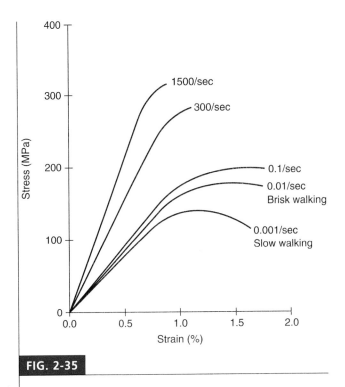

FIG. 2-35

Rate dependency of cortical bone is demonstrated at five strain rates. Both stiffness (modulus) and strength increase considerably at increased strain rates. *Adapted from McElhaney, J.H. (1966). Dynamic response of bone and muscle tissue.* J Appl Physiol, 21, 1231–1236.

walking. At very high strain rates (>1 per second) representing impact trauma, the bone becomes more brittle. In a full range of experimental testing for ultimate tensile strength and elasticity of cortical bone, the strength increases by a factor of three and the modulus by a factor of two (Keaveny & Hayes, 1993).

The loading rate is clinically significant because it influences both the fracture pattern and the amount of soft tissue damage at fracture. When a bone fractures, the stored energy is released. At a low loading rate, the energy can dissipate through the formation of a single crack; the bone and soft tissues remain relatively intact, with little or no displacement of the bone fragments. At a high loading rate, however, the greater energy stored cannot dissipate rapidly enough through a single crack, and comminution of bone and extensive soft tissue damage result. Figure 2-36 shows a human tibia tested in vitro in torsion at a high loading rate; numerous bone fragments

were produced, and displacement of the fragments was pronounced.

Clinically, bone fractures fall into three general categories based on the amount of energy released at fracture: low-energy, high-energy, and very high-energy. A low-energy fracture is exemplified by the simple torsional ski fracture; a high-energy fracture is often sustained during automobile accidents; and a very high-energy fracture is produced by very high-muzzle velocity gunshot.

FATIGUE OF BONE UNDER REPETITIVE LOADING

Bone fractures can be produced by a single load that exceeds the ultimate strength of the bone or by repeated applications of a load of lower magnitude. A fracture caused by a repeated load application is called a fatigue fracture and is typically produced either by few repetitions of a high load or by many repetitions of a relatively normal load (Case Study 2-1).

The interplay of load and repetition for any material can be plotted on a fatigue curve (Fig. 2-37). For some materials (some metals, for example), the fatigue curve is asymptotic, indicating that if the load is kept below a certain level, theoretically the material will remain intact no matter how many repetitions. For bone tested in vitro, the curve is not asymptotic. When bone is subjected to repetitive low loads, it may sustain microfractures. Testing of bone in vitro also reveals that bone fatigues rapidly when the load or deformation approaches its yield strength; that is, the number of repetitions needed to produce a fracture diminishes rapidly.

In repetitive loading of living bone, the fatigue process is affected not only by the amount of load and the number of repetitions but also by the number of applications of the load within a given time (frequency of loading). Because living bone is self-repairing, a fatigue fracture results only when the remodeling process is outpaced by the fatigue process—that is, when loading is so frequent that it precludes the remodeling necessary to prevent failure.

Fatigue fractures are usually sustained during continuous strenuous physical activity, which causes the muscles to become fatigued and reduces their ability to contract. As a result, they are less able to store energy and thus to neutralize the stresses imposed on the bone. The resulting alteration of the stress distribution in the bone causes

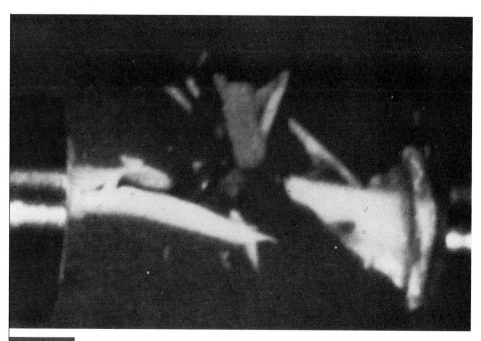

FIG. 2-36

Human tibia experimentally tested to failure in torsion at a high loading rate. Displacement of the numerous fragments was pronounced.

CASE STUDY 2-1

Bone Overloading

A 23-year-old military recruit was exposed to an intensive heavy physical training regime that included repetitive continuous crawling in an awkward position for several weeks (Case Study Fig. 2-1-1A). The repeated application of loads (high repetitions) and the number of applications of a load during a short period of time (high frequency of loading) surpassed the time for the bone remodeling process to prevent failure. Muscle fatigue occurred as a result of the abnormal loading pattern and the intensive training. It affected the muscle function in the neutralization of the stress imposed, leading to abnormal loading and altered stress distribution (Case Study Fig. 2-1-1B).

After 4 weeks of strenuous physical activity, the damage accumulation from fatigue at the femoral shaft lead to an oblique fracture.

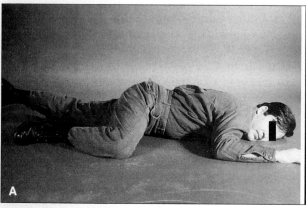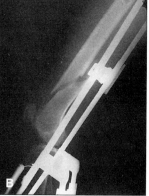

Case Study Figure 2-1-1A. Abnormal loads at the femoral shaft occurred.

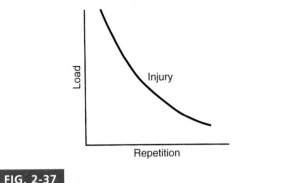

FIG. 2-37

The interplay of load and repetition is represented on a fatigue curve.

abnormally high loads to be imposed, and a fatigue damage accumulation occurs that may lead to a fracture. Bone may fail on the tensile side, on the compressive side, or on both sides. Failure on the tensile side results in a transverse crack, and the bone proceeds rapidly to complete fracture. Fatigue fractures on the compressive side appear to be pro-

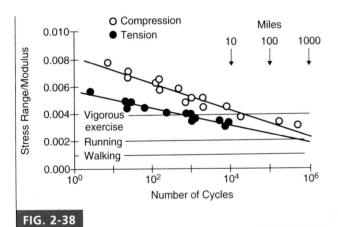

FIG. 2-38

Fatigue testing showing the number of cycles (x-axis) and strain range (y-axis) expressed as stress range/modulus in human cortical bone specimens loaded in tension and compression. Typical strain ranges are shown for walking, running, and vigorous exercises. Note that resistance to fatigue fracture is greater in compressive loading. Ten miles represent approximately 5,000 cycles, corresponding to the number of steps running during that distance. *Adapted from Carter, D.R., Cater, W.E., Spengler, D.M., Frankel, V.H. (1981). Fatigue behavior of adult cortical bone: the influence of mean strain and strain range.* Acta Orthop Scand, *52, 481–490.*

duced more slowly; the remodeling is less easily outpaced by the fatigue process and the bone may not proceed to complete fracture.

This theory of muscle fatigue as a cause of fatigue fracture in the lower extremities is outlined in the schema in Flowchart 2-1 on p. 41.

Figure 2-38 shows typical strain ranges for human femoral cortical bone during different activities and distances. Resistance to fatigue behavior is greater in compression than in tension (Keaveny & Hayes, 1993). On average, approximately 5,000 cycles of experimental loading correspond to the number of steps in 10 miles of running. One million cycles corresponds to approximately 1,000 miles. A total distance of less than 1,000 miles could cause a fracture of the cortical bone tissue. This is consistent with stress fractures reported among military recruits undergoing strenuous training of up to 1,000 miles of running over a short period of time (6 weeks). Fractures of individual trabeculae in cancellous bone have been observed in postmortem human specimens and may be caused by fatigue accumulation. Common sites are the lumbar vertebrae, the femoral head, and the proximal tibia. It has been suggested that these fractures may play a role in bone remodeling as well as in age-related fractures, collapse of subchondral bone, degenerative joint diseases, and other bone disorders.

INFLUENCE OF BONE GEOMETRY ON BIOMECHANICAL BEHAVIOR

The geometry of a bone greatly influences its mechanical behavior. In tension and compression, the load to failure and the stiffness are proportional to the cross-sectional area of the bone. The larger the area, the stronger and stiffer the bone. In bending, both the cross-sectional area and the distribution of bone tissue around a neutral axis affect the bone's mechanical behavior. The quantity that takes into account these two factors in bending is called the area moment of inertia. A larger moment of inertia results in a stronger and stiffer bone. Figure 2-39 shows the influence of the area moment of inertia on the load to failure and the stiffness of three rectangular structures that have the same area but different shapes. In bending, beam III is the stiffest of the three and can withstand the highest load because the greatest amount of material is distributed at a distance from the neutral axis. For rectangular cross-sections, the formula for the area moment of

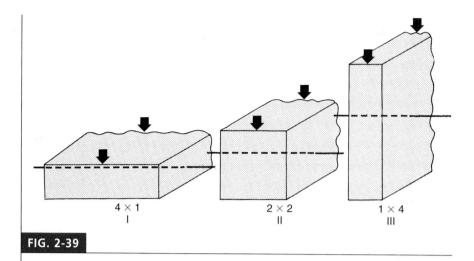

4 × 1   2 × 2   1 × 4
I   II   III

FIG. 2-39

Three beams of equal area but different shapes subjected to bending. The area moment of inertia for beam I is 4/12; for beam II, 16/12; and for beam III, 64/12. *Adapted from Frankel, V.H., & Burstein, A.H. (1970).* Orthopaedic Biomechanics. *Philadelphia: Lea & Febiger.*

inertia is the width (B) multiplied by the cube of the height (H^3) divided by 12:

$$\frac{B \cdot H^3}{12}$$

Because of its large area moment of inertia, beam III can withstand four times more load in bending than can beam I.

A third factor, the length of the bone, influences the strength and stiffness in bending. The longer the bone, the greater the magnitude of the bending moment caused by the application of a force. In a rectangular structure, the magnitude of the stresses produced at the point of application of the bending moment is proportional to the length of the structure. Figure 2-40 depicts the forces acting on two beams with the same width and height but different lengths: beam B is twice as long as beam A. The bending moment for the longer beam is twice that for the shorter beam; consequently, the stress magnitude throughout the beam is twice as high. Because of their length, the long bones of the skeleton are subjected to high bending moments and, therefore, to high tensile and compressive stresses. Their tubular shape gives them the ability to resist bending moments in all directions. These bones have a large area moment of inertia because much of the bone tissue is distributed at a distance from the neutral axis.

The factors that affect bone strength and stiffness in torsion are the same that operate in bending: the cross-sectional area and the distribution of bone tissue around a neutral axis. The quantity that takes into account these two factors in torsional loading is the polar moment of inertia. The larger the polar moment of inertia, the stronger and stiffer the bone.

Figure 2-41 shows distal and proximal cross-sections of a tibia subjected to torsional loading. Although the proximal section has a slightly smaller bony area than does the distal section, it has a much higher polar moment of inertia because much of the bone tissue is distributed at a distance from the neutral axis. The distal section, while it has a larger bony area, is subjected to much higher shear stress because much of the bone tissue is distributed close to the neutral axis. The magnitude of the shear stress in the distal section is approximately double that in the proximal section. Clinically, torsional fractures of the tibia commonly occur distally.

When bone begins to heal after fracture, blood vessels and connective tissue from the periosteum migrate into the region of the fracture, forming a cuff of dense fibrous tissue, or callus (woven bone), around the fracture site, stabilizing that area (Fig. 2-42A). The callus significantly increases the area and polar moments of inertia, thereby increasing the strength and stiffness of the bone in bending and torsion during the healing period. As the frac-

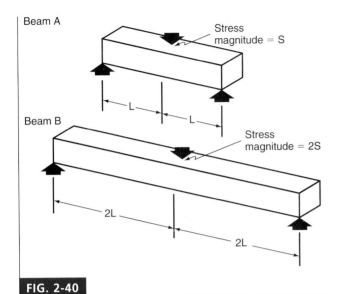

FIG. 2-40

Beam B is twice as long as beam A and sustains twice the bending moment. Hence, the stress magnitude throughout beam B is twice as high. *Adapted from Frankel, V.H., & Burstein, A.H. (1970).* Orthopaedic Biomechanics. *Philadelphia: Lea & Febiger.*

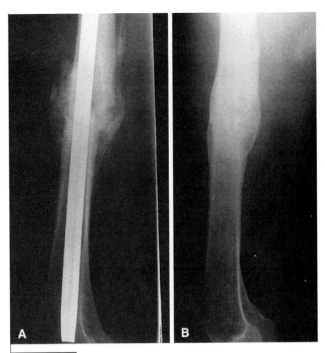

FIG. 2-42

A, Early callus formation in a femoral fracture fixed with an intramedullary nail. **B,** Nine months after injury, the fracture has healed and most of the callus cuff has been resorbed. *Courtesy of Robert A. Winquist, M.D.*

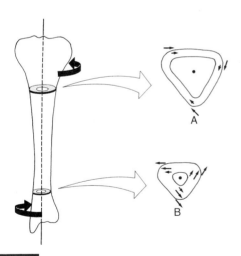

FIG. 2-41

Distribution of shear stress in two cross-sections of a tibia subjected to torsional loading. The proximal section **(A)** has a higher moment of inertia than does the distal section **(B)** because more bony material is distributed away from the neutral axis. *Adapted from Frankel, V.H., & Burstein, A.H. (1970).* Orthopaedic Biomechanics. *Philadelphia: Lea & Febiger.*

ture heals and the bone gradually regains its normal strength, the callus cuff is progressively resorbed and the bone returns to as near its normal size and shape as possible (Fig. 2-42*B*).

Certain surgical procedures produce defects that greatly weaken the bone, particularly in torsion. These defects fall into two categories: those whose length is less than the diameter of the bone (stress raisers) and those whose length exceeds the bone diameter (open section defects).

A stress raiser is produced surgically when a small piece of bone is removed or a screw is inserted. Bone strength is reduced because the stresses imposed during loading are prevented from being distributed evenly throughout the bone and instead become concentrated around the defect. This defect is analogous to a rock in a stream, which diverts the water, producing high water turbulence around it. The weakening effect of a stress raiser is particularly marked under torsional loading; the total decrease in bone strength in this loading mode can reach 60%.

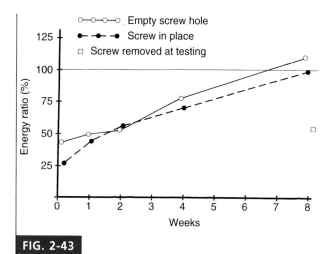

FIG. 2-43

Effect of screws and of empty screw holes on the energy storage capacity of rabbit femora. The energy storage for experimental animals is expressed as a percentage of the total energy storage capacity for control animals. When screws were removed immediately before testing, the energy storage capacity decreased by 50%. *Adapted from Burstein, A.H., et al. (1972). Bone strength: The effect of screw holes.* J Bone Joint Surg, 54A, 1143.

raiser effect produced by the screws and by the holes without screws had disappeared completely because the bone had remodeled: bone had been laid down around the screws to stabilize them, and the empty screw holes had been filled in with bone. In femora from which the screws had been removed immediately before testing, however, the energy storage capacity of the bone decreased by 50%, mainly because the bone tissue around the screw sustained microdamage during screw removal (Fig. 2-43).

An open section defect is a discontinuity in the bone caused by the surgical removal of a piece of bone longer than the bone's diameter (e.g., by the cutting of a slot during a bone biopsy). Because the outer surface of the bone's cross-section is no longer continuous, its ability to resist loads is altered, particularly in torsion.

In a normal bone subjected to torsion, the shear stress is distributed throughout the bone and acts to resist the torque. This stress pattern is illustrated in the cross-section of a long bone shown in Figure 2-44A. (A cross-section with a continuous outer surface is called a closed section.) In a bone with an

Burstein and associates (1972) showed the effect of stress raisers produced by screws and by empty screw holes on the energy storage capacity of rabbit bones tested in torsion at a high loading rate. The immediate effect of drilling a hole and inserting a screw in a rabbit femur was a 74% decrease in energy storage capacity. After 8 weeks, the stress

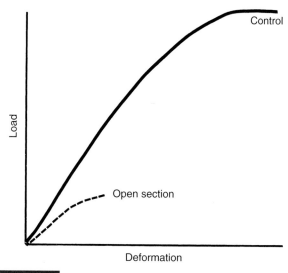

FIG. 2-45

Load-deformation curves for human adult tibiae tested in vitro under torsional loading. The control curve represents a tibia with no defect; the open section curve represents a tibia with an open section defect. *Adapted from Frankel, V.H., & Burstein, A.H. (1970). Orthopaedic Biomechanics.* Philadelphia: Lea & Febiger.

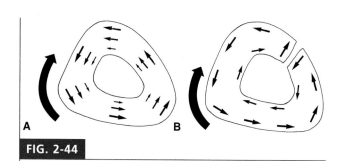

FIG. 2-44

Stress pattern in an open and closed section under torsional loading. **A,** In the closed section, all the shear stress resists the applied torque. **B,** In the open section, only the shear stress at the periphery of the bone resists the applied torque.

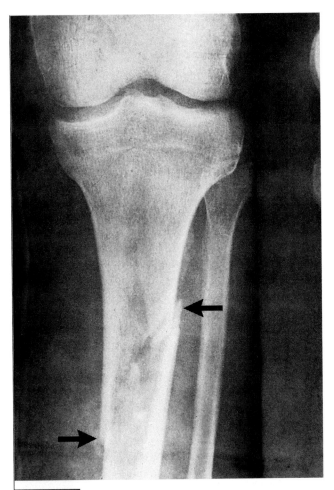

FIG. 2-46

A patient sustained a tibial fracture through a surgically produced open section defect when she tripped a few weeks after the biopsy.

graft was removed for use in an arthrodesis of the hip. A few weeks after operation, the patient tripped while twisting and the bone fractured through the defect.

Bone Remodeling

Bone has the ability to remodel, by altering its size, shape, and structure, to meet the mechanical demands placed on it (Buckwalter et al., 1995). This phenomenon, in which bone gains or loses cancellous and/or cortical bone in response to the level of stress sustained, is summarized as Wolff's law, which states that the remodeling of bone is influenced and modulated by mechanical stresses (Wolff, 1892).

Load on the skeleton can be accomplished by either muscle activity or gravity. A positive correlation exists between bone mass and body weight. A greater body weight has been associated with a larger bone mass (Exner et al., 1979). Conversely, a prolonged condition of weightlessness, such as that experienced during space travel, has been found to result in decreased bone mass in weight-bearing bones. Astronauts experience a fast loss of calcium and consequent bone loss (Rambaut & Johnston, 1979; Whedon, 1984). These changes are not completely reversible.

open section defect, only the shear stress at the periphery of the bone resists the applied torque. As the shear stress encounters the discontinuity, it is forced to change direction (Fig. 2-44B). Throughout the interior of the bone, the stress runs parallel to the applied torque, and the amount of bone tissue resisting the load is greatly decreased.

In torsion tests in vitro of human adult tibiae, an open section defect reduced the load to failure and energy storage to failure by as much as 90%. The deformation to failure was diminished by approximately 70% (Frankel & Burstein, 1970) (Fig. 2-45).

Clinically, the surgical removal of a piece of bone can greatly weaken the bone, particularly in torsion. Figure 2-46 is a radiograph of a tibia from which a

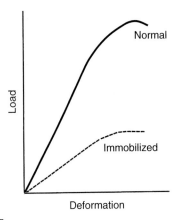

FIG. 2-47

Load-deformation curves for vertebral segments L5 to L7 from normal and immobilized Rhesus monkeys. Note the extensive loss of strength and stiffness in the immobilized specimens. *Adapted from Kazarian, L.L., & Von Gierke, H.E. (1969) Bone loss as a result of immobilization and chelation. Preliminary results in Macaca mulatta. Clin Orthop, 65, 67.*

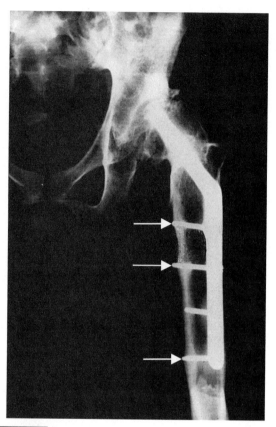

FIG. 2-49

Roentgenogram of a fractured femoral neck to which a nail plate was applied. Loads are transmitted from the plate to the bone via the screws. Bone has been laid down around the screws to bear these loads.

CASE STUDY 2-2

Bone Remodeling

A 30-year-old man who had a surgical removal of an ulna plate after stabilization of a displaced ulnar fracture. Figure 2-48 shows anteroposterior (A) and lateral (B) roentgenograms of the ulna after late plate removal.

The implant is used to stabilize the fracture for rapid healing. However, in situations such as this, the late plate removal decreased the amount of mechanical stresses necessary for bone remodeling. It is of concern when the plate carries most or all of the mechanical load and remains after fracture healing. Thus, according to Wolff's law, it will promote localized osseous resorption as a result of decreased mechanical stress and stimulus of the bone under the plate, resulting in a decrease in strength and stiffness of the bone.

Disuse or inactivity has deleterious effects on the skeleton. Bed rest induces a bone mass decrease of approximately 1% per week (Jenkins & Cochran, 1969; Krolner & Toft, 1983). In partial or total immobilization, bone is not subjected to the usual mechanical stresses, which leads to resorp-

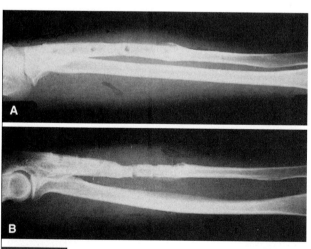

FIG. 2-48

Anteroposterior (A) and lateral (B) roentgenograms of an ulna after plate removal show a decreased bone diameter caused by resorption of the bone under the plate. Cancellization of the cortex and the presence of screw holes also weaken the bone. *Courtesy of Marc Martens, M.D.*

tion of the periosteal and subperiosteal bone and a decrease in the mechanical properties of bone (i.e., strength and stiffness). This decrease in bone strength and stiffness was shown by Kazarian and Von Gierke (1969), who immobilized Rhesus monkeys in full-body casts for 60 days. Subsequent compressive testing in vitro of the vertebrae from the immobilized monkeys and from controls showed up to a threefold decrease in load to failure and energy storage capacity in the vertebrae that had been immobilized; stiffness was also significantly decreased (Fig. 2-47).

An implant that remains firmly attached to a bone after a fracture has healed may also diminish the strength and stiffness of the bone. In the case of a plate fixed to the bone with screws, the plate and the bone share the load in proportions deter-

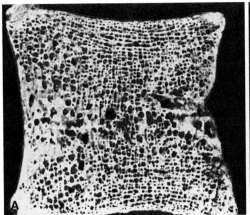 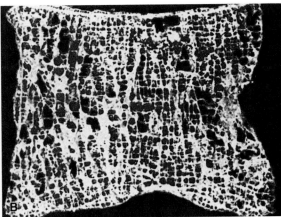 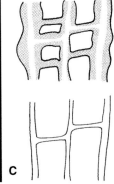

FIG. 2-50

Vertebral cross-sections from autopsy specimens of young **(A)** and old **(B)** bone show a marked reduction in cancellous bone in the latter. *Reprinted with permission from Nordin, B.E.C. (1973).* Metabolic Bone and Stone Disease. *Edinburgh: Churchill Livingstone.* **C**, Bone reduction with aging is schematically depicted. As normal bone *(top)* is subjected to absorption *(shaded area)* during the aging process, the longitudinal trabeculae become thinner and some transverse trabeculae disappear *(bottom)*. *Adapted from Siffert, R.S., & Levy, R.N. (1981).* Trabecular patterns and the internal architecture of bone. *Mt. Sinai J Med, 48, 221.*

mined by the geometry and material properties of each structure (Case Study 2-2). A large plate, carrying high loads, unloads the bone to a great extent; the bone then atrophies in response to this diminished load. (The bone may hypertrophy at the bone-screw interface in an attempt to reduce the micromotion of the screws.)

Bone resorption under a plate is illustrated in Figure 2-48. A compression plate made of a material approximately 10 times stiffer than the bone was applied to a fractured ulna and remained after the fracture had healed. The bone under the plate carried a lower load than normal; it was partially resorbed, and the diameter of the diaphysis became markedly smaller. A reduction in the size of the bone diameter greatly decreases bone strength, particularly in bending and torsion, as it reduces the area and polar moments of inertia. A 20% decrease in bone diameter may reduce the strength in torsion by 60%. Changes in bone size and shape illustrated in Figure 2-48 suggest that rigid plates should be removed shortly after a fracture has healed and before the bone has markedly diminished in size. Such a decrease in bone size is usually accompanied by secondary osteoporosis, which further weakens the bone (Slätis et al., 1980).

An implant may cause bone hypertrophy at its attachment sites. An example of bone hypertrophy around screws is illustrated in Figure 2-49. A nail plate was applied to a femoral neck fracture and the bone hypertrophied around the screws in response to the increased load at these sites. Hypertrophy may also result if bone is repeatedly subjected to high mechanical stresses within the normal physiological range. Hypertrophy of normal adult bone in response to strenuous exercise has been observed (Dalén & Olsson, 1974; Huddleston et al., 1980; Jones et al., 1977), as has an increase in bone density (Nilsson & Westlin, 1971).

Degenerative Changes in Bone Associated With Aging

A progressive loss of bone density has been observed as part of the normal aging process. The longitudinal trabeculae become thinner, and some of the transverse trabeculae are resorbed (Siffert & Levy, 1981) (Fig. 2-50). The result is a marked reduction in the amount of cancellous bone and a thinning of cortical bone. The relationship between bone mass, age, and gender is shown in Figure 2-51. The decrease in bone tissue and the slight decrease in the size of the bone reduce bone strength and stiffness.

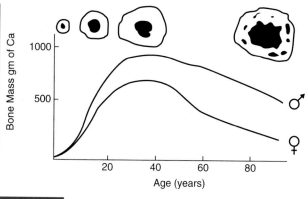

FIG. 2-51

Graph showing the relationship between bone mass, age, and gender. On the top of the figure, a cross-section of the diaphysis of the femur and the bone mass configuration is shown. *Reprinted with permission from Kaplan, F.S., Hayes, W.C., Keaveny, T.M., et al (1994). Form and function of bone. In S.R. Simon (ed.) Orthopaedic Basic Science (p. 167). Rosemont, IL:AAOS.*

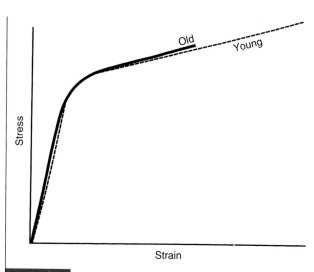

FIG. 2-52

Stress-strain curves for samples of adult young and old human tibiae tested in tension. Note that the bone strength is comparable but that the old bone is more brittle and has lost its ability to deform. *Adapted from Burstein, A.H., Reilly, D.T., & Martens, M. (1976). Aging of bone tissue: Mechanical properties. J Bone Joint Surg, 58A, 82.*

Stress-strain curves for specimens from human adult tibiae of two widely differing ages tested in tension are shown in Figure 2-52. The ultimate stress was approximately the same for the young and the old bone. The old bone specimen could withstand only half the strain that the young bone could, indicating greater brittleness and a reduction in energy storage capacity. The reduction in bone density, strength, and stiffness results in increased bone fragility. Age-related bone loss depends on a number of factors, including gender, age, postmenopause, endocrine abnormality, inactivity, disuse, and calcium deficiency. Over several decades, the skeletal mass may be reduced to 50% of original trabecular and 25% of cortical mass. In the fourth decade, women lose approximately 1.5 to 2% a year while men lose only approximately half that rate (0.5 to 0.75%) yearly. Regular physical activity and exercise (Zetterbarg et al., 1990), calcium, and possibly estrogen intake may decrease the rate of bone mineral loss during aging.

Summary

1 Bone is a complex two-phase composite material. One phase is composed of inorganic mineral salts and the other is an organic matrix of collagen and ground substance. The inorganic component makes bone hard and rigid, whereas the organic component gives bone its flexibility and resilience.

2 Microscopically, the fundamental structural unit of bone is the osteon, or haversian system, composed of concentric layers of a mineralized matrix surrounding a central canal containing blood vessels and nerve fibers.

3 Macroscopically, the skeleton is composed of cortical and cancellous (trabecular) bone. Cortical bone has high density while trabecular bone varies in density over a wide range.

4 Bone is an anisotropic material, exhibiting different mechanical properties when loaded in different directions. Mature bone is strongest and stiffest in compression.

5 Bone is subjected to complex loading patterns during common physiological activities such as walking and jogging. Most bone fractures are produced by a combination of several loading modes.

6 Muscle contraction affects stress patterns in bone by producing compressive stress that partially or totally neutralizes the tensile stress acting on the bone.

7 Bone is stiffer, sustains higher loads before failing, and stores more energy when loaded at higher physiological strain rates.

8 Living bone fatigues when the frequency of loading precludes the remodeling necessary to prevent failure.

9 The mechanical behavior of a bone is influenced by its geometry (length, cross-sectional area, and distribution of bone tissue around the neutral axis).

10 Bone remodels in response to the mechanical demands placed on it; it is laid down where needed and resorbed where not needed.

11 With aging comes a marked reduction in the amount of cancellous bone and a decrease in the thickness of cortical bone. These changes diminish bone strength and stiffness.

REFERENCES

Bassett, C.A.L. (1965). Electrical effects in bone. *Sci Am, 213,* 18.

Bonefield, W., & Li, C.H. (1967). Anisotropy of nonelastic flow in bone. *J Appl Physics, 38,* 2450.

Buckwalter, J.A., Glimcher, M.J., Cooper, R.R., et al. (1995). Bone biology. Part I: Structure, blood supply, cells, matrix and mineralization. Part II: Formation, form, remodelling and regulation of cell function. (Instructional Course Lecture). *J Bone Joint Surg, 77A,* 1256–1289.

Burstein, A.H., Reilly, D.T., & Martens, M. (1976). Aging of bone tissue: Mechanical properties. *J Bone Joint Surg, 58A,* 82

Burstein, A.H., et al. (1972). Bone strength: The effect of screw holes. *J Bone Joint Surg, 54A,* 1143.

Carter, D.R. (1978). Anisotropic analysis of strain rosette information from cortical bone. *J Biomech, 11,* 199.

Carter, D.R., & Hayes, W.C. (1977). Compact bone fatigue damage: A microscopic examination. *Clin Orthop, 127,* 265.

Dalen, N., & Olsson, K.E. (1974). Bone mineral content and physical activity. *Acta Orthop Scand, 45,* 170.

Exner, G.U., et al. (1979). Bone densitometry using computed tomography. Part 1: Selective determination of trabecular bone density and other bone mineral parameters. Normal values in children and adults. *Br J Radiol, 52,* 14.

Frankel, V.H., & Burstein, A.H. (1970). *Orthopaedic Biomechanics.* Philadelphia: Lea & Febiger.

Huddleston, A.L., Rockwell, D., Kulund, D.N., et al. (1980). Bone mass in lifetime tennis athletes. *JAMA, 244,* 1107.

International Society of Biomechanics (1987). *Quantities and Units of Measurements in Biomechanics* (unpublished).

Jenkins, D.P., & Cochran, T.H. (1969). Osteoporosis: The dramatic effect of disuse of an extremity. *Clin Orthop, 64,* 128.

Jones, H., Priest, J., Hayes, W., et al. (1977). Humeral hypertrophy in response to exercise. *J Bone Joint Surg, 59A,* 204.

Kaplan, F.S., Hayes, W.C., Keaveny, T.M., et al. (1994). Form and function of bone. In S.R. Simon (Ed.). *Orthopaedic Basic Science* (pp.127–184). Rosemont, IL: AAOS.

Kazarian, L.L., & Von Gierke, H.E. (1969) Bone loss as a result of immobilization and chelation. Preliminary results in Macaca mulatta. *Clin Orthop, 65,* 67.

Keaveny, T.M., & Hayes, W.C. (1993). Mechanical properties of cortical and trabecular bone. *Bone, 7,* 285–344.

Krolner, B., & Toft, B. (1983). Vertebral bone loss: An unheeded side effect of bedrest. *Clin Sci, 64,* 537–540.

Kummer, J.K. (1999). Implant Biomaterials. In: J.M. Spivak, P.E. DiCesare, D.S. Feldman, K.J. Koval, A.S. Rokito, & J.D. Zuckerman (Eds.). *Orthopaedics: A Study Guide* (pp. 45–48). New York: McGraw-Hill.

Lanyon, L.E., & Bourn, S. (1979). The influence of mechanical function on the development and remodeling of the tibia: An experimental study in sheep. *J Bone Joint Surg, 61A,* 263.

Lanyon, L.E., Hampson, W.G.J., Goodship, A.E., et al. (1975). Bone deformation recorded in vivo from strain gauges attached to the human tibial shaft. *Acta Orthop Scand, 46,* 256.

Nilsson, B.E., & Westlin, N.E. (1971). Bone density in athletes. *Clin Orthop, 77,* 179.

Özkaya, N., & Nordin, M. (1999). *Fundamentals of Biomechanics: Equilibrium, Motion, and Deformation* (2nd ed.) New York: Springer-Verlag.

Rambaut, P.C., & Johnston, R.S. (1979). Prolonged weightlessness and calcium loss in man. *Acta Astronautica, 6,* 1113.

Siffert, R.S., & Levy, R.N. (1981). Trabecular patterns and the internal architecture of bone. *Mt. Sinai J Med, 48,* 221.

Slätis, P., Paavolainen, P., Karaharju, E., et al. (1980). Structural and biomechanical changes in bone after rigid plate fixation. *Can J Surg, 23,* 247.

Whedon, G.D. (1984) Disuse osteoporosis: Physiological aspects. *Calcif Tissue Int, 36,* 146–150.

Wolff, J. (1892). *Das Gesetz der Transformation der Knochen.* Berlin: Hirschwald.

Zetterberg C., Nordin, M., Skovron, M.L., et al. (1990). Skeletal effects of physical activity. *Geri-Topics, 13*(4), 17–24.

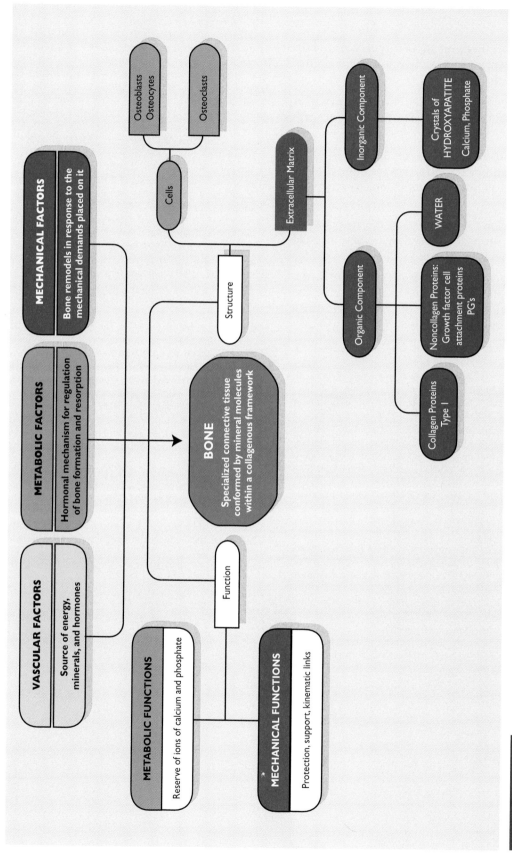

FLOW CHART 2-2 Bone composition, structure, and functions.* (*PG's*, proteoglycans)

*This flow chart is designed for classroom or group discussion. Flow chart is not meant to be exhaustive.

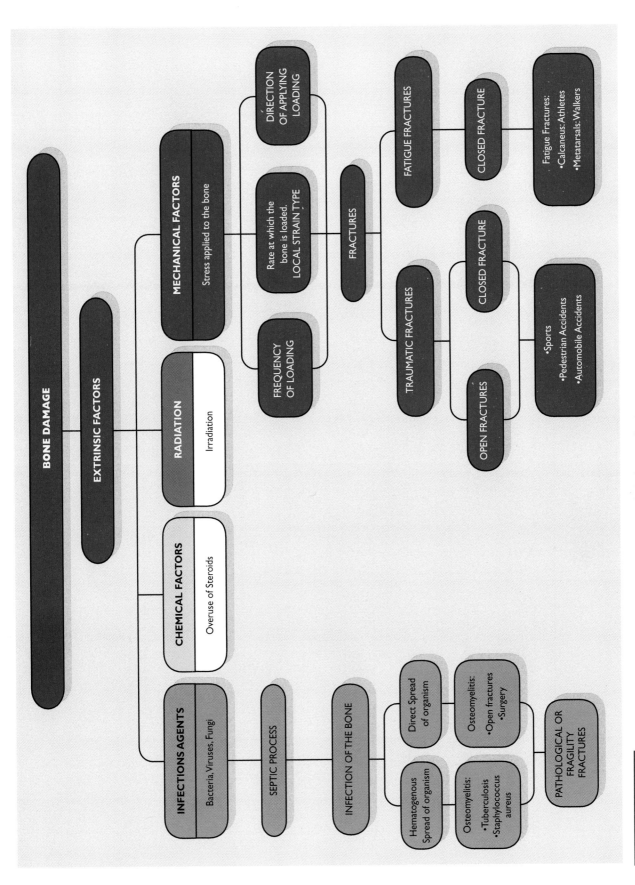

FLOW CHART 2-3   Extrinsic factors associated with bone damage. Clinical examples.*

*This flow chart is designed for classroom or group discussion. Flow chart is not meant to be exhaustive.

FLOW CHART 2-4 Intrinsic factors associated with bone damage. Clinical examples.*

*This flow chart is designed for classroom or group discussion. Flow chart is not meant to be exhaustive.

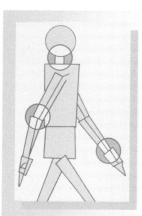

CHAPTER 3

Biomechanics of Articular Cartilage

Van C. Mow, Clark T. Hung

Introduction

Three types of joints exist in the human body: fibrous, cartilaginous, and synovial. Only one of these, the synovial, or diarthrodial, joint, allows a large degree of motion. In young normal joints, the articulating bone ends of diarthrodial joints are covered by a thin (1–6 mm), dense, translucent, white connective tissue called hyaline articular cartilage (Box 3-1). Articular cartilage is a highly specialized tissue precisely suited for withstanding the highly loaded joint environment without failure during an average individual's lifetime. Physiologically, however, it is virtually an isolated tissue, devoid of blood vessels, lymphatic channels, and neurological innervation. Furthermore, its cellular density is less than that of any other tissue (Stockwell, 1979).

In diarthrodial joints, articular cartilage has two primary functions: (1) to distribute joint loads over a wide area, thus decreasing the stresses sustained by the contacting joint surfaces (Ateshian et al., 1995; Helminen et al., 1987) and (2) to allow relative movement of the opposing joint surfaces with minimal friction and wear (Mow & Ateshian, 1997). In this chapter, we will describe how the biomechanical properties of articular cartilage, as determined by its composition and structure, allow for the optimal performance of these functions.

BOX 3-1   Hyaline Articular Cartilage

A notable exception to the definition of hyaline articular cartilage is the temporomandibular joint, a synovial joint in which fibrocartilage is found covering the bone ends. Fibrocartilage and a third type of cartilage, elastic cartilage, are closely related to hyaline cartilage embryologically and histologically but are vastly different in mechanical and biochemical properties. Fibrocartilage represents a transitional cartilage found at the margins of some joint cavities, in the joint capsules, and at the insertions of ligaments and tendons into bone.

Fibrocartilage also forms the menisci interposed between the articular cartilage of some joints and composes the outer covering of the intervertebral discs, the anulus fibrosus. Elastic cartilage is found in the external ear, in the cartilage of the eustachian tube, in the epiglottis, and in certain parts of the larynx.

Composition and Structure of Articular Cartilage

Chondrocytes, the sparsely distributed cells in articular cartilage, account for less than 10% of the tissue's volume (Stockwell, 1979). Schematically, the zonal arrangement of chondrocytes is shown in Figure 3-1. Despite their sparse distribution, chondrocytes manufacture, secrete, organize, and maintain the organic component of the extracellular matrix (ECM) (Fosang & Hardingham, 1996; Muir, 1983). The organic matrix is composed of a dense network of fine collagen fibrils (mostly type II collagen, with minor amounts of types V, VI, IX, and XI) that are enmeshed in a concentrated solution of proteoglycans (PGs) (Bateman et al., 1996; Eyre, 1980; Muir, 1983). In normal articular cartilage the collagen content ranges from 15 to 22% by wet weight and the PG content from 4 to 7% by wet weight; the remaining 60 to 85% is water, inorganic salts, and small amounts of other matrix proteins, glycoproteins, and lipids (Mow & Ratcliffe, 1997). Collagen fibrils and PGs, each being capable of forming structural networks of significant strength (Broom & Silyn-Roberts, 1990; Kempson et al., 1976; Schmidt et al., 1990; Zhu et al., 1991, 1993), are the structural components supporting the internal mechanical stresses that result from loads being applied to the articular cartilage. Moreover, these structural components, together with water, determine the biomechanical behavior of this tissue (Ateshian et al., 1997; Maroudas, 1979; Mow et al., 1980, 1984; Mow & Ateshian, 1997).

COLLAGEN

Collagen is the most abundant protein in the body (Bateman et al., 1996; Eyre, 1980). In articular cartilage, collagen has a high level of structural organization that provides a fibrous ultrastructure (Clark, 1985; Clarke, 1971; Mow & Ratcliffe, 1997). The basic biological unit of collagen is tropocollagen, a structure composed of three procollagen polypeptide chains (alpha chains) coiled into left-handed helixes (Fig. 3-2A) that are further coiled about each other into a right-handed triple helix (Fig. 3-2B). These rod-like tropocollagen molecules, 1.4 nanometers (nm) in diameter and 300 nm long (Fig. 3-2, C & D), polymerize into larger collagen fibrils (Bateman et al., 1996; Eyre, 1980). In articular cartilage, these fibrils have an average diameter of 25 to 40 nm (Fig.3-2E, Box 3-2); however, this is highly variable.

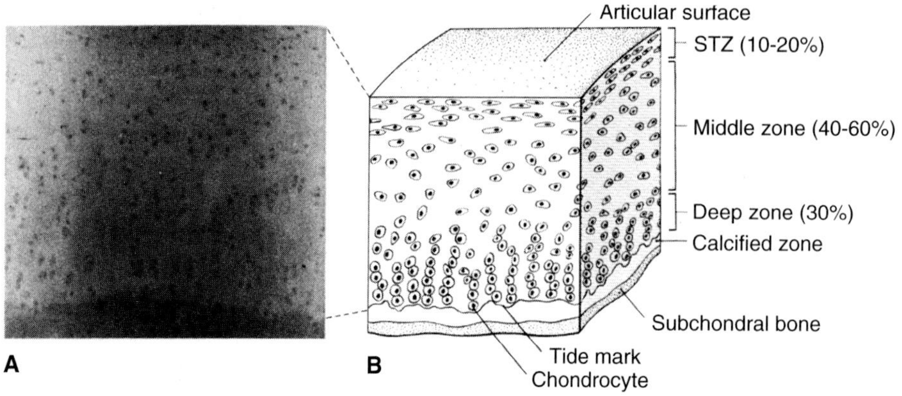

FIG. 3-1

Photomicrograph (**A**) and schematic representation (**B**) of the chondrocyte arrangement throughout the depth of noncalcified articular cartilage. In the superficial tangential zone, chondrocytes are oblong with their long axes aligned parallel to the articular surface. In the middle zone, the chondrocytes are "round" and randomly distributed. Chondrocytes in the deep zone are arranged in a columnar fashion oriented perpendicular to the tidemark, the demarcation between the calcified and noncalcified tissue.

Scanning electron microscopic studies, for instance, have described fibers with diameters ranging up to 200 nm (Clarke, 1971). Covalent cross-links form between these tropocollagen molecules, adding to the fibrils high tensile strength (Bateman et al., 1996).

The collagen in articular cartilage is inhomogeneously distributed, giving the tissue a layered character (Lane & Weiss, 1975; Mow & Ratcliffe, 1997). Numerous investigations using light, transmission electron, and scanning electron microscopy have identified three separate structural zones. For example, Mow et al. (1974) proposed a zonal arrangement for the collagen network shown schematically in Figure 3-3A. In the superficial tangential zone, which represents 10 to 20% of the total thickness, are sheets of fine, densely packed fibers randomly woven in planes parallel to the articular surface (Clarke, 1971; Redler & Zimny, 1970; Weiss et al., 1968). In the middle zone (40 to 60% of the total thickness), there are greater distances between the randomly oriented and homogeneously dispersed fibers. Below this, in the deep zone (approximately 30% of the total thickness), the fibers come together, forming larger, radially oriented fiber bundles (Redler et al., 1975). These bundles then cross the tidemark, the interface between articular cartilage and the calcified cartilage beneath it, to enter the calcified cartilage, thus forming an interlocking "root" system anchoring the cartilage to the underlying bone (Bullough & Jagannath, 1983; Redler et al., 1975). This anisotropic fiber orientation is mirrored by the inhomogeneous zonal variations in the collagen content, which is highest at the surface and then remains relatively constant throughout the deeper zones (Lipshitz et al., 1975). This compositional layering appears to provide an important biomechanical function by distributing the stress more uniformly across the loaded regions of the joint tissue (Setton et al., 1995).

Cartilage is composed primarily of type II collagen. In addition, an array of different collagen (types V, VI, IX, XI) can be found in quantitatively minor amounts within articular cartilage. Type II collagen is present primarily in articular cartilage, the nasal septum, and sternal cartilage, as well as in

BOX 3-2 Differences in Collagen Types

Differences in tropocollagen alpha chains in various body tissues give rise to specific molecular species, or types of collagen. The collagen type in hyaline cartilage, type II collagen, differs from type I collagen found in bone, ligament, and tendon. Type II collagen forms a thinner fibril than that of type I, permitting maximum dispersion of collagen throughout the cartilage tissue.

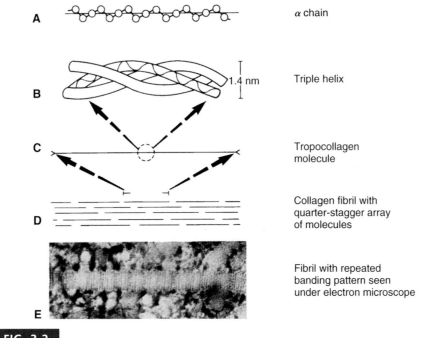

A   α chain

B   1.4 nm   Triple helix

C   Tropocollagen molecule

D   Collagen fibril with quarter-stagger array of molecules

E   Fibril with repeated banding pattern seen under electron microscope

FIG. 3-2

Molecular features of collagen structure from the alpha chain (α) to the fibril. The flexible amino acid sequence in the alpha chain (**A**) allows these chains to wind tightly into a right-handed triple helix configuration (**B**), thus forming the tropocollagen molecule (**C**). This tight triple helical arrangement of the chains contributes to the high tensile strength of the collagen fibril. The parallel alignment of the individual tropocollagen molecules, in which each molecule overlaps the other by about one quarter of its length (**D**), results in a repeating banded pattern of the collagen fibril seen by electron microscopy (×20,000) (**E**). *Reprinted with permission from Donohue, J.M., Buss, D., Oegema, T.R., et al. (1983). The effects of indirect blunt trauma on adult canine articular cartilage.* J Bone Joint Surg, 65A, 948.

the inner regions of the intervertebral disc and meniscus. For reference, type I is the most abundant collagen in the human body and can be found in bone and soft tissues such as intervertebral discs (mainly in the annulus fibrosis), skin, meniscus, tendons, and ligaments. The most important mechanical properties of collagen fibers are their tensile stiffness and their strength (Fig. 3-4A). Although a single collagen fibril has not been tested in tension, the tensile strength of collagen can be inferred from tests on structures with high collagen content. Tendons, for example, are about 80% collagen (dry weight) and have a tensile stiffness of 10^3 MPa and a tensile strength of 50 MPa (Akizuki et al., 1986; Kempson, 1976, 1979; Woo et al., 1987, 1997). Steel, by comparison, has a tensile stiffness of approximately 220×10^3 MPa. Although strong in tension, collagen fibrils offer little resistance to compression

because their large slenderness ratio, the ratio of length to thickness, makes it easy for them to buckle under compressive loads (Fig. 3-4B).

Like bone, articular cartilage is anisotropic; its material properties differ with the direction of loading (Akizuki et al., 1986; Kempson, 1979; Mow & Ratcliffe, 1997; Roth & Mow, 1980; Woo et al., 1987). It is thought that this anisotropy is related to the varying collagen fiber arrangements within the planes parallel to the articular surface. It is also thought, however, that variations in collagen fiber cross-link density, as well as variations in collagen-PG interactions, also contribute to articular cartilage tensile anisotropy. In tension, this anisotropy is usually described with respect to the direction of the articular surface split lines. These split lines are elongated fissures produced by piercing the articular surface with a small round awl (Fig. 3-5;

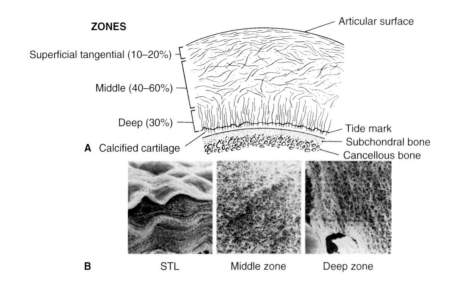

ZONES

Superficial tangential (10–20%)

Middle (40–60%)

Deep (30%)

A Calcified cartilage

Articular surface

Tide mark
Subchondral bone
Cancellous bone

B   STL   Middle zone   Deep zone

FIG. 3-3

A, Schematic representation. *(Reprinted with permission from Mow V.C. et al. [1974]. Some surface characteristics of articular cartilages. A scanning electron microscopy study and a theoretical model for the dynamic interaction of synovial fluid and articular cartilage. J Biomechanics, 7, 449).* **B,** Photomicrographs (×3000; provided through the courtesy of Dr. T. Takei, Nagano, Japan) of the ultrastructural arrangement of the collagen network throughout the depth of articular cartilage. In the superficial tangential zone (STZ), collagen fibrils are tightly woven into sheets arranged parallel to the articular surface. In the middle

zone, randomly arrayed fibrils are less densely packed to accommodate the high concentration of proteoglycans and water. The collagen fibrils of the deep zone form larger radially oriented fiber bundles that cross the tidemark, enter the calcified zone, and anchor the tissue to the underlying bone. Note the correspondence between this collagen fiber architecture and the spatial arrangement of the chondrocytes shown in Figure 3-1. In the above photomicrographs (**B**), the STZ is shown under compressive loading while the middle and deep zones are unloaded.

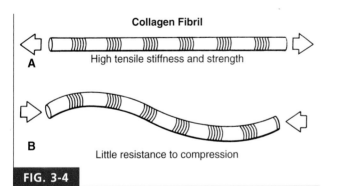

Collagen Fibril

A

High tensile stiffness and strength

B

Little resistance to compression

FIG. 3-4

Illustration of the mechanical properties of collagen fibrils: (**A**) stiff and strong in tension, but (**B**) weak and buckling easily with compression. *Adapted from Myers, E.R., Lai, W.M., & Mow, V.C. (1984). A continuum theory and an experiment for the ion-induced swelling behavior cartilage. J Biomech Eng, 106(2), 151–158.*

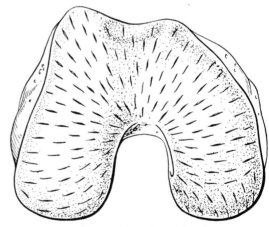

Human femoral condyles

FIG. 3-5

Diagrammatic representation of a split line pattern on the surface of human femoral condyles. *Reprinted with permission from Hultkrantz, W. (1898). Ueber die Spaltrichtungen der Gelenkknorpel. Verhandlungen der Anatomischen Gesellschaft, 12, 248.*

Hultkrantz, 1898). The origin of the pattern is related to the directional variation of the tensile stiffness and strength characteristics of articular cartilage described above. To date, however, the exact reasons as to why articular cartilage exhibits such pronounced anisotropies in tension is not known, nor is the functional significance of this tensile anisotropy.

PROTEOGLYCAN

Many types of PGs are found in cartilage. Fundamentally, it is a large protein-polysaccharide molecule composed of a protein core to which one or more glycosaminoglycans (GAGs) are attached (Fosang & Hardingham, 1996; Muir, 1983; Ratcliffe & Mow, 1996). Even the smallest of these molecules, biglycan and decorin, are quite large (approximately 1×10^4 mw), but they comprise less than 10% of all PGs present in the tissue. Aggrecans are much larger (1–4×10^6 mw), and they have the remarkable capability to attach to a hyaluronan molecule (HA: 5×10^5 mw) via a specific HA-binding region (HABR). This binding is stabilized by a link protein (LP) (40–48×10^6 mw). Stabilization is crucial to the function of normal cartilage; without it, the components of the PG molecule would rapidly escape from the tissue (Hardingham & Muir, 1974; Hascall, 1977; Muir, 1983).

Two types of GAGs comprise aggrecan: chondroitin sulfate (CS) and keratan sulfate (KS). Each CS chain contains 25 to 30 disaccharide units, while the shorter KS chain contains 13 disaccharide units (Muir, 1983). Aggrecans (previously referred to as subunits in the American literature or as monomers in the UK and European literature) consist of an approximately 200-nanometer-long protein core to which approximately 150 GAG chains, and both O-linked and N-linked oligosaccharides, are covalently attached (Fosang & Hardingham, 1996; Muir, 1983). Furthermore, the distribution of GAGs along the protein core is heterogeneous; there is a region rich in KS and O-linked oligosaccharides and a region rich in CS (Fig. 3-6A). Figure 3-6A depicts the famous "bottle-brush" model for an aggrecan (Muir, 1983). Also shown in Figure 3-6A is the heterogeneity of the protein core that contains three globular regions: G_1, the HABR located at the N-terminus that contains a small amount of KS (Poole, 1986) and a few N-linked oligosaccharides, G_2, located between the HABR- and the KS-rich region (Hardingham et al., 1987), and G_3, the core protein C-terminus. A 1:1 stoichiometry exists between the LP and the $G1$

binding region in cartilage. More recently, the other two globular regions have been extensively studied (Fosang & Hardingham, 1996), but their functional significance has not yet been elucidated. Figure 3-6B is the accepted molecular conformation of a PG aggregate; Rosenberg et al. (1975) were the first to obtain an electron micrograph of this molecule (Fig. 3-6C).

In native cartilage, most aggrecans are associated with HA to form the large PG aggregates (Fig. 3-6C). These aggregates may have up to several hundred aggrecans noncovalently attached to a central HA core via their HABR, and each site is stabilized by an LP. The filamentous HA core molecule is a nonsulfated disaccharide chain that may be as long as 4 μm in length. PG biochemists have dubbed the HA an "honorary" PG, as it is so intimately involved in the structure of the PG aggregate in articular cartilage. The stability afforded by the PG aggregates has a major functional significance. It is accepted now that PG aggregation promotes immobilization of the PGs within the fine collagen meshwork, adding structural stability and rigidity to the ECM (Mow et al., 1989b; Muir, 1983; Ratcliffe et al., 1986). Furthermore, two additional forms of dermatan sulfate PG have been identified in the ECM of articular cartilage (Rosenberg et al., 1985). In tendon, dermatan sulfate PGs have been shown to bind noncovalently to the surfaces of collagen fibrils (Scott & Orford, 1981); however, the role of dermatan sulfate in articular cartilage is unknown, biologically and functionally.

Although aggrecans generally have the basic structure as described above, they are not structurally identical (Fosang & Hardingham, 1996). Aggrecans vary in length, molecular weight, and composition in a variety of ways; in other words, they are polydisperse. Studies have demonstrated two distinct populations of aggrecans (Buckwalter et al., 1985; Heinegard et al., 1985). The first population is present throughout life and is rich in CS; the second contains PGs rich in KS and is present only in adult cartilage. As articular cartilage matures, other age-related changes in PG composition and structure occur. With cartilage maturation, the water content (Armstrong & Mow, 1982; Bollet & Nance, 1965; Linn & Sokoloff, 1965; Maroudas, 1979; Venn, 1978) and the carbohydrate/protein ratio progressively decrease (Garg & Swann, 1981; Roughley & White, 1980). This decrease is mirrored by a decrease in the CS content. Conversely, KS, which is present only in small amounts at birth, increases throughout development and aging. Thus, the

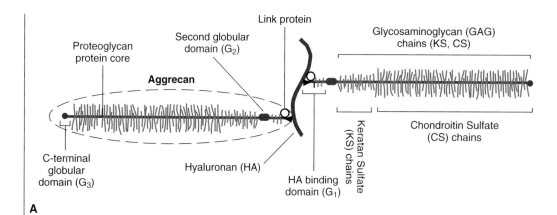

A

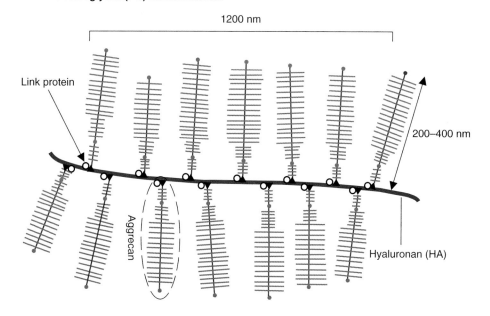

Proteoglycan (PG) Macromolecule

B

FIG. 3-6

A, Schematic depiction of aggrecan, which is composed of keratan sulfate and chondroitin sulfate chains bound covalently to a protein core molecule. The proteoglycan protein core has three globular regions as well as keratan sulfate-rich and chondroitin sulfate-rich regions. **B,** Schematic representation of a proteoglycan macromolecule. In the matrix, aggrecan noncovalently binds to HA to form a macromolecule with a molecular weight of approximately 200×106. Link protein stabilizes this interaction between the binding region of the aggrecan and the HA core molecule. **C,** Dark field electron micrograph of a proteoglycan aggregate from bovine humeral articular cartilage ($\times 120,000$). *Horizontal line* at lower right represents 0.5μm. *Reprinted with permission from Rosenberg, L., Hellmann, W., & Kleinschmidt, A.K. (1975). Electron microscopic studies of proteoglycan aggregates from bovine articular cartilage.* J Biol Chem, *250, 1877.*

CS/KS ratio, which is approximately 10:1 at birth, is only approximately 2:1 in adult cartilage (Roughley & White, 1980; Sweet et al., 1979; Thonar et al., 1986). Furthermore, sulfation of the CS molecules, which can occur at either the 6 or the 4 position, also undergoes age-related changes. In utero, chondroitin-6-sulfate and chondroitin-4-sulfate are present in equal molar amounts; however, by maturity, the chondroitin-6-sulfate:chondroitin-4-sulfate ratio has increased to approximately 25:1 (Roughley et al., 1981). Other studies have also documented an age-related decrease in the hydrodynamic size of the aggrecan. Many of these early changes seen in articular cartilage may reflect cartilage maturation, possibly as a result of increased functional demand with increased weight-bearing. However, the functional significance of these changes, as well as those occurring later in life, is as yet undetermined.

WATER

Water, the most abundant component of articular cartilage, is most concentrated near the articular surface (~80%) and decreases in a near-linear fashion with increasing depth to a concentration of approximately 65% in the deep zone (Lipshitz et al., 1976; Maroudas, 1979). This fluid contains many free mobile cations (e.g., Na^+, K^+, and Ca^{2+}) that greatly influence the mechanical and physicochemical behaviors of cartilage (Gu et al., 1998; Lai et al., 1991; Linn & Sokoloff, 1965; Maroudas, 1979). The fluid component of articular cartilage is also essential to the health of this avascular tissue because it permits gas, nutrient, and waste product movement back and forth between chondrocytes and the surrounding nutrient-rich synovial fluid (Bollet & Nance, 1965; Linn & Sokoloff, 1965; Mankin & Thrasher, 1975; Maroudas, 1975, 1979).

A small percentage of the water in cartilage resides intracellularly, and approximately 30% is strongly associated with the collagen fibrils (Maroudas et al., 1991; Torzilli et al., 1982). The interaction between collagen, PG, and water, via Donnan osmotic pressure, is believed to have an important function in regulating the structural organization of the ECM and its swelling properties (Donnan, 1924; Maroudas, 1968, 1975). Most of the water thus occupies the interfibrillar space of the ECM and is free to move when a load or pressure gradient or other electrochemical motive forces are applied to the tissue (Gu et al., 1998; Maroudas, 1979). When loaded by a compressive force, approximately 70% of the water may be moved. This interstitial fluid movement is important in controlling cartilage mechanical behavior and joint lubrication (Ateshian et al., 1997, 1998; Hlavacek, 1995; Hou et al., 1992; Mow et al., 1980; Mow & Ateshian, 1997).

STRUCTURAL AND PHYSICAL INTERACTION AMONG CARTILAGE COMPONENTS

The chemical structure and physical interactions of the PG aggregates influence the properties of the ECM (Ratcliffe & Mow, 1996). The closely spaced (5–15 angstroms) sulfate and carboxyl charge groups on the CS and KS chains dissociate in solution at physiological pH (Fig. 3-7), leaving a high concentration of fixed negative charges that create strong intramolecular and intermolecular charge-charge repulsive forces; the colligative sum of these forces (when the tissue is immersed in a physiological saline solution) is equivalent to the Donnan osmotic pressure (Buschmann & Grodzinsky, 1995; Donnan, 1924; Gu et al., 1998; Lai et al., 1991). Structurally, these charge-charge repulsive forces tend to extend and stiffen the PG macromolecules into the interfibrillar space formed by the surrounding collagen network. To appreciate the magnitude of this force, according to Stephen Hawkings (1988), this electrical repulsion is one million, million, million, million, million, million, million times (42 zeros) greater than gravitational forces.

In nature, a charged body cannot persist long without discharging or attracting counter-ions to maintain electroneutrality. Thus, the charged sulfate and carboxyl groups fixed along the PGs in articular cartilage must attract various counter-ions and co-ions (mainly Na^+, Ca^{2+}, and Cl^-) into the tissue to maintain electroneutrality. The total concentration of these counter-ions and co-ions is given by the well-known Donnan equilibrium ion distribution law (Donnan, 1924). Inside the tissue, the mobile counter-ions and co-ions form a cloud surrounding the fixed sulfate and carboxyl charges, thus shielding these charges from each other. This charge shielding acts to diminish the very large electrical repulsive forces that otherwise would exist. The net result is a swelling pressure given by the Donnan osmotic pressure law (Buschmann & Grodzinsky, 1995; Donnan, 1924; Gu et al., 1998; Lai et al., 1991; Schubert & Hamerman, 1968). The Donnan osmotic pressure theory has been extensively used to calculate the

Aggregate Domain

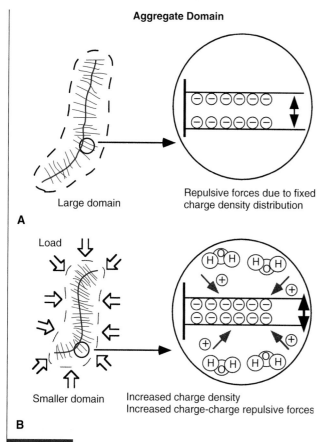

Large domain

Repulsive forces due to fixed charge density distribution

A

Load

Smaller domain

Increased charge density
Increased charge-charge repulsive forces

B

FIG. 3-7

A, Schematic representation of a proteoglycan aggregate solution domain (*left*) and the repelling forces associated with the fixed negative charge groups on the GAGs of aggrecan (*right*). These repulsive forces cause the aggregate to assume a stiffly extended conformation, occupying a large solution domain. **B,** Applied compressive stress decreases the aggregate solution domain (*left*), which in turn increases the charge density and thus the intermolecular charge repulsive forces (*right*).

swelling pressures of articular cartilage and the intervertebral disc (Maroudas, 1979; Urban & McMullin, 1985). By Starling's law, this swelling pressure is, in turn, resisted and balanced by tension developed in the collagen network, confining the PGs to only 20% of their free solution domain (Maroudas, 1976; Mow & Ratcliffe, 1997; Setton et al., 1995). Consequently, this swelling pressure subjects the collagen network to a "pre-stress" of sig-

nificant magnitude even in the absence of external loads (Setton et al., 1995, 1998).

Cartilage PGs are inhomogeneously distributed throughout the matrix, with their concentration generally being highest in the middle zone and lowest in the superficial and deep zones (Lipshitz et al., 1976; Maroudas, 1968, 1979; Venn, 1978). The biomechanical consequence of this inhomogeneous swelling behavior of cartilage (caused by the varying PG content throughout the depth of the tissue) has recently been quantitatively assessed (Setton et al., 1998). Also, results from recent finite element calculations based on models incorporating an inhomogeneous PG distribution show that it has a profound effect on the interstitial counter-ion distribution throughout the depth of the tissue (Sun et al., 1998).

When a compressive stress is applied to the cartilage surface, there is an instantaneous deformation caused primarily by a change in the PG molecular domain, Figure 3-7B. This external stress causes the internal pressure in the matrix to exceed the swelling pressure and thus liquid will begin to flow out of the tissue. As the fluid flows out, the PG concentration increases, which in turn increases the Donnan osmotic swelling pressure or the charge-charge repulsive force and bulk compressive stress until they are in equilibrium with the external stress. In this manner, the physicochemical properties of the PG gel trapped within the collagen network enable it to resist compression. This mechanism complements the role played by collagen that, as previously described, is strong in tension but weak in compression. The ability of PGs to resist compression thus arises from two sources: (1) the Donnan osmotic swelling pressure associated with the tightly packed fixed anionic groups on the GAGS and (2) the bulk compressive stiffness of the collagen-PG solid matrix. Experimentally, the Donnan osmotic pressure ranges from 0.05 to 0.35 MPa (Maroudas, 1979), while the elastic modulus of the collagen-PG solid matrix ranges from 0.5 to 1.5 MPa (Armstrong & Mow, 1982; Athanasiou et al., 1991; Mow & Ratcliffe, 1997).

It is now apparent that collagen and PGs also interact and that these interactions are of great functional importance. A small portion of the PGs have been shown to be closely associated with collagen and may serve as a bonding agent between the collagen fibrils, spanning distances that are too great for collagen cross-links to develop (Bateman et al., 1996; Mow & Ratcliffe, 1997; Muir, 1983).

PGs are also thought to play an important role in maintaining the ordered structure and mechanical properties of the collagen fibrils (Muir, 1983; Scott & Orford, 1981). Recent investigations show that in concentrated solutions, PGs interact with each other to form networks of significant strength (Mow et al., 1989b; Zhu et al., 1991, 1996). Moreover, the density and strength of the interaction sites forming the network were shown to depend on the presence of LP between aggrecans and aggregates, as well as collagen. Evidence suggests that there are fewer aggregates, and more biglycans and decorins than aggrecans, in the superficial zone of articular cartilage. Thus, there must be a difference in the interaction between these PGs and the collagen fibrils from the superficial zone than from those of the deeper zones (Poole et al., 1986). Indeed, the interaction between PG and collagen not only plays a direct role in the organization of the ECM but also contributes directly to the mechanical properties of the tissue (Kempson et al., 1976; Schmidt et al., 1990; Zhu et al., 1993).

The specific characteristics of the physical, chemical, and mechanical interactions between collagen and PG have not yet been fully determined. Nevertheless, as discussed above, we know that these structural macromolecules interact to form a porous-permeable, fiber-reinforced composite matrix possessing all the essential mechanical characteristics of a solid that is swollen with water and ions and that is able to resist the high stresses and strains of joint articulation (Andriacchi et al., 1997; Hodge et al., 1986; Mow & Ateshian, 1997; Paul, 1976). It has been demonstrated that these collagen-PG interactions involve an aggrecan, an HA filament, type II collagen, other minor collagen types, an unknown bonding agent, and possibly smaller cartilage components such as collagen type IX, recently identified glycoproteins, and/or polymeric HA (Poole et al., 1986). A schematic diagram depicting the structural arrangement within a small volume of articular cartilage is shown in Figure 3-8.

When articular cartilage is subjected to external loads, the collagen-PG solid matrix and interstitial fluid function together in a unique way to protect against high levels of stress and strain developing in the ECM. Furthermore, changes to the biochemical composition and structural organization of the ECM, such as during osteoarthritis (OA), are paralleled by changes to the biomechanical proper-

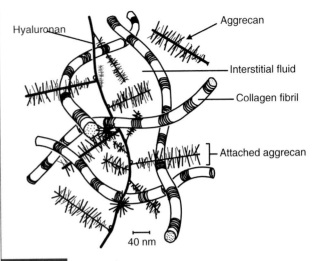

FIG. 3-8

Schematic representation of the molecular organization of cartilage. The structural components of cartilage, collagen, and proteoglycans, interact to form a porous composite fiber-reinforced organic solid matrix that is swollen with water. Aggrecans bind covalently to HA to form large proteoglycan macromolecules.

ties of cartilage. In the following section, the behavior of articular cartilage under loading and the mechanisms of cartilage fluid flow will be discussed in detail.

Biomechanical Behavior of Articular Cartilage

The biomechanical behavior of articular cartilage can best be understood when the tissue is viewed as a multiphasic medium. In the present context, articular cartilage will be treated as biphasic material consisting of two intrinsically incompressible, immiscible, and distinct phases (Bachrach et al., 1998; Mow et al., 1980): an interstitial fluid phase and a porous-permeable solid phase (i.e., the ECM). For explicit analysis of the contribution of the PG charges and ions, one would have to consider three distinct phases: a fluid phase, an ion phase, and a charged solid phase (Gu et al., 1998; Lai et al., 1991). For understanding how the water contributes to its mechanical properties, in the present context, articular cartilage may be considered as a fluid-filled porous-permeable (uncharged) biphasic medium, with each constituent playing a role in the functional behavior of cartilage.

During joint articulation, forces at the joint surface may vary from almost zero to more than ten times body weight (Andriacchi et al., 1997; Paul, 1976). The contact areas also vary in a complex manner and typically they are only of the order of several square centimeters (Ahmed & Burke, 1983; Ateshian et al., 1994). It is estimated that the peak contact stress may reach 20 MPa in the hip while rising from a chair and 10 MPa during stair climbing (Hodge et al., 1986; Newberry et al., 1997). Thus, articular cartilage, under physiological loading conditions, is a highly stressed material. To understand how this tissue responds under these high physiological loading conditions, its intrinsic mechanical properties in compression, tension, and shear must be determined. From these properties, one can understand the load-carrying mechanisms within the ECM. Accordingly, the following subsections will characterize the tissue behavior under these loading modalities.

NATURE OF ARTICULAR CARTILAGE VISCOELASTICITY

If a material is subjected to the action of a constant (time-independent) load or a constant deformation and its response varies with time, then the mechanical behavior of the material is said to be viscoelastic. In general, the response of such a material can be theoretically modeled as a combination of the response of a viscous fluid (dashpot) and an elastic solid (spring), hence viscoelastic.

The two fundamental responses of a viscoelastic material are creep and stress relaxation. Creep occurs when a viscoelastic solid is subjected to the action of a constant load. Typically, a viscoelastic solid responds with a rapid initial deformation followed by a slow (time-dependent), progressively increasing deformation known as creep until an equilibrium state is reached. Stress relaxation occurs when a viscoelastic solid is subjected to the action of a constant deformation. Typically, a viscoelastic solid responds with a rapid, high initial stress followed by a slow (time-dependent), progressively decreasing stress required to maintain the deformation; this phenomenon is known as stress relaxation.

Creep and stress relaxation phenomena may be caused by different mechanisms. For single-phase solid polymeric materials, these phenomena are the result of internal friction caused by the motion of the long polymeric chains sliding over each other within the stressed material (Fung, 1981). The viscoelastic behavior of tendons and ligaments is primarily caused by this mechanism (Woo et al., 1987, 1997). For bone, the long-term viscoelastic behavior is thought to be caused by a relative slip of lamellae within the osteons along with the flow of the interstitial fluid (Lakes & Saha, 1979). For articular cartilage, the compressive viscoelastic behavior is primarily caused by the flow of the interstitial fluid and the frictional drag associated with this flow (Ateshian et al., 1997; Mow et al., 1980, 1984). In shear, as in single-phase viscoelastic polymers, it is primarily caused by the motion of long polymer chains such as collagen and PGs (Zhu et al., 1993, 1996). The component of articular cartilage viscoelasticity caused by interstitial fluid flow is known as the biphasic viscoelastic behavior (Mow et al., 1980), and the component of viscoelasticity caused by macromolecular motion is known as the flow-independent (Hayes & Bodine, 1978) or the intrinsic viscoelastic behavior of the collagen-PG solid matrix.

Although the deformational behavior has been described in terms of a linear elastic solid (Hirsch, 1944) or viscoelastic solid (Hayes & Mockros, 1971), these models fail to recognize the role of water in the viscoelastic behavior of and the significant contribution that fluid pressurization plays in joint load support and cartilage lubrication (Ateshian et al., 1998; Elmore et al., 1963, Mow & Ratcliffe, 1997; Sokoloff, 1963). Recently, experimental measurements have determined that interstitial fluid pressurization supports more than 90% of the applied load to the cartilage surface (Soltz & Ateshian, 1998) immediately following loading. This effect can persist for more than 1,000 seconds and thus shields the ECM and chondrocytes from the crushing deformations of the high stresses (20 MPa) resulting from joint loading.

CONFINED COMPRESSION EXPLANT LOADING CONFIGURATION

The loading of cartilage in vivo is extremely complex. To achieve a better understanding of the deformational behavior of the tissue under load, an explant loading configuration known as confined compression (Mow et al., 1980) has been adopted by researchers. In this configuration, a cylindrical cartilage specimen is fitted snugly into a cylindrical, smooth-walled (ideally frictionless) confining ring that prohibits motion and fluid loss in the radial direction. Under an axial loading condition via a rigid porous-permeable loading platen (Fig. 3-9A), fluid will flow from the tissue into the porous-permeable platen, and, as this occurs, the cartilage sample will compress in creep. At any time the amount of compression equals the volume of fluid loss because both the water and the ECM are each intrinsically incompressible (Bachrach et al., 1998). The advantage of the confined compression test is that it creates a uniaxial, one-dimensional flow and deformational field within the tissue, which does not depend on tissue anisotropy or properties in the radial direction. This greatly simplifies the mathematics needed to solve the problem.

It should be emphasized that the stress-strain, pressure, fluid, and ion flow fields generated within the tissue during loading can only be calculated; however, these calculations are of idealized models and testing conditions. There are many confounding factors, such as the time-dependent nature and magnitude of loading and alterations in the natural state of pre-stress (acting within the tissue), that arise from disruption of the collagen network during specimen harvesting. Despite limitations in determining the natural physiological states of stress and strain within the tissue in vivo, a number of researchers have made gains toward an understanding of potential mechanosignal transduction mechanisms in cartilage through the use of explant loading studies (Bachrach et al., 1995; Buschmann et al., 1992; Kim et al., 1994; Valhmu et al., 1998) based on the biphasic constitutive law for soft hydrated tissues (Mow et al., 1980).

BIPHASIC CREEP RESPONSE OF ARTICULAR CARTILAGE IN COMPRESSION

The biphasic creep response of articular cartilage in a one-dimensional confined compression experiment is depicted in Figure 3-9. In this case, a constant compressive stress (σ_0) is applied to the tissue at time t_0 (point A in Fig. 3-9B) and the tissue is allowed to creep to its final equilibrium strain (ϵ^∞). For articular cartilage, as illustrated in the top diagrams, creep is caused by the exudation of the interstitial fluid. Exudation is most

rapid initially, as evidenced by the early rapid rate of increased deformation, and it diminishes gradually until flow cessation occurs. During creep, the load applied at the surface is balanced by the compressive stress developed within the collagen-PG solid matrix and the frictional drag generated by the flow of the interstitial fluid during exudation. Creep ceases when the compressive stress developed within the solid matrix is sufficient to balance the applied stress alone; at this point no fluid flows and the equilibrium strain ϵ^∞ is reached.

Typically, for relatively thick human and bovine articular cartilages, 2 to 4 mm, it takes 4 to 16 hours to reach creep equilibrium. For rabbit cartilage, which is generally less than 1.0 mm thick, it takes approximately 1 hour to reach creep equilibrium. Theoretically, it can be shown that the time it takes to reach creep equilibrium varies inversely with the square of the thickness of the tissue (Mow et al., 1980). Under relatively high loading conditions, >1.0 MPa, 50% of the total fluid content may be squeezed from the tissue (Edwards, 1967). Furthermore, in vitro studies demonstrate that if the tissue is immersed in physiological saline, this exuded fluid is fully recoverable when the load is removed (Elmore et al., 1963; Sokoloff, 1963).

Because the rate of creep is governed by the rate of fluid exudation, it can be used to determine the permeability coefficient of the tissue (Mow et al., 1980, 1989a). This is known as the indirect measurement for tissue permeability (k). Average values of normal human, bovine, and canine patellar groove articular cartilage permeability k obtained in this manner are 2.17×10^{-15} M^4/N·s, 1.42×10^{-15} M^4/N·s, and 0.9342×10^{-15} M^4/N·s, respectively (Athanasiou et al., 1991). At equilibrium, no fluid flow occurs and thus the equilibrium deformation can be used to measure the intrinsic compressive modulus (H_A) of the collagen-PG solid matrix (Armstrong & Mow, 1982; Mow et al., 1980). Average values of normal human, bovine, and canine patellar groove articular cartilage compressive modulus H_A are 0.53, 0.47, and 0.55 megapascal (MPa; note 1.0 MPa = 145 lb/in^2), respectively. Because these coefficients are a measure of the intrinsic material properties of the solid matrix, it is therefore meaningful to determine how they vary with matrix composition. It was determined that k varies directly, while H_A varies inversely with water content and varies directly with PG content (Mow & Ratcliffe, 1997).

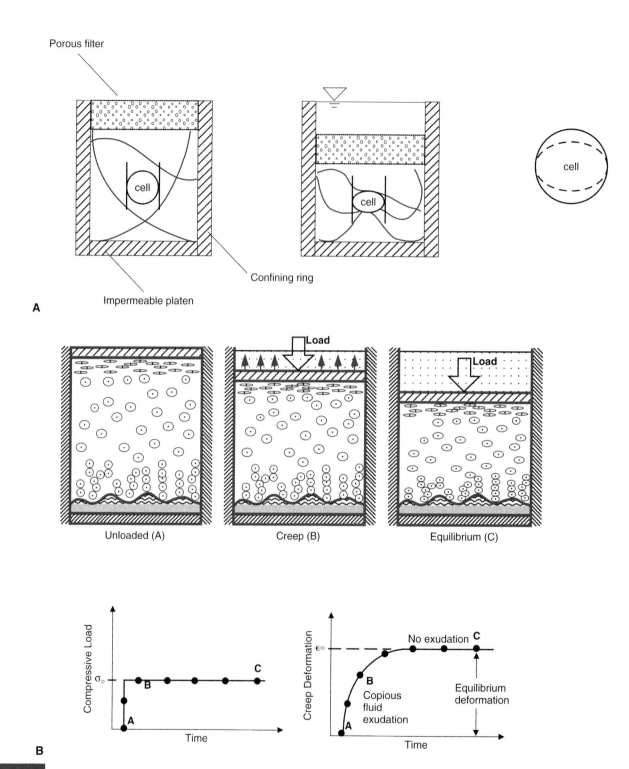

Porous filter

cell

cell

cell

Confining ring

Impermeable platen

A

Load

Load

Unloaded (A)   Creep (B)   Equilibrium (C)

Compressive Load

σ_o

A

B

C

Time

Creep Deformation

ϵ_∞

A

B
Copious
fluid
exudation

No exudation C

Equilibrium
deformation

Time

B

FIG. 3-9

A, A schematic of the confined compression loading configuration. A cylindrical tissue specimen is positioned tightly into an impermeable confining ring that does not permit deformation (or fluid flow) in the radial direction. Under loading, fluid exudation occurs through the porous platen in the vertical direction. **B,** A constant stress σ_o applied to a sample of articular cartilage (*bottom left*) and creep response of the sample under the constant applied stress (*bottom right*). The

drawings of a block of tissue above the curves illustrate that creep is accompanied by copious exudation of fluid from the sample and that the rate of exudation decreases over time from points A to B to C. At equilibrium (ϵ_∞), fluid flow ceases and the load is borne entirely by the solid matrix (point C). *Adapted from Mow, V.C., Kuei, S.C., Lai, W.M., et al. (1980). Biphasic creep and stress relaxation of articular cartilage in compression: Theory and experiments.* J Biomech Eng, 102, 73–84.

BIPHASIC STRESS-RELAXATION RESPONSE OF ARTICULAR CARTILAGE IN COMPRESSION

The biphasic viscoelastic stress-relaxation response of articular cartilage in a 1D compression experiment is depicted in Figure 3-10. In this case, a constant compression rate (line t_0-A-B of lower left figure) is applied to the tissue until u_0 is reached; beyond point B, the deformation u_0 is maintained. For articular cartilage, the typical stress response caused by this imposed deformation is shown in the lower right figure (Holmes et al., 1985; Mow et al.,

1984). During the compression phase, the stress rises continuously until σ_0 is reached, corresponding to u_0, while during the stress-relaxation phase, the stress continuously decays along the curve B-C-D-E until the equilibrium stress ($\sigma\infty$) is reached.

The mechanisms responsible for the stress rise and stress relaxation are depicted in the lower portion of Figure 3-10. As illustrated in the top diagrams, the stress rise in the compression phase is associated with fluid exudation, while stress relaxation is associated with fluid redistribution within the porous solid matrix. During the compressive phase,

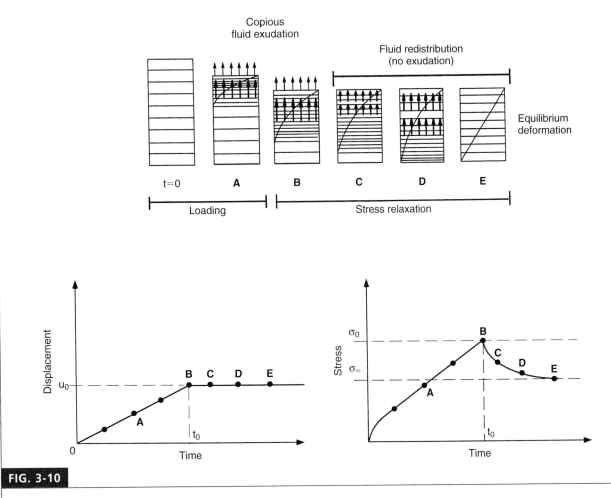

FIG. 3-10

Controlled ramp displacement curve imposed on a cartilage specimen commencing at t_0 (*bottom left*) and the stress-response curve of the cartilage in this uniaxial confined-compression experiment (*bottom right*). The sample is compressed to point B and maintained over time (points B to E). The history of the stress and response shows a characteristic stress that rises during the compressive phase (points t_0 to B) and then decreases during the relaxation phase (points B to D) until an equilibrium is reached (point E). Above these two curves, schematics illustrate interstitial fluid flow (represented by *arrows*) and solid matrix deformation during this compressive process. Fluid exudation gives rise to the peak stress (point B), and fluid redistribution gives rise to the stress-relaxation phenomena.

the high stress is generated by forced exudation of the interstitial fluid and the compaction of the solid matrix near the surface. Stress relaxation is in turn caused by the relief or rebound of the high compaction region near the surface of the solid matrix. This stress-relaxation process will cease when the compressive stress developed within the solid matrix reaches the stress generated by the intrinsic compressive modulus of the solid matrix corresponding to u_0 (Holmes et al., 1985; Mow et al., 1980, 1984). Analysis of this stress-relaxation process leads to the conclusion that under physiological loading conditions, excessive stress levels are difficult to maintain because stress relaxation will rapidly attenuate the stress developed within the tissue; this must necessarily lead to the rapid spreading of the contact area in the joint during articulation (Ateshian et al., 1995, 1998; Mow & Ateshian, 1997).

Recently, much focus has been on the inhomogeneity of HA with cartilage depth (Schinagl et al., 1996, 1997). Based on this data, from an analysis of the stress-relaxation experiment it was found that an inhomogeneous tissue would relax at a faster rate than would the uniform tissue (Wang & Mow, 1998). Moreover, the stress, strain, pressure, and fluid flow fields within the tissue were significantly altered as well. Thus it seems that the variations in biochemical and structural composition in the layers of cartilage provide another challenge to understanding the environment of chondrocytes in situ.

PERMEABILITY OF ARTICULAR CARTILAGE

Fluid-filled porous materials may or may not be permeable. The ratio of fluid volume (V^f) to the total volume (V^T) of the porous material is known as the porosity ($\beta = V^f/V^T$); thus, porosity is a geometric concept. Articular cartilage is therefore a material of high porosity (approximately 80%). If the pores are interconnected, the porous material is permeable. Permeability is a measure of the ease with which fluid can flow through a porous material, and it is inversely proportional to the frictional drag exerted by the fluid flowing through the porous-permeable material. Thus, permeability is a physical concept; it is a measure of the resistive force that is required to cause the fluid to flow at a given speed through the porous-permeable material. This frictional resistive force is generated by the interaction of the interstitial fluid and the pore walls of the porous-permeable material. The permeability coefficient k is related to the frictional drag coefficient K

by the relationship $k = \beta^2/K$ (Lai & Mow, 1980). Articular cartilage has a very low permeability and thus high frictional resistive forces are generated when fluid is caused to flow through the porous solid matrix.

In the previous sections on cartilage viscoelasticity we discussed the process of fluid flow through articular cartilage induced by solid matrix compression and how this process influences the viscoelastic behavior of the tissue. This process also provides an indirect method to determine the permeability of the tissue. In this section, we discuss the experimental method used to directly measure the permeability coefficient. Such an experiment is depicted in Figure 3-11A. Here, a specimen of the tissue is held fixed in a chamber subjected to the action of a pressure gradient; the imposed upstream pressure P_1 is greater than the downstream pressure P_2. The thickness of the specimen is denoted by h and the cross-sectional area of permeation is defined by A. Darcy's law, used to determine the permeability k from this simple experimental setup, yields $k = Qh/A(P_1-P_2)$, where Q is the volumetric discharge per unit time through the specimen whose area of permeation is A (Mow & Ratcliffe, 1997). Using low pressures, approximately 0.1 MPa, this method was first used to determine the permeability of articular cartilage (Edwards, 1967; Maroudas, 1975). The value of k obtained in this manner ranged from 1.1×10^{-15} m^4/N·s to 7.6×10^{-15} m^4/N·s. In addition, using a uniform straight tube model, the average "pore diameter" has been estimated at 6 nm (Maroudas, 1979). Thus, the "pores" within articular cartilage are of molecular size.

The permeability of articular cartilage under compressive strain and at high physiological pressures (3 MPa) was first obtained by Mansour and Mow (1976) and later analyzed by Lai and Mow (1980). The high pressure and compressive strain conditions examined in these studies more closely resemble those conditions found in diarthrodial joint loading. In these experiments, k was measured as a function of two variables: the pressure gradient across the specimen and the axial compressive strain applied to the sample. The results from these experiments are shown in Figure 3-11B. Permeability decreased exponentially as a function of both increasing compressive strain and increasing applied fluid pressure. It was later shown, however, that the dependence of k on the applied fluid pressure derives from compaction of the solid matrix that, in turn, results from the frictional drag caused by the permeating fluid (Lai & Mow, 1980). From the point of view of pore

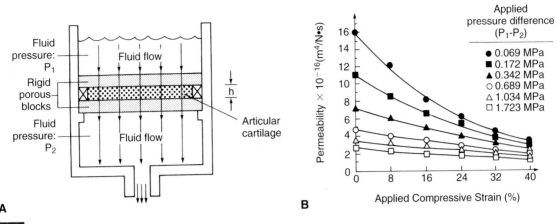

FIG. 3-11

A, Experimental configuration used in measuring the permeability of articular cartilage, involving the application of a pressure gradient $(P_1–P_2)/h$ across a sample of the tissue (h = tissue thickness). Because the fluid pressure (P_1) above the sample is greater than that beneath it (P_2), fluid will flow through the tissue. The permeability coefficient k in this experiment is given by the expression $Qh/A(P_1–P_2)$, where Q is the volumetric discharge per unit time and A is the area of permeation. *Adapted from Torzilli, P.A., & Mow, V.C. (1976). On the fundamental fluid transport mechanisms through normal and* *pathologic cartilage during function. I. The formulation.* J Biomech, 9(8), *541–552.* **B,** Experimental curves for articular cartilage permeability show its strong dependence on compressive strain and applied pressure. Measurements were taken at applied pressure differential $(P_1–P_2)$ and applied strains. The permeability decreased in an exponential manner as a function of both increasing applied compressive strain and increasing applied pressure. *Adapted from Lai, W.M., & Mow, V.C. (1980). Drag-induced compression of articular cartilage during a permeation experiment.* J Biorheology, 17, 111.

structure, compaction of the solid matrix decreases the porosity and hence the average "pore diameter" within the solid matrix; thus, solid matrix compaction increases frictional resistance (Mow et al., 1984).

The nonlinear permeability of articular cartilage demonstrated in Figure 3-11*B* suggests that the tissue has a mechanical feedback system that may serve important purposes under physiological conditions. When subjected to high loads through the mechanism of increased frictional drag against interstitial fluid flow, the tissue will appear stiffer and it will be more difficult to cause fluid exudation. Recent analyses of articular cartilage compressive stress-relaxation behavior have validated this concept and its importance in the capacity of the interstitial fluid to support load (Ateshian et al., 1998; Soltz & Ateshian, 1998). Moreover, this mechanism also is important in joint lubrication.

BEHAVIOR OF ARTICULAR CARTILAGE UNDER UNIAXIAL TENSION

The mechanical behavior of articular cartilage in tension is highly complex. In tension, the tissue is strongly anisotropic (being stiffer and stronger for specimens harvested in the direction parallel to the split line pattern than those harvested perpendicular to the split line pattern) and strongly inhomogeneous (for mature animals, being stiffer and stronger for specimens harvested from the superficial regions than those harvested deeper in the tissue) (Kempson, 1979; Roth & Mow, 1980). Interestingly, articular cartilage from immature bovine knee joints does not exhibit these layered inhomogeneous variations; however, the superficial zones of both mature and immature bovine cartilage appear to have the same tensile stiffness (Roth & Mow, 1980). These anisotropic and inhomogeneous characteristics in mature joints are believed to be caused by the varying collagen and PG structural organization of the joint surface and the layering structural arrangements found within the tissue. Thus, the collagen-rich superficial zone appears to provide the joint cartilage with a tough wear-resistant protective skin (Setton et al., 1993) (Fig. 3-3*A*).

Articular cartilage also exhibits viscoelastic behavior in tension (Woo et al., 1987). This viscoelastic behavior is attributable to both the internal friction associated with polymeric motion and the flow of the interstitial fluid. To examine the intrinsic mechanical response of the collagen-PG solid matrix in tension, it is necessary to negate the biphasic fluid flow effects. To do this, one must perform slow, low strain-rate experiments (Akizuki et al., 1986; Roth & Mow, 1980; Woo et al., 1987) or perform an incremental strain experiment in which stress relaxation is allowed to progress toward equilibration at each increment of strain (Akizuki et al., 1986). Typically, in a low strain-rate (or near-equilibrium tensile) experiment, a displacement rate of 0.5 cm/minute is used and the specimens usually are pulled to failure. Unfortunately, using these procedures to negate the effect of interstitial fluid flow also negates the manifestation of the intrinsic viscoelastic behavior of the solid matrix. Thus, only the equilibrium intrinsic mechanical properties of the solid matrix may be determined from these tensile tests. The intrinsic viscoelastic properties of the solid matrix must be determined from a pure shear study.

The "equilibrium" stress-strain curve for a specimen of articular cartilage tested under a constant low strain-rate condition is shown in Figure 3-12. Like other fibrous biological tissues (tendons and ligaments), articular cartilage tends to stiffen with increasing strain when the strain becomes large. Thus, over the entire range of strain (up to 60%) in tension, articular cartilage cannot be described by a single Young's modulus. Rather, a tangent modulus, defined by the tangent to the stress-strain curve, must be used to describe the tensile stiffness of the tissue. This fundamental result has given rise to the wide range of Young's modulus, 3 to 100 MPa, reported for articular cartilage in tension (Akizuki et al., 1986; Kempson, 1979; Roth & Mow, 1980; Woo et al., 1987). At physiological strain levels, however, less than 15% (Armstrong et al., 1979) of the linear Young's modulus of articular cartilage ranges between 5 and 10 MPa (Akizuki et al., 1986).

Morphologically, the cause for the shape of the tensile stress-strain curve for large strains is depicted in the diagrams on the right of Figure 3-12. The initial toe region is caused by collagen fiber pull-out and realignment during the initial portion of the tensile experiment, and the final linear region is caused by the stretching of the straightened-aligned collagen fibers. Failure occurs when all the collagen fibers contained within the specimen are ruptured. Figure 3-13A depicts an unstretched articular cartilage specimen, while Figure 3-13B depicts a stretched specimen. Figure 3-14, A & B shows scanning electron micrographs of cartilage blocks under 0 and 30% stretch (right) and the corresponding histograms of collagen fiber orientation

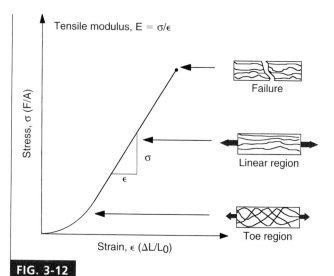

FIG. 3-12

Typical tensile stress-strain curve for articular cartilage. The drawings on the right of the curve show the configuration of the collagen fibrils at various stages loading. In the toe region, collagen fibril pull-out occurs as the fibrils align themselves in the direction of the tensile load. In the linear region, the aligned collagen fibers are stretched until failure occurs.

determined from the scanning electron micrograph pictures (left). Clearly it can be seen that the collagen network within cartilage responds to tensile stress and strain (Wada & Akizuki, 1987).

If the molecular structure of collagen, the organization of the collagen fibers within the collagenous network, or the collagen fiber cross-linking is altered (such as that occurring in mild fibrillation or OA), the tensile properties of the network will change. Schmidt et al. (1990) have shown a definitive relationship between collagen hydroxypyridinium cross-linking and tensile stiffness and strength of normal bovine cartilage. Akizuki et al. (1986) showed that progressive degradation of human knee joint cartilage, from mild fibrillation to OA, yields a progressive deterioration of the intrinsic tensile properties of the collagen-PG solid matrix. Similar results have been observed recently in animal models of OA (Guilak et al., 1994; Setton et al., 1994). Together, these observations support the belief that disruption of the collagen network is a key factor in the initial events leading to the development of OA. Also, loosening of the collagen network is generally believed to be responsible for the increased swelling, hence water content, of osteoarthritic cartilage (Mankin & Thrasher, 1975; Maroudas, 1979). We have already discussed how increased water content leads

Unloaded

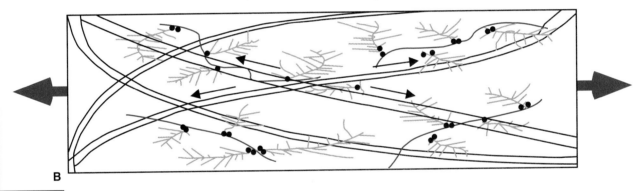

Uniaxial tensile loading

FIG. 3-13

Schematic depiction of the main components of articular cartilage when the tissue is unloaded (**A**) and when a tensile load is applied (**B**). Loading would result in an alignment of collagen fibrils along the axis of tension. *Adapted from Myers,* *E.R., Lai, W.M., & Mow, V.C. (1984). A continuum theory and an experiment for the ion-induced swelling behavior cartilage.* J Biomech Eng, 106(2), *151–158.*

to decreased compressive stiffness and increased permeability of articular cartilage.

BEHAVIOR OF ARTICULAR CARTILAGE IN PURE SHEAR

In tension and compression, only the equilibrium intrinsic properties of the collagen-PG solid matrix can be determined. This is because a volumetric change always occurs within a material when it is subjected to uniaxial tension or compression. This volumetric change causes interstitial fluid flow and induces biphasic viscoelastic effects within the tissue. If, however, articular cartilage is tested in pure shear under infinitesimal strain conditions, no pressure gradients or volumetric changes will be produced within the material; hence, no interstitial fluid flow will occur (Hayes & Bodine, 1978; Zhu et al. 1993) (Fig. 3-15). Thus, a steady dynamic pure shear experiment can be used to assess the

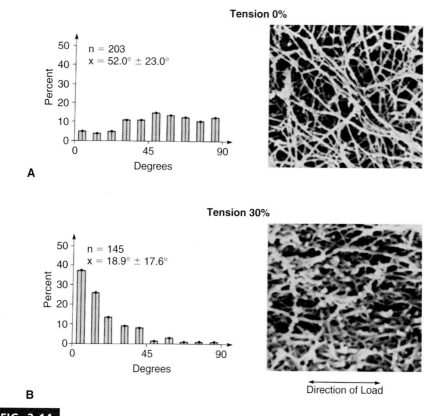

FIG. 3-14

Collagen fibril alignment is clearly demonstrated by the scanning electron micrographs (×10,000) (*right*) of cartilage blocks under 0% stretch (**A**) and 30% stretch (**B**). The histograms (*left*), calculated from the micrographs, represent the percent of collagen fibers oriented in the direction of the applied tension. At 0% stretch the fibers have a random orientation; however, at 30% they are aligned in the direction of the applied tension. *Reprinted with permission from Wada, T., & Akizuki, S. (1987). An ultrastructural study of solid matrix in articular cartilage under uniaxial tensile stress. J Jpn Orthop Assn, 61.*

intrinsic viscoelastic properties of the collagen-PG solid matrix.

In a steady dynamic shear experiment, the viscoelastic properties of the collagen-PG solid matrix are determined by subjecting a thin circular wafer of tissue to a steady sinusoidal torsional shear, shown in Figure 3-16. In an experiment of this type, the tissue specimen is held by a precise amount of compression between two rough porous platens. The lower platen is attached to a sensitive torque transducer and the upper platen is attached to a precision mechanical spectrometer with a servo-controlled dc motor. A sinusoidal excitation signal may be provided by the motor in a frequency of excitation range of 0.01 to 20 hertz (Hz). For shear strain magnitudes ranging from 0.2 to 2.0%, the viscoelastic properties are equivalently defined by the elastic storage modulus G'; the viscous loss modulus G" of the collagen-PG solid matrix may be determined as a function of frequency (Fung, 1981; Zhu et al., 1993).

Sometimes it is more convenient to determine the magnitude of the dynamic shear modulus |G*| given by:

$$|G^*|^2 = (G')^2 + (G'')^2$$

and the phase shift angle given by:

$$\delta = \tan^{-1}(G''/G')$$

The magnitude of the dynamic shear modulus is a measure of the total resistance offered by the viscoelastic material. The value of δ, the angle between

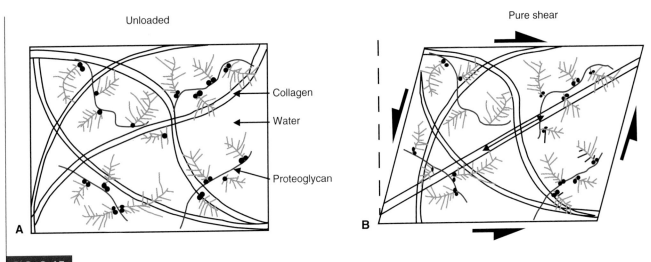

Unloaded

Pure shear

Collagen

Water

Proteoglycan

A

B

FIG. 3-15

Schematic depiction of unloaded cartilage (**A**), and cartilage subjected to pure shear (**B**). When cartilage is tested in pure shear under infinitesimal strain conditions, no volumetric changes or pressure gradients are produced; hence, no interstitial fluid flow occurs. This figure also demonstrates the functional role of collagen fibrils in resisting shear deformation.

the steady applied sinusoidal strain and the steady sinusoidal torque response, is a measure of the total frictional energy dissipation within the material. For a pure elastic material with no internal frictional dissipation, the phase shift angle δ is zero; for a pure viscous fluid, the phase shift angle δ is 90°.

The magnitude of the dynamic shear modulus for normal bovine articular cartilage has been measured to range from 1 to 3 MPa, while the phase shift angle has been measured to range from 9 to 20° (Hayes & Bodine, 1978; Zhu et al., 1993). The intrinsic transient shear stress-relaxation behavior of the collagen-PG solid matrix along with the steady dynamic shear properties also has been measured (Zhu et al., 1986). With both the steady dynamic and the transient results, the latter investigators showed that the quasilinear viscoelasticity theory proposed by Fung (1981) for biological materials provides an accurate description of the flow-independent viscoelastic behavior of the collagen-PG solid matrix. Figure 3-17 depicts a comparison of the theoretical prediction of the transient stress-relaxation phenomenon in shear with the results from Fung's 1981 quasilinear viscoelasticity theory.

From these shear studies, it is possible to obtain some insight as to how the collagen-PG solid matrix functions. First, we note that measurements of PG solutions at concentrations similar to those found in articular cartilage in situ yield a magnitude of shear modulus to be of the order of 10 Pa and phase shift angle ranging up to 70° (Mow et al., 1989b; Zhu et al., 1991, 1996). Therefore, it appears that the magnitude of the shear modulus of concentrated PG so-

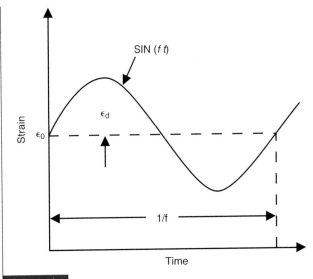

Strain

ϵ_0

ϵ_d

SIN ($f\,t$)

1/f

Time

FIG. 3-16

Steady sinusoidal torsional shear imposed on a specimen in pure shear. The fluctuating strain in the form of a sine wave with a strain amplitude ϵ_d and frequency f.

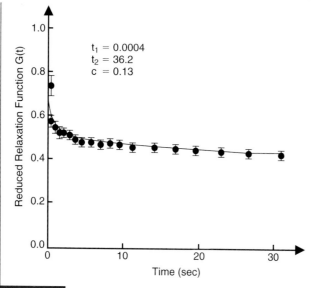

$t_1 = 0.0004$
$t_2 = 36.2$
$c = 0.13$

FIG. 3-17

Typical stress-relaxation curve after a step change in shear strain, expressed in terms of the mean of ten cycles of stress relaxation normalized by the initial stress. The *solid line* represents the theoretical prediction of the quasilinear viscoelasticity theory. *Adapted from Zhu, W.B., Lai, W.M., & Mow, V.C. (1986). Intrinsic quasi-linear viscoelastic behavior of the extracellular matrix of cartilage.* Trans Orthop Res Soc, 11, 407.

lution is one hundred thousand times less and the phase angle is six to seven times greater than that of articular cartilage solid matrix. This suggests that PGs do not function in situ to provide shear stiffness for articular cartilage. The shear stiffness of articular cartilage must therefore derive from its collagen content, or from the collagen-PG interaction (Mow & Ratcliffe, 1997). From this interpretation, an increase in collagen, which is a much more elastic element than PG and the predominant load-carrying element of the tissue in shear, would decrease the frictional dissipation and hence the observed phase angle.

SWELLING BEHAVIOR OF ARTICULAR CARTILAGE

The Donnan osmotic swelling pressure, associated with the densely packed fixed anionic groups (SO_3^- and COO^-) on the GAG chains as well as the bulk compressive stiffness of the PG aggregates entangled

in the collagen network, permits the PG gel in the collagen network to resist compression (Donnan, 1924; Maroudas, 1979; Mow & Ratcliffe, 1997). To account for such Fixed Charge Density (FCD) effects in cartilage, a triphasic mechano-electrochemical, multi-electrolyte theory was developed that models cartilage as a mixture of three miscible phases: a charged solid phase representing the collagen-PG network, a fluid phase representing the interstitial water, and an ion phase comprising the monovalent cation Na^+ and anion Cl^- as well as other multivalent species such as Ca^{2+} (Gu et al., 1998; Lai et al.,1991). In this theory, the total stress is given by the sum of two terms: $\sigma^{total} = \sigma^{solid} + \sigma^{fluid}$, where σ^{solid} and σ^{fluid} are the solid matrix stress and interstitial fluid pressure, respectively. At equilibrium, σ^{fluid} is given by the Donnan osmotic pressure, π (see discussion below). Derived from all of the fundamental laws of mechanics and thermodynamics rather than through the ad hoc combination of existing specialized theories (e.g., Frank & Grodzinsky, 1987a,b), this triphasic theory provides a set of thermodynamically permissible constitutive laws to describe the time-dependent physicochemical, mechanical, and electrical properties of charged-hydrated soft tissues. Moreover, the triphasic multi-electrolyte theory has been shown to be entirely consistent with the specialized classical osmotic pressure theory for charged polymeric solutions, phenomenological transport theories, and the biphasic theory (Donnan, 1924; Katchalsky & Curran, 1975; Mow et al., 1980; Onsager, 1931), all of which have been frequently used to study specific facets of articular cartilage.

The triphasic theory has been used successfully to describe many of the mechano-electrochemical behaviors of articular cartilage. These include the prediction of free swelling under chemical load; nonlinear dependence of hydraulic permeability with FCD; nonlinear dependence of streaming potentials with FCD; curling of cartilage layers; pre-stress; osmotic and negative osmotic flows; swelling and electrical responses of cells to osmotic shock loading; and the influence of inhomogeneous fixed charge density (Gu et al., 1993, 1997, 1998; Lai et al., 1991; Mow et al., 1998; Setton et al., 1998; Sun et al., 1998). Providing more versatility, the triphasic theory has been generalized to include multi-electrolytes in the tissue (Gu et al., 1998).

From analysis using the triphasic theory, it becomes clear that the swelling behavior of the tissue can be responsible for a significant fraction of the compressive load-bearing capacity of articular cartilage at equilibrium (Mow & Ratcliffe, 1997). For example, the triphasic theory predicts for confined-compression at equilibrium that the total stress (σ^{total}) acting on the cartilage specimen is the sum of the stress in the solid matrix (σ^{solid}) and the Donnan osmotic pressure ($\sigma^{fluid} = \pi$). The Donnan osmotic pressure is the swelling pressure caused by the ions in association with the FCD and represents the physicochemical motive force for cartilage swelling (Fig. 3-18). From the classical theory for osmotic pressure, the Donnan osmotic pressure caused by the excess of ion particles inside the tissue is given by:

$$\pi = RT[\phi(2c+c^F)-2\phi^*c^*] + P\infty$$

where c is the interstitial ion concentration, c^* is the external ion concentration, c^F is the FCD, R is the universal gas constant, T is the absolute temperature, ϕ and ϕ^* are osmotic coefficients, and $P\infty$ is the osmotic pressure caused by the concentration of PG particles in the tissue, usually assumed to be negligible (Lai et al., 1991). For a lightly loaded tissue, the swelling pressure may contribute significantly to the load support. But for highly loaded tissues, such as those found under physiological conditions and certainly for dynamically loaded tissues, the interstitial fluid pressurization (σ^{fluid}) would dominate; the contribution of this swelling pressure to load support would be less than 5% (Soltz & Ateshian, 1998).

As with the biphasic theory, the triphasic mechano-electrochemical theory can be used to elucidate potential mechanosignal transduction mechanisms in cartilage. For example, because of their potential effects on chondrocyte function, it is important to describe and predict electrokinetic phenomena such as streaming potentials and streaming currents (Gu et al., 1993, 1998; Katchalsky & Curran, 1975; Kim et al., 1994) that arise from ion movement caused by the convection of interstitial fluid flow past the FCD of the solid matrix. As a second example, the pressure produced in the interstitial fluid by polyethylene glycol-induced osmotic loading of cartilage explants (Schneiderman et al., 1986) was recently shown to be theoretically nonequivalent to the pressure produced in any other commonly used mechanically loaded explant experiment or by hydrostatic loading (Lai et al., 1998). In light of this finding, earlier interpretations of biological data from studies making such an assumption of equivalency should be revisited.

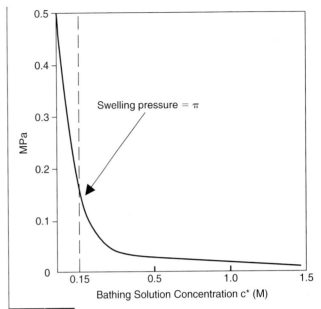

FIG. 3-18

Swelling pressure of articular cartilage versus bathing solution concentration (c*). At equilibrium, the interstitial fluid pressure is equal to the swelling pressure, which is defined by the tissue Donnan osmotic pressure (π).

Lubrication of Articular Cartilage

As already discussed, synovial joints are subjected to an enormous range of loading conditions, and under normal circumstances the cartilage surface sustains little wear. The minimal wear of normal cartilage associated with such varied loads indicates that sophisticated lubrication processes are at work within the joint and within and on the surface of the tissue. These processes have been attributed to a lubricating fluid-film forming between the articular cartilage surface and to an adsorbed boundary lubricant on the surface during motion and loading. The variety of joint demands also suggests that a number of mechanisms are responsible for diarthrodial joint lubrication. To understand diarthrodial joint lubrication, one should use basic engineering lubrication concepts.

From an engineering perspective, there are two fundamental types of lubrication. One is boundary lubrication, which involves a single monolayer of lubricant molecules adsorbed on each bearing surface.

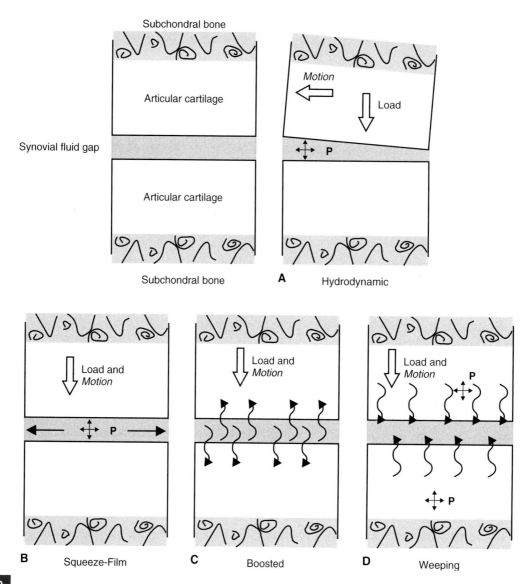

FIG. 3-19

A, In hydrodynamic lubrication, viscous fluid is dragged into a convergent channel, causing a pressure field to be generated in the lubricant. Fluid viscosity, gap geometry, and relative sliding speed determine the load-bearing capacity. **B,** As the bearing surfaces are squeezed together, the viscous fluid is forced from the gap into the transverse direction. This squeeze action generates a hydrodynamic pressure in the fluid for load support. The load-bearing capacity depends on the size of the surfaces, velocity of approach, and fluid viscosity. **C,** The direction of fluid flow under squeeze-film lubrication in the boosted mode for joint lubrication. **D,** Depicts the Weeping lubrication hypothesis for the uniform exudation of interstitial fluid from the cartilage. The driving mechanism is a self-pressurization of the interstitial fluid when the tissue is compressed.

The other is fluid-film lubrication, in which a thin fluid-film provides greater surface-to-surface separation (Bowden & Tabor, 1967). Both lubrication types appear to occur in articular cartilage under varying circumstances. Intact synovial joints have an extremely low coefficient of friction, approximately 0.02 (Dowson, 1966/1967; Linn, 1968; McCutchen, 1962; Mow & Ateshian, 1997). Boundary-lubricated surfaces typically have a coefficient of friction one or two orders of magnitude higher than surfaces lubricated by a fluid-film, suggesting that synovial joints are lubricated, at least in part, by the fluid-film mechanism. It is quite possible that synovial joints use the mechanism that will most effectively provide lubrication at a given loading condition. Unresolved, though, is the manner by which synovial joints generate the fluid lubricant film.

FLUID-FILM LUBRICATION

Fluid-film lubrication utilizes a thin film of lubricant that causes a bearing surface separation. The load on the bearing is then supported by the pressure that is developed in this fluid-film. The fluid-film thickness associated with engineering bearings is usually less than 20 μm. Fluid-film lubrication requires a minimum fluid-film thickness (as predicted by a specific lubrication theory) to exceed three times the combined statistical surface roughness of cartilage (e.g., 4 to 25 μm; Clarke, 1971; Walker et al., 1970). If fluid-film lubrication is unachievable because of heavy and prolonged loading, incongruent gap geometry, slow reciprocating-grinding motion, or low synovial fluid viscosity, boundary lubrication must exist (Mow & Ateshian, 1997).

The two classical modes of fluid-film lubrication defined in engineering are hydrodynamic and squeeze-film lubrication (Fig. 3-19, *A & B*). These modes apply to rigid bearings composed of relatively undeformable material such as stainless steel. Hydrodynamic lubrication occurs when nonparallel rigid bearing surfaces lubricated by a fluid-film move tangentially with respect to each other (i.e., slide on each other), forming a converging wedge of fluid. A lifting pressure is generated in this wedge by the fluid viscosity as the bearing motion drags the fluid into the gap between the surfaces, as shown in Figure 3-19*A*. In contrast, squeeze-film lubrication occurs when the bearing surfaces move perpendicularly toward each other. A pressure is generated in the fluid-film as a result of the viscous resistance of the fluid that acts to impede its escape from the gap (Fig. 3-19*B*). The squeeze-film mechanism is sufficient to carry high loads for short durations. Eventually, however, the fluid-film becomes so thin that contact between the asperities (peaks) on the two bearing surfaces occurs.

Calculations of the relative thickness of the fluid-film layer and the surface roughness are valuable in establishing when hydrodynamic lubrication may exist. In hydrodynamic and squeeze-film lubrication, the thickness and extent of the fluid-film, as well as its load-carrying capacity, are characteristics independent of the (rigid) bearing surface material properties. These lubrication characteristics are instead determined by the lubricant's properties, such as its rheological properties, viscosity and elasticity, the film geometry, the shape of the gap between the two bearing surfaces, and the speed of the relative surface motion.

Cartilage is unlike any man-made material with respect to its near frictionless properties. Classical theories developed to explain lubrication of rigid and impermeable bearings (e.g., steel) cannot fully explain the mechanisms responsible for lubrication of the natural diarthrodial joint. A variation of the hydrodynamic and squeeze-film modes of fluid-film lubrication, for example, occurs when the bearing material is not rigid but instead relatively soft, such as with the articular cartilage covering the joint surface. This type of lubrication, termed elastohydrodynamic, operates when the relatively soft bearing surfaces undergo either a sliding (hydrodynamic) or squeeze-film action and the pressure generated in the fluid-film substantially deforms the surfaces (Fig. 3-19, *A & B*). These deformations tend to increase the surface area and congruency, thus beneficially altering film geometry. By increasing the bearing contact area, the lubricant is less able to escape from between the bearing surfaces, a longer-lasting lubricant film is generated, and the stress of articulation is lower and more sustainable. Elastohydrodynamic lubrication enables bearings to greatly increase their load-carrying capacity (Dowson, 1966/1967, 1990).

Note that several studies have shown that hyaluronidase treatment of synovial fluid, which decreases its viscosity (to that of saline) by causing depolymerization of HA, has little effect on lubrication (Linn, 1968; Linn & Radin, 1968). Because fluid-film lubrication is highly dependent on lubricant viscosity, these results strongly suggest that an alternative mode of lubrication is the primary mechanism responsible for the low frictional coefficient of joints.

BOUNDARY LUBRICATION

During diarthrodial joint function, relative motion of the articulating surfaces occurs. In boundary lubrication, the surfaces are protected by an adsorbed layer of boundary lubricant, which prevents direct, surface-to-surface contact and eliminates most of the surface wear. Boundary lubrication is essentially independent of the physical properties of either the lubricant (e.g., its viscosity) or the bearing material (e.g., its stiffness), instead depending almost entirely on the chemical properties of the lubricant (Dowson, 1966/67). In synovial joints, a specific glycoprotein, "lubricin," appears to be the synovial fluid constituent responsible for boundary lubrication (Swann et al., 1979, 1985). Lubricin (25×10^4 mw) is adsorbed as a macromolecular monolayer to each articulating surface (Fig. 3-20). These two layers, ranging in combined thickness from 1 to 100 nm, are able to carry loads and appear to be effective in reducing friction (Swann et al., 1979). More recently, Hills (1989) suggested that the boundary lubricant found in synovial fluid was more likely to be a phospholipid named dipalmitoyl phosphatidylcholine. Although experiments demonstrate that a boundary lubricant can account for a reduction of the friction coefficient by a factor of threefold to sixfold (Swann et al., 1985; Williams et al., 1993), this reduction is quite modest compared with the much greater range (e.g., up to 60-fold) reported earlier (McCutchen, 1962). Even so, these results do suggest that boundary lubrication exists as a complementary mode of lubrication.

MIXED LUBRICATION

There are two joint lubrication scenarios that can be considered a combination of fluid-film and boundary lubrication or simply mixed lubrication (Dowson, 1966). The first case refers to the temporal coexistence of fluid-film and boundary lubrication at spatially distinct locations, whereas the second case, termed "boosted lubrication," is characterized by a

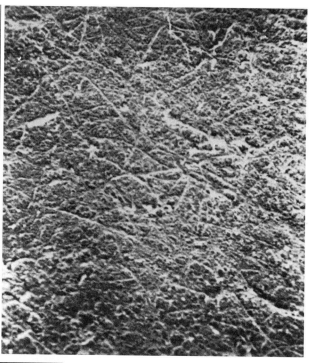

FIG. 3-21

Scanning electron micrograph of the surface of human articular cartilage from a normal young adult showing the typical irregularities characteristic of this tissue (×3,000). *Adapted from Armstrong, C.G., & Mow, V.C. (1980). Friction, lubrication and wear of synovial joints. In: R. Owen, J. Goodfellow, and P. Bullough (Eds.). Scientific Foundations of Orthopaedics and Traumatology (pp. 223–232). London: William Heinermann.*

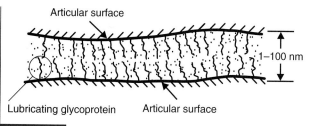

FIG. 3-20

Boundary lubrication of articular cartilage. The load is carried by a monolayer of the lubricating glycoprotein (LGP), which is adsorbed onto the articular surfaces. The monolayer effectively serves to reduce friction and helps to prevent cartilaginous wear. *Adapted from Armstrong, C.G., & Mow, V.C. (1980). Friction, lubrication and wear of synovial joints. In: R. Owen, J. Goodfellow, and P. Bullough (Eds.). Scientific Foundations of Orthopaedics and Traumatology (pp. 223–232). London: William Heinermann.*

shift of fluid-film to boundary lubrication with time over the same location (Walker et al., 1970).

The articular cartilage surface, like all surfaces, is not perfectly smooth; asperities project out from the surface (Clarke, 1971; Gardner & McGillivray, 1971; Redler & Zimny, 1970) (Figs. 3-3*B* and 3-21). In synovial joints, situations may occur in which the fluid-film thickness is of the same order as the mean articular surface asperity (Walker et al., 1970). During such instances, boundary lubrication between the asperities may come into play. If this occurs, a mixed mode of lubrication is operating, with the joint surface load sustained by both the fluid-film pressure in areas of noncontact and by the boundary lubricant lubricin in the areas of asperity contact (shown in Figure 3-22). In this mode of mixed lubrication, it is probable that most of the friction (which is still extremely low) is generated in the

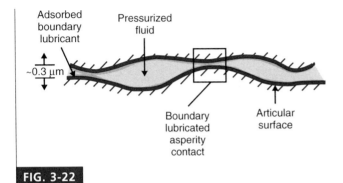

Adsorbed boundary lubricant

Pressurized fluid

~0.3 μm

Boundary lubricated asperity contact

Articular surface

FIG. 3-22

Schematic depiction of mixed lubrication operating in articular cartilage. Boundary lubrication occurs when the thickness of the fluid-film is on the same order as the roughness of the bearing surfaces. Fluid-film lubrication takes place in areas with more widely separated surfaces. *Adapted from Armstrong, C.G., & Mow, V.C. (1980). Friction, lubrication and wear of synovial joints. In: R. Owen, J. Goodfellow, and P. Bullough (Eds.).* Scientific Foundations of Orthopaedics and Traumatology *(pp. 223–232). London: William Heinermann.*

boundary lubricated areas while most of the load is carried by the fluid-film (Dowson, 1966/1967, 1990).

The second mode of mixed lubrication (boosted lubrication) proposed by Walker et al. (1968, 1970) and Maroudas (1966/1967) is based on the movement of fluid from the gap between the approaching articular surfaces into the articular cartilage (Fig. 3-19C). Specifically, in boosted lubrication, articular surfaces are believed to be protected during joint loading by the ultrafiltration of the synovial fluid through the collagen-PG matrix. This ultrafiltration permits the solvent component of the synovial fluid (water and small electrolytes) to pass into the articular cartilage during squeeze-film action, yielding a concentrated gel of HA protein complex that coats and lubricates the bearing surfaces (Lai & Mow, 1978). According to this theory, it becomes progressively more difficult, as the two articular surfaces approach each other, for the HA macromolecules in the synovial fluid to escape from the gap between the bearing surfaces because they are physically too large (0.22–0.65 μm), as shown in Figure 3-23. The water and small solute molecules can still escape into the articular cartilage through the cartilage surface and/or laterally into the joint space at the periphery of the joint. Theoretical results by Hou et al. (1992) predict that fluid entry into the cartilage-bearing surface is possible, leading them to suggest that boosted lubrication may occur. The role of this HA gel in joint lubrication remains unclear, how-

ever, particularly in view of the findings by Linn (1968), which demonstrated that purified HA acts as a poor lubricant.

To summarize, in any bearing, the effective mode of lubrication depends on the applied loads and on the relative velocity (speed and direction of motion) of the bearing surfaces. Adsorption of the synovial fluid glycoprotein, lubricin, to articular surfaces seems to be most important under severe loading conditions, that is, contact surfaces with high loads, low relative speeds, and long duration. Under these conditions, as the surfaces are pressed together, the boundary lubricant monolayers interact to prevent direct contact between the articular surfaces. Conversely, fluid-film lubrication operates under less severe conditions, when loads are low and/or oscillate in magnitude and when the contacting surfaces are moving at high relative speeds. In light of the varied demands on diarthrodial joints during normal function, it is unlikely that only a single mode of lubrication exists. As yet, it is impossible to state definitely under which conditions a particular lubrication mechanism may operate. Nevertheless, using the human hip as an example, some general statements are possible.

1. Elastohydrodynamic fluid-films of both the sliding (hydrodynamic) and the squeeze type probably play an important role in lubricating the joint. During the swing phase of walking, when loads on the joint are minimal, a substantial layer of synovial fluid-film is probably maintained. After the first peak force, at heel strike, a supply of fluid lubricant is generated by articular cartilage. However, this fluid-film thickness will begin to decrease under the high load of stance phase; as a result, squeeze-film action occurs. The second peak force during the walking cycle, just before the toe leaves the ground, occurs when the joint is swinging in the opposite direction. Thus, it is possible that a fresh supply of fluid-film could be generated at toe-off, thereby providing the lubricant during the next swing phase.

2. With high loads and low speeds of relative motion, such as during standing, the fluid-film will decrease in thickness as the fluid is squeezed out from between the surfaces (fluid film). Under these conditions, the fluid exuded from the compressed articular cartilage could become the main contributor to the lubricating film.

3. Under extreme loading conditions, such as during an extended period of standing follow-

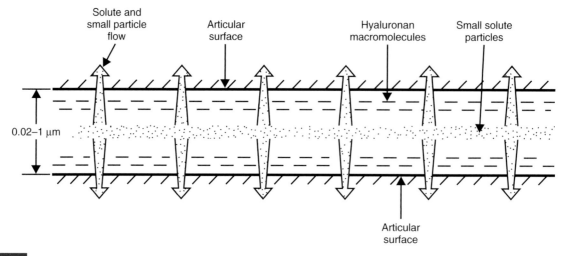

FIG. 3-23

Ultrafiltration of the synovial fluid into a highly viscous gel. As the articular surfaces come together, the small solute molecules escape into the articular cartilage and into the lateral joint space, leaving the large HA macromolecules that, be-cause of their size, are unable to escape. These HA macro-molecules form a concentrated gel less than 1 μm thick that lubricates the articular surfaces. This hypothesized lubrication mode is termed "boosted lubrication."

ing impact, the fluid-film may be eliminated, allowing surface-to-surface contact. The surfaces, however, will probably still be protected, either by a thin layer of ultrafiltrated synovial fluid gel (boosted lubrication) or by the adsorbed lubricin monolayer (boundary lubrication).

ROLE OF INTERSTITIAL FLUID PRESSURIZATION IN JOINT LUBRICATION

During joint articulation, loads transmitted across a joint may be supported by the opposing joint surfaces via solid-to-solid contact, through a fluid-film layer, or by a mixture of both. Although fluid-film lubrication is achievable, its contribution to joint lubrication is transient, a consequence of the rapid dissipation of the fluid-film thickness by joint loads. With this caveat, Ateshian (1997), adopting the theoretical framework of the biphasic theory (Mow et al., 1980), proposed a mathematical formulation of a boundary friction model of articular cartilage to describe the underlying mechanism behind diarthrodial joint lubrication, in particular, the time-dependence of the friction coefficient for cartilage reported during creep and stress-relaxation experiments (Malcolm, 1976; McCutchen, 1962).

Although load is partitioned between the solid and fluid phases of a biphasic material (Mow et al., 1980), Ateshian (1997) derived an expression for the effective (or measured) coefficient of friction that was dependent solely on the proportion of the load supported by the solid matrix (e.g., the difference between total load and that supported by hydrostatic pressure in the fluid). The implication of such an expression is that the frictional properties of cartilage vary with time during applied loading, a reflection of the interstitial fluid and collagen-PG matrix interactions that give rise to the flow-dependent viscoelastic properties of the tissue described earlier and shown in Figures 3-9 and 3-10.

To validate his model, Ateshian developed a novel loading experiment that superimposed a frictional torque load on a cartilage explant undergoing creep loading in a confined compression configuration (Fig. 3-24A) (Ateshian et al., 1998). More specifically, a cylindrical biphasic cartilage plug was compressed in a confining ring (e.g., prohibiting radial motion and fluid exudation) under a constant applied load generated by an impermeable rigid platen that was rotating at a prescribed angular speed. The surface of the plug opposite the platen was pressed against a fixed rigid porous filter whereby the interdigitation of the cartilage with the rough surface of the porous filter prevented it from rotating. In this

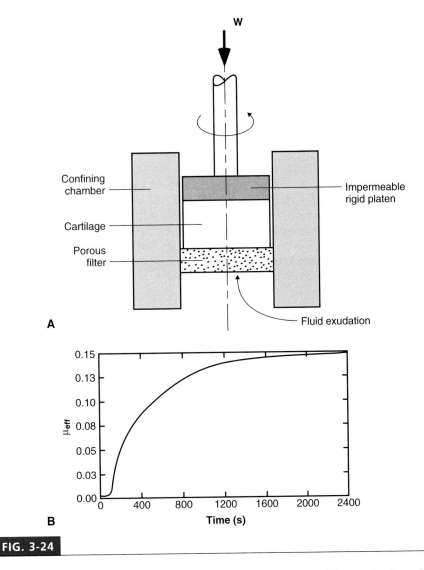

FIG. 3-24

Experimental configuration superimposing a frictional torque with creep loading of an articular cartilage explant in confined compression (Ateshian et al., 1998). **A,** Note that fluid exudation occurs on the opposite face of the tissue exposed to the frictional load, indicating that the frictional properties of cartilage are not dependent on the weeping of interstitial fluid to the lubricating boundary. **B,** Note that effective friction coefficient (μ_{eff}) varies with increasing proportion of load on the solid matrix, as can be seen from the theoretical curve for μ_{eff} as a function of time during the experiment. *Adapted from Mow, V.C., & Ateshian, G.A. (1997). Lubrication and wear of diarthrodial joints. In V.C. Mow & W.C. Hayes (Eds.),* Basic Biomechanics *(2nd ed., pp. 275–315). Philadelphia: Lippincott-Raven.*

manner, a frictional torque was developed in the tissue. Because the application of a torque load that yields pure shear, under infinitesimal deformations, induces no volume change in the tissue or associated fluid exudation, the load generated by the frictional torque is independent of the biphasic creep behavior of the tissue. Theoretical predictions, which closely match experimental results, show that during initial loading, when interstitial pressurization is high, the friction coefficient can be very low (Fig. 3-24B). As creep equilibrium is reached and the load is transferred to the solid matrix, the friction coefficient becomes high (e.g., 0.15). The time constant for this transient response is in excellent agreement with observed experimental results (Malcolm, 1976; McCutchen, 1962). Another important result of this work is that fluid pressurization can function in joint lubrication without concomitant fluid exudation to the lubricating boundary as is proposed for weeping lubrication (McCutchen, 1962) (Fig. 3-19D). Equally significant, this lubrication theory is capable of explaining the observed decrease of the effective friction coefficient with increasing rolling and sliding joint velocities and with increasing joint load (Linn, 1968).

Recently, the interstitial fluid pressurization within cartilage during uniaxial creep and stress relaxation experiments was successfully measured (Soltz & Ateshian, 1998). As predicted by the biphasic theory, they found that interstitial fluid pressurization supported more that 90% of the load for several hundred seconds following loading in confined compression (Ateshian & Wang, 1995). The close agreement of their measurements with biphasic theoretical predictions represents a major advancement in the understanding of diarthrodial joint lubrication and provides compelling evidence for the role of interstitial fluid pressurization as a fundamental mechanism underlying the load-bearing capacity in cartilage. It is emphasized that while the collagen-PG matrix is subjected to hydrostatic pressure in the surrounding interstitial fluid, it does not expose the solid matrix (nor encased chondrocytes) to deformation, presumably causing no mechanical damage.

Wear of Articular Cartilage

Wear is the unwanted removal of material from solid surfaces by mechanical action. There are two components of wear: interfacial wear resulting from the interaction of bearing surfaces and fatigue wear resulting from bearing deformation under load.

Interfacial wear occurs when bearing surfaces come into direct contact with no lubricant film (boundary or fluid) separating them. This type of wear can take place in either of two ways: adhesion or abrasion. Adhesive wear arises when, as the bearings come into contact, surface fragments adhere to each other and are torn off from the surface during sliding. Abrasive wear, conversely, occurs when a soft material is scraped by a harder one; the harder material can be either an opposing bearing or loose particles between the bearings. The low rates of interfacial wear observed in articular cartilage tested in vitro (Lipshitz & Glimcher, 1979) suggest that di-

rect surface-to-surface contact between the asperities of the two cartilage surfaces rarely occurs. Abrasive wear in these experiments, however, was not ruled out. The multiple modes of effective lubrication working in concert are the mechanisms making interfacial wear of articular cartilage unlikely. Nevertheless, adhesive and abrasive wear may take place in an impaired or degenerated synovial joint. Once the cartilage surface sustains ultrastructural defects and/or decreases in mass, it becomes softer and more permeable (Akizuki et al., 1986; Armstrong & Mow, 1982; Setton et al., 1994). Thus, fluid from the lubricant film separating the bearing surfaces may leak away more easily through the cartilage surface. This loss of lubricating fluid from between the surfaces increases the probability of direct contact between the asperities and exacerbates the abrasion process.

Fatigue wear of bearing surfaces results not from surface-to-surface contact but from the accumulation of microscopic damage within the bearing material under repetitive stressing. Bearing surface failure may occur with the repeated application of high loads over a relatively short period or with the repetition of low loads over an extended period even though the magnitude of those loads may be much lower than the material's ultimate strength. This fatigue wear, resulting from cyclically repeated deformation of the bearing materials, can take place even in well-lubricated bearings.

In synovial joints, the cyclical variation in total joint load during most physiological activities causes repetitive articular cartilage stressing (deformation). In addition, during rotation and sliding, a specific region of the articular surface "moves in and out" of the loaded contact area, repetitively stressing that articular region. Loads imposed on articular cartilage are supported by the collagen-PG matrix and by the resistance generated by fluid movement throughout the matrix. Thus, repetitive joint movement and loading will cause repetitive stressing of the solid matrix and repeated exudation and imbibition of the tissue's interstitial fluid (Mow & Ateshian, 1997). These processes give rise to two possible mechanisms by which fatigue damage may accumulate in articular cartilage: disruption of the collagen-PG solid matrix and PG "wash out."

First, repetitive collagen-PG matrix stressing could disrupt the collagen fibers, the PG macromolecules, and/or the interface between these two components. A popular hypothesis is that cartilage fatigue is the result of a tensile failure of the collagen fiber network (Freeman, 1975). Also, as discussed above, pronounced changes in the articular cartilage PG population have been observed with age and disease (Buckwalter et al., 1985; Muir, 1983; Roughley et al., 1980; Sweet et al., 1979). These PG changes could be considered as part of the accumulated tissue damage. These molecular structural changes would result in lower PG-PG interaction sites and thus lower network strength (Mow et al., 1989b; Zhu et al., 1991, 1996). Second, repetitive and massive exudation and imbibition of the interstitial fluid may cause the degraded PGs to "wash out" from the ECM, with a resultant decrease in stiffness and increase in permeability of the tissue that in turn defeats the stress-shielding mechanism of interstitial fluid-load support and establishes a vicious cycle of cartilage degeneration.

A third mechanism of damage and resultant articular wear is associated with synovial joint impact loading—that is, the rapid application of a high load. With normal physiological loading, articular cartilage undergoes surface compaction during the compression with the lubricating fluid being exuded through this compacted region, as shown in Figure 3-10. As described above, however, fluid redistribution within the articular cartilage occurs over time, which relieves the stress in this compacted region. This process of stress relaxation takes place quickly; the stress may decrease by 63% within 2 to 5 seconds (Ateshian et al., 1998; Mow et al., 1980). If, however, loads are supplied so quickly that there is insufficient time for internal fluid redistribution to relieve the compacted region, the high stresses produced in the collagen-PG matrix may induce damage (Newberry et al., 1997, Thompson et al., 1991). This phenomenon could well explain why Radin and Paul (1971) found dramatic articular cartilage damage with repeated impact loads.

These mechanisms of wear and damage may be the cause of the commonly observed large range of structural defects observed in articular cartilage (Bullough & Goodfellow, 1968; Meachim & Fergie, 1975) (Fig. 3-25, A–C). One such defect is the splitting of the cartilage surface. Vertical sections of cartilage exhibiting these lesions, known as fibrillation, show that they eventually extend through the full depth of the articular cartilage. In other specimens, the cartilage layer appears to be eroded rather than split. This erosion is known as smooth-surfaced destructive thinning.

Considering the variety of defects noted in articular cartilage, it is unlikely that a single wear mechanism is responsible for all of them. At any given site, the stress history may be such that fatigue is the initiating failure mechanism. At another, the lubrication conditions may be so unfavorable that interfacial wear dominates the progression of cartilage failure. As yet, there is little experimental information on the type of defect produced by any given wear mechanism.

Once the collagen-PG matrix of cartilage is disrupted, damage resulting from any of the three wear mechanisms mentioned becomes possible: (1) further disruption of the collagen-PG matrix as a result of repetitive matrix stressing; (2) an increased "washing out" of the PGs as a result of violent fluid movement and thus impairment of articular cartilage's interstitial fluid load support capacity; and (3) gross alteration of the normal load carriage mechanism in cartilage, thus increasing frictional shear loading on the articular surface.

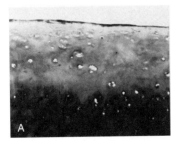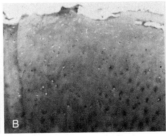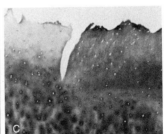

FIG. 3-25

Photomicrographs of vertical sections through the surface of articular cartilage showing a normal intact surface (**A**), an eroded articular surface (**B**), and a vertical split or fibrillation of the articular surface that will eventually extend through the full depth of the cartilage (**C**). *Photomicrographs provided through the courtesy of Dr. S. Akizuki, Nagano, Japan.*

All these processes will accelerate the rate of interfacial and fatigue wear of the already disrupted cartilage microstructure.

Hypotheses on the Biomechanics of Cartilage Degeneration

ROLE OF BIOMECHANICAL FACTORS

Articular cartilage has only a limited capacity for repair and regeneration, and if subjected to an abnormal range of stresses can quickly undergo total failure (Fig. 3-26). It has been hypothesized that failure progression relates to the following: (1) the magnitude of the imposed stresses; (2) the total number of sustained stress peaks; (3) the changes in the intrinsic molecular and microscopic structure of the collagen-PG matrix; and (4) the changes in the intrinsic mechanical property of the tissue. The most important failure-initiating factor appears to be the "loosening" of the collagen network that allows abnormal PG expansion and thus tissue swelling (Maroudas, 1976; McDevitt & Muir, 1976). Associated with this change is a decrease in cartilage stiffness and an increase in cartilage permeability (Altman et al., 1984; Armstrong & Mow, 1982; Guilak et al., 1994, Setton et al., 1994), both of which alter cartilage function in a diarthrodial joint during joint motion, as shown in Figure 3-27 (Mow & Ateshian, 1997).

The magnitude of the stress sustained by the articular cartilage is determined by both the total load on the joint and how that load is distributed over the articular surface contact area (Ahmed & Burke, 1983; Armstrong et al., 1979; Paul, 1976). Any intense stress concentration in the contact area will play a primary role in tissue degeneration. A large number of well-known conditions cause excessive stress concentrations in articular cartilage and result in cartilage failure. Most of these stress concentrations are caused by joint surface incongruity, resulting in an abnormally small contact area. Examples of conditions causing such joint incongruities include OA subsequent to congenital acetabular dysplasia, a slipped capital femoral epiphysis, and intra-articular fractures. Two further examples are knee joint meniscectomy, which eliminates the load-distributing function of the meniscus (Mow et al., 1992), and ligament rupture, which allows excessive movement and the generation of abnormal mechanical stresses in the affected joint (Altman et al., 1984; Guilak et al, 1994; McDevitt & Muir, 1976; Setton et al., 1994). In all the above cases, abnormal joint articulation increases the stress acting on the joint surface, which appears to predispose the cartilage to failure.

Macroscopically, stress localization and concentration at the joint surfaces have a further effect. High contact pressures between the articular surfaces decrease the probability of fluid-film lubrication (Mow & Ateshian, 1997). Subsequent actual surface-to-surface contact of asperities will cause microscopic stress concentrations that are responsible for further tissue damage (Ateshian et al., 1995, 1998; Ateshian & Wang, 1995) (Case Study 3-1).

The high incidence of specific joint degeneration in individuals with certain occupations, such as football players' knees and ballet dancers' ankles, can be explained by the increase in high and abnormal load frequency and magnitude sustained by the joints of these individuals. It has been suggested

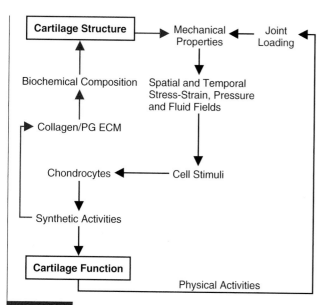

FIG. 3-26

Flow diagram of the events mediating the structure and function of articular cartilage. Physical activities result in joint loads that are transmitted to the chondrocyte via the extracellular matrix (ECM). The chondrocyte varies its cellular activities in response to the mechano-electrochemical stimuli generated by loading of its environment. The etiology of osteoarthritis is unclear but may be traced to intrinsic changes to the chondrocyte or to an altered ECM (e.g., resulting from injury or gradual wear) that leads to abnormal chondrocyte stimuli and cell activities.

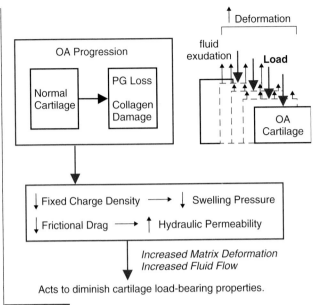

FIG. 3-27

A figure illustrating how osteoarthritic changes to the collagen-PG network can compromise the ability of articular cartilage to maintain interstitial fluid pressurization, which underlies the tissue's load-bearing and joint lubrication capacity. Loss of PG and damage to the collagen fibers result in an increased hydraulic permeability (decreased resistance to fluid flow) and supra-normal loads and strains on the solid matrix (and chondrocyte).

that, in some cases, OA may be caused by deficiencies in the mechanisms that act to minimize peak forces on the joints. Examples of these mechanisms include the active processes of joint flexion and muscle lengthening and the passive absorption of shocks by the subchondral bone (Radin, 1976) and meniscus (Mow et al., 1992).

Degenerative changes to the structure and composition of articular cartilage could lead to abnormal tissue swelling and functionally inferior biomechanical properties. In this weakened state, the cartilage ultrastructure will then be gradually destroyed by stresses of normal joint articulation (Fig. 3-27). OA may also arise secondarily from insult to the intrinsic molecular and microscopic structure of the collagen-PG matrix. Many conditions may promote such a breakdown in matrix integrity; these include degeneration associated with rheumatoid arthritis, joint space hemorrhage associated with hemophilia, various collagen metabolism disorders, and tissue degradation by proteolytic enzymes. The presence of soluble mediators such as cytokines

(e.g., interleukin-1) (Ratcliffe et al., 1986) and growth factors (e.g., transforming growth factor-beta 1) also appear to play an important role in OA. Another contributing factor to the etiology of OA may be age-related changes to the chondrocyte (Case Study 3-2).

IMPLICATIONS ON CHONDROCYTE FUNCTION

The ECM modulates the transmission of joint loads to the chondrocyte, acting as a transducer that converts mechanical loading to a plethora of environmental cues that mediate chondrocyte function. In healthy articular cartilage, loads from normal joint function motion result in the generation of

CASE STUDY 3-1

Knee Meniscectomy

Forty-year-old man who had a meniscectomy 10 years ago in his right knee. Currently, he is suffering pain associated with movement, swelling, and limitations of knee motion (Fig. 3-1-1).

The history of knee meniscectomy not only implies an alteration in joint surface congruence but also the elimination of the load-distribution function of the meniscus. The effect is an abnormal joint, characterized by an increase in the stress acting on the joint surface that results in cartilage failure. Most of these stress concentrations are caused by joint surface incongruity, resulting in an abnormally small contact area. This small contact area will suffer high contact pressure, decreasing the probability of fluid-film lubrication, and thus the actual surface-to-surface contact will cause microscopic stress concentrations that lead to damage.

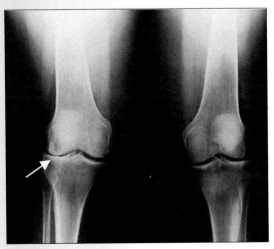

Case Study Figure 3-1-1.

CASE STUDY 3-2

Osteoarthritis

Seventy-year-old woman, overweight, with OA of the right hip joint with associated symptoms of pain, limitation of motion, joint deformity, and abnormal gait (Fig. 3-2-1).

OA is characterized by erosive cartilage lesions, cartilage loss and destruction, subchondral bone sclerosis and cysts, and large osteophyte formation at the margins of the joint (Mow & Ratcliffe, 1997). In this case, roentgenograms of the right hip of the patient show a decrease in the interarticular space and changes in bone surfaces as sclerotic and osteophyte formations. The most severe alterations are found at the point of maximum pressure against the opposing cartilage surface, in this case at the superior aspect of the femoral head.

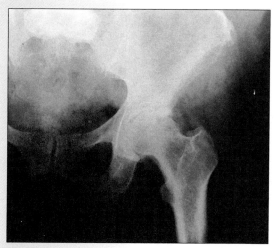

Case Study Figure 3-2-1.

mechano-electrochemical stimuli (e.g., hydrostatic pressure, stress and strain fields, streaming potentials) that promote normal cartilage maintenance (by the chondrocytes) and normal tissue function (Fig. 3-26). However, when the integrity of the collagen-PG network (the transducer) of articular cartilage is compromised, such as from trauma or disease, normal joint articulation leads to abnormal mechano-electrochemical stimuli, with ensuing abnormal ECM remodeling by the chondrocytes and debilitated tissue function.

In the absence of joint loading, the normal environment of the chondrocyte is characterized by the pre-stress established by the balance between tension in the collagen fibers and the Donnan osmotic pressure. During joint loading, by virtue of the tissue's low permeability, the normal environment of the chondrocyte is dominated by hydrostatic pressure in the interstitial fluid. Various phenomena originating from interstitial fluid flow exist as well. Implicated in enhancing nutrient diffusion, interstitial fluid flow (i.e., of unbound water) gives rise to cellular stimuli of an electrical nature, namely streaming potentials and currents (Frank & Grodzinsky, 1987; Gu et al., 1993, 1998). In addition, interstitial fluid flow through the small pores associated with the solid matrix (~50 nm) of normal cartilage, which offer considerable resistance to fluid flow (Maroudas, 1979; McCutchen, 1962; Mow et al., 1984), can give rise to a mechanical phenomena termed fluid-induced matrix compaction (Lai & Mow, 1980). The frictional interaction between interstitial fluid and solid are a result of drag resistance to forced flow through the porous-permeable cartilage matrix and a viscous shear stress exerted by the interstitial fluid. Given the nominal flow rates of the interstitial fluid mentioned earlier and the low permeability of the cartilage matrix, chondrocyte perception of this frictional interaction force is likely to be dominated by the drag resistance of flow through the matrix rather than by direct viscous shear stress on the cell. This frictional drag force can produce solid matrix deformation on the order of 15 to 30%.

From the discussion above, chondrocyte deformation can be considered to be governed by three coupled loading mechanisms: direct ECM deformation; flow-induced compaction; and fluid pressurization. In OA, the increased tissue permeability diminishes cartilage's normal fluid pressure load-support mechanism. Thus, there is a shift of load support onto the solid matrix, causing supranormal stresses and strains to be imposed on the chondrocytes (Fig. 3-27). These abnormally high stress and strain levels, and other mechano-electrochemical changes that are manifested with OA, can trigger an imbalance of chondrocyte anabolic and catabolic activities, further contributing to a vicious cycle of progressive cartilage degeneration. Indeed, changes to the biochemical composition and structure of cartilage can have a profound impact on tissue and chondrocyte function. With multidisciplinary collaborations and an appropriate theoretical framework, such as the biphasic theory, insights into the factors that govern chondrocyte function, cartilage structure and function, and the etiology of OA can be obtained.

Summary

1 The function of articular cartilage in diarthrodial joints is to increase the area of load distribution (thereby reducing the stress) and provide a smooth, wear-resistant bearing surface.

2 Biomechanically, articular cartilage should be viewed as a multiphasic material. In terms of a biphasic material, articular cartilage is comprised of a porous-permeable collagen-PG solid matrix (approximately 25% by wet weight) filled by the freely movable interstitial fluid (approximately 75% by wet weight). In addition to solid and fluid there exists an additional ion phase when considering articular cartilage as a triphasic medium. The ion phase is necessary to describe the swelling and other electromechanical behaviors of the tissue.

3 Important biomechanical properties of articular cartilage are the intrinsic material properties of the solid matrix and the frictional resistance to the flow of interstitial fluid through the porous-permeable solid matrix (a parameter inversely proportional to the tissue permeability). Together, these parameters define the level of interstitial fluid pressurization, a major determinant of the load-bearing and lubrication capacity of the tissue, which can be generated in cartilage.

4 Damage to articular cartilage, from whatever cause, can disrupt the normal interstitial fluid load-bearing capacity of the tissue and thus the normal lubrication process operating within the joint. Therefore, lubrication insufficiency may be a primary factor in the etiology of OA.

5 When describing articular cartilage in the context of a rigorous theoretical framework such as the biphasic, triphasic, or multiphasic theories, it is possible to accurately predict the biomechanical behaviors of articular cartilage under loading and to elucidate the underlying mechanisms that govern its load-bearing and lubrication function. Furthermore, insights into the temporal and spatial nature of the physical stimuli that may affect chondrocyte function in situ can be gained.

ACKNOWLEDGMENTS

This work was sponsored by the National Institutes of Health grants AR41913 and AR42850.

REFERENCES

Ahmed, A.M., & Burke, D.L. (1983). In vitro measurement of static pressure distribution in synovial joints—Part 1: Tibial surface of the knee. *J Biomech Eng, 105*, 216.

Akizuki, S., Mow, V.C., Muller, F., et al. (1986). Tensile properties of knee joint cartilage: 1. Influence of ionic condition, weight bearing, and fibrillation on the tensile modulus. *J Orthop Res, 4*, 379.

Altman, R.D., Tenebaum, J., Latta, L., et al. (1984). Biomechanical and biochemical properties of dog cartilage in experimentally induced osteoarthritis. *Ann Rheum Dis, 43*, 83.

Andriacchi, T.P., Natarajan, R.N., & Hurwitz, D.E. (1997). Musculoskeletal dynamics, locomotion, and clinical application. In V.C. Mow & W.C. Hayes (Eds.). *Basic Orthopaedic Biomechanics* (2nd ed.) (pp. 31–68). Philadelphia: Lippincott-Raven.

Armstrong, C.G., Bahrani, A.S., & Bardner, D.L. (1979). In vitro measurement of articular cartilage deformations in the intact human hip joint under load. *J Bone Joint Surg, 61A*, 744.

Armstrong, C.G., & Mow, V.C. (1980). Friction, lubrication and wear of synovial joints. *In* Owen, R., Goodfellow, J. & Bullough, P. (Eds.). *Scientific Foundations of Orthopaedics and Traumatology* (pp 223–232). London: William Heinermann.

Armstrong, C.G., & Mow, V.C. (1982). Variations in the intrinsic mechanical properties of human articular cartilage with age, degeneration, and water content. *J Bone Joint Surg, 64A*, 88.

Ateshian, G.A. (1997). Theoretical formulation for boundary friction in articular cartilage. *J Biomech Eng, 119*, 81.

Ateshian, G.A., Kwak, S.D., Soslowsky, L.J., et al. (1994). A new stereophotogrammetry method for determining in situ contact areas in diarthrodial joints: A comparison study. *J Biomechanics, 27*, 111.

Ateshian, G.A., Lai, W.M., Zhu, W.B., et al. (1995). An asymptotic solution for the contact of two biphasic cartilage layers. *J Biomechanics, 27*, 1347.

Ateshian, G.A., & Wang, H. (1995). A theoretical solution for the frictionless rolling contact of cylindrical biphasic articular cartilage layers. *J Biomechanics, 28*, 1341.

Ateshian, G.A., Wang, H., & Lai, W.M. (1998). The role of interstitial fluid in pressurization and surface porosities on the boundary friction of articular cartilage. *J Tribology, 120*, 241.

Ateshian, G.A., Warden, W.H., Kim, J.J., et al. (1997). Finite deformation biphasic material properties of bovine articular cartilage from confined compression experiments. *J Biomechanics, 30*, 1157.

Athanasiou, K.A., Rosenwasser, M.P., Buckwalter, J.A., et al. (1991). Interspecies comparison of in situ mechanical properties of distal femoral cartilage. *J Orthop Res, 9*, 330.

Bachrach, N.M., Valhmu, W.B., Stazzone, E.J., et al. (1995). Changes in proteoglycan synthesis rates of chondrocytes in articular cartilage are associated with the time dependent changes in the mechanical environment. *J Biomechanics, 28*, 1561.

Bachrach, N.M., Mow, V.C., & Guilak, F. (1998). Incompressibility of the solid matrix of articular cartilage under high hydrostatic pressure. *J Biomechanics, 31*, 445.

Bateman, J.F., Lamande, S.R., & Ramshaw, J.A.M. (1996). Collagen superfamily. In W.D. Comper (Ed.). *Extracellular Matrix* (Vol. 2, p. 2267). Amsterdam: Harwood Academic Pubs.

Bollet, A.J., & Nance, J.L. (1965). Biochemical findings in normal and osteoarthritic articular cartilage, II: Chondroitin sulfate concentration and chain length, and water and ash content. *J Clin Invest, 45,* 1170.

Bowden, F.P., & Tabor, D. (1967). *Friction and Lubrication.* London: Methuen Pubs.

Broom, N.D., & Silyn-Roberts, H. (1990). Collagen-collagen versus collagen-proteoglycan interactions in the determination of cartilage strength. *Arthritis Rheum, 33,* 1512.

Buckwalter, J.A., Kuettner, K.E., & Thonar, E.J.-M.A. (1985). Age-related changes in articular cartilage proteoglycans: Electron microscopic studies. *J Orthop Res, 3,* 251.

Bullough, P.G., & Goodfellow, J. (1968). The significance of the fine structures of articular cartilage. *J Bone Joint Surg 50B,* 852.

Bullough, P.G., & Jagannath, A. (1983). The morphology of the calcification front in articular cartilage. *J Bone Joint Surg, 65B,* 72.

Buschmann, M.D., Gluzband, Y.A., Grodzinsky, A.J., et al. (1992). Chondrocytes in agarose culture synthesize a mechanically functional extracellular matrix. *J Orthop Res, 10,* 745.

Buschmann, M.D., & Grodzinsky, A.J. (1995). A molecular model of proteoglycan-associated electrostatic forces in cartilage mechanics. *J Biomech Eng, 117,* 170.

Clark, J.M. (1985). The organization of collagen in cryofractured rabbit articular cartilage: A scanning electron microscopy study. *J Orthop Res, 3,* 17.

Clarke, I.C. (1971). Articular cartilage: A review and scanning electron microscope study—l. The interterritorial fibrillar architecture. *J Bone Joint Surg, 53B,* 732.

Donohue, J.M., Buss, D., Oegema, T.R., et al. (1983). The effects of indirect blunt trauma on adult canine articular cartilage. *J Bone Joint Surg, 65A,* 948.

Donnan, F.G. (1924). The theory of membrane equilibria. *Chemical Review, 1,* 73.

Dowson, D. (1966/1967). Modes of lubrication in human joints. *Proc Inst Mech Eng, 181J,* 45.

Dowson, D. (1990). Bio-tribology of natural and replacement joints. In V.C. Mow, A. Ratcliffe, S-L.Y. Woo (Eds.) *Biomechanics of Diarthrodial Joints* (pp. 305–345). New York: Springer-Verlag.

Edwards, J. (1967). Physical characteristics of articular cartilage. *Proc Inst Mech Eng, 181J,* 16.

Elmore, S.M., Sokoloff, L., Norris, G., et al. (1963). Nature of "imperfect" elasticity of articular cartilage. *J Applied Physiol, 18,* 393.

Eyre, D.R. (1980). Collagen: Molecular diversity in the body's protein scaffold. *Science, 207,* 1315.

Fosang, A.J., & Hardingham, T.E. (1996). Matrix proteoglycans. In W.D. Comper (Ed.) *Extracellular Matrix* (Vol. 2, pp. 200–229). Amsterdam: Harwood Academic Pubs.

Frank, E.H., & Grodzinsky, A.J. (1987a). Cartilage electromechanics—I. Electrokinetic transduction and effects of pH and ionic strength. *J Biomechanics, 30,* 615.

Frank, E.H., & Grodzinsky, A.J. (1987b). Cartilage electromechanics—II. A continuum model of cartilage electrokinetics and correlation with experiments. *J Biomechanics, 20,* 629.

Freeman, M.A.R. (1975). The fatigue of cartilage in the pathogenesis of osteoarthrosis. *Acta Orthop Scand, 46,* 323.

Fung, Y.C. (1981). Quasi-linear viscoelasticity of soft tissues. In *Biomechanics: Mechanical Properties of Living Tissues* (p. 226). New York: Springer-Verlag.

Gardner, S.L., & McGillivray, D.C. (1971). Living articular cartilage is not smooth. The structure of mammalian and avian joint surfaces demonstrated in vivo by immersion incident light microscopy. *Ann Rheum Dis, 30,* 3.

Garg, H.G., & Swann, D.A. (1981). Age-related changes in the chemical composition of bovine articular cartilage. *Biochem J, 193,* 459.

Gu, W.Y., Lai, W.M., & Mow, V.C. (1993). Transport of fluid and ions through a porous-permeable charged-hydrated tissue, and streaming potential data on normal bovine articular cartilage. *J Biomechanics, 26,* 709.

Gu, W.Y., Lai, W.M., & Mow, V.C. (1997). A triphasic analysis of negative osmotic flows through charged hydrated soft tissues. *J Biomechanics, 30,* 71.

Gu, W.Y., Lai, W.M., & Mow, V.C. (1998). A mixture theory for charged hydrated soft tissues containing multi-electrolytes: Passive transport and swelling behaviors. *J Biomech Eng, 102,* 169.

Guilak, F., Ratcliffe, A., Lane, N., et al. (1994). Mechanical and biochemical changes in the superficial zone of articular cartilage in a canine model of osteoarthritis. *J Orthop Res, 12,* 474.

Hardingham, T.M., & Muir, H. (1974). Hyaluronic acid in cartilage and proteoglycan aggregation. *Biochem J, L39,* 565.

Hardingham, T.E., Beardmore-Garg, M., & Dunham, D.G. (1987). Protein domain structure of the aggregating proteoglycan from cartilage. *Trans Orthop Res Soc, 12,* 61.

Hascall, V.C. (1977). Interactions of cartilage proteoglycans with hyaluronic acid. *J Supramol Structure, 7,* 101.

Hayes, W.C., & Bodine, A.J. (1978). Flow-independent viscoelastic properties of articular cartilage matrix. *J Biomechanics, 11,* 407.

Hayes, W.C., & Mockros, L.F. (1971).Viscoelastic properties of human articular cartilage. *J Appl Physiol, 31,* 562.

Hawkings, S.W. (1988). *A Brief History of Time: From the Big Bang to Black Holes.* New York: Bantam Books.

Heinegard, D., Wieslander, J., Sheehan, J., et al. (1985). Separation and characterization of two populations of aggregating proteoglycans from cartilage. *Biochem J, 225,* 95.

Helminen, H.J., Kiviranta, I., Tammi, M., et al. (Eds.) (1987). *Joint Loading: Biology and Health of Articular Structures.* Bristal, U.K: Wright & Sons, Pubs.

Hills, B.A. (1989). Oligolamellar lubrication of joints by surface active phospholipid. *J Rheum, 1–6,* 82–91.

Hirsch, C. (1944). The pathogenesis of chondromalacia of the patella. *Acta Chir Scand, 83* (Suppl), 1.

Hlavacek, M. (1995). The role of synovial fluid filtration by cartilage in lubrication of synovial joints: IV. Squeeze-film lubrication for axial symmetry under high loading conditions. *J Biomechanics, 28,* 1199.

Hodge, W.A., Fijan, R.S., Carlson, K., et al. (1986). Contact pressure in the human hip joint measured in vivo. *Proc Natl Acad Sci, USA, 83,* 2879.

Holmes, M.H., Lai, W.M., & Mow, V.C. (1985). Singular perturbation analysis on the nonlinear, flow-dependent, compressive stress-relaxation behavior of articular cartilage. *J Biomech Eng, 107,* 206.

Hou, J.S., Mow, V.C., Lai, W.M., et al. (1992). An analysis of the squeeze-film lubrication mechanism for articular cartilage. *J Biomechanics, 25,* 247.

Hultkrantz, W. (1898). Ueber die Spaltrichtungen der Gelenkknorpel. *Verhandlungen der Anatomischen Gesellschaft, 12,* 248.

Katchalsky, A., & Curran, P.F. (1975). *Nonequilibrium Thermodynamics in Biophysics* (4th ed.). Cambridge: Harvard University Press.

Kempson, G.E., Tuke, M.A., Dingle, J.T., et al. (1976). The effects of proteolytic enzymes on the mechanical properties of adult human articular cartilage. *Biochem Biophys Acta, 428*, 741.

Kempson, G.E. (1979). Mechanical properties of articular cartilage. In M.A.R. Freeman (Ed.), *Adult Articular Cartilage* (2nd ed., pp. 333–414). Tunbridge Wells, U.K.: Pitman Medical.

Kim, Y.J., Sah, R.L., Grodzinsky, A.J., et al. (1994). Mechanical regulation of cartilage biosynthetic behavior: Physical stimuli. *Arch Biochem Biophys, 311*, 1.

Lai, W.M., Gu, W.Y., & Mow, V.C. (1998). On the conditional equivalence of chemical loading and mechanical loading on articular cartilage. *J Biomechanics 31(12)*, 1181-1185.

Lai, W.M., & Mow, V.C. (1978). Ultrafiltration of synovial fluid by cartilage. *J Eng Mech Div ASCE, 104*, 79.

Lai, W.M., & Mow, V.C. (1980). Drag-induced compression of articular cartilage during a permeation experiment. *J Biorheology, 17*, 111.

Lai, W.M., Hou, J.S., & Mow, V.C. (1991). A triphasic theory for the swelling and deformation behaviors of articular cartilage. *J Biomech Eng, 113*, 245.

Lakes, R., & Saha, S. (1979). Cement line motion in bone. *Science, 204*, 501.

Lane, J.M., & Weiss, C. (1975). Review of articular cartilage collagen research. *Arthritis Rheum, 18*, 553.

Linn, F.C. (1968). Lubrication of animal joints: 1. The mechanism. *J Biomechanics, 1*, 193.

Linn, F.C., & Radin, E.L. (1968). Lubrication of animal joints: III. The effect of certain chemical alterations of the cartilage and lubricant. *Arthritis Rheum, 11*, 674.

Linn, F.C., & Sokoloff, L. (1965). Movement and composition of interstitial fluid of cartilage. *Arthritis Rheum, 8*, 481.

Lipshitz, H., Etheredge, R., & Glimcher, M.J. (1975). In vitro wear of articular cartilage. I: Hydroxyproline, hexosamine, and amino acid composition of bovine articular cartilage as a function of depth from the surface; hydroxyproline content of the lubricant and the wear debris as a measure of wear. *J Bone Joint Surg, 57A*, 527.

Lipshitz, H., Etheredge, R., & Glimcher, M.J. (1976). Changes in the hexosamine content and swelling ratio of articular cartilage as functions of depth from the surface. *J Bone Joint Surg, 58A*, 1149.

Lipshitz, H., & Glimcher, M.J. (1979). In vitro studies of the wear of articular cartilage. *Wear, 52*, 297.

Malcolm, L.L. (1976). *An experimental investigation of the frictional and deformational responses of articular cartilage interfaces to static and dynamic loading.* Doctoral thesis, University of California, San Diego.

Mankin, H.A., & Thrasher, A.Z. (1975). Water content and binding in normal and osteoarthritic human cartilage. *J Bone Joint Surg, 57A*, 76.

Mansour, J.M., & Mow, V.C. (1976). The permeability of articular cartilage under compressive strain and at high pressures. *J Bone Joint Surg, 58A*, 509.

Maroudas, A. (1966/1967). Hyaluronic acid films. *Proc Inst Mech Eng, London, 181J*, 122.

Maroudas, A. (1968). Physicochemical properties of cartilage in light of ion-exchange theory. *Biophys J, 8*, 575.

Maroudas, A. (1975). Biophysical chemistry of cartilaginous tissues with special reference to solute and fluid transport. *Biorheology, 12*, 233.

Maroudas, A. (1976). Balance between swelling pressure and collagen tension in normal and degenerate cartilage. *Nature, 260*, 808.

Maroudas, A. (1979). Physicochemical properties of articular cartilage. In M.A.R. Freeman (Ed.), *Adult Articular Cartilage* (2nd ed., pp. 215–290). Tunbridge Wells, England: Pitman Medical.

Maroudas, A., Wachtel, E., Grushko, G., et al. (1991). The effect of osmotic and mechanical pressures on water partitioning in articular cartilage. *Biochem Biophys Acta, 1073*, 285.

McCutchen, C.W. (1962). The frictional properties of animal joints. *Wear, 5*, 1.

McDevitt, C.A., & Muir, H. (1976). Biochemical changes in the cartilage of the knee in experimental and natural osteoarthritis in the dog. *J Bone Joint Surg, 58B*, 94.

Meachim, G., & Fergie, I.A. (1975). Morphological patterns of articular cartilage fibrillation. *J Pathol, 115*, 231.

Mow, V.C., Amoczky, S.P., & Jackson, D.W. (1992). *Knee Meniscus: Basic and Clinical Foundations.* New York: Raven Press.

Mow, V.C., & Ateshian, G.A. (1997). Lubrication and wear of diarthrodial joints. In V.C. Mow & W.C. Hayes (Eds.), *Basic Biomechanics* (2nd ed., pp. 275–315). Philadelphia: Lippincott-Raven.

Mow, V.C., Ateshian, G.A., Lai, W.M., et al. (1998). Effects of fixed charges on the stress-relaxation behavior of hydrated soft tissues in a confined compression problem. *Int J Solids & Structures, 35*, 4945–4962.

Mow, V.C., Gibbs, M.C., Lai, W.M., et al. (1989a). Biphasic indentation of articular cartilage–Part II. A numerical algorithm and an experimental study. *J Biomechanics, 22*, 853.

Mow, V.C., Holmes, M.H., & Lai, W.M. (1984). Fluid transport and mechanical properties of articular cartilage: A review. *J Biomechanics, 17*, 377.

Mow, V.C., Kuei, S.C., Lai, W.M., et al. (1980). Biphasic creep and stress relaxation of articular cartilage in compression: Theory and experiments. *J Biomech Eng, 102*, 73.

Mow, V.C., Lai, W.M., & Redler, I. (1974). Some surface characterisics of articular cartilages. A scanning electron microscopy study and a theoretical model for the dynamic interaction of synovial fluid and articular cartilage. *J Biomechanics, 7*, 449.

Mow, V.C., & Ratcliffe, A. (1997). Structure and function of articular cartilage and meniscus. In V.C. Mow & W.C. Hayes (Eds.), *Basic Orthopaedic Biomechanics* (2nd ed., pp. 113–177). Philadelphia: Lippincott-Raven.

Mow, V.C., Zhu, W.B., Lai, W.M., et al. (1989b). The influence of link protein stabilization on the viscoelastic properties of proteoglycan aggregates. *Biochem Biophys Acta, 992*, 201.

Muir, H. (1983). Proteoglycans as organizers of the extracellular matrix. *Biochem Soc Trans, 11*, 613.

Myers, E.R., Lai, W.M., & Mow, V.C. (1984). A continuum theory and an experiment for the ion-induced swelling behavior cartilage. *J Biomech Eng, 106(2)*, 151–158.

Newberry, W.N., Zukosky, D.K., & Haut, R.C. (1997). Subfracture insult to a knee joint causes alterations in the bone and in the functional stiffness of overlying cartilage. *J Orthop Res, 15*, 450.

Onsager, L. (1931). Reciprocal relations in irreversible processes. I. *Phys Rev 37*, 405.

Paul, J.P. (1976). Force actions transmitted by joints in the human body. *Proc Roy Soc Lond, 192B*, 163.

Poole, A.R. (1986). Proteoglycans in health and disease: Structure and function. *Biochem J, 236*, 1.

Radin, E.L., and Paul, I.L. (1971). Response of joints to impact loading. I. In vitro wear. *Arthritis Rheum, 14*, 356.

Radin, E.L. (1976). Aetiology of osteoarthrosis. *Clin Rheum Dis, 2*, 509.

Ratcliffe, A., & Mow, V.C. (1996). Articular cartilage. In W.D. Comper (Ed.), *Extracellular Matrix* (Vol. 1, pp. 234–302). Amsterdam: Harwood Academic Pubs.

Ratcliffe, A., Tyler, J., & Hardingham, T.E. (1986). Articular cartilage culture with interleukin 1: Increased release of link protein, hyaluronate-binding region and other proteoglycan fragments. *Biochem J, 238*, 571.

Redler, I., & Zimny, M.L. (1970). Scanning electron microscopy of normal and abnormal articular cartilage and synovium. *J Bone Joint Surg, 52A*, 1395.

Redler, I., Zimny, M.L., Mansell, J., et al. (1975). The ultrastructure and biomechanical significance of the tidemark of articular cartilage. *Clin Orthop Rel Res, 112*, 357.

Rosenberg, L., Choi, H.U., Tang, L.-H., et al. (1985). Isolation of dermatan sulfate proteoglycans from mature bovine articular cartilage. *J Biol Chem, 260*, 6304.

Rosenberg, L., Hellmann, W., & Kleinschmidt, A.K. (1975). Electron microscopic studies of proteoglycan aggregates from bovine articular cartilage. *J Biol Chem, 250*, 1877.

Roth, V., & Mow, V.C. (1980). The intrinsic tensile behavior of the matrix of bovine articular cartilage and its variation with age. *J Bone Joint Surg, 62A*, 1102.

Roughley, P.J., & White, R.J. (1980). Age-related changes in the structure of the proteoglycan subunits from human articular cartilage. *J Biol Chem, 255*, 217.

Roughley, P.J., White, R.J., & Santer, V. (1981). Comparison of proteoglycans extracted from high- and low-weight bearing human articular cartilage, with particular reference to sialic acid content. *J Biol Chem, 256*, 12699.

Schinagl, R.M., Gurskis, D., Chen, A.C., et al. (1997). Depth-dependent confined compression modulus of full-thickness bovine articular cartilage. *J Orthop Res, 15*, 499.

Schinagl, R.M., Ting, M.K., Price, J.H., et al. (1996). Video microscopy to quantitate the inhomogeneous equilibrium strain within articular cartilage during confined compression. *Ann Biomed Eng, 24*, 500.

Schmidt, M.B., Mow, V.C., Chun, L.E., et al. (1990). Effects of proteoglycan extraction on the tensile behavior of articular cartilage. *J Orthop Res, 8*, 353.

Schneiderman, R., Keret, D., & Maroudas, A. (1986). Effects of mechanical and osmotic pressure on the rate of glycosaminoglycan synthesis in adult femoral head cartilage: An in vitro study. *J Orthop Res, 4*, 393.

Schubert, M., & Hamerman, D. (1968). *A Primer on Connective Tissue Biochemistry*. Philadelphia: Lea & Febiger.

Scott, J.E., & Orford, C.R. (1981). Dermatan sulphate-rich proteoglycan associates with rat tail-tendon collagen at the d band in the gap region. *Biochem J, 197*, 213.

Setton, L.A., Gu, W.Y., Lai, W.M., et al. (1995). Predictions of the swelling induced pre-stress in articular cartilage. In A.P.S. Selvadurai (Ed.), *Mechanics of Porous Media* (pp. 299–322). Kluwer Academic Pubs. Dordrecht, the Netherlands.

Setton, L.A., Mow, V.C., Muller, F.J., et al. (1994). Mechanical properties of canine articular cartilage are significantly altered following transaction of the anterior cruciate ligament. *J Orthop Res, 12*, 451.

Setton, L.A., Tohyama, H., & Mow, V.C. (1998). Swelling and curling behavior of articular cartilage. *J Biomech Eng, 120*, 355.

Setton, L.A., Zhu, W.B., & Mow, V.C. (1993). The biphasic poroviscoelastic behavior of articular cartilage in compression: Role of the surface zone. *J Biomechanics, 26*, 581.

Sokoloff, L. (1963). Elasticity of articular cartilage: Effect of ions and viscous solutions. *Science, 141*, 1055.

Soltz, M.A., & Ateshian, G.A. (1998). Experimental verification and theoretical prediction of cartilage interstitial fluid pressurization at an impermeable contact interface in confined compression. *J Biomechanics*, Oct 31 (10), 927–934

Stockwell, R.S. (1979). *Biology of Cartilage Cells*. Cambridge: Cambridge University Press.

Sun, D.N., Gu, W.Y., Guo, X.E., et al. (1998). The influence of inhomogeneous fixed charge density on cartilage mechano-electrochemical behaviors. *Trans Orthop Res Soc, 23*, 484.

Swann, D.A., Radin, E.L., & Hendren, R.B. (1979). The lubrication of articular cartilage by synovial fluid glycoproteins. *Arthritis Rhein, 22*, 665.

Swann, D.A., Silver, F.H., Slayter, H.S., et al. (1985). The molecular structure and lubricating activity of lubricin from bovine and human synovial fluids. *Biochem J, 225*, 195.

Sweet, M.B.E., Thonar, E.J.-M.A., & Marsh, J. (1979). Age-related changes in proteoglycan structure. *Arch Biochem Biophys, 198*, 439–448.

Thompson, R.C., Oegema, T.R., Lewis, J.L., et al. (1991). Osteoarthrotic changes after acute transarticular load. An animal model. *J Bone Joint Surg, 73A*, 990.

Thonar, E.J.-M.A., Bjornsson, S., & Kuettner, K.E. (1986). Age-related changes in cartilage proteoglycans. In K. Kuettner, R.S., Schleyerbach, & V. C. Hascall (Eds.). *Articular Cartilage Biochemistry* (pp. 273–287). New York: Raven Press.

Torzilli, P.A., & Mow, V.C. (1976). On the fundamental fluid transport mechanisms through normal and pathologic cartilage during function. I. The formulation. *J Biomech, 9(8)*, 541–552.

Torzilli, P.A., Rose, D.E., & Dethemers, S.A. (1982). Equilibrium water partition in articular cartilage. *Biorheology, 19*, 519.

Urban, J.P.G., & McMullin, J.F. (1985). Swelling pressure of the intervertebral disc: Influence of collagen and proteoglycan content. *Biorheology, 22*, 145.

Valhmu, W.B., Stazzone, E.J., Bachrach, N.M., et al. (1998). Load-controlled compression of articular cartilage induces a transient stimulation of aggrecan gene expression. *Arch Biochem Biophys 353*, 29.

Venn, M.F. (1978). Variation of chemical composition with age in human femoral head cartilage. *Ann Rheum Dis, 37*, 168.

Wada, T., & Akizuki, S. (1987). An ultrastructural study of solid matrix in articular cartilage under uniaxial tensile stress. *J Jpn Orthop Assn*, 61.

Walker, P.S., Dowson, D., Longfeild, M.D., et al. (1968). "Boosted lubrication" in synovial joints by fluid entrapment and enrichment. *Ann Rheum Dis, 27*, 512.

Walker, P.S., Unsworth, A., Dowson, D., et al. (1970). Mode of aggregation of hyaluronic acid protein complex on the surface of articular cartilage. *Ann Rheum Dis, 29,* 591.

Wang, C.B., & Mow, V.C. (1998). Inhomogeneity of aggregate modulus affects cartilage compressive stress-relaxation behavior. *Trans Orthop Res Soc, 23*(1), 481.

Weiss, C., Rosenberg, L., & Helfet, A.J. (1968). An ultrastructural study of normal young adult human articular cartilage. *J Bone Joint Surg, 50A,* 663.

Williams, P.F., Powell, G.L., & Laberge, M. (1993). Sliding friction analysis of phosphatidylcholine as a boundary lubricant for articular cartilage. Proc *Inst Mech Engrs, 207,* 59.

Woo, S.L.-Y., Mow, V.C., & Lai, W.M. (1987). Biomechanical properties of articular cartilage. In *Handbook of Bioengineering* (pp. 4.1–4.44). New York: McGraw-Hill.

Woo, S.L.Y., Levesay G.A., Runco, T.J., et al. (1997). Structure and function of tendons and ligaments. In V.C. Mow & W.C. Hayes (Eds.), *Basic Orthopaedic Biomechanics* (2nd ed., pp. 209–251). Philadelphia: Lippincott-Raven.

Zhu, W.B., Iatridis, J.C., Hlibczjk, V., et al. (1996). Determination of collagen-proteoglycan interactions in vitro. *J Biomechanics, 29,* 773.

Zhu, W.B., Lai, W.M., & Mow, V.C. (1986). Intrinsic quasi-linear viscoelastic behavior of the extracellular matrix of cartilage. *Trans Orthop Res Soc, 11,* 407.

Zhu, W.B., Lai, W.M., & Mow, V.C. (1991). The density and strength of proteoglycan-proteoglycan interaction sites in concentrated solutions. *J Biomechanics, 24,* 1007.

Zhu, W.B., Mow, V.C., Koob, T.J., et al. (1993). Viscoelastic shear properties of articular cartilage and the effects of glycosidase treatments. *J Orthop Res, 11,* 771.

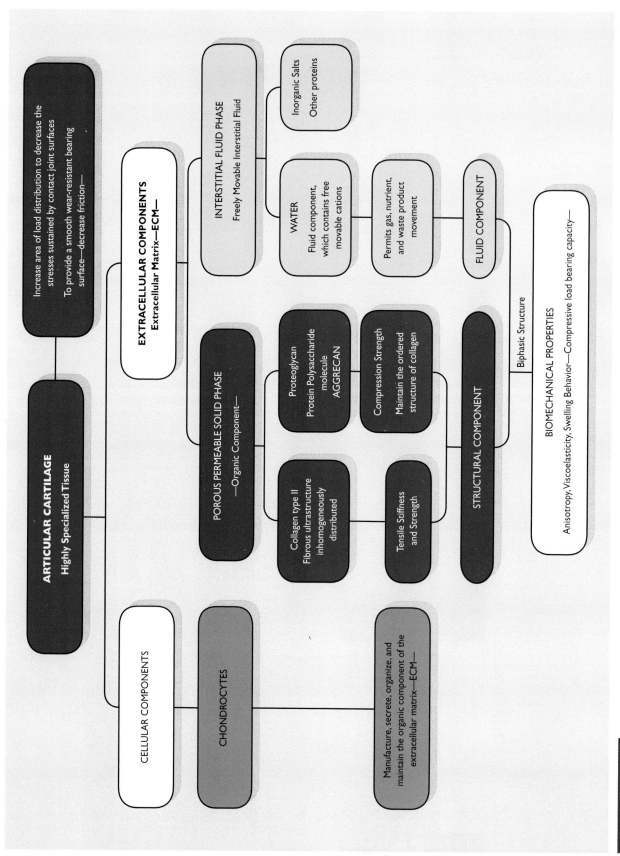

FLOW CHART 3-1 Articular cartilage structure and biomechanical properties.*

*This flow chart is designed for classroom or group discussion. Flow chart is not meant to be exhaustive.

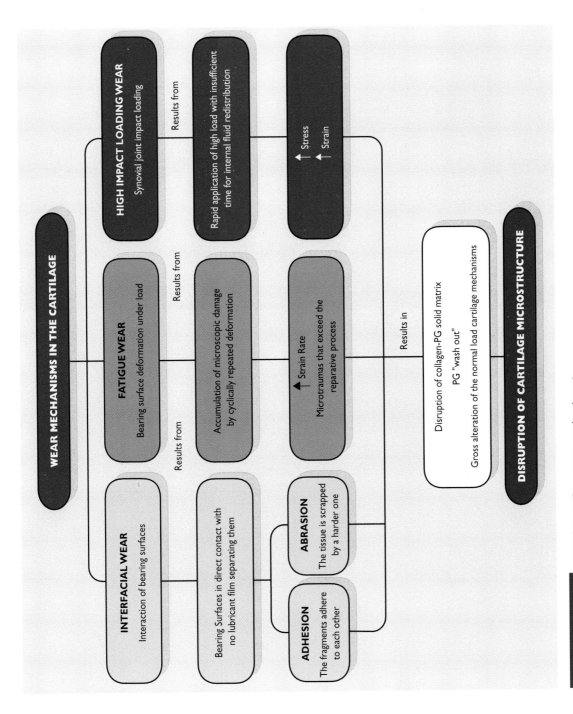

FLOW CHART 3-2   Articular cartilage wear mechanisms.*

*This flow chart is designed for classroom or group discussion. Flow chart is not meant to be exhaustive.

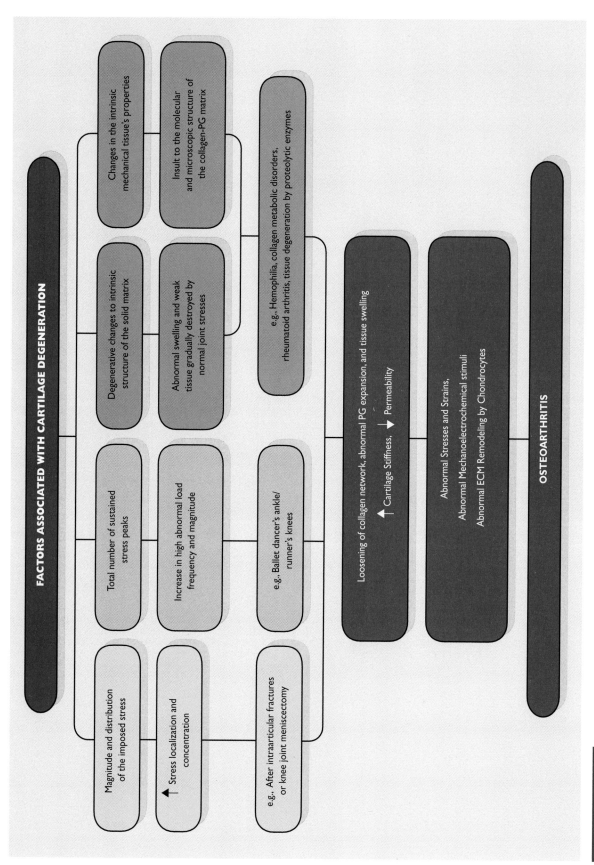

FLOW CHART 3-3 Factors associated with cartilage degeneration.* (*PG*, proteoglycan; *ECM*, extracellular matrix)

*This flow chart is designed for classroom or group discussion. Flow chart is not meant to be exhaustive.

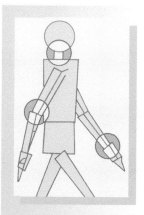

CHAPTER 4

Biomechanics of Tendons and Ligaments

Margareta Nordin, Tobias Lorenz, Marco Campello

Introduction

The three principal structures that closely surround, connect, and stabilize the joints of the skeletal system are tendons, ligaments, and joint capsules. Although these structures are passive (i.e., they do not actively produce motion as do the muscles), each plays an essential role in joint motion.

The role of the ligaments and joint capsules, which connect bone with bone, is to augment the mechanical stability of the joints, to guide joint motion, and to prevent excessive motion. Ligaments and joint capsules act as static restraints. The function of the tendons is to attach muscle to bone and to transmit tensile loads from muscle to bone, thereby producing joint motion, or to maintain the body posture. The tendons and the muscles form the muscle-tendon unit, which acts as a dynamic restraint. The tendon also enables the muscle belly to be at an optimal distance from the joint on which it acts without requiring an extended length of muscle between origin and insertion.

Tendon and ligament injuries and derangements are common. Proper management of these disorders requires an understanding of the mechanical properties and function of tendons and ligaments and their capacity for self-repair. This chapter discusses the following:

1. Composition and structure of tendons and ligaments
2. Biomechanical properties and behavior of normal tendon and ligament tissue
3. Biomechanical properties and behavior of injured tendon and ligament tissue

Several factors that affect the biomechanical function of tendons and ligaments are aging, pregnancy, mobilization and immobilization, diabetes, nonsteroidal anti-inflammatory drug (NSAID) use, and the effects of hemodialysis. Biomechanical considerations regarding grafts are also given.

Composition and Structure of Tendons and Ligaments

Tendons and ligaments are dense connective tissues known as parallel-fibered collagenous tissues. These sparsely vascularized tissues are composed largely of collagen, a fibrous protein constituting approximately one third of the total protein in the body (White, Handler, & Smith, 1964). Collagen constitutes a large portion of the organic matrix of bone and cartilage and has a unique mechanical supportive function in other connective tissues such as blood vessels, heart, ureters, kidneys, skin, and liver. The great mechanical stability of collagen gives the tendons and ligaments their characteristic strength and flexibility.

Like other connective tissues, tendons and ligaments consist of relatively few cells (fibroblasts) and an abundant extracellular matrix. In general, the cellular material occupies approximately 20% of the total tissue volume, while the extracellular matrix accounts for the remaining 80%. Approximately 70% of the matrix consists of water, and approximately 30% is solids. These solids are collagen, ground substance, and a small amount of elastin. The collagen content is generally over 75% and is somewhat greater in tendons than in ligaments (Kasser, 1996); in extremity tendons, the solid material may consist almost entirely of collagen (up to 99% of the dry weight) (Table 4-1).

The structure and chemical composition of ligaments and tendons are identical in humans and in many animal species such as rats, rabbits, dogs, and monkeys. Hence, extrapolations regarding these structures in humans can be made from the results of studies on these animal species.

COLLAGEN

The collagen molecule is synthesized by the fibroblast within the cell as a larger precursor (procollagen), which is then secreted and cleaved extracellularly to become collagen (Fitton-Jackson, 1965) (Fig. 4-1). Tendons and ligaments, like bone, are composed of the most common collagen molecule,

TABLE 4-1		
Structural Composition of Tendons and Ligaments		
Component	Ligament	Tendon
Cellular Material: Fibroblast	20%	20%
Extracellular Matrix:	80%	80%
Water	60–80%	60–80%
Solids:	20–40%	20–40%
Collagen:	70–80%	slightly higher
Type 1	90%	95–99%
Type 3	10%	1–5%
Ground substance	20–30%	slightly lesser

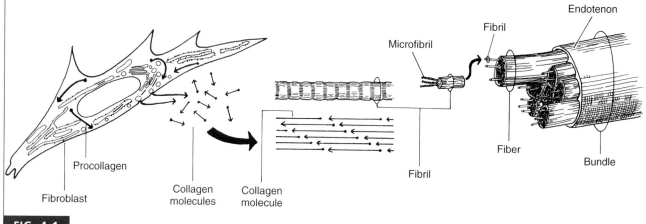

FIG. 4-1

Schematic representation of collagen fibrils, fibers, and bundles in tendons and collagenous ligaments (not drawn to scale). Collagen molecules, triple helices of coiled polypeptide chains, are synthesized and secreted by the fibroblasts. These molecules (depicted with "heads" and "tails" to represent positive and negative polar charges) aggregate in the extracellular matrix in a parallel arrangement to form microfibrils and then fibrils. The staggered array of the molecules, in which each overlaps the other, gives a banded appearance to the collagen fibrils under the electron microscope. The fibrils aggregate further into fibers, which come together into densely packed bundles.

type I collagen. This molecule consists of three polypeptide chains (α chains), each coiled in a left-handed helix with approximately 100 amino acids, which give it a total molecular weight of approximately 340,000 daltons (Rich & Crick, 1961) (Fig. 4-2). Two of the peptide chains (called α-1 chains) are identical, and one differs slightly (the α-2 chain). The three α-chains are combined in a right-handed triple helix, which gives the collagen molecule a rod-like shape. The length of the molecule is approximately 280 nanometers (nm), and its diameter is approximately 1.5 nm.

Almost two thirds of the collagen molecule consists of three amino acids: glycine (33%), proline (15%), and hydroxyproline (15%) (Ramachandran, 1963). Every third amino acid in each α chain is glycine, and this repetitive sequence is essential for the proper formation of the triple helix. The small size of this amino acid allows the tight helical packing of the collagen molecule. Moreover, glycine enhances the stability of the molecule by forming hydrogen bonds among the three chains of the superhelix. Hydroxyproline and proline form hydrogen bonds, or hydrogen-bonded water bridges, within each chain. The intra- and interchain bonding, or cross-linking, between specific groups on the chains is essential to the stability of the molecule.

Cross-links are also formed between collagen molecules and are essential to aggregation at the fibril level. It is the cross-linked character of the collagen fibrils that gives strength to the tissues they compose and allows these tissues to function under mechanical stress. Within the fibrils, the molecules are apparently cross-linked by "head-to-tail" interactions (Fig. 4-1), but interfibrillar cross-linking of a more complex nature also may occur.

In newly formed collagen, the cross-links are relatively few and are reducible; the collagen is soluble in neutral salt solutions and in acid solutions, and the cross-links are fairly easily denatured by heat. As collagen ages, the total number of reducible cross-links decreases to a minimum as a large number of stable, nonreducible cross-links are formed. Mature collagen is not soluble in neutral salt solutions or in acid solutions, and it survives a higher denaturation temperature. (For a review of cross-linkage in collagen, see Viidik, Danielsen, & Oxlund, 1982.)

A fibril is formed by the aggregation of several collagen molecules in a quaternary structure. This structure, in which each molecule overlaps the other, is responsible for the repeating bands observed on the fibrils under the electron microscope (Fig. 4-2; see also Fig. 3-3). The quaternary structure of collagen relates to the organization of collagen molecules into a stable, low energetic biological unit based on a regular association of adjacent molecules' basic and acidic amino acids. By arranging adjacent collagen molecules in a quarter-stagger, op-

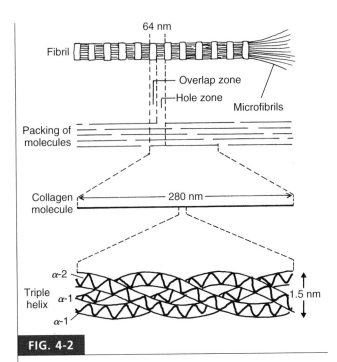

FIG. 4-2

Schematic drawing of collagen microstructure. The collagen molecule consists of three alpha chains in a triple helix (*bottom*). Several collagen molecules are aggregated into a staggered parallel array. This staggering, which creates hole zones and overlap zones, causes the cross-striation (banding pattern) visible in the collagen fibril under the electron microscope. *Adapted from Prockop, D.J., & Guzman, N.A. (1977). Collagen diseases and the biosynthesis of collagen. Hosp Pract, Dec, 61–68.*

positely charged amino acids are aligned. This stable structure will require a great amount of energy and force to separate its molecules, thus contributing to the strength of the structure. In this way, organized collagen molecules (five) form units of microfibrils, subfibrils, and fibrils (Fig. 4-3) (Simon, 1994). The fibrils aggregate further to form collagen fibers, which are visible under the light microscope. These fibers, which range from 1 to 20 μm in diameter, do not branch and may be many centimeters long. They reflect a 64-nm periodicity of the fibrils and have a characteristic undulated form. The fibers aggregate further into bundles. Fibroblasts are aligned in rows between these bundles and are elongated along an axis in the direction of ligament or tendon function (Fig. 4-4).

The arrangement of the collagen fibers differs somewhat in the tendons and ligaments and is suited to the function of each structure. The fibers composing the tendons have an orderly, parallel arrangement, which equips the tendons to handle the high unidirectional (uniaxial) tensile loads to which they are subjected during activity (Fig. 4-4*A*). The ligaments generally sustain tensile loads in one predominant direction but may also bear smaller tensile loads in other directions; their fibers may not be completely parallel but are closely interlaced with one another (Fig. 4-4*B*). The specific orientation of the fiber bundles varies to some extent among the ligaments and is dependent on the function of the ligament (Amiel et al., 1984).

The metabolic turnover of collagen may be studied by tritium labeling of hydroxyproline or glycine and by autoradiographic methods. Studies in animals have shown that the half-life of collagen in mature animals is very long: the same collagen molecules may exist throughout the animal's adult life; however, in young animals and in physically altered (e.g., injured or immobilized) tissue, the turnover is accelerated. Rabbit studies have shown metabolic activity to be somewhat greater in ligaments than in tendons, probably because of different stress patterns (Amiel et al., 1984).

ELASTIN

The mechanical properties of tendons and ligaments are dependent not only on the architecture and properties of the collagen fibers but also on the proportion of elastin that these structures contain. The protein elastin is scarcely present in tendons and extremity ligaments, but in elastic ligaments such as the ligamentum flavum, the proportion of elastic fibers is substantial. Nachemson and Evans (1968) found a 2 to 1 ratio of elastic to collagen fibers in the ligaments flava. These ligaments, which connect the laminae of adjacent vertebrae, appear to have a specialized role, which is to protect the spinal nerve roots from mechanical impingement, to pre-stress (preload) the motion segment (the functional unit of the spine), and to provide some intrinsic stability to the spine.

GROUND SUBSTANCE

The ground substance in ligaments and tendons consists of proteoglycans (PGs) (up to approximately 20% of the solids) along with structural glycoproteins, plasma proteins, and a variety of small molecules. The PG units, macromolecules composed of various sulfated polysaccharide chains (glycosaminoglycans) bonded to a core protein, bind to a long hyaluronic acid (HA) chain to form an extremely high molecular

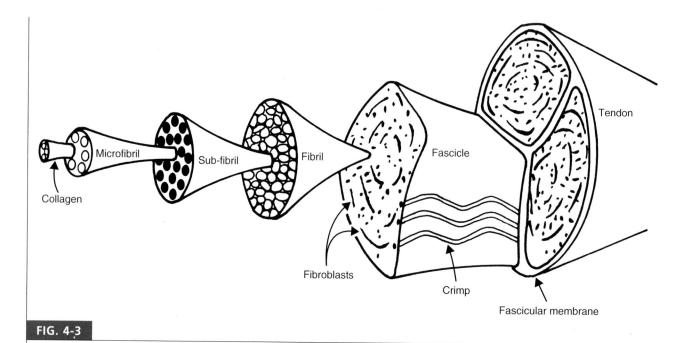

FIG. 4-3

Schematic representation of the microarchitecture of a tendon.

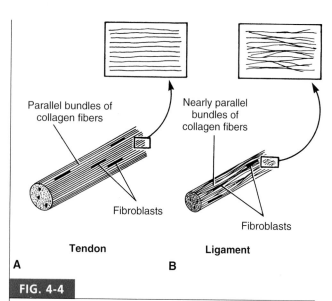

FIG. 4-4

Schematic diagram of the structural orientation of the fibers of tendon (**A**) and ligament (**B**); *insets* show longitudinal sections. In both structures the fibroblasts are elongated along an axis in the direction of function. *Adapted from Snell, R.S. (1984).* Clinical and Functional Histology for Medical Students. *Boston: Little, Brown.*

weight PG aggregate like that found in the ground substance of articular cartilage (see Fig. 3-6).

The PG aggregates bind most of the extracellular water of the ligament and tendon, making the matrix a highly structured gel-like material rather than an amorphous solution. Furthermore, by acting as a cement-like substance between the collagen microfibrils, they may help stabilize the collagenous skeleton of tendons and ligaments and contribute to the overall strength of these composite structures. Only a small number of these molecules exist in tendons, however, and their importance for its biomechanical properties has been questioned.

VASCULARIZATION

Tendons and ligaments have a limited vascularization, which affects directly their healing process and metabolic activity. Tendons receive their blood supply directly from vessels in the perimysium, the periosteal insertion, and the surrounding tissue via vessels in the paratenon or mesotenon. Tendons surrounded by paratenon have been referred to as vascular tendons, and those surrounded by a tendon sheath as avascular tendons. In tendons surrounded by a paratenon, vessels enter from many points on the periphery and anastomose with a longitudinal system of capillaries (Fig. 4-5).

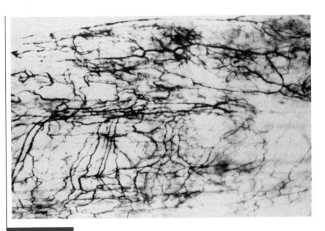

FIG. 4-5

India ink-injected (Spalteholz technique) into the calcaneal tendon of a rabbit, illustrating the vasculature of a paratenon-covered tendon. Vessels enter from many points on the periphery and anastomose with a longitudinal system of capillaries. *Reprinted with permission from Woo, S.L.Y., An, K.N., Arnoczky, D.V.M., et al. (1994). Anatomy, biology, and biomechanics of the tendon, ligament, and meniscus. In S.R. Simon (Ed.). Orthopaedic Basic Science (p. 52). Rosemont, IL: AAOS.*

The vascular pattern for tendons surrounded by a tendon sheath is different. Here the mesotenons are reduced to vincula (Fig. 4-6). This avascular region led a variety of researchers to propose a dual pathway for tendon nutrition: a vascular pathway, and, for the avascular regions, a synovial (diffusion) pathway. The concept of diffusional nutrition is of primary clinical significance in that it implies that tendon healing and repair can occur in the absence of adhesions (i.e., a blood supply). Conversely, ligaments in comparison with surrounding tissue appear to be hypovascular. However, histological studies reveal that throughout the ligament substance there is a uniform multivascularity, which originates from the insertion sites of the ligament. Despite the small size and limited blood flow of this vascular system, it is of primary importance in the maintenance of the ligament. Specifically, by providing nutrition for the cellular population, this vascular system maintains the continued process of matrix synthesis and repair. In its absence, damage from normal activities accumulates (fatigue) and the ligament is at risk for rupture (Woo et al., 1994).

Ligaments and tendons have been shown in both human and animal studies to have a variety of specialized nerve endings and mechanoreceptors. They play an important role in proprioception and nociception, which are directly related to the functionality of joints.

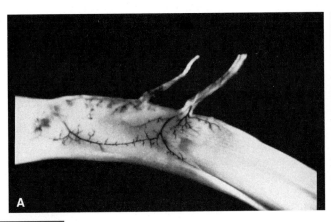
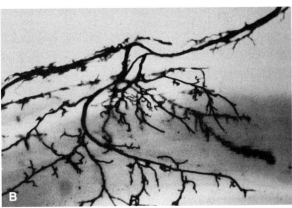

FIG. 4-6

A, India ink-injected specimen illustrating the vascular supply of the flexor digitorum profundus in a human through the vinculum longus. **B,** Close-up specimen (Spalteholz technique) showing the extent of the blood supply from the vinculum longus. The vessels in the vinculum divide into the dorsal, proximal, and distal branches, giving off vascular loops into the tendon substance. *Reprinted with permission from Woo, S.L.Y., An, K.N., Arnoczky, D.V.M., et al. (1994). Anatomy, biology, and biomechanics of the tendon, ligament, and meniscus. In S.R. Simon (Ed.). Orthopaedic Basic Science (p. 52). Rosemont, IL: AAOS.*

OUTER STRUCTURE AND INSERTION INTO BONE

Certain similarities are found in the outer structure of tendons and ligaments, but there are also important differences related to function. Both tendons and ligaments are surrounded by a loose areolar connective tissue. In ligaments, this tissue has no specific name, but in tendons it is referred to as the paratenon. More structured than the connective tissue surrounding the ligaments, the paratenon forms a sheath that protects the tendon and enhances gliding. In some tendons, such as the flexor tendons of the digits, the sheath runs the length of the tendons, and in others the sheath is found only at the point where the tendon bends in concert with a joint.

In locations where the tendons are subjected to particularly high friction forces (e.g., in the palm, in the digits, and at the level of the wrist joint), a parietal synovial layer is found just beneath the paratenon; this synovium-like membrane, called the epitenon, surrounds several fiber bundles. The synovial fluid produced by the synovial cells of the epitenon facilitates gliding of the tendon. In locations where tendons are subjected to lower friction forces, they are surrounded by the paratenon only.

Each fiber bundle is bound together by the endotenon (Fig. 4-1), which continues at the musculotendinous junction into the perimysium. At the tendo-osseous junction, the collagen fibers of the endotenon continue into the bone as Sharpey's perforating fibers and become continuous with the periosteum (Woo et al., 1988).

The structure of the insertions into bone is similar in ligaments and tendons and consists of four zones; Figure 4-7 illustrates these zones in a tendon. At the end of the tendon (zone 1), the collagen fibers intermesh with fibrocartilage (zone 2). This fibrocartilage gradually becomes mineralized fibrocartilage (zone 3) and then merges into cortical bone (zone 4). The change from more tendinous to more bony material produces a gradual alteration in the mechanical properties of the tissue (i.e., increased stiffness), which results in a decreased stress concentration effect at the insertion of the tendon into the stiffer bone (Cooper & Misol, 1970).

Mechanical Behavior of Tendons and Ligaments

Tendons and ligaments are viscoelastic structures with unique mechanical properties. Tendons are

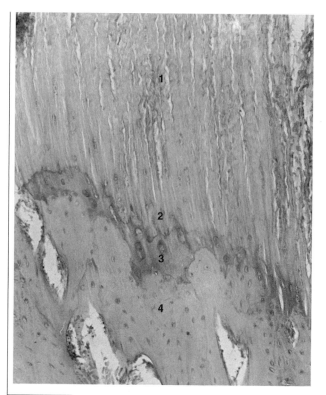

FIG. 4-7

Electron micrograph of a patellar tendon insertion from a dog, showing four zones (×25,000). *Zone 1,* parallel collagen fibers; *zone 2,* unmineralized fibrocartilage; *zone 3,* mineralized fibrocartilage; *zone 4,* cortical bone. The ligament-bone junction (not pictured) has a similar appearance. *Reprinted with permission from Cooper, R.R. & Misol, S. (1970). Tendon and ligament insertion. A light and electron microscopic study.* J Bone Joint Surg, *52A, I.*

strong enough to sustain the high tensile forces that result from muscle contraction during joint motion yet are sufficiently flexible to angulate around bone surfaces and to deflect beneath retinacula to change the final direction of muscle pull. The ligaments are pliant and flexible, allowing natural movements of the bones to which they attach, but are strong and inextensible so as to offer suitable resistance to applied forces.

Analysis of the mechanical behavior of tendons and ligaments provides important information for the understanding of injury mechanisms. Both structures sustain chiefly tensile loads during normal and excessive loading. When loading leads to injury, the degree of damage is affected by the rate of impact as well as the amount of load.

BIOMECHANICAL PROPERTIES

One means of analyzing the biomechanical properties of tendons and ligaments is to subject specimens to tensile deformation using a constant rate of elongation. The tissue is elongated until it ruptures, and the resulting force, or load (P), is plotted. The resulting load-elongation curve has several regions that characterize the behavior of the tissue (Fig. 4-8).

The first region of the load-elongation curve is called the "toe" region. The elongation reflected in this region is believed to be the result of a change in the wavy pattern of the relaxed collagen fibers. In this region, the tissue stretches easily, without much force, and the collagen fibers become straight and lose their wavy appearance as the loading progresses (Hirsch, 1974; Woo et al., 1994) (Fig. 4-9, *A & B*). Some data suggest, however, that this elongation may be caused mainly by interfibrillar sliding

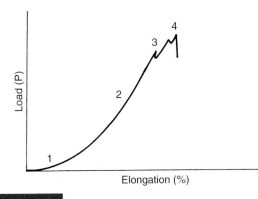

FIG. 4-8

Load-elongation curve for rabbit tendon tested to failure in tension. The numbers indicate the four characteristic regions of the curve. (1) Primary or "toe" region, in which the tissue elongated with a small increase in load as the wavy collagen fibers straightened out. (2) Secondary or "linear" region, in which the fibers straightened out and the stiffness of the specimen increased rapidly. Deformation of the tissue began and had a more or less linear relationship with load. (3) End of secondary region. The load value at this point is designated as P_{lin}. Progressive failure of the collagen fibers took place after P_{lin} was reached, and small force reductions (dips) occurred in the curve. (4) Maximum load (P_{max}) reflecting the ultimate tensile strength of the tissue. Complete failure occurred rapidly, and the specimen lost its ability to support loads. *Adapted from Carlstedt, C.A. (1987). Mechanical and chemical factors in tendon healing: Effects of indomethacin and surgery in the rabbit.* Acta Orthop Scand Suppl, 224.

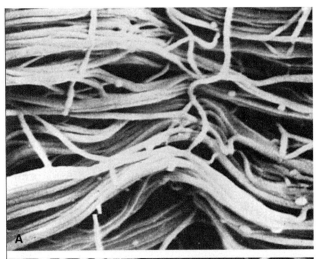

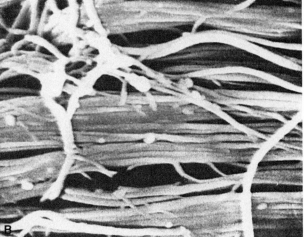

FIG. 4-9

Scanning electron micrographs of unloaded (relaxed) and loaded collagen fibers of human knee ligaments ($\times$10,000). **A,** The unloaded collagen fibers have a wavy configuration. **B,** The collagen fibers have straightened out under load. *Reprinted with permission from Kennedy, J.C., Hawkins, R.J., Willis, R.B., et al. (1976). Tension studies of human knee ligaments. Yield point, ultimate failure, and disruption of the cruciate and tibial collateral ligaments.* J Bone Joint Surg, 58A, 350.

and shear of the interfibrillar gel (ground substance) (for review, see Viidik, Danielson, & Oklund, 1982).

As loading continues, the stiffness of the tissue increases and progressively greater force is required to produce equivalent amounts of elongation. The elongation is often expressed as strain (ϵ), which is the deformation of the tissue calculated as a percentage of the original length of the specimen. If strains are increased (strain values of between 1.5 and 4% [Viidik, 1973]), a linear region will follow the toe region. This sudden increase in slope represents the second region in the diagram and corresponds to the response of the tissue to further elongation (Diamant et al., 1972).

Following the linear region, at large strains the stress-strain curve can end abruptly or curve downward as a result of irreversible changes (failure) (Woo et al., 1994). Where the curve levels off toward the strain axis, the load value is designated as P_{lin}. The point at which this value is reached is the yield point for the tissue. The energy uptake to P_{lin} is represented by the area under the curve up to the end of the linear region.

When the linear region is surpassed, major failure of fiber bundles occurs in an unpredictable manner. With the attainment of maximum load that reflects the ultimate tensile strength of the specimen, complete failure occurs rapidly, and the load-supporting ability of the tendon or ligament is substantially reduced.

The modulus of elasticity for tendons and ligaments has been determined in several investigations (Fung, 1967, 1972; Viidik, 1968). This parameter is based on a linear relationship between load and deformation (elongation), or stress and strain; that is, the stress (force per unit area) is proportional to the strain:

$$E = \sigma/\epsilon$$

where E = modulus of elasticity

$$\sigma = \text{stress}$$
$$\epsilon = \text{strain}$$

In the toe portion of the load-elongation curve (or stress-strain curve), the modulus of elasticity is not constant but increases gradually. The modulus stabilizes in the fairly linear secondary region of the curve.

The load-elongation curve depicted in Figure 4-8 generally applies to tendons and extremity ligaments. The curve for the ligamentum flavum, with its high proportion of elastic fibers, is entirely different (Fig. 4-10). In tensile testing of a human ligamentum flavum, elongation of the specimen reached 50% before the stiffness increased appreciably. Beyond this point, the stiffness increased greatly with additional loading and the ligament failed abruptly (reached P_{max}), with little further deformation (Nachemson & Evans, 1968).

The proportion of elastic proteins in ligaments and capsules is extremely important for the small

elastic deformation that they endure under tensile strain and the storage and loss of energy. During loading and unloading of a ligament between two limits of elongation, the elastic fibers allow the material to return to its original shape and size after being deformed. Meanwhile, part of the energy spent is stored; what is left will represent the energy loss during the cycle and is called hysteresis. The area enclosed by the loop represents the energy loss (Fig. 4-11).

PHYSIOLOGICAL LOADING OF TENDONS AND LIGAMENTS

The ultimate tensile strength (P_{max},) of ligaments and tendons is of limited interest from a functional standpoint because under normal physiological conditions in vivo these structures are subjected to a stress magnitude that is only approximately one third of this value. The upper limit for physiological strain in tendons and ligaments (when running and jumping, for example) is from 2 to 5% (Fung, 1981).

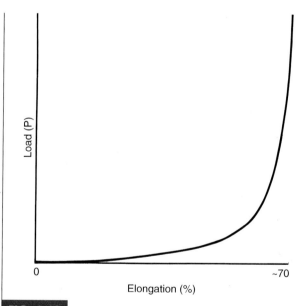

FIG. 4-10

Load-elongation curve for a human ligamentum flavum (60 to 70% elastic fibers) tested in tension to failure. At 70% elongation the ligament exhibited a great increase in stiffness with additional loading and failed abruptly without further deformation. *Adapted from Nachemson, A.L., & Evans, J.H. (1968). Some mechanical properties of the third human lumbar interlaminar ligament (ligamentum flavum). J Biomech, 1, 211–220.*

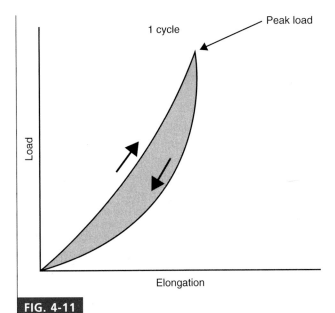

FIG. 4-11

Typical loading (*top*) and unloading curves (*bottom*) from tensile testing of knee ligaments. The two nonlinear curves form a hysteresis loop. The area between the curves, called the area of hysteresis, represents the energy losses within the tissue.

Few studies of loading of tendons or ligaments in vivo have been performed. Kear and Smith (1975), using the strain gauge method, measured the maximal strain in the lateral digital extensor tendons of sheep. The strain reached 2.6% while the sheep were trotting rapidly and decreased when the trotting speed decreased. This maximal strain occurred for only 0.1 second during each stride. The maximal load imposed on the entire tendon was approximately 45 newtons (N). These results suggest that during normal activity, a tendon in vivo is subjected to less than one fourth of its ultimate stress.

VISCOELASTIC BEHAVIOR (RATE DEPENDENCY) IN TENDONS AND LIGAMENTS

Ligaments and tendons exhibit viscoelastic, or rate-dependent (time-dependent), behavior under loading; their mechanical properties change with different rates of loading. When ligament and tendon specimens are subjected to increased strain rates (loading rates), the linear portion of the stress-strain curve becomes steeper, indicating greater stiffness of the tissue at higher strain rates. With higher strain rates, ligaments and tendons in isolation

store more energy, require more force to rupture, and undergo greater elongation (Kennedy, Hawkins, Willis, & Danylchuk, 1976).

During cyclic testing of ligaments and tendons, where loads are applied and released at specific intervals, the stress-strain curve is displaced to the right along the deformation (strain) axis with each loading cycle, revealing the presence of a nonelastic (plastic) component; the amount of permanent (nonrecoverable) deformation is progressively greater with every loading cycle. As cyclic loading progresses, the specimen also shows an increase in elastic stiffness as a result of plastic deformation (molecular displacement). Microfailure can occur within the physiological range if frequent loading is imposed on an already damaged structure where the stiffness has decreased.

Two standard tests that reveal the viscoelasticity of ligaments and tendons are the stress-relaxation test and the creep test (Fig. 4-12). During a stress-relaxation test, loading is halted safely below the linear region of the stress-strain curve and the strain is kept constant over an extended period. The stress decreases rapidly at first and then more slowly. When the stress-relaxation test is repeated cyclically, the decrease in stress gradually becomes less pronounced.

During a creep test, loading is halted safely below the linear region of the stress-strain curve and the stress is kept constant over an extended period. The strain increases relatively quickly at first and then more and more slowly. When this test is performed cyclically, the increase in strain gradually becomes less pronounced.

The clinical application of a constant low load to the soft tissues over a prolonged period, which takes advantage of the creep response, is a useful treatment for several types of deformities. One example is the manipulation of a child's clubfoot by subjecting it to constant loads by means of a plaster cast. Another example is the treatment of idiopathic scoliosis with a brace, whereby constant loads are applied to the spinal area to elongate the soft tissues surrounding the abnormally curved spine.

More complex viscoelastic behavior is observed in the entire bone-ligament-bone complex. Anterior cruciate ligaments (ACLs) in knee specimens taken from 30 primates were tested in tension to failure at a slow and a fast loading rate (Noyes et al., 1976). At the slow loading rate (60 seconds), much slower than that of an injury mechanism in vivo, the bony insertion of the ligament was the weakest component of the bone-ligament-bone complex, and a tibial spine

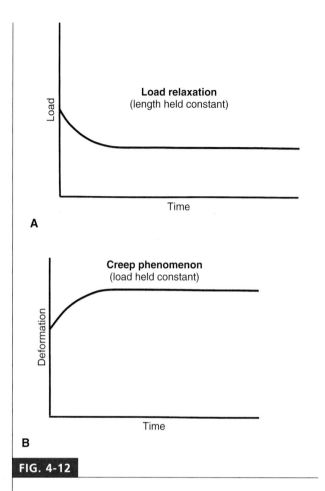

FIG. 4-12

The viscoelasticity (rate dependency, or time dependency) of ligaments and tendons can be demonstrated by two standard tests: the load-relaxation test and the creep test. **A,** Load relaxation is demonstrated when the loading of a specimen is halted safely below the linear region of the load-deformation curve and the specimen is maintained at a constant length over an extended period (i.e., the amount of elongation is constant). The load decreases rapidly at first (i.e., during the first 6 to 8 hours of loading) and then gradually more slowly, but the phenomenon may continue at a low rate for months. **B,** The creep response takes place when loading of a specimen is halted safely below the linear region of the load-deformation curve and the amount of load remains constant over an extended period. The deformation increases relatively quickly at first (within the first 6 to 8 hours of loading) but then progressively more slowly, continuing at a low rate for months.

avulsion was produced. At the fast loading rate (0.6 seconds), which simulated an injury mechanism in vivo, the ligament was the weakest component in two thirds of the specimens tested. At the slower rate, the load to failure decreased by 20%, and 30% less energy was stored to failure, but the stiffness of the

bone-ligament-bone complex was nearly the same. These results suggest that as the loading rate is increased, bone shows a greater increase in strength than does ligament.

Ligament Failure and Tendon Injury Mechanisms

Injury mechanisms are similar for ligaments and tendons, therefore the following description of ligament injury and failure is generally applicable to tendons. When a ligament in vivo is subjected to loading that exceeds the physiological range, microfailure takes place even before the yield point (P_{lin}) is reached. When P_{lin} is exceeded, the ligament begins to undergo gross failure and simultaneously the joint begins to displace abnormally. This displacement can also result in damage to the sur-

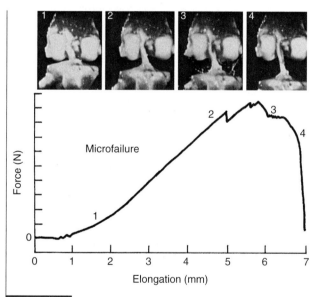

FIG. 4-13

Progressive failure of the anterior cruciate ligament from a cadaver knee tested in tension to failure at a physiological strain rate. The joint was displaced 7 mm before the ligament failed completely. The force-elongation curve generated during this experiment is correlated with various degrees of joint displacement recorded photographically; photos correspond to similarly numbered points on the curve. *Reprinted with permission from Noyes, F.R., and Grood, E.S. (1976). The strength of the anterior cruciate ligament in humans and Rhesus monkeys. Age-related and species-related changes. J Bone Joint Surg, 58A, 1074–1082.*

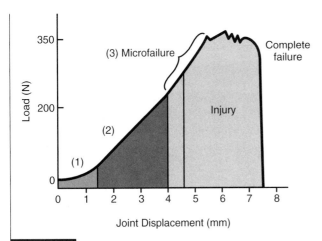

FIG. 4-14

The curve produced during tensile testing of a human anterior cruciate ligament in vitro (20) (see Fig. 4-13) has been converted to a load-displacement curve and divided into three regions correlating with clinical findings: (1) the load imposed on the anterior cruciate ligament during the anterior drawer test; (2) that placed on the ligament during physiological activity; and (3) that imposed on the ligament from partial injury to complete rupture. It should be noted that the divisions shown here represent a generalization. Microfailure is shown to begin toward the end of the physiological loading region, but it may take place well before this point in any given ligament.

rounding structures, such as the joint capsule, the adjacent ligaments, and the blood vessels that supply these structures.

Noyes (1977) demonstrated the progressive failure of the ACL and displacement of the tibiofemoral joint by applying a clinical test, the anterior drawer test, to a cadaver knee up to the point of ACL failure (Fig. 4-13). At maximum load, the joint had displaced several millimeters. The ligament was still in continuity even though it had undergone extensive macro- and microfailure and extensive elongation. In Figure 4-13, the force-elongation curve generated during the experiment, indicating where microfailure of the ligament began, is compared with various stages of joint displacement recorded photographically.

Correlation of the results of this test in vitro with clinical findings sheds light on the microevents that take place in the ACL during normal daily activity and during injuries of various degrees of severity. In Figure 4-14, the curve for the experimental study on cadaver knees that was presented in Figure 4-13 has been converted into a load-displacement curve and divided into three regions, corresponding re-

spectively to (1) the load placed on the ACL during tests of knee joint stability performed clinically, (2) the load placed on this ligament during physiological activity, and (3) that imposed on the ligament during injury from the beginning of microfailure to complete rupture. Microfailure begins even before the physiological loading range is exceeded and can occur throughout the physiological range in any given ligament. In fact, under experimental testing, the ultimate tensile loads—or the load at failure for human ACL—is between 340 and 390 N (Case Study 4-1).

ACL Failure: Failure of the ACL Associated With High Strain and Stress

A 25-year-old male occasional soccer player injured his ACL as a result of an abnormal torque in rotation of the knee. The player locked his foot on the ground and pivoted on his lower limb to produce a high rotational torque on the knee, which increased tensile loads on the ACL.

The first region of the load-displacement curve shows a normal physiological loading response. In the microfailure region, the increase in strain deformation leads to high internal stress and finally a complete rupture. Experimental testing in vitro in human ACL yielded a point of failure between 340 and 390 N.

The knee with the ACL injury will increase intra-articular joint motion, producing abnormally high stresses on other joint structures such as cartilage, which can lead to osteoarthritis. A deficiency in joint stability that results from ACL impairments will increase the likelihood of experiencing the "giving way" sensation or functional instability, thus affecting activities of daily living such as gait, jogging, and squatting (Case Study Fig 4-1-1).

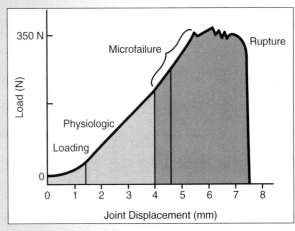

Case Study Figure 4-1-1.

Ligament injuries are categorized clinically in three ways according to degree of severity. Injuries in the first category produce negligible clinical symptoms. Some pain is felt, but no joint instability can be detected clinically, even though microfailure of the collagen fibers may have occurred.

Injuries in the second category produce severe pain and some joint instability can be detected clinically. Progressive failure of the collagen fibers has taken place, resulting in partial ligament rupture. The strength and stiffness of the ligament may have decreased by 50% or more, mainly because the amount of undamaged tissue has been reduced. The joint instability produced by the partial rupture of a ligament is often masked by muscle activity, and thus the clinical test for joint stability is usually performed with the patient under anesthesia.

Injuries in the third category produce severe pain during the course of trauma with less pain after injury. Clinically, the joint is found to be completely unstable. Most collagen fibers have ruptured, but a few may still be intact, giving the ligament the appearance of continuity even though it is unable to support any loads.

Loading of a joint that is unstable as a result of ligament or joint capsule rupture produces abnormally high stresses on the articular cartilage. This abnormal loading of the articular cartilage in the knee has been correlated with early osteoarthritis in humans and in animals.

Although injury mechanisms are generally comparable in ligaments and tendons, two additional factors become important in tendons because of their attachment to muscles: the amount of force produced by contraction of the muscle to which the tendon is attached and the cross-sectional area of the tendon in relation to that of its muscle. A tendon is subjected to increasing stress as its muscle contracts (see Fig. 6-10). When the muscle is maximally contracted, the tensile stress on the tendon reaches high levels. This stress can be increased further if rapid eccentric contraction of the muscle takes place; for example, rapid dorsiflexion of the ankle, which does not allow for reflex relaxation of the gastrocnemius and soleus muscles, increases the tension on the Achilles tendon. The load imposed on the tendon under these circumstances may exceed the yield point, causing Achilles tendon rupture (Case Study 4-2).

The strength of a muscle depends on its physiological cross-sectional area. The larger the cross-sectional area of the muscle, the higher the magnitude of the force produced by the contraction and

thus the greater the tensile loads transmitted through the tendon. Similarly, the larger the cross-sectional area of the tendon, the greater the loads it can bear. Although the maximal stress to failure for a muscle has been difficult to compute accurately, such measurements have shown that the tensile strength of a healthy tendon may be more than twice that of its muscle (Elliot, 1967). This finding is supported clinically by the fact that muscle ruptures are more common than are ruptures through a tendon.

Large muscles usually have tendons with large cross-sectional areas. Examples are the quadriceps

---

CASE STUDY 4-2

Tendon Injuries: Achilles Tendon Injuries in Runners, Which Result From a High Strain Rate

A middle-aged male marathoner engaged in a strenuous running activity experienced pain and a popping sensation in his posterior calf. An overuse injury is diagnosed.

The first region of the load-deformation curve shows a normal physiological toe-loading response. In the linear region, high load is producing a higher deformation within the tendon structure. When the Achilles tendon is subjected to higher strain rates during frequent loading cycles and insufficient time is allowed for the healing process, the result is an overuse injury. Histological studies of these injuries reveal a pathological pattern described as "angiofibrotic hyperplasia," which suggests a degenerative process. This failure in tendon remodeling frequently occurs before the abrupt rupture of the tendon. Relative avascularity, inflammatory disease, and other local factors also contribute to midsubstance ruptures (Case Study 4-2-1).

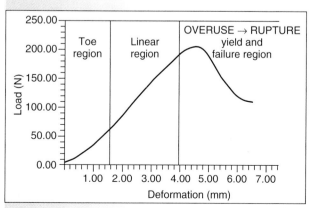

Case Study Figure 4-2-1.

muscle with its patellar tendon and the triceps surae muscle with its Achilles tendon. Some small muscles have tendons with large cross-sectional areas; such as the plantaris, which is a tiny muscle with a large tendon.

Factors That Affect the Biomechanical Properties of Tendons and Ligaments

Numerous factors affect the biomechanical properties of tendons and ligaments. The most common are aging, pregnancy, mobilization and immobilization, diabetes, steroids, NSAID use, and hemodialysis. The biomechanical properties of grafts are also discussed because reconstruction, particularly of the anterior and posterior knee ligaments, is common.

MATURATION AND AGING

The physical properties of collagen and of the tissues it composes are closely associated with the number and quality of the cross-links within and between the collagen molecules. During maturation (up to 20 years of age), the number and quality of cross-links increases, resulting in increased tensile strength of the tendon and ligament (Viidik, Danielsen, & Oxlund, 1982). An increase in collagen fibril diameter is also observed (Parry et al., 1978) with high variability in size (range 20–180 nm) (Strocchi, et al., 1996) noted in the young (<20 years). The diameter in adults (20–60 years) and in the elderly (>60 years) decreases remarkably (120 and 110 nm) but with a more even distribution. Strocchi et al. (1996) investigated age-related changes in human ACL collagen fibrils and reports an increase of fibril concentration from 68 fibrils/mu² in the young to 140 fibrils/mu² in the elderly. However, Amiel (1991) reports that the water content and the collagen concentration decreases significantly in the medial cruciate ligament of 2-, 12-, and 39-month-old rabbits.

After maturation, as aging progresses, collagen reaches a plateau with respect to its mechanical properties, after which the tensile strength and stiffness of the tissue begin to decrease. This may be the result of an increase in small collagen fibrils. Conversely, when the ACL of younger donors (average age 30 years) was compared with the ACL of older donors (average age 64.7 years), the material properties (strain, elastic modules, and maximum stress)

did not differ significantly (Kasperczyk et al., 1991). This may be due to the fact that only the ACL was taken from donors in whom no vascular or cardiopulmonary disease and no osteoarthritis of the knee was found on autopsy.

PREGNANCY AND THE POSTPARTUM PERIOD

A common clinical observation is the increased laxity of the tendons and ligaments in the pubic area during later stages of pregnancy and the postpartum period. This observation has been confirmed in animal studies. Rundgren (1974) found that the tensile strength of the tendons and the pubic symphysis in rats decreased at the end of pregnancy and during the postpartum period. Stiffness of these structures decreased in the early postpartum period but was later restored.

MOBILIZATION AND IMMOBILIZATION

Living tissues are dynamic and change their mechanical properties in response to stress, which leads to functional adaptation and optimal operation of the tissue.

Like bone, ligament and tendon appear to remodel in response to the mechanical demands placed on them; they become stronger and stiffer when subjected to increased stress and weaker and less stiff when the stress is reduced (Noyes et al., 1977a).

Physical training has been found to increase the tensile strength of tendons and of the ligament-bone interface (Woo et al., 1981). Tipton and coworkers (1970) compared the strength and stiffness of medial collateral ligaments from dogs that were exercised strenuously for 6 weeks with the values for ligaments from a control group of animals. The ligaments of the exercised dogs were stronger and stiffer than those of the control dogs, and the collagen fiber bundles had larger diameters.

Immobilization has been found to decrease the tensile strength of ligaments (Newton et al., 1995; Walsh et al., 1993). Noyes (1977a) demonstrated a reduction in the mechanical properties of the bone-ligament-bone complex in knees of primates immobilized in body casts for 8 weeks. When tested in tension to failure, the ACLs from these animals showed a 39% decrease in maximum load to failure and a 32% decrease in energy stored to failure compared with ligaments from a control group of animals (Fig. 4-15A). The immobilized ligaments also displayed more elongation and were significantly less stiff than the control specimens (Fig. 4-15B).

Amiel and coworkers (1982) showed a similar decrease in the strength and stiffness of lateral collateral ligaments in rabbits immobilized for 9 weeks. As the cross-sectional area of the specimens did not change significantly, the degeneration of mechanical properties was attributed to changes in the ligament substance itself. The tissue metabolism was noted to increase, leading to proportionally more immature collagen with a decrease in the amount and quality of the cross-links between collagen molecules. Newton et al. (1995) reported that the cross-sectional area of ligaments in immobilized rabbit knees was 74% of the control value.

In Noyes' (1977a) experiment, assessment of the effects of a reconditioning program initiated directly after the 8-week immobilization period demonstrated that considerable time was needed for the immobilized ligaments to regain their former strength and stiffness. After 5 months, the reconditioned ligaments still showed considerably less stiffness and 20% less strength than did ligaments from control animals. At 12 months, the reconditioned ligaments had strength and stiffness values comparable to those of control group liga-

ments (Fig. 4-15A). Woo et al. (1987) found that the stress-strain characteristics after remobilization return to normal but that the energy-absorbing capabilities of the bone-ligament complex improved but did not return to normal.

DIABETES MELLITUS

The term diabetes refers to disorders characterized by excessive urine excretion. Diabetes mellitus is a metabolic disorder in which the ability to oxidize carbohydrates is more or less completely lost. This is usually caused by pancreas insufficiency and a disturbance of the normal insulin mechanism, resulting in hyperglycemia, glycosuria, and polyuria. Diabetes mellitus is known to cause musculoskeletal disorders. Diabetics compared with nondiabetics show higher rates of tendon contracture (29 vs. 9%), tenosynovitis (59 vs. 7%), joint stiffness (40 vs. 9%), and capsulitis (16 vs. 1%). Diabetes also causes osteoporosis (Carvallo et al., 1991; Lancaster et al., 1994).

Duquette (1996) examined the effects of diabetes on the properties of the collateral knee ligament in rats. The tissue elastic properties did not differ between the diabetic and the control group. The vis-

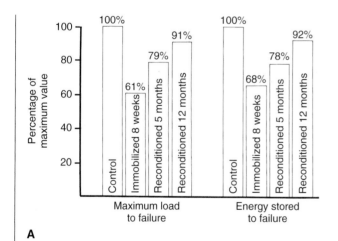

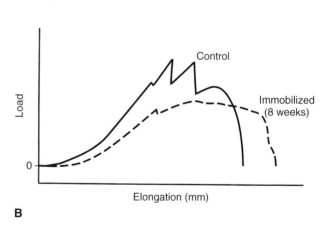

FIG. 4-15

A, Maximal load to failure and energy stored to failure for primate anterior cruciate ligaments tested in tension to failure. Values are shown as a percentage of control values for three groups of experimental animals: (1) those immobilized in body casts for 8 weeks; (2) those immobilized for 8 weeks and given a reconditioning program for 5 months; and (3) those immobilized for 8 weeks and given a reconditioning program for 12 months. **B,** Compared with controls, ligaments immobilized for 8 weeks were significantly less stiff (as indicated by the slope of the curve) and underwent greater elongation. *Adapted from Noyes, F.R. (1977a). Functional properties of knee ligaments and alterations induced by immobilization.* Clin Orthop, 123, 210–242.

cous component of the tissue response, however, was increased in the hyperglycemic group. Insulin therapy seems to lessen such alterations. Lancaster, et al. (1994) examined the changes in the mechanical properties of the patellar tendon in diabetic dogs. The results showed the stiffness of the canine patellar tendon-tibia complex in a physiological range of loading was 13% greater than in the control group. There was no difference in the strength of the tendon between the groups, but the mode of failure was different. In the control group, failure was caused by substance and avulsion failure, whereas failure of the tendon in the diabetic group was caused by tensile fractures of the patella (Lancaster et al., 1994).

STEROIDS

Corticosteroids, when applied immediately after injury, may cause significant impairment of the biomechanical and histological properties in ligaments. Corticosteroids also are known to inhibit collagen synthesis in vitro (Walsh et al., 1995). Wiggins et al. (1994) described these results in rabbits and implied that an acute injured ligament treated with corticosteroid injections may not withstand the mechanical loads of an early, vigorous rehabilitation. Noyes et al. (1977b) reported decreased ligament stiffness, failure load, and energy absorption in monkey ligaments after injection of long-acting corticosteroids. These findings were time- and dosage-dependent. After application of a dosage that was approximately 10 times an equivalent human dose, only minimal changes were found after 6 weeks, but after 15 weeks the maximum failure load (20%), energy absorption prior to failure (11%), and linear stiffness (11%) decreased significantly. After application of a dosage equivalent to the human dose, the maximum failure load (9%) and the energy absorption (8%) decreased significantly.

Campbell et al. (1996), however, showed that a single injection of long-acting corticosteroid does not cause histological differences in rats with acute injured ligaments as compared with rats with acute ligament injury and no injection of corticosteroids. Mechanical testing showed no significant difference in ultimate load or ultimate stress in the two groups. Oxlund et al. (1980) reports that local injections of corticosteroids every 3 days for 24 days increase the tensile strength and maximum load stiffness of muscle tendons but decrease the strength of the bone attachments of ligaments.

Laboratory investigations established the presence of estrogen receptors in human ACLs. Liu et al. (1997) reports that physiological levels of estrogen reduce the collagen production by 40% and at pharmacological levels of estrogen, collagen production is decreased by more than 50%. Estrogen fluctuations may alter ligament metabolism and may change the composition of ligament, rendering it more susceptible to injury.

NONSTEROIDAL ANTI-INFLAMMATORY DRUGS

NSAIDs (which include aspirin, acetaminophen, and indomethacin) are frequently used in the treatment of various painful conditions of the musculoskeletal system. NSAIDs are also widely used in the treatment of soft tissue injuries such as inflammatory disorders and partial ruptures of tendons and ligaments. Vogel (1977) found that treatment with indomethacin resulted in increased tensile strength in rat tail tendons. An increase in the proportion of insoluble collagen and in the total collagen content also was observed. Ohkawa (1982) found increased tensile strength in the periodontium of rats after indomethacin treatment. Carlstedt and associates (1986a, 1986b) found that indomethacin treatment increased the tensile strength in developing and healing plantaris longus tendons in the rabbit and noted that the mechanism for this increase was probably an increased cross-linkage of collagen molecules. These animal studies suggest that short-term administration of NSAIDs would not be deleterious for tendon healing but instead would increase the rate of biomechanical restoration of the tissue.

HEMODIALYSIS

Tendinous failure resulting from chronic renal failure does occur, with tendon rupture reaching 36% among individuals receiving hemodialysis. Hyperlaxity of tendons and ligaments was found in 74%, patellar tendon elongation in 49%, and articular hypermobility in 51% of individuals receiving long-term hemodialysis (Rillo et al., 1991). Dialysis-related amyloidosis may cause the deposition of amyloid in the synovium of tendons. The major constituent of the amyloid fibrils is the beta 2-microglobulin (Morita et al., 1995; Honda et al., 1990; Bardin et al., 1985).

GRAFTS

Reconstruction of torn ligaments, especially of the anterior and posterior cruciate ligament, is now a frequent procedure. The need for reconstruction is related to age, activity level, and associated injuries.

Grafts derived from different individuals of the same species are called allografts; grafts derived from the same individual are called autografts. Allograft tissue preservation is done through freeze-drying and low-dose irradiation to reduce rates of rejection and infection and to limit effects on the structural properties. Bone-patellar, tendon-bone, and Achilles tendon are usually used as allograft tissue, whereas the central tissue of the patellar tendon is commonly used as autograft tissue.

Shino et al. (1995) used fresh-frozen allogenic Achilles, tibialis anterior or posterior, and peroneus longus or brevis tendons for ACL reconstruction in humans. Specimens were procured during second-look arthroscopy. Several years after reconstruction, the allografts had collagen fibril profiles that did not resemble normal tendon grafts or normal ACL.

Strocchi et al. (1992) used patellar tendons that had been autografted to reconstruct torn ACLs. Follow-up biopsies were performed 6, 12, and 24 months after surgery. During this time, the autograft underwent considerable changes, and after 24 months the autograft had the appearance of normal ligament tissue. Strocchi suggested that the patellar tendon autograft is a valid functional ACL substitution for patients who desire to perform normal mechanical activity.

Corsetti et al. (1996) reports that replacement tissue undergoes extensive biological remodeling and incorporation. However, even a fully incorporated graft will never duplicate the native ACL but works instead as a check reign that increases the knee function. Tohayama et al. (1996) stated that the graft elongation at the time of implantation influences the long-term outcome of ACL reconstructions, at least in the canine model. They compared those cases where the graft elongation behavior was within the 95% confidence limit of normal ACL (group 1) with those cases where the graft elongation behavior was more than the 95% confidence limit of the normal ACL (group 2). Group 2 had significantly less inner stiffness of the graft than did group 1. Group 2 showed a significantly increased anteroposterior laxity, but there was no difference in ultimate failure load and absorbed energy.

Summary

1 Tendons and extremity ligaments are composed largely of collagen, whose mechanical stability gives these structures their characteristic strength and flexibility. The ligaments flava of the spine have a substantial proportion of elastin, which lends these structures their great elasticity.

2 The arrangement of the collagen fibers is nearly parallel in tendons, equipping them to withstand high unidirectional loads. The less parallel arrangement of the collagen fibers in ligaments allows these structures to sustain predominant tensile stresses in one direction and smaller stresses in other directions.

3 At the insertion of ligament and tendon into stiffer bone, the gradual change from a more fibrous to a more bony material results in a decreased stress concentration effect.

4 Tendons and ligaments undergo deformation before failure. When the ultimate tensile strength of these structures is surpassed, complete failure occurs rapidly, and their load-bearing ability is substantially decreased.

5 Studies suggest that during normal activity, a tendon in vivo is subjected to less than one fourth of its ultimate stress.

6 Injury mechanisms in a tendon are influenced by the amount of force produced by the contraction of the muscle to which the tendon is attached and the cross-sectional area of the tendon in relation to that of its muscle.

7 The biomechanical behavior of ligaments and tendons is viscoelastic, or rate-dependent, so that these structures display an increase in strength and stiffness with an increased loading rate.

8 An additional effect of rate dependency is the slow deformation, or creep, that occurs when tendons and ligaments are subjected to a constant low load over an extended period; stress relaxation takes place when these structures sustain a constant elongation over time.

9 Aging results in a decline in the mechanical properties of tendons and ligaments, that is, their strength, stiffness, and ability to withstand deformation.

10 Pregnancy, immobilization, diabetes, steroids, NSAID use, and hemodialysis affect the biomechanical properties of ligaments and tendons.

11 Allografts and autografts are useful in ligament reconstruction but material properties do not return completely to normal levels.

12 Ligaments and tendons remodel in response to the mechanical demands placed on them.

REFERENCES

Amiel, D., Kuiper. S.D., Wallace, C.D., Harwood, F. Vandeberg, J.S. (1991). Age-related properties of medial collateral ligament and anterior cruciate ligament: A morphologic and collagen maturation study in the rabbit. *J Gerontol, 46*(4), B156–B165.

Amiel, D., Frank, C., Harwood, F., et al. (1984). Tendons and ligaments: A morphological and biochemical comparison. *J Orthop Res, 1,* 257.

Amiel, D., Woo, S.L.Y., Harwood, F.L., et al. (1982). The effect of immobilization on collagen turnover in connective tissue. A biochemical-biomechanical correlation. *Acta Orthop Scand, 53,* 325.

Bardin, T., Kuntz, S., Zingraff, J., Voisin, M.C., Zelmar, A. (1985). Synovial amyloidosis in patients undergoing long-term hemodialysis. *Arthritis Rheum, 28*(9), 1052–1058.

Campbell, R.B., Wiggins, M.E., Cannistra, L.M., Fadale, P.P., Akelman, E. (1996). Influence of steroid injection in ligament healing in the rat. *Clin Orthop, 332,* 242–253.

Carlstedt, C.A. (1987). Mechanical and chemical factors in tendon healing: Effects of indomethacin and surgery in the rabbit. *Acta Orthop Scand Suppl, 224.*

Carlstedt, C.A., Madson, K., & Wredmark, T. (1986a). The influence of indomethacin on collagen synthesis during tendon healing in the rabbit. *Prostaglandins, 32,* 353.

Carlstedt, C.A., Madson, K., & Wredmark, T. (1986b). The influence of indomethacin on tendon healing. A biomechanical and biochemical study. *Arch Orthop Trauma Surg, 105,* 332.

Carvallo, A., Ordonez, M.A., Garcia, H., Tapia, J.C., Bekavac, J., Valencia, J., Moreira, M. (1991). Adult non-insulin-dependent diabetic: Limitation of articular mobility and soft tissue involvement. *Rev Med Chil,119*(9), 1016–1021.

Cooper, R.R., & Misol, S. (1970). Tendon and ligament insertion. A light and electron microscopic study. *J Bone Joint Surg, 52A,* l.

Corsetti, J.R., Jackson, D.W. (1996). Failure of anterior cruciate ligament reconstruction: The biologic basis. *Clin Orthop, 325,* 42–49.

Diamant, J., Keller, A., Baer, A., Litt, M., Arridge, R.G. (1972). Collagen: Ultrastructure and its relations to mechanical properties as a function of aging. *Proc R Soc Lond [Biol],180,* 293.

Duquette, J.J., Grigg, P., & Hoffman, A.H. (1996). The effect of diabetes on the viscoelastic properties of rat knee ligaments. *J Biomech Eng, 118*(4), 557–564.

Elliott, D.H. (1967). The biomechanical properties of tendon in relation to muscular strength. *Ann Phys Med, 9,* 1.

Fitton-Jackson, S. (1965). Antecedent phases in matrix formation. In *Structure and Function of Connective and Skeletal Tissues* (p. 277). London: Butterworth.

Fung, Y.C.B. (1981). *Biomechanics: Mechanical Properties of Living Tissues* (p. 222). New York: Springer-Verlag.

Fung, Y.C.B. (1967). Elasticity of soft tissues in simple elongation. *Am J Physiol, 213,* 1532.

Fung, Y.C.B. (1972). Stress-strain-history relations of soft tissues in simple elongation. In Y.C. Fung, N. Perrone, & M. Anliker (Eds.). *Biomechanics: Its Foundations and Objectives* (pp. 181–208). Englewood Cliffs, NJ: Prentice-Hall.

Hirsch, C. (1974). Tensile properties during tendon healing. *Acta Orthop Scand, Suppl 153.*

Honda, K., Hara, M., Ogura, Y., Nihei, H., Mimura, N. (1990). Beta-2-microglobulin amyloidosis in hemodialysis patients. An autopsy study of intervertebral disks and posterior ligaments. *Acta Pathol Jpn, 40*(11), 820–826.

Kasperczyk, W. J., Rosocha, S., Bosch, U., Oestern, J.J., Tscherne, H. (1991). Age activity and strength of knee ligaments. *Unfallchirurg, 94*(7), 372–375.

Kasser, J. (Ed.) (1996). *Orthopaedic Knowledge Update 5: Home Study Syllabus.* Park Ridge, IL: American Academy of Orthopaedic Surgeons.

Kear, M., & Smith, R.N. (1975). A method for recording tendon strain in sheep during locomotion. *Acta Orthop Scand, 46,* 896.

Kennedy, J.C., Hawkins, R.J., Willis, R.B., et al. (1976). Tension studies of human knee ligaments. Yield point, ultimate failure, and disruption of the cruciate and tibial collateral ligaments. *J Bone Joint Surg, 58A,* 350.

Lancaster, R.L., Haut, R.C., DeCamp, C.E. (1994). Changes in the mechanical properties of patellar tendon preparations of spontaneously diabetic dogs under long-term insulin therapy. *J Biomech, 27*(8), 1105–1108.

Liu, S.H., Al-Shaikh, R.A., Panossian, V., Finerman, G.A., Lane, J.M. (1997). Estrogen affects the cellular metabolism of the anterior cruciate ligament. A potential explanation for female athletic injury. *Am J Sports Med, 25*(5), 704–709.

Morita, H., Shinzaato, T., Cai, Z., David, G., Mizutani, A., Habuchi, H., Ito, M., Asai, J. et al. (1995). Basic fibroblast growth factor-hepatin sulphate complex in the human dialysis-related amyloidosis. *Virchows Arch, 427*(4), 395–400.

Nachemson, A.L., & Evans, J.H. (1968). Some mechanical properties of the third human lumbar interlaminar ligament (ligamentum flavum). *J Biomech, 1,* 211–220.

Newton, P.O., Woo, S.L., Mackenna, D.A., Akeson, W.H. (1995). Immobilization of the knee joint alters the mechanical and ultrastructural properties of the rabbit anterior cruciate ligament. *J Orthop Res, 13*(2), 191–200.

Noyes, F.R., et al. (1977a). Functional properties of knee ligaments and alterations induced by immobilization. *Clin Orthop, 123,* 210–242.

Noyes, F.R., Grood, E.S., Nussbaum N.S., Cooper, S.M (1977b). Effect of intra-articular corticosteroids on ligament properties: A biomechanical and histological study in Rhesus knees. *Clin Orthop, 123,* 197–209.

Noyes, F.R., and Grood, E.S. (1976). The strength of the anterior cruciate ligament in humans and Rhesus monkeys. Age-related and species-related changes. *J Bone Joint Surg, 58A,* 1074–1082.

Ohkawa, S. (1982). Effects of orthodontic forces and anti-inflammatory drugs on the mechanical strength of the periodontium in the rat mandibular first molar. *Am J Orthod, 81,* 498–502.

Oxlund, H. (1980). The influence of a local injection of cortisol on the mechanical properties of tendons and ligaments and the indirect effect on skin. *Acta Orthop Scand, 51*(2), 231–238.

Parry, D.A.D., Barnes, G.R.G., and Craig, A.S. (1978). A comparison of the size distribution of collagen fibrils in connective tissues as a function of age and possible relation between fibril size and mechanical properties. *Proc R Soc Lond, 203,* 305–321.

Prockop, D.J., & Guzman, N.A. (1977). Collagen diseases and the biosynthesis of collagen. *Hosp Pract,* Dec, 61–68.

Ramachandran, G.N. (1963). Molecular structure of collagen. *Int Rev Connect Tissue Res, 1,* 127.

Rich, A., Crick, F.H.C. (1961). The molecular structure of collagen. *J Mol Biol, 3,* 483.

Rillo, O.L., Babini, S.M., Basnak, A., Wainer, E., Balbachan, E., Cocco, J.A. (1991). Tendinous and ligamentous hyperlaxity in patients receiving long-term hemodialysis. *J Rheumatol, 18*(8), 1227–1231.

Rundgren, A. (1974). Physical properties of connective tissue as influenced by single and repeated pregnancies in the rat. *Acta Physiol Scand, Suppl.,* 417.

Shino, K., Oakes, B.W., Horibe, S., Nakata, K., Nakamura, N. (1995). Collagen fibril populations in human anterior cruciate ligament allografts. Electron microscopic analysis. *Am J Sports Med, 23*(2), 203–208.

Simon, S.R. (1994). *Orthopedic Basic Science.* Rosemont, IL: AAOS.

Snell, R.S. (1984). *Clinical and Functional Histology for Medical Students.* Boston: Little, Brown.

Strocchi, R., De Pasquale, V., Facchini, A., Raspanti, M., Zaffagnini, S., Marcacci, M. (1996). Age-related changes in human anterior cruciate ligament (ACL) collagen fibrils. *Ital Anat Embryol, 101*(4), 213–220.

Strocchi, R., DePasquale, V., Guizzardi, S., Marcacci, M., Ruggeri, A. (1992). Ultrastructural modifications of patellar tendon fibres used as anterior cruciate ligament (ACL) replacement. *Ital J Anat Embryol, 97*(4), 221–228.

Tipton, C.M., James, S.L., Mergner, W., et al. (1970). Influence of exercise on strength of medial collateral ligaments of dogs. *Am J Physiol, 218,* 894.

Tohayama, H., Beynnon, B. D., Johnson, R.J., Renstrom, P.A., Arms S.W. (1996). The effect of anterior cruciate ligament graft elongation at the time of implantation on the biomechanical behavior of the graft and knee. *Am J Sports Med, 24*(5), 608–614.

Viidik, A. (1968). Elasticity and tensile strength of the anterior cruciate ligament in rabbits as influenced by training. *Acta Physiol Scand, 74,* 372.

Viidik, A. (1973). Functional properties of collagenous tissues. *Int Rev Connect Tissue Res, 6,* 127.

Viidik, A., Danielsen, C.C., Oxlund, H. (1982). Fourth International Congress of Biorheology Symposium on Mechanical Properties of Living Tissues: On fundamental and phenomenological models, structure and mechanical properties of collagen, elastic and glycosaminoglycan complexes. *Biorheology, 19,* 437.

Vogel, H.C. (1977). Mechanical and chemical properties of various connective tissue organs in rats as influenced by nonsteroidal antirheumatic drugs. *Connect Tissue Res, 5,* 91.

Walsh, W.R., Wiggins, M.E., Fadale, P.D., Ehrlich, M.G. (1995). Effects of delayed steroid injection on ligament healing using a rabbit medial collateral ligament model. *Biomaterials, 16*(12), 905–910.

Walsh, S., Frank, C., Shrive, N., Hart, D. (1993). Knee immobilization inhibits biomechanical maturation of the rabbit medial collateral ligament. *Clin Orthop, 297,* 253–261.

White, A., Handler, P., & Smith, E.L. (1964). *Principles of Biochemistry.* New York: McGraw-Hill.

Wiggins, M.E., Fadale, P.D., Barrach, H., Ehrilich, M.G., Walsh, W.R. (1994). Healing characteristics of a type I collagenous structure treated with corticosteroids. *Am J Sports Med, 22*(2), 279–288.

Woo, S.L.Y., An, K.N., Arnoczky, D.V.M., Fithian, D., & Myers B. (1994). Anatomy, biology, and biomechanics of the tendon, ligament, and meniscus. In S.R. Simon (Ed.). *Orthopaedic Basic Science* (p. 52). Rosemont, IL: AAOS.

Woo, S.L.Y., Gomez, M.A., Sites, T.J., et al. (1987). The biomechanical and morphological changes in the medial collateral ligament of the rabbit after immobilization and remobilization. *J Bone Joint Surg, 69A*(8), 1200–1211.

Woo, S.L.Y., Gomez, M.A., Amiel, D., Ritter, M.A., Gelberman, R.H., Akeson, W.H. (1981). The effects of exercise on the biomechanical and biochemical properties of swine digital flexor tendons. *J Biomech Eng, 103,* 51.

Woo, S.L.Y. (1988). Ligament, tendon, and joint capsule insertions to bone. In S.L.Y. Woo, & J. Buckwalter (Eds.), *Injury and Repair of the Musculoskeltal Soft Tissues* (pp. 133–166). Park Ridge, Il. American Academy of Orthopaedic Surgeons.

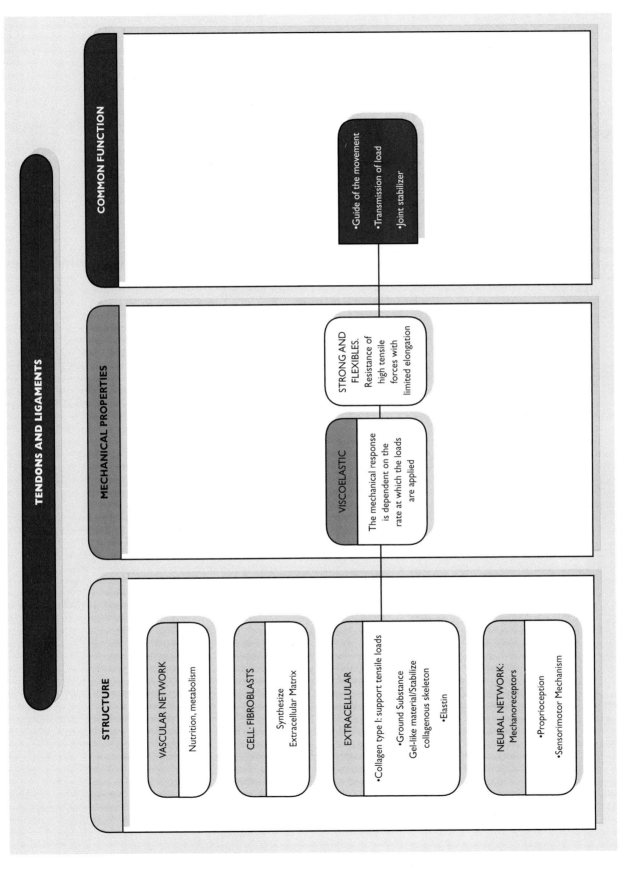

FLOW CHART 4-1   Common structure and mechanical properties of tendons and ligaments.*

*This flow chart is designed for classroom or group discussion. Flow chart is not meant to be exhaustive.

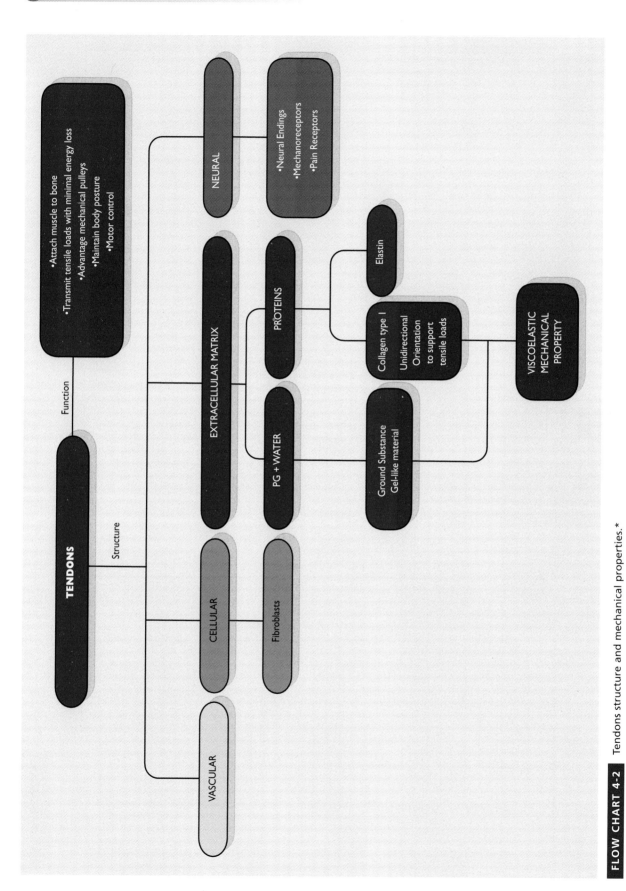

FLOW CHART 4-2 Tendons structure and mechanical properties.*

*This flow chart is designed for classroom or group discussion. Flow chart is not meant to be exhaustive.

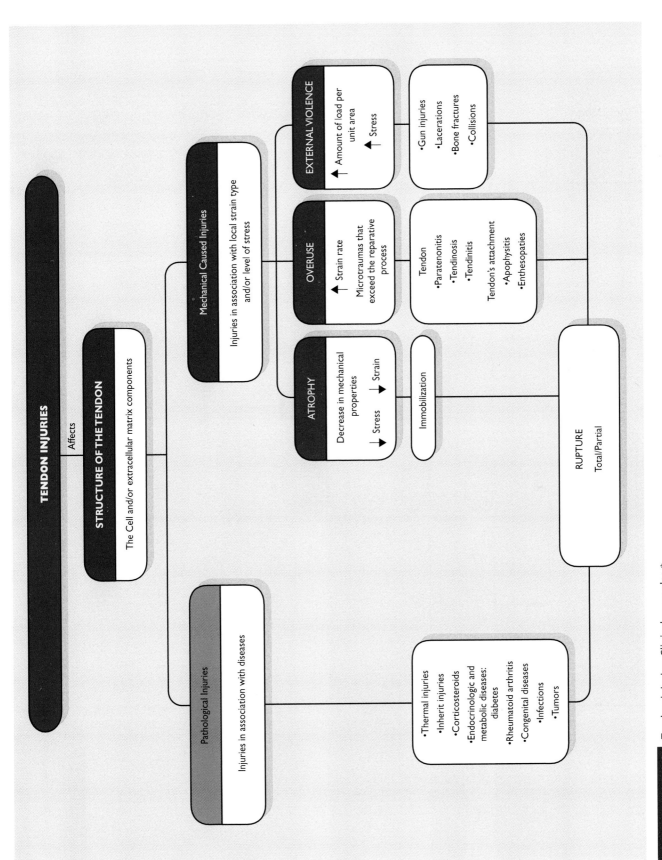

FLOW CHART 4-3   Tendon injuries. Clinical examples.*

*This flow chart is designed for classroom or group discussion. Flow chart is not meant to be exhaustive.

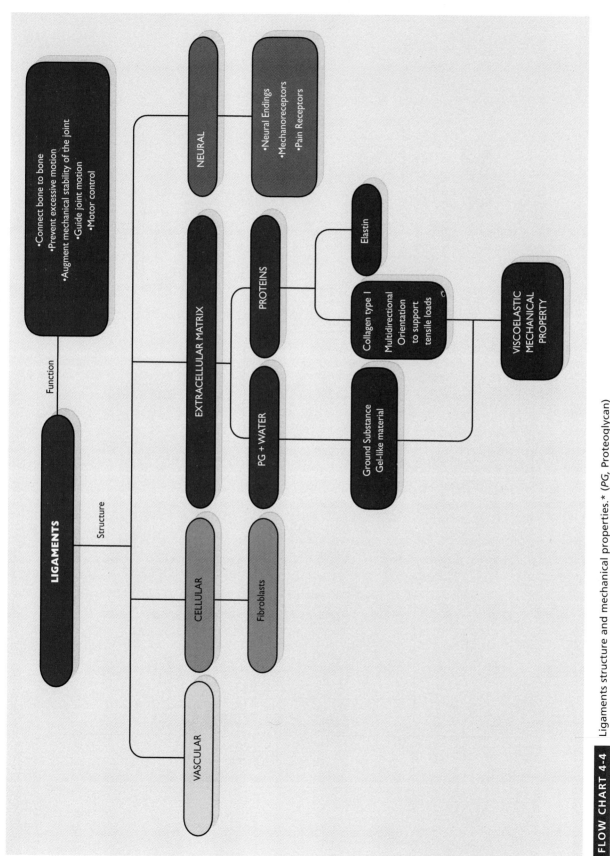

FLOW CHART 4-4 Ligaments structure and mechanical properties.* (*PG*, Proteoglycan)

*This flow chart is designed for classroom or group discussion. Flow chart is not meant to be exhaustive.

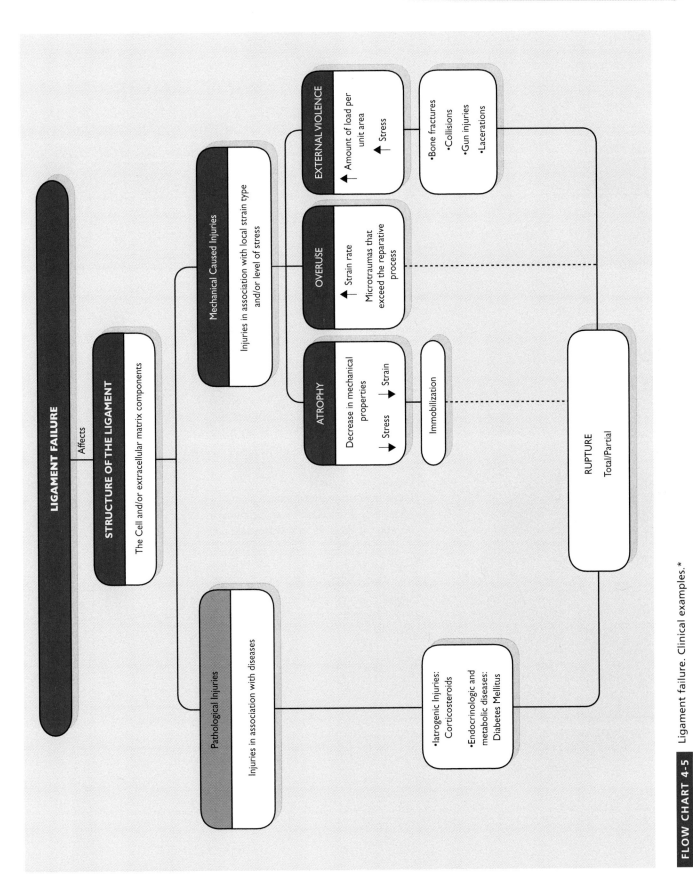

FLOW CHART 4-5 Ligament failure. Clinical examples.*

*This flow chart is designed for classroom or group discussion. Flow chart is not meant to be exhaustive.

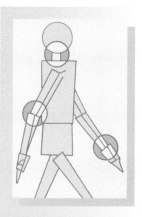

CHAPTER 5

Biomechanics of Peripheral Nerves and Spinal Nerve Roots

Bjorn Rydevik, Goran Lundborg, Kjell Olmarker, Robert R. Myers

Introduction

The nervous system serves as the body's control center and communications network. As such, it has three broad roles: it senses changes in the body and in the external environment, it interprets these changes, and it responds to this interpretation by initiating action in the form of muscle contraction or gland secretion.

For descriptive purposes, the nervous system can be divided into two parts: the central nervous system, consisting of the brain and spinal cord, and the peripheral nervous system, composed of the various nerve processes that extend from the brain and spinal cord. These peripheral nerve processes provide input to the central nervous system from sensory receptors in skin, joints, muscles, tendons, viscera, and sense organs and provide output from it to effectors (muscles and glands). The peripheral nervous system includes 12 pairs of cranial nerves and their branches and 31 pairs of spinal nerves and their branches (Fig. 5-1A). These branches are called peripheral nerves.

Each spinal nerve is connected to the spinal cord through a posterior (dorsal) root and an anterior (ventral) root, which unite to form the spinal nerve at the intervertebral foramen (Fig. 5-1, B–D). The posterior roots contain fibers of sensory neurons (those conducting sensory information from receptors in the skin, muscles, tendons, and joints to the central nervous system) and the anterior roots contain mainly fibers of motor neurons (those that conduct impulses from the central nervous system to distal targets such as muscle fibers).

Shortly after the spinal nerves leave their intervertebral foramina, they divide into two main branches: the dorsal rami, which innervate the muscles and skin of the head, neck, and back, and the generally larger and more important ventral rami, which innervate the ventral and lateral parts of these structures as well as the upper and lower extremities. Except in the thoracic region, the ventral rami do not run directly to the structures that they innervate but first form interlacing networks, or plexuses, with adjacent nerves (Fig. 5-1A).

This chapter focuses on both the peripheral nerves and spinal nerve roots, which contain not only nerve fibers but also connective tissue elements and vascular structures that encompass the nerve fibers. The nerves possess some special anatomical properties that may serve to protect the nerve from mechanical damage, for instance, stretching (tension) and compression. In this chapter, the basic microanatomy of the peripheral nerves and the spinal nerve roots are reviewed with special reference to these built-in mechanisms of protection. The mechanical behavior of peripheral nerves that are subjected to tension and compression is also described in some detail.

Anatomy and Physiology of Peripheral Nerves

The peripheral nerves are complex composite structures consisting of nerve fibers, connective tissue, and blood vessels. Because the three tissue elements that make up these nerves react to trauma in different ways and may each play distinct roles in the functional deterioration of the nerve after injury, each element is described separately.

THE NERVE FIBERS: STRUCTURE AND FUNCTION

The term nerve fiber refers to the elongated process (axon) extending from the nerve cell body along with its myelin sheath and Schwann cells (Figs. 5-2 and 5-3). The nerve fibers of sensory neurons conduct impulses from the skin, skeletal muscles, and joints to the central nervous system. The nerve fibers of the motor neurons convey impulses from the central nervous system to the skeletal muscles, causing muscle contraction. (A detailed description of the mechanics of muscle contraction is given in Chapter 6.)

The nerve fibers not only transmit impulses but also serve as an anatomical connection between the nerve cell body and its end organs. This connection is maintained by axonal transport systems, through which various substances synthesized within the cell body (e.g., proteins) are transported from the cell body to the periphery and in the opposite direction. The axonal transport takes place at speeds that vary from approximately 1 to approximately 400 mm per day.

Most axons of the peripheral nervous system are surrounded by multilayered, segmented coverings known as myelin sheaths (Fig. 5-3). Fibers with this covering are said to be myelinated, whereas those without it (mainly small sensory fibers conducting impulses for pain from the skin) are unmyelinated. The myelin sheath of the axons of the peripheral nerves is produced by flattened cells called Schwann cells arranged along the axon (Fig. 5-3). A sheath is formed as the Schwann cell encircles the axon and

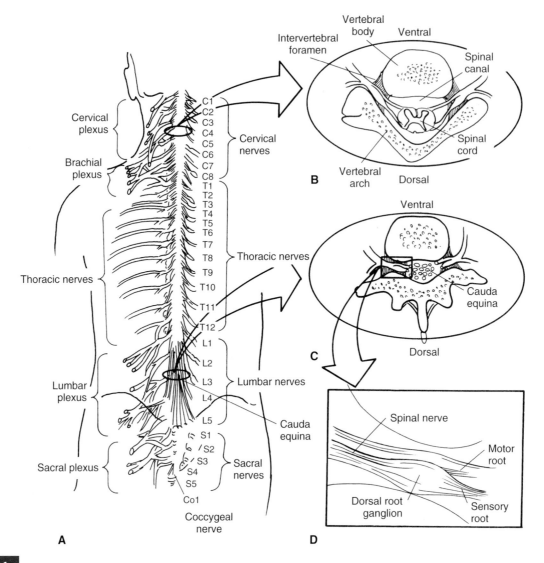

FIG. 5-1

A, Schematic drawing of the spinal cord and the spinal nerves (posterior view). The spinal nerves emerge from the spinal canal through the intervertebral foramina. There are 8 pairs of cervical nerves, 12 pairs of thoracic nerves, 5 pairs of lumbar nerves, 5 pairs of sacral nerves, and 1 pair of coccygeal nerves. Except in the region of the 2nd to the 11th thoracic vertebrae (T2–T11), the nerves form complex networks called plexuses after exiting the intervertebral foramina. Only the main branch of each nerve, the ventral ramus, is depicted. *Adapted from Tortora, G.J. & Anagnostakos, N.P. (1984). Principles of Anatomy and Physiology (4th ed.). New York: Harper & Row.* **B,** Cross-section of the cervical spine showing the spinal cord in the spinal canal and the nerve roots exiting through the intervertebral foramina. **C,** Cross-section of the lumbar spine showing the nerve roots of the cauda equina in the spinal canal. **D,** Each exiting nerve root complex in the intervertebral foramen consists of a motor root, a sensory root, and a dorsal root ganglion.

winds around it many times, pushing its cytoplasm and nucleus to the outside layer. Unmyelinated gaps called nodes of Ranvier lie between the segments of the myelin sheath at approximately 1 to 2 mm apart.

The myelin sheath increases the speed of the conduction of nerve impulses, and insulates and maintains the axon. Impulses are propagated along the unmyelinated nerve fibers in a slow, continuous way, whereas in the myelinated nerve fibers the impulses "jump" at a higher speed from one node of Ranvier to the next in a process called saltatory conduction. The conduction velocity of a myelinated nerve is directly proportional to the diameter of the fiber, which usually ranges from 2 to 20 μm. Motor fibers that innervate skeletal muscle have large diameters, as do sensory fibers that relay impulses associated with touch, pressure, heat, cold, and kinesthetic sense, such as skeletal muscle tension and joint position. Sensory fibers that conduct impulses for dull, diffuse pain (as opposed to sharp, immediate pain) have the smallest diameters. Nerve fibers are packed closely in fascicles, which are further arranged into bundles that make up the nerve itself. The fascicles are the functional subunits of the nerve.

INTRANEURAL CONNECTIVE TISSUE OF PERIPHERAL NERVES

Successive layers of connective tissue surround the nerve fibers—called the endoneurium, perineurium, and epineurium—and protect the fibers' continuity (Fig. 5-4). The protective function of these connec-

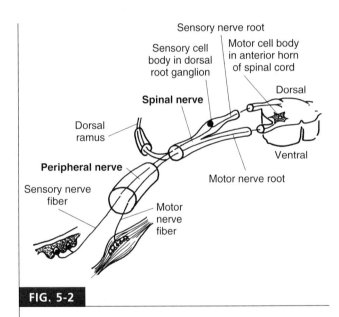

FIG. 5-2

Schematic representation of the arrangement of a typical spinal nerve as it emerges from its dorsal and ventral nerve roots. The peripheral nerve begins after the dorsal ramus branches off. (For the sake of simplicity, the nerve is not shown entering a plexus.) Spinal nerves and most peripheral nerves are mixed nerves: they contain both sensory (afferent) and motor (efferent) nerve fibers. The cell body and its nerve fibers make up the neuron. The cell bodies of the motor neurons are located in the anterior horn of the spinal cord, and those of the sensory neurons are found in the dorsal root ganglia. Here, a motor nerve fiber is shown innervating muscle and a sensory nerve fiber is depicted innervating skin. *Adapted from Rydevik, B., Brown, M.D., & Lundborg, G. (1984). Pathoanatomy and pathophysiology of nerve root compression. Spine, 9, 7.*

tive tissue layers is essential because nerve fibers are extremely susceptible to stretching and compression.

The outermost layer, the epineurium, is located between the fascicles and superficially in the nerve. This rather loose connective tissue layer serves as a cushion during movements of the nerve, protecting the fascicles from external trauma and maintaining the oxygen supply system via the epineural blood vessels. The amount of epineural connective tissue varies among nerves and at different levels within the same nerve. Where the nerves lie close to bone or pass joints, the epineurium is often more abundant than elsewhere, as the need for protection may be greater in these locations. The spinal nerve roots are devoid of both epineurium and perineurium, and the nerve fibers in the nerve root may therefore be more susceptible to trauma (Rydevik et al., 1984).

The perineurium is a lamellar sheath that encompasses each fascicle. This sheath has great mechanical strength as well as a specific biochemical barrier. Its strength is demonstrated by the fact that the fascicles can be inflated by fluid to a pressure of approximately l000 mm of mercury (Hg) before the perineurium ruptures.

The barrier function of the perineurium chemically isolates the nerve fibers from their surroundings, thus preserving an ionic environment of the interior of the fascicles, a special milieu interieur. The endoneurium, the connective tissue inside the fascicles, is composed principally of fibroblasts and collagen.

The interstitial tissue pressure in the fascicles, the endoneurial fluid pressure, is normally slightly elevated ($+1.5 \pm 0.7$ mm Hg [Myers & Powell, 1981]) compared with the pressure in surrounding tissues such as subcutaneous tissue (-4.7 ± 0.8 mm Hg) and muscle tissue (-2 ± 2 mm Hg). The elevated endoneurial fluid pressure is illustrated by the phenomenon whereby incision of the perineurium results in herniation of nerve fibers. The endoneurial fluid pressure may increase further as a result of trauma to the nerve, with subsequent edema. Such a pressure increase may affect the microcirculation and the function of the nerve.

THE MICROVASCULAR SYSTEM OF PERIPHERAL NERVES

The peripheral nerve is a well-vascularized structure containing vascular networks in the epineurium, the perineurium, and the endoneurium. Because both impulse propagation and axonal transport depend

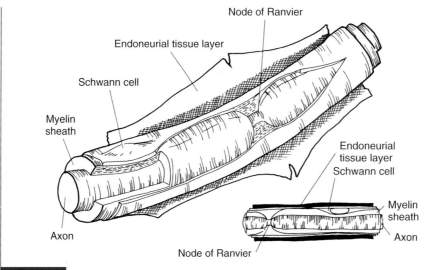

FIG. 5-3

Schematic drawings of the structural features of a myelinated nerve fiber. *Adapted from Sunderland, S. (1978).* Nerves and Nerve Injuries *(2nd ed.). Edinburgh: Churchill Livingstone.*

on a local oxygen supply, it is natural that the microvascular system has a large reserve capacity.

The blood supply to the peripheral nerve as a whole is provided by large vessels that approach the nerve segmentally along its course. When these local nutrient vessels reach the nerve, they divide into ascending and descending branches. These vessels run longitudinally and frequently anastomose with the vessels in the perineurium and endoneurium. Within the epineurium, large arterioles and venules, 50 to 100 μm in diameter, constitute a longitudinal vascular system (Fig. 5-4).

Within each fascicle lies a longitudinally oriented capillary plexus with loop formations at various levels. The capillary system is fed by arterioles 25 to 150 μm in diameter that penetrate the perineurial membrane. These vessels run an oblique course through the perineurium, and it is believed that because of this structural peculiarity, they are easily closed like valves in the event that tissue pressure inside the fascicles increases (Lundborg, 1975; Myers et al., 1986). This phenomenon may explain why even a limited increase in endoneurial fluid pressure is associated with a reduction in intrafascicular blood flow.

The built-in safety system of longitudinal anastomoses provides a wide margin of safety if the regional segmental vessels are transected. In an ex-

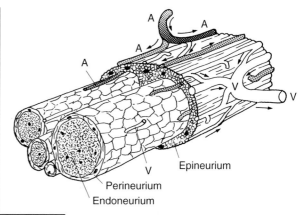

FIG. 5-4

Schematic drawing of a segment of a peripheral nerve. The individual nerve fibers are located within the endoneurium. They are closely packed in fascicles, each of which is surrounded by a strong sheath, the perineurium. A bundle of fascicles is embedded in a loose connective tissue, the epineurium. Blood vessels are present in all layer of the nerve. *A,* arterioles *(shaded); V,* venules *(unshaded).* The *arrows* indicated the direction of blood flow. *Adapted from Dahlin, L.B., Rydevik, B., & Lundborg, G. (1986). The pathophysiology of nerve entrapments and nerve compression injuries. In A.R. Hargens (Ed.).* Effects of Mechanical Stress on Tissue Viability. *New York: Springer-Verlag.*

perimental animal in vivo model, it is extremely difficult to induce complete ischemia to a nerve by local surgical procedures. For example, if the whole sciatic-tibial nerve complex of a rabbit (15 cm long) is surgically separated from its surrounding structures and the regional nutrient vessels are cut, there is no detectable reduction in the intrafascicular blood flow as studied by intravital microscopic techniques. Even if such a mobilized nerve is cut distally or proximally, the intraneural longitudinal vascular systems can maintain the microcirculation at least 7 to 8 cm from the cut end. If a nonmobilized nerve is cut, there is still perfect microcirculation even at the very tip of the nerve; this phenomenon demonstrates the sufficiency of the intraneural vascular collaterals. However, other studies in rats indicate that stripping the epineural circulation from nerve bundles causes demyelination of subperineural nerve fibers.

Anatomy and Physiology of Spinal Nerve Roots

In the early embryological developmental stages, the spinal cord has the same length as the spinal column. However, in the fully grown individual, the spinal cord ends as the conus medullaris, approximately at the level of the first lumbar vertebra. A nerve root that leaves the spinal canal through an intervertebral foramen in the lumbar or sacral spine therefore has to pass from the point where it leaves the spinal cord, which is in the lower thoracic spine, to the point of exit from the spine (Fig. 5-5). Because the spinal cord is not present below the first lumbar vertebra, the nervous content of the spinal canal is only comprised of the lumbosacral nerve roots. This "bundle" of nerve roots within the lumbar and sacral part of the spinal canal has been suggested to resemble the tail of a horse and is therefore often called the cauda equina, that is, tail of horse.

Two different types of nerve roots are found within the lumbosacral spine, ventral/motor roots and dorsal/sensory roots. The cell bodies of the motor axons are located in the anterior horns of the gray matter in the spinal cord, and because these nerve roots leave the spinal cord from the ventral aspect, they are also called ventral roots. The other type of nerve root is the sensory, or dorsal root. As the name suggests, these nerve roots mainly comprise sensory (i.e., afferent) axons and reach the spinal cord at the dorsal region of the spinal cord. The cell bodies of the sensory axons are located in a

"swelling" of the most caudal part of the respective dorsal nerve root, called the dorsal root ganglion. The dorsal root ganglia are located in or close to the intervertebral foramen. Unlike the nerve roots, the dorsal root ganglia are not enclosed by cerebrospinal fluid and the meninges. Instead, they are enclosed by both a multilayered connective tissue sheath, similar to the perineurium of the peripheral

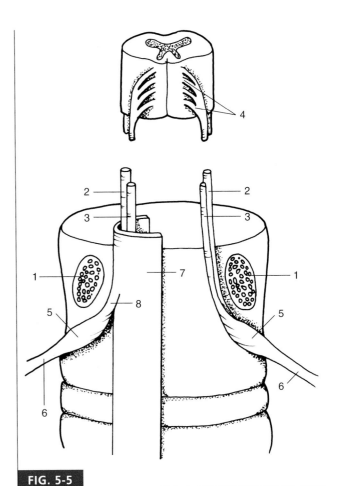

FIG. 5-5

The intraspinal nervous structures as seen from behind. The vertebral arches are removed by cutting the pedicles (1). A ventral (2) and a dorsal (3) nerve root leave the spinal cord as small rootlets (4). Before leaving the spinal canal, the dorsal root forms a swelling called the dorsal root ganglion (5), which contains the sensory cell bodies, before forming the spinal nerve (6) together with the ventral nerve root. The nerve roots are covered by a central dural sac (7) or with extensions of this sac called nerve root sleeves (8). *Reproduced with permission from Olmarker, K. (1991). Spinal nerve root compression. Acute compression of the cauda equina studied in pigs. Acta Orthop Scand, 62, Suppl 242.*

nerve, and a loose connective tissue layer called epineurium.

When the nerve root approaches the intervertebral foramen, the root sleeve gradually encloses the nerve tissue more tightly. The subarachnoid space and the amount of cerebrospinal fluid surrounding each nerve root pair will thus become gradually reduced in the caudal direction. Compression injury of a nerve root may induce an increase in the permeability of the endoneurial capillaries, resulting in edema formation (Olmarker et al., 1989b; Rydevik & Lundborg, 1977). This can lead to an increase of the intraneural fluid and subsequent impairment of the nutritional transport to the nerve (Myers & Powell, 1981; Myers, 1998). Such a mechanism might be particularly important at locations where the nerve roots are tightly enclosed by connective tissue. Thus there is a more pronounced risk for an "entrapment syndrome" within the nerve roots at the intervertebral foramen than more central in the cauda equina (Rydevik et al., 1984). The dorsal root ganglion, with its content of sensory nerve cell bodies, tightly enclosed by meninges, might be particularly susceptible to edema formation.

MICROSCOPIC ANATOMY OF SPINAL NERVE ROOTS

There are two microscopically different regions of the nerve roots. Closest to the spinal cord is a central glial segment comprised of glial cells and therefore resembles the microscopic organization of central nervous structures at the spinal cord or the brain. This glial segment is transferred to a nonglial segment in a "dome-shaped" junction a few millimeters from the spinal cord. This nonglial segment is organized in the same manner as the endoneurium of the peripheral nerves, that is, with Schwann cells instead of glia cells. However, some small islets of glia cells also are found in this otherwise "peripherally" organized endoneurium.

MEMBRANOUS COVERINGS OF SPINAL NERVE ROOTS

The axons in the endoneurium are separated from the cerebrospinal fluid by a thin layer of connective tissue called the root sheath. This root sheath is the structural analogue to the pia mater that covers the spinal cord. There are usually 2 to 5 cellular layers in the root sheath, but as many as 12 layers have been identified. The cells of the proximal part of the

outer layers of the root sheath are similar to the pia cells of the spinal cord, and the cells in the distal part are more similar to the arachnoid cells of the spinal dura. The inner layers of the root sheath are comprised of cells that show similarities to the cells of the perineurium of peripheral nerves. An interrupted basement membrane encloses these cells separately. The inner layers of the root sheath constitute a diffusion barrier between the endoneurium of the nerve roots and the cerebrospinal fluid. This barrier is considered to be relatively weak and may only prevent the passage of macromolecules.

The spinal dura encloses the nerve roots and the cerebrospinal fluid. When the two layers of the cranial dura enter the spinal canal, the outer layer blends with the periosteum of the part of the laminae of the cervical vertebrae facing the spinal canal. The inner layers join the arachnoid and become the spinal dura. In contrast to the root sheath, the spinal dura is an effective diffusion barrier. The barrier properties are located in a connective tissue sheath between the dura and the arachnoid called the neurothelium. Similar to the inner layer of the root sheath, this neurothelium resembles the perineurium of the peripheral nerves. It is suggested that these two layers in fact form the perineurium when the nerve root is transformed to a peripheral nerve upon leaving the spinal.

THE MICROVASCULAR SYSTEM OF SPINAL NERVE ROOTS

Information about the vascular anatomy of the nerve roots has mainly been derived from studies on the vascularization of the spinal cord. Therefore, the nomenclature of the various vessels has been somewhat confusing. A summary of the existing knowledge on nerve root vasculature will be presented below.

The segmental arteries generally divide into three branches when approaching the intervertebral foramen: (1) an anterior branch that supplies the posterior abdominal wall and lumbar plexus, (2) a posterior branch that supplies the paraspinal muscles and facet joints, and (3) an intermediate branch that supplies the contents of the spinal canal. A branch of the intermediate branch joins the nerve root at the level of the dorsal root ganglion. There are usually three branches from this vessel: one to the ventral root, one to the dorsal root, and one to the vasa corona of the spinal cord.

The branches to the vasa corona of the spinal cord, called medullary arteries, are inconsistent. Only 7 to 8 remain of the 128 from the embryological period of life, and each supplies more than one segment of the spinal cord. The main medullary artery in the thoracic region of the spine was discovered by Adamkiewicz in 1881 and still bears his name. The medullary arteries run parallel to the nerve roots (Fig. 5-6). In humans, there are no connections between these vessels and the vascular network of the nerve roots. Because the medullary feeder arteries only occasionally supply the nerve roots with blood, they have been referred to as the extrinsic vascular system of the cauda equina.

The vasculature of the nerve roots is formed by branches from the intermediate branch of the segmental artery distally and by branches from the vasa corona of the spinal cord proximally. As opposed to the medullary arteries, this vascular network has been named the intrinsic vascular system of the cauda equina. The distal branch to the dorsal root first forms the ganglionic plexus within the dorsal root ganglion. The vessels run within the outer layers of the root sheath, called epi-pial tissue. As there are vessels coming from both distal and proximal directions, the nerve roots are supplied by two separate vascular systems. The two systems anastomose at approximately two thirds of the nerve root length from the spinal cord. This location demonstrates a region of a less-developed vascular network and has been suggested to be a particularly vulnerable site of the nerve roots.

The arteries of the intrinsic system send branches down to the deeper parts of the nerve tissue in a T-like manner. To compensate for elongation of the nerve roots, the arteries are coiled both longitudinally and in the steep running branches between the different fascicles (Fig. 5-6). Unlike peripheral nerves, the venules do not course together with the arteries in the nerve roots but instead usually have a spiraling course in the deeper parts of the nerve.

There is a barrier of the endoneurial capillaries in peripheral nerves called the blood-nerve barrier, which is similar to the blood-brain barrier of the central nervous system (Lundborg, 1975; Rydevik & Lundborg, 1977). The presence of a corresponding barrier in nerve roots has been questioned. If present, a blood-nerve barrier in nerve roots does not seem to be as well developed as in endoneurial capillaries of peripheral nerve, which implies that edema may be formed more easily in nerve roots than in peripheral nerves (Rydevik et al., 1984).

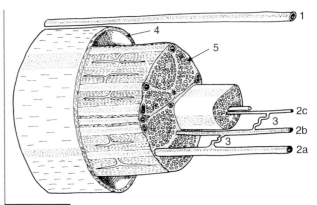

FIG. 5-6

Schematic presentation of some anatomical features of the intrinsic arteries of the spinal nerve roots. The arterioles within the cauda equina may be referred to either the extrinsic (1) or the intrinsic (2) vascular system. From the superficial intrinsic arterioles are branches that continue almost at right angles down between the fascicles. These vessels often run in a spiraling course, thus forming vascular "coils" (3). When reaching a specific fascicle they branch in a T-like manner, with one branch running cranially and one caudally, forming interfascicular arterioles (2b). From these interfascicular arterioles are small branches that enter the fascicles, where they supply the endoneurial capillary networks (2c). Arterioles of the extrinsic vascular system run outside the spinal dura (4) and have no connections with the intrinsic system by local vascular branches. The superficial intrinsic arterioles (2a) are located within the root sheath (5). *Reproduced with permission from Olmarker, K. (1991). Spinal nerve root compression. Acute compression of the cauda equina studied in pigs.* Acta Orthop Scand, 62, *Suppl 242.*

Biomechanical Behavior of Peripheral Nerves

External trauma to the extremities and nerve entrapment may produce mechanical deformation of the peripheral nerves that results in the deterioration of nerve function. If the mechanical trauma exceeds a certain degree, the nerves' built-in mechanisms of protection may not be sufficient, resulting in changes in nerve structure and function. Common modes of nerve injury are stretching and compression, which may be inflicted, respectively, by rapid extension and crushing.

STRETCHING (TENSILE) INJURIES OF PERIPHERAL NERVES

Nerves are strong structures with considerable tensile strength. The maximal load that can be sustained by the median and ulnar nerves is in the range of 70 to 220 newtons (N) and 60 to 150 N, respectively. These figures are of academic interest only because severe intraneural tissue damage is produced by tension long before a nerve breaks.

A discussion of the elasticity and biomechanical properties of nerves is complicated by the fact that nerves are not homogeneous isotropic materials but, instead, composite structures, with each tissue component having its own biomechanical properties. The connective tissues of the epineurium and perineurium are primarily longitudinal structures.

When tension is applied to a nerve, initial elongation of the nerve under a very small load is followed by an interval in which stress and elongation show a linear relationship characteristic of an elastic material (Fig. 5-7). As the limit of the linear region is approached, the nerve fibers start to rupture inside the endoneurial tubes and inside the intact perineurium. The perineurial sheaths rupture at approximately 25 to 30% elongation (ultimate strain) above in vivo length (Rydevik et al., 1990). After this point, there is a disintegration of the elastic properties, and the nerve behaves more like a plastic material (i.e., its response to the release of loads is incomplete recovery).

Although variations exist in the tensile strength of various nerves, the maximal elongation at the elastic limit is approximately 20%, and complete structural failure seems to occur at a maximum elongation of approximately 25 to 30%. These values are for normal nerves; injury to a nerve may induce changes in its mechanical properties, namely increased stiffness and decreased elasticity.

Stretching, or tensile, injuries of peripheral nerves are usually associated with severe accidents, such as when high-energy tension is applied to the brachial plexus in association with a birth-related injury, as a result of high-speed vehicular collision, or after a fall from a height. Such plexus injuries may result in partial or total functional loss of some or all of the nerves in the upper extremity, and the consequent functional deficits represent a considerable disability in terms of sensory and motor loss. The outcome depends on which tissue components of the nerves are damaged as well as on the extent of the tissue injury. Of clinical importance is the observation that there can be considerable structural damage (perineurial sheath injuries) induced by stretching with no visible injury on the surface of the nerve (Case Study 5-1).

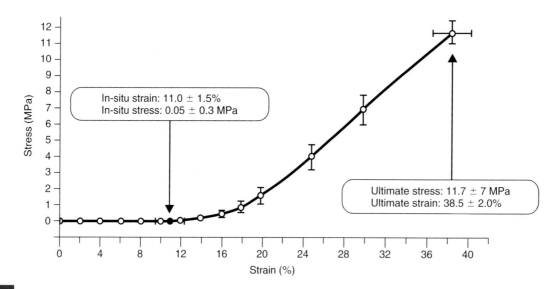

FIG. 5-7

The stress-strain behavior of a rabbit tibial nerve. The nerve exhibits a low stiffness toe region of approximately 15 % and begins to retain significant tension as the strain increases beyond 20%. *Reproduced with permission from Rydevik, B.L.,*

Kwan, M.K., Myers, R.R., et al. (1990). An in vitro mechanical and histological study of acute stretching on rabbit tibial nerve. J Orthop Res, 8, 694–701.

CASE STUDY 5-1

Brachial Plexus Palsy

During the birth process, a newborn suffered a traction injury in his left brachial plexus. A few months later, he presents with the upper left arm in a static position of adduction, internal rotation of the shoulder, extension of the elbow, pronation of the forearm, and flexion of the wrist. He does not respond to sensory stimulus in his shoulder and presents biceps and brachioradialis areflexia. A sudden deformation and high tensile stress injuries in the C5–C6 nerve roots affected the mixed (motor and sensory) neural functions, mainly the muscles responsible for the scapulohumeral rhythm (see Chapter 12).

An Erb's palsy is diagnosed. The sudden elongation suffered during the traction can lead to structural damage and reduction in the transverse fascicular cross-sectional area, producing impairment of the intraneural vascular flow and impulse transmission.

In less severe cases, functional restoration may occur within weeks or months. In more severe cases, healing may take place during the first 2 to 3 years, but if the structural nerve injury is severe, considerable long-term functional disability can result. If structural derangement of the nerve trunk has taken place, nerve grafting may be required.

High-energy plexus injuries represent an extreme type of stretching lesion caused by sudden violent trauma. A different stretching situation of considerable clinical interest is the suturing of the two ends of a cut nerve under moderate tension. This situation occurs when a substantial gap exists in the continuity of a nerve trunk and the restoration of the continuity requires the application of tension to bring the nerve ends back together. The moderate, gradual tension applied to the nerve in these cases may stretch and angulate local feeding vessels. It may also be sufficient to reduce the transverse fascicular cross-sectional area and impair the intraneural nutritive capillary flow (Fig. 5-8).

As the sutured nerve is stretched, the perineurium tightens; as a result, the endoneurial fluid pressure is increased and the intrafascicular capillaries may be obliterated. Also, the flow is impaired in the segmental, feeding, and draining vessels, as it is in larger vessels in the epineurium, and at a certain stage the intraneural microcirculation ceases. Intravital observations of intraneural blood flow in rabbit tibial nerves (Lundborg & Rydevik, 1973) showed that an elongation of 8% induced impaired venular flow and that even greater tension produced continuous impairment of capillary and arteriolar flow until, at 15% elongation, all intraneural microcirculation ceased completely. For the same nerve, an elongation (strain) of 6% induced a reduction of nerve action potential amplitude by 70% at 1 hour with recovery to

normal values during 1-hour restitution. At 12% elongation, conduction was completely blocked by 1 hour and showed minimal recovery (Wall et al., 1992). Such data have clinical implication in nerve repair, limb trauma, and limb lengthening.

A situation of even more gradual stretching, applied over a long time, is the growth of intraneural tumors such as schwannomas. In this situation, the nerve fibers are forced into a circumferential course around the gradually expanding tumor. Functional changes in cases of such very gradual stretching are often minimal or nonexistent.

COMPRESSION INJURIES OF PERIPHERAL NERVES

It has long been known that compression of a nerve can induce symptoms such as numbness, pain, and muscle weakness. The biological basis for the functional changes has been investigated extensively (Rydevik & Lundborg, 1977; Rydevik et al., 1981). In these investigations (Fig. 5-9), even mild compression was observed to induce structural and functional changes, and the significance of mechanical

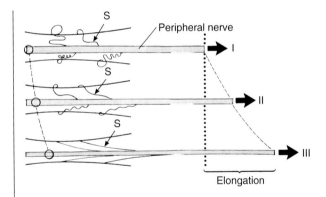

FIG. 5-8

Schematic representation of a peripheral nerve and its blood supply at three stages during stretching. Stage I: The segmental blood vessels (S) are normally coiled to allow for the physiological movements of the nerve. Stage II: Under gradually increasing elongation, these regional vessels become stretched and the blood flow in them is impaired. Stage III: The cross-sectional area of the nerve (represented within the circle) is reduced during stretching and the intraneural blood flow is further impaired. Complete cessation of all blood flow in the nerve usually occurs at approximately 15% elongation. *Adapted from Lundborg, G. & Rydevik, B. (1973). Effects of stretching the tibial nerve of the rabbit: A preliminary study of the intraneural circulation and the barrier function of the perineurium.* J Bone Joint Surg, 55B, 390.

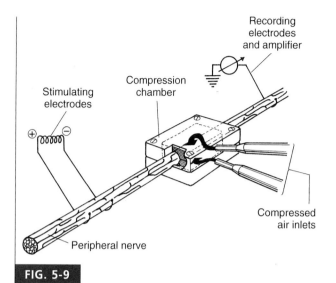

FIG. 5-9

Schematic drawing of an experimental setup for studying deterioration of nerve function during compression.
Adapted from Dahlin, L.B., Rydevik, B., & Lundborg, G. (1986). The pathophysiology of nerve entrapments and nerve compression injuries. In A.R. Hargens (Ed.). Effects of Mechanical Stress on Tissue Viability. New York: Springer-Verlag.

factors such as pressure level and mode of compression became apparent.

Critical Pressure Levels

Experimental and clinical observations have revealed some data on the critical pressure levels at which disturbances occur in intraneural blood flow, axonal transport, and nerve function. Certain pressure levels seem to be well defined with respect to structural and functional changes induced in the nerve. The duration of the compression also influences the development of these changes.

At 30 mm Hg of local compression, functional changes may occur in the nerve, and its viability may be jeopardized during prolonged compression (4 to 6 hours) at this pressure level (Lundborg et al., 1982). Such changes appear to be caused by impairment of the blood flow in the compressed part of the nerve (Rydevik et al., 1981). Corresponding pressure levels (approximately 32 mm Hg) were recorded close to the median nerve in the carpal tunnel in patients with carpal tunnel syndrome, while in a group of control subjects the pressure in the carpal tunnel averaged only 2 mm Hg. Long-standing or intermittent compression at low pressure levels (approximately 30 to 80 mm Hg) may induce intraneural edema, which in turn may become organized into a fibrotic scar in the nerve (Rydevik & Lundborg, 1977).

Compression at approximately 30 mm Hg also brings about changes in the axonal transport systems, and long-standing compression may thus lead to depletion of axonally transported proteins distal to the compression site. Such blockage of axonal transport induced by local compression (pinching) may cause the axons to be more susceptible to additional compression distally, the so-called double-crush syndrome.

Slightly higher pressure (80 mm Hg, for example) causes complete cessation of intraneural blood flow; the nerve in the locally compressed segment becomes completely ischemic. Yet, even after 2 hours or more of compression, blood flow is rapidly restored when the pressure is released (Rydevik et al., 1981). Even higher levels of pressure (200 to 400 mm Hg, for example) applied directly to a nerve can induce structural nerve fiber damage and rapid deterioration of nerve function, with incomplete recovery after even shorter periods of compression. Hence, the magnitude of the applied pressure and the severity of the induced compression lesion appear to be correlated.

Mode of Pressure Application

The pressure level is not the only factor that influences the severity of nerve injury brought about by compression. Experimental and clinical evidence indicates that the mode of pressure application is also of major significance. Its importance is illustrated by the fact that direct compression of a nerve at 400 mm Hg by means of a small inflatable cuff around the nerve induces a more severe nerve injury than does indirect compression of the nerve at 1000 mm Hg via a tourniquet applied around the extremity. Even though the hydrostatic pressure acting on the nerve in the former situation is less than half that in the latter, the nerve lesion is more severe, probably because direct compression causes a more pronounced deformation of the nerve (especially at its edges) than does indirect compression, in which the tissue layers between the compression device and the nerve "bolster" the nerve. One may also conclude that the nerve injury caused by compression is not directly related to the high hydrostatic pressure in the center of the compressed nerve segment but instead is more dependent on the specific mechanical deformation induced by the applied pressure.

Mechanical Aspects of Nerve Compression

Electron microscopic analysis of the deformation of the nerve fibers in the peroneal nerve of the baboon hind limb induced by tourniquet compression demonstrated the so-called edge effect; that is, a specific lesion was induced in the nerve fibers at both edges of the compressed nerve segment: the nodes of Ranvier were displaced toward the noncompressed parts of the nerve. The nerve fibers in the center of the compressed segment, where the hydrostatic pressure is highest, generally were not affected acutely. The large-diameter nerve fibers were usually affected, but the thinner fibers were spared. This finding confirms theoretical calculations that indicate larger nerve fibers undergo a relatively greater deformation than do thinner fibers at a given pressure. It is also known clinically that a compression lesion of a nerve first affects the large fibers (e.g., those that carry motor function), while the thin fibers (e.g., those that mediate pain sensation) are often preserved. The intraneural blood vessels have also been shown to be injured at the edges of the compressed segment (Rydevik & Lundborg, 1977). Basically, the lesions of nerve fibers and blood vessels seem to be consequences of the pressure gradient, which is maximal just at the edges of the compressed segment.

In considering the mechanical effects on nerve compression, keep in mind that the effect of a given pressure depends on the way in which it is applied, its magnitude and duration. Although pressure may be applied with a variety of spatial distributions, two basic types of pressure applications are generally encountered in experimental settings and in pathological conditions. One type is uniform pressure applied around the entire circumference of a longitudinal segment of a nerve or extremity. This is the kind of purely radial pressure that is applied by the common pneumatic tourniquet. It has also been used in miniature apparatus to produce controlled compression of individual nerves (Rydevik & Lundborg, 1977) (Fig. 5-9). Clinically, this type of loading on a nerve probably occurs when the pressure on the median nerve is elevated in the carpal tunnel, producing a characteristic syndrome.

Another type of mechanical action takes place when the nerve is compressed laterally. This is the kind of deformation that occurs if a nerve or extremity is placed between two parallel flat rigid surfaces that are then moved toward each other, squeezing the nerve or extremity. This type of deformation occurs if a sudden blow by a rigid object squeezes a nerve against the surface of an underlying bone. It may also occur when a spinal nerve is compressed by a herniated disc (Case Study 5-2).

The details of the deformation of a nerve may be quite different in these two cases of loading. In uniform circumferential compression like that applied

---

CASE STUDY 5-2

Sciatic Pain

A 35-year-old male construction worker has chronic low back pain radiating below the left knee that is more severe with lifting activities and prolonged positions. After a careful examination, certain neurological signs were found. Positive straight leg raising and L5 motor and sensory functions were affected.

A MRI shows a herniated disc at level L4-L5 with posterolateral protrusion, which laterally compresses the left L5 nerve root. Compression of the nerve deforms it toward a more elliptical shape, increasing strain and stress loads. The effects of the pressure and mechanical deformation resultant from the load affects the nerve tissue, its nutrition, and the transmission function. Inflammation of the nerve root, induced by the nucleus pulposus, may sensitize the nerve root so that mechanical nerve root deformation causes sciatic pain (Case Study Fig 5-2-1).

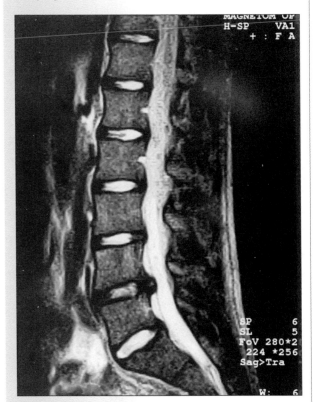

Case Study Figure 5-2-1.

by a pneumatic tourniquet (Fig. 5-10), the cross-section of the nerve or extremity tends to remain circular but decreases in diameter in the loaded region. Because the material of the tissues is relatively incompressible, this radial compression requires a squeezing out of the tissue under the tourniquet, moving it outward from the center-line toward each of the free edges. It can be seen readily that the displacement of the tissue builds up from zero at the center-line to a maximum at the edge of the tourniquet. It is this large displacement, along with accompanying shear stresses, that is believed to cause the edge effect mentioned, that is observed in experiments in vivo. This region sustains both the maximum pressure gradient and the maximum displacement.

Lateral compression does not necessarily produce any axial motion of material, but it may simply deform the cross-section from nearly circular to more elliptical, as shown in Figure 5-11. In this kind of compression it is clear that in the direction perpendicular to the direction of compression (x), the nerve must be extended. This extension is illustrated by the movement of point G to G' during compres-

sion. At the same time point A moves to A', indicating shortening or compression, in the direction of loading. The degree of compression can be measured by the maximum extension ratio (l), which is defined as the maximum diameter divided by the initial diameter of the nerve. The theoretically computed shapes are shown for l values of 1.1, 1.3, and 1.5. The theoretical results shown in the figure are based on the theory of elasticity. Point B moves to B', C moves to C', and so on during the deformation.

The effects of a deformation such as that shown in Figure 5-11 on the functioning of the axoplasm and the neural membrane are not known. It seems likely that the initial degeneration of function would be associated with damage to the membrane. It can be shown that if the cross-sectional area of the nerve shown in Figure 5-11 remains constant during the deformation, the perimeter must increase in moving from the initial circular shape to the final elliptical shape. This increase indicates that there must be stretching of the membrane, which is likely to affect its permeability and electrical properties. This deformation is similar to that of a Pacinian corpuscle, which senses pressure applied to the skin. It may be

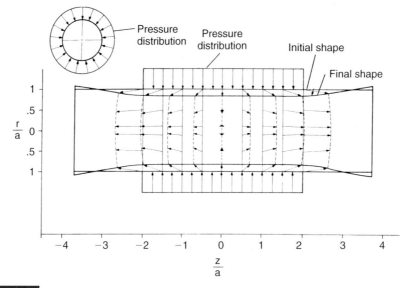

FIG. 5-10

Theoretical displacement field under a pressure cuff applied to a model cylindrical nerve of radius (a). Displacements in the radial (r) and longitudinal (z) directions are computed on the basis of isotropic material properties and elastic theory, so the deformation is proportional to the pressure. The *arrows* represent displacement vectors.

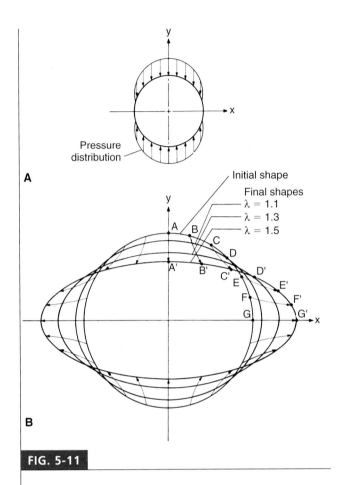

FIG. 5-11

A, Theoretical displacement field under lateral compression as a result of uniform clamping pressure. **B,** The original and deformed cross-sections are shown for maximum elongation in the x direction of 10, 30, and 50%. The vectors shown from A to A', B to B', and so forth, indicate the paths followed by the particular points A, B, and so forth during the deformation.

factor at both high and low pressures, but ischemia plays a dominant role in longer-duration compression. This phenomenon is illustrated by the fact that direct nerve compression at 30 mm Hg for 2 to 4 hours produces reversible changes, whereas prolonged compression above this time period at this pressure level may cause irreversible damage to the nerve (Lundborg et al., 1982; Rydevik et al., 1981). Compression at 400 mm Hg causes a much more severe nerve injury after 2 hours than after 15 minutes. Such information indicates that even high pressure has to "act" for a certain period of time for injury to occur. These data also give some information about the viscoelastic (time-dependent) properties of peripheral nerve tissue. Sufficient time must elapse for permanent deformation to develop.

Biomechanical Behavior of Spinal Nerve Roots

The nerve roots in the thecal sac lack epineurium and perineurium, but under tensile loading they exhibit both elasticity and tensile strength. The ultimate load for ventral spinal nerve roots from the thecal sac is between 2 and 22 N, and for dorsal nerve roots from the thecal sac the load is between 5 and 33 N. The length of the nerve roots from the spinal cord to the foramina varies from approximately 60 mm at the L1 level to approximately 170 mm at the S1 level. The mechanical properties of human spinal nerve roots are different for any given nerve root at its location in the central spinal canal and in the lateral intervertebral foramina. The ultimate load for the intrathecal portion of human S1 nerve roots at the S1 level is approximately 13 N, and that for the foraminal portion is approximately 73 N. For human nerve roots at the L5 level, the corresponding values are 16 N and 71 N, respectively (Fig. 5-12). Thus, the values for ultimate load are approximately five times higher for the foraminal segment of the spinal nerve roots than for the intrathecal portion of the same nerve roots under tensile loading. However, the cross-sectional area of the nerve root in the intervertebral foramen is significantly larger than that of the same nerve root in the thecal sac; thus, the ultimate tensile stress was more comparable for the two locations. The ultimate strain under tensile loading is 13 to 19% for the human nerve root at the L5–S1 level (Fig. 5-13).

The nerve roots in the spine are not static structures; they move relative to the surrounding tissues

that this kind of deformation can trigger firing of nerves, resulting in a sensation of pain when the nerve fibers are laterally compressed. The details of such deformation of nerves and their functional consequences have not been studied extensively and require further research for their elucidation.

Duration of Pressure Versus Pressure Level

Knowledge is limited regarding the relative importance of pressure and time, respectively, in the production of nerve compression lesions. Mechanical factors seem to be relatively more important at higher than at lower pressures. Time is a significant

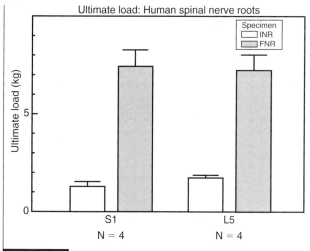

Diagram illustrating values for ultimate load obtained for human spinal nerve roots under tensile loading. *INR,* intrathecal nerve roots; *FNR,* foraminal nerve root. Note the marked difference in ultimate load for the intrathecal and the foraminal portions of the nerve roots. Error bars indicate standard deviation. *Reproduced with permission from Weinstein, J.N., LaMotte, R., Rydevik, B., et al. (1989). Nerve. In J.W. Frymoyer & S.L. Gordon (Eds.).* New Perspectives on Low Back Pain *(Chapter 4, pp. 35–130). Park Ridge, IL: AAOS. [Based on a workshop arranged by the National Institutes of Health (NIH) in Airlie, Virginia, USA, May 1988.]*

with every spinal motion. To allow for such motion the nerve roots in the intervertebral foramina, for example, must have the capacity to glide. Chronic irritation with subsequent fibrosis around the nerve roots, in association with conditions such as disc herniation and/or foraminal stenosis, can thus impair the gliding capacity of the nerve roots. This produces repeated "microstretching" injuries of the nerve roots even during normal spinal movements, which might be speculated to induce yet further tissue irritation in the nerve root components. The normal range of movements of nerve roots in the human lumbar spine has been measured in cadaver experiments. It was found that straight leg raising moved the nerve roots at the level of the intervertebral foramina approximately 2 to 5 mm.

Certain biomechanical factors are obviously involved in the pathogenesis of various symptoms induced by nerve root deformation in association with disc herniation and spinal stenosis and resulting in radiating pain. In disc herniation, only one nerve root is usually compressed. Because individual nerve

roots normally adhere to the surrounding tissues above and below the intervertebral disc they traverse, compression may give rise to intraneural tension. Spencer and associates (1984) measured the contact force between a simulated disc herniation and a deformed nerve root in cadavers. Taking the area of contact into account, they assumed a contact pressure of approximately 400 mm Hg. With reduced disc height, the contact force and pressure between the experimental disc herniation and the nerve root was reduced. They suggested that these findings may explain in part why sciatic pain is relieved after chemonucleolysis, and as disc degeneration progresses over time and the disc height thereby decreases.

In central spinal stenosis, the mechanics of nerve root compression are completely different. Under these conditions, the pressure is applied circumferentially around the nerve roots in the cauda equina at a slow, gradual rate. These different deformation factors, together with the fact that the nerve roots centrally within the cauda equina differ completely from the nerve roots located more laterally, close to the discs, may explain some of the different symptoms found in spinal stenosis and disc herniation.

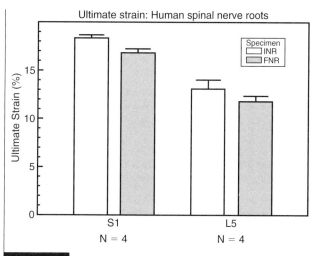

Ultimate strain for human spinal nerve roots under tensile loading. INR, intrathecal nerve root; FNR, foraminal nerve root. *Reproduced with permission from Weinstein, J.N., LaMotte, R., Rydevik, B., et al. (1989). Nerve. In J.W. Frymoyer & S.L. Gordon (Eds.).* New Perspectives on Low Back Pain *(Chapter 4, pp. 35–130). Park Ridge, IL: AAOS. [Based on a workshop arranged by the National Institutes of Health (NIH) in Airlie, Virginia, USA, May 1988.]*

EXPERIMENTAL COMPRESSION OF SPINAL NERVE ROOTS

There has been moderate interest in the past to study nerve root compression in experimental models. Early studies in the 1950s and 1970s found that nerve roots seemed to be more susceptible to compression than did peripheral nerves. During recent years, however, the interest in nerve root pathophysiology has increased considerably and a number of studies have been performed that are reviewed below.

Some years ago, a model was presented to evaluate the effects of compression of the cauda equina in pigs, which for the first time allowed for experimental, graded compression of cauda equina nerve roots at known pressure levels (Olmarker, 1991) (Fig. 5-14). In this model, the cauda equina was compressed by an inflatable balloon that was fixed to the spine. The cauda equina could also be observed through the translucent balloon. This model made it possible to study the flow in the intrinsic nerve root blood vessels at various pressure levels (Olmarker et al., 1989a). The experiment was designed in a way that the pressure in the compression balloon was increased by 5 mm Hg every 20 seconds. Blood flow and vessel diameters of the intrinsic vessels could simultaneously be observed through the balloon using a vital microscope. The average occlusion pressure for the arterioles was found to be slightly below and directly related to the systolic blood pressure, and the blood flow in the capillary networks was intimately dependent on the blood flow of the adjacent venules. This corroborates the assumption that venular stasis may induce capillary stasis and thus changes in the microcirculation of the nerve tissue and is in accordance with previous studies in which such a mechanism has been suggested as involved in carpal tunnel syndrome. The mean occlusion pressures for the venules demonstrated large variations. However, a pressure of 5 to 10 mm Hg was found to be sufficient for inducing venular occlusion. Because of retrograde stasis, it is not unlikely to assume that the capillary blood flow will be affected as well in such situations.

In the same experimental set-up, the effects of gradual decompression, after initial acute compression was maintained for only a short while, were studied. The average pressure for starting the blood flow was slightly lower at decompression than at compression for arterioles, capillaries, and venules.

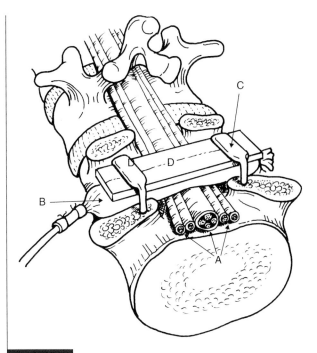

FIG. 5-14

Schematic drawing of an experimental model. The cauda equina (**A**) is compressed by an inflatable balloon (**B**) that is fixed to the spine by two L-shaped pins (**C**) and a plexiglass plate (**D**). *Reproduced with permission from Olmarker, K., Rydevik, B., & Holm, S. (1989a). Edema formation in spinal nerve roots induced by experimental, graded compression. An experimental study on the pig cauda equina with special reference to differences in effects between rapid and slow onset of compression. Spine, 14, 579.*

However, with this protocol a full restoration of the blood flow did not occur until the compression was lowered from 5 to 0 mm Hg. This observation further supports the previous hypothesis that vascular impairment is present even at low pressure levels.

A compression-induced impairment of the vasculature may thus be one mechanism for nerve root dysfunction because the nutrition of the nerve root will be affected. However, the nerve roots will also derive a considerable nutritional supply via diffusion from the cerebrospinal fluid. To assess the compression-induced effects on the total contribution to the nerve roots, an experiment was designed in which ^{3}H-labeled methyl-glucose was allowed to be transported to the nerve tissue in the compressed segment via both the blood vessels and the cerebrospinal fluid diffusion after systemic injection. The results showed that no compensatory mechanism from cerebrospinal fluid diffusion could be expected at the low pressure levels. On the contrary, 10 mm Hg compression was sufficient to induce a 20 to 30% reduction of the transport of methyl-glucose to the nerve roots, as compared with the control.

We know from experimental studies on peripheral nerves that compression may also induce an increase in the vascular permeability, leading to an intraneural edema formation. Such edema may increase the endoneurial fluid pressure, which in turn may impair the endoneurial capillary blood flow and jeopardize the nutrition of the nerve roots. Because the edema usually persists for some time after the removal of a compressive agent, edema may negatively affect the nerve root for a longer period than the compression itself. The presence of intraneural edema is also related to the subsequent formation of intraneural fibrosis and may therefore contribute to the slow recovery seen in some patients with nerve compression disorders. To assess if intraneural edema also may form in nerve roots as the result of compression, the distribution of Evan's blue-labeled albumin in the nerve tissue was analyzed after compression at various pressures and at various durations (Olmarker et al., 1989b). The study showed that edema was formed even at low pressure levels. The predominant location was at the edges of the compression zone.

The function of the nerve roots has been studied by direct electrical stimulation and recordings either on the nerve itself or in the corresponding muscular segments. During a 2- hour compression period, a critical pressure level for inducing a reduction of MAP-amplitude seems to be located between 50 and 75 mm Hg. Higher pressure levels (100–200 mm Hg) may induce a total conduction block with varying degrees of recovery after compression release. To study the effects of compression on sensory nerve fibers, electrodes in the sacrum were used to record a compound nerve action potential after stimulating the sensory nerves in the tail, that is, distal to the compression zone. The results showed that the sensory fibers are slightly more susceptible to compression than are the motor fibers. Also, the nerve roots are more susceptible to compression injury if the blood pressure is lowered pharmacologically. This further indicates the importance of the blood supply to maintain the functional properties of the nerve roots.

ONSET RATE OF COMPRESSION

One factor that has not been fully recognized in compression trauma of nerve tissue is the onset rate of the compression. The onset rate, that is, the time from start to full compression, may vary clinically from fractions of seconds in traumatic conditions to months or years in association with degenerative processes. Even in the clinically rapid-onset rates, there may be a wide variation of onset rates. With the presented model, it was possible to vary the onset time of the applied compression. Two onset rates have been investigated. Either the pressure is present and compression is started by flipping the switch of the compressed-air system used to inflate the balloon or the compression pressure level is slowly increased during 20 seconds. The first onset rate was measured at 0.05 to 0.1 seconds, thus providing a rapid inflation of the balloon and a rapid compression onset.

Such a rapid-onset rate has been found to induce more pronounced effects on edema formation, methyl-glucose transport, and impulse propagation than the slow-onset rate (Olmarker, 1991). Regarding methyl-glucose transport, the results show that the levels within the compression zone are more pronounced at the rapid than at the slow onset rate at corresponding pressure levels. There was also a striking difference between the two onset rates when considering the segments outside the compression zones. In the slow-onset series, the levels approached baseline values closer to the compression zone than in the rapid-onset series. This may indicate the presence of a more pronounced edge-zone edema in the rapid-onset series, with a subsequent reduction of the nutritional transport in the nerve tissue adjacent to the compression zone.

For the rapid-onset compression, which is likely to be more closely related to spine trauma or disc herniation than to spinal stenosis, a pressure of 600 mm Hg maintained for only 1 second is sufficient to induce a gradual impairment of nerve conduction during the 2 hours studied after the compression was ended. Overall, the mechanisms for these pronounced differences between the different onset rates are not clear but may be related to differences in the displacement rates of the compressed nerve tissue toward the uncompressed parts, as a result of the viscoelastic properties of the nerve tissue. Such phenomena may lead not only to structural damage to the nerve fibers but also to structural changes in the blood vessels with subsequent edema formation.

The gradual formation of intraneural edema may also be closely related to observations of a gradually increasing difference in nerve conduction impairment between the two onset rates (Olmarker et al., 1989b).

MULTIPLE LEVELS OF SPINAL NERVE ROOT COMPRESSION

Patients with double or multiple levels of spinal stenosis seem to have more pronounced symptoms than do patients with stenosis only at one level. The presented model was modified to address this interesting clinical question. Using two balloons at two adjacent disc levels, which resulted in a 10-mm uncompressed nerve segment between the balloons, induced a much more pronounced impairment of nerve impulse conduction than previously had been found at corresponding pressure levels (Olmarker & Rydevik, 1992). For instance, a pressure of 10 mm Hg in two balloons induced a 60% reduction of nerve impulse amplitude during 2 hours of compression, whereas 50 mm Hg in one balloon showed no reduction.

The mechanism for the difference between single and double compression may not simply be based on the fact that the nerve impulses have to pass more than one compression zone at double-level compression. There may also be a mechanism based on the local vascular anatomy of the nerve roots. Unlike for peripheral nerves, there are no regional nutritive arteries from the surrounding structures to the intraneural vascular system in spinal nerve roots. Compression at two levels might therefore induce a nutritionally impaired region between the two compression sites. In this way, the segment affected by the compression would be widened from one balloon diameter (10 mm) to two balloon diameters including the interjacent nerve segment (30 mm). This hypothesis was partly confirmed in an experiment on continuous analyses of the total blood flow in the uncompressed nerve segment located between two compression balloons (Takahashi et al., 1993). The results showed that a 64% reduction of total blood flow in the uncompressed segment was induced when both balloons were inflated to 10 mm Hg. At a pressure close to the systemic blood pressure there was complete ischemia in the nerve segment. Thus, experimental evidence shows that the blood supply to the nerve segment located between two compression sites in nerve roots is severely impaired although this nerve segment itself is uncompressed. Regarding nerve conduction, the effects were much enhanced if the distance between the compression balloons was increased from one vertebral segment to two vertebral segments (Olmarker & Rydevik, 1992). This indicates that the functional impairment may be directly related to the distance between the two compression sites.

CHRONIC NERVE ROOT COMPRESSION IN EXPERIMENTAL MODELS

The discussion of compression-induced effects on nerve roots has dealt primarily with acute compression, that is, compression that lasts for some hours and with no survival of the animal. To better mimic various clinical situations, compression must be applied over longer periods of time. There are probably many changes in the nerve tissue, such as adaptation of axons and vasculature, that will occur in patients but cannot be studied in experimental models using only 1 to 6 hours of compression. Another important factor in this context is the onset rate that was discussed previously. In clinical syndromes with nerve root compression, the onset time may in many cases be quite slow. For instance, a gradual remodeling of the vertebrae to induce a spinal stenosis probably leads to an onset time of many years. It will of course be difficult to mimic such a situation in an experimental model. It will also be impossible to have control over the pressure acting on the nerve roots in chronic models because of the remodeling and adaptation of the nerve tissue to the applied pressure. However, knowledge of the exact pressures is probably of less importance in chronic than in acute compression situations. Instead, chronic models should induce a controlled compression with a slow onset time that is easily reproducible. Such models may be well suited for studies on pathophysiological events as well as intervention by surgery or drugs. Some attempts have been made to induce such compression.

Delamarter and collaborators (1990) presented a model on dog cauda equina in which they applied a constricting plastic band. The band was tightened around the thecal sac to induce a 25, 50, or 75% reduction of the cross-sectional area. The band was left in place for various times. Analyses were performed and showed both structural and functional changes that were proportional to the degree of constriction.

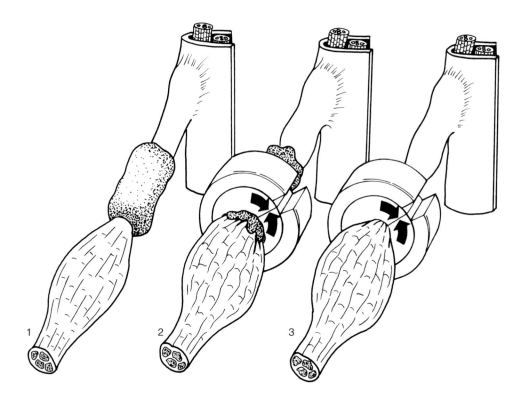

FIG. 5-15

Experimental study to analyze the effects on nerve conduction velocity of nucleus pulposus (1), the combination of nucleus pulposus and compression (2), and compression only (3). The nucleus pulposus and the constrictor were applied to the first sacral nerve root in pigs. The contralateral nerve root served as a control. *Reproduced with permission from Cornefjord, M., Sato, K., Olmarker, K., et al. (1997). A model for chronic nerve root compression studies. Presentation of a porcine model for controlled slow-onset compression with analyses of anatomic aspects, compression onset rate, and morphologic and neurophysiologic effects. Spine, 22, 946–957.*

To induce a slower onset and more controlled compression, Cornefjord and collaborators (1997) used a constrictor to compress the nerve roots in the pig (Fig. 5-15). The constrictor was initially intended for inducing vascular occlusion in experimental ischemic conditions in dogs. The constrictor consists of an outer metal shell that on the inside is covered with a material called amaroid that expands when in contact with fluids. Because of the metal shell, the amaroid expands inwards with a maximum expansion after 2 weeks, resulting in compression of a nerve root placed in the central opening of the constrictor. Compression of the first sacral nerve root in the pig resulted in a significant reduction of nerve conduction velocity and axonal injuries using a constrictor with a defined original diameter. An increase in substance P in the nerve root and the dorsal root ganglion following such compression also has been found. Substance P is a neurotransmitter that is related to pain transmission. The study may thus provide experimental evidence that compression of nerve roots produces pain.

The constrictor model has also been used to study blood flow changes in the nerve root vasculature. It could then be observed that the blood flow is not reduced just outside the compression zone but significantly reduced in parts of the nerve roots located inside the constrictor. In this context, note that in case of disc herniation, the nerve root may become sensitized by substances from the disc tissue (nucleus pulposus) so that mechanical root deformation can induce pronounced sciatic pain.

Summary

1 The peripheral nerves are composed of nerve fibers, layers of connective tissue, and blood vessels.

2 The nerve fibers are extremely susceptible to trauma but because they are surrounded by successive layers of connective tissue (the epineurium and perineurium), they are mechanically protected.

3 Stretching induces changes in intraneural blood flow and nerve fiber structure before the nerve trunk ruptures.

4 Compression of a nerve can cause injury to both nerve fibers and blood vessels in the nerve, mainly at the edges of the compressed nerve segment, but also by ischemic mechanisms.

5 Pressure level, duration of compression, and mode of pressure application are significant variables in the development of nerve injury.

6 Spinal nerve roots are anatomically different from peripheral nerves and therefore react differently to mechanical deformation.

7 Spinal nerve roots are more susceptible than peripheral nerves to mechanical deformation, mainly because of the lack of protective connective tissue layers in nerve roots.

REFERENCES

Cornefjord, M., Sato, K., Olmarker, K., et al. (1997). A model for chronic nerve root compression studies. Presentation of a porcine model for controlled slow-onset compression with analyses of anatomic aspects, compression onset rate, and morphologic and neurophysiologic effects. *Spine, 22,* 946–957.

Dahlin, L.B., Rydevik, B., & Lundborg, G. (1986). The pathophysiology of nerve entrapments and nerve compression injuries. In A.R. Hargens (Ed.). *Effects of Mechanical Stress on Tissue Viability.* New York: Springer-Verlag.

Delamarter, R.B., Bohlman, H.H., Dodge, L.D., et al. (1990). Experimental lumbar spinal stenosis. Analysis of the cortical evoked potentials, microvasculature and histopathology. *J Bone Joint Surg, 72A,* 110–120.

Lundborg, G., & Rydevik, B. (1973). Effects of stretching the tibial nerve of the rabbit: A preliminary study of the intraneural circulation and the barrier function of the perineurium. *J Bone Joint Surg, 55B,* 390.

Lundborg, G. (1975). Structure and function of the intraneural microvessels as related to trauma, edema formation and nerve function. *J Bone Joint Surg, 57A,* 938.

Lundborg, G., et al. (1982). Median nerve compression in the carpal tunnel: The functional response to experimentally induced controlled pressure. *J Hand Surg, 7,* 252.

Myers, R.R. (1998). Morphology of the peripheral nervous system and its relationship to neuropathic pain. In T.L. Yaksh, C. Lynch III, W.M. Zapol, M. Maze, J.F. Biebuyck, & L.J. Saidman (Eds.). *Anesthesia: Biologic Foundations* (pp. 483–514). Philadelphia: Lippincott-Raven.

Myers, R.R., Murakami, H., & Powell, H.C. (1986). Reduced nerve blood flow in edematous neuropathies—A biomechanical mechanism. *Microvascular Res, 32,* 145–151.

Myers, R.R., & Powell, H.C. (1981). Endoneurial fluid pressure in peripheral neuropathies. In A.R. Hargens (Ed.). *Tissue Fluid Pressure and Composition* (p. 193). Baltimore: Williams & Wilkins.

Olmarker, K., Rydevik, B., & Holm, S. (1989a). Edema formation in spinal nerve roots induced by experimental, graded compression. An experimental study on the pig cauda equina with special reference to differences in effects between rapid and slow onset of compression. *Spine, 14,* 579.

Olmarker, K., Rydevik, B., Holm, S., et al. (1989b). Effects of experimental graded compression on blood flow in spinal nerve roots. A vital microscopic study on the porcine cauda equina. J Orthop Res, 7,817.

Olmarker, K. (1991). Spinal nerve root compression. Acute compression of the cauda equina studied in pigs. *Acta Orthop Scand, 62,* Suppl 242.

Olmarker, K. & Rydevik, B. (1992). Single versus double level compression. An experimental study on the porcine cauda equina with analyses of nerve impulse conduction properties. *Clin Orthop, 279,* 3539.

Olmarker, K. & Hasue, M. (1995). Classification and pathophysiology of spinal pain syndromes. In J.N. Weinstein & B. Rydevik (Eds.), *Essentials of the Spine.* Raven Press, New York, NY.

Rydevik, B.L., Kwan, M.K., Myers, R.R., et al. (1990). An in vitro mechanical and histological study of acute stretching on rabbit tibial nerve. *J Orthop Res, 8,* 694–701.

Rydevik, B. & Lundborg, G. (1977). Permeability of intraneural microvessels and perineurium following acute, graded experimental nerve compression. *Scand J Plast Reconstr Surg, 11,* 179.

Rydevik, B., Lundborg, G., & Bagge, U. (1981). Effects of graded compression on intraneural blood flow. An in vivo study on rabbit tibial nerve. *J Hand Surg, 6,* 3.

Rydevik, B., Brown, M.D., & Lundborg, G. (1984). Pathoanatomy and pathophysiology of nerve root compression. *Spine, 9,* 7.

Rydevik, B.L., Kwan, M.K., Myers R.R., et al. (1990). An in vitro mechanical and histological study of acute stretching on rabbit tibial nerve. *J Orthop Res, 8,* 694.

Spencer, D.L., Miller, J.A., & Bertolini, J.E. (1984). The effects of intervertebral disc space narrowing on the contact force between the nerve root and a simulated disc protrusion. *Spine 9,* 422.

Sunderland, S. (1978). *Nerves and Nerve Injuries* (2nd ed.). Edinburgh: Churchill Livingstone.

Takahashi, K., Olmarker, K., Holm, S., et al. (1993). Double-level cauda equina compression. An experimental study with continuous monitoring of intraneural blood flow. *J Orthop Res,11,* 104.

Tortora, G.J., & Anagnostakos, N.P. (1984). *Principles of Anatomy and Physiology* (4th ed.). New York: Harper & Row.

Wall, E.J., Massie, J.B., Kwan, M.K., et al. (1992). Experimental stretch neuropathy. Changes in nerve conduction under tension. *J Bone Joint Surg, 74-B,* 126.

Weinstein, J.N., LaMotte, R., Rydevik, B. et al., (1989). Nerve. In J.W. Frymoyer & S.L. Gordon (Eds.). *New Perspectives on Low Back Pain* (Chapter 4, pp. 35–130). Park Ridge, IL: AAOS. [Based on a workshop arranged by the National Institutes of Health (NIH) in Airlie, Virginia, USA, May 1988.]

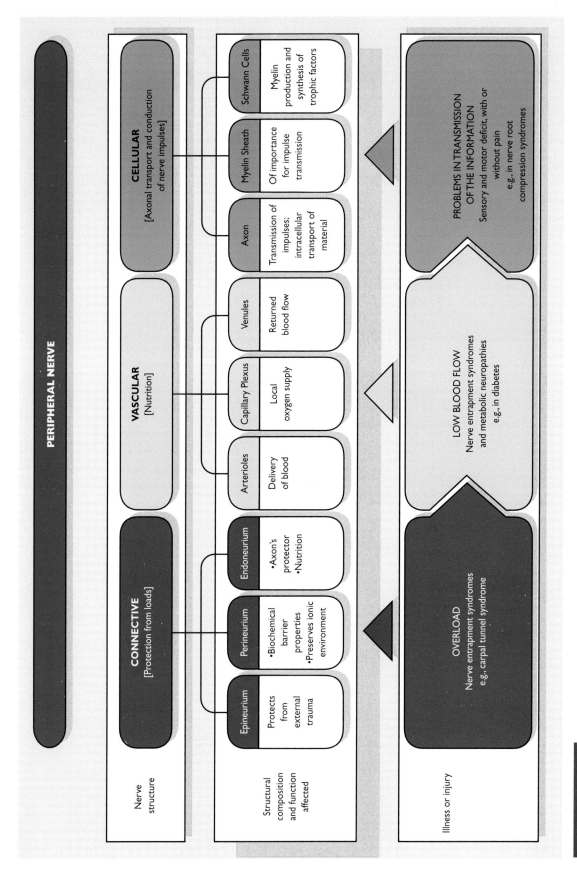

FLOW CHART 5-1 Peripheral nerve's structure and alteration. Clinical examples.*

*This flow chart is designed for classroom or group discussion. Flow chart is not meant to be exhaustive.

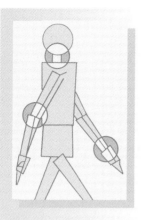

CHAPTER 6

Biomechanics of Skeletal Muscle

Tobias Lorenz, Marco Campello adapted from
Mark I. Pitman, Lars Peterson

Introduction

The muscular system consists of three muscle types: the cardiac muscle, which composes the heart; the smooth (nonstriated or involuntary) muscle, which lines the hollow internal organs; and the skeletal (striated or voluntary) muscle, which attaches to the skeleton via the tendons. The focus of this chapter is the role and function of skeletal muscle.

Skeletal muscle is the most abundant tissue in the human body, accounting for 40 to 45% of the total body weight. The human body has more than 430 skeletal muscles, found in pairs on the right and left sides of the body. The most vigorous movements are produced by fewer than 80 pairs. The muscles provide strength and protection to the skeleton by distributing loads and absorbing shock; they enable the bones to move at the joints and provide the maintenance of body posture against force. Such abilities usually represent the action of muscle groups, not of individual muscles.

The skeletal muscles perform both dynamic and static work. Dynamic work permits locomotion and the positioning of the body segments in space. Static work maintains body posture or position. In this chapter we describe the composition and structure of skeletal muscle, the mechanics of muscle contraction, force production in muscle, muscle fiber differentiation, and muscle remodeling.

Composition and Structure of Skeletal Muscle

An understanding of the biomechanics of muscle function requires knowledge of the gross anatomical structure and function of the musculotendinous unit and the basic microscopic structure and chemical composition of the muscle fiber.

STRUCTURE AND ORGANIZATION OF MUSCLE

The structural unit of skeletal muscle is the muscle fiber, a long cylindrical cell with many hundreds of nuclei. Muscle fibers range in thickness from approximately 10 to 100 μm and in length from approximately 1 to 30 cm. A muscle fiber consists of many myofibrils, which are invested by a delicate plasma membrane called the sarcolemma. The sarcolemma is connected via vinculin- and dystrophin-rich costameres with the sarcometric Z lines, which represent a part of the extramyofibrillar cytoskeleton. The myofibril is made up of several sarcomeres that contain thin (actin), thick (myosin), elastic (titin), and inelastic (nebulin) filaments. Actin and myosin are the contractile part of the myofibrils, whereas titin and nebulin are part of the intramyofibrillar cytoskeleton (Stromer et al., 1998). The myofibrils are the basic unit of contraction.

Each fiber is encompassed by a loose connective tissue called the endomysium and the fibers are organized into various-sized bundles, or fascicles (Fig. 6-1, A & B), which are in turn encased in a dense connective tissue sheath known as the perimysium. The muscle is composed of several fascicles surrounded by a fascia of fibrous connective tissue called the epimysium.

In general, each end of a muscle is attached to bone by tendons, which have no active contractile properties. The muscles form the contractile component and the tendons the series elastic component. The collagen fibers in the perimysium and epimysium are continuous with those in the tendons; together these fibers act as a structural framework for the attachment of bones and muscle fibers. The perimysium, endomysium, epimysium, and sarcolemma act as parallel elastic components. The forces produced by the contracting muscles are transmitted to bone through these connective tissues and tendons (Kasser, 1996).

Each muscle fiber is composed of a large number of delicate strands, the myofibrils. These are the contractile elements of muscle. Their structure and function have been studied exhaustively by light and electron microscopy, and their histochemistry and biochemistry have been explained elsewhere (Arvidson et al., 1984; Guyton, 1986). Approximately 1 μm in diameter, the myofibrils lie parallel to each other within the cytoplasm (sarcoplasm) of the muscle fiber and extend throughout its length. They vary in number from a few to several thousand depending on the diameter of the muscle fiber, which depends in turn on the type of muscle fiber.

The transverse banding pattern in striated muscles repeats itself along the length of the muscle fiber, each repeat being known as a sarcomere (Fig. 6-1C). These striations are caused by the individual myofibrils, which are aligned continuously throughout the muscle fiber. The sarcomere is the functional unit of the contractile system in muscle, and the events that take place in one sarcomere are duplicated in the others. Various sarcomere build a myofibril, various myofibrils build the muscle fiber, and various muscle fibers build the muscle.

FIG. 6-1

Schematic drawings of the structural organization of muscle. **A,** A fibrous connective tissue fascia, the epimysium, surrounds the muscle, which is composed of many bundles, or fascicles. The fascicles are encased in a dense connective tissue sheath, the perimysium. **B,** The fascicles are composed of muscle fibers, which are long, cylindrical, multinucleated cells. Between the individual muscle fibers are capillary blood vessels. Each muscle fiber is surrounded by a loose connective tissue called the endomysium. Just beneath the endomysium lies the sarcolemma, a thin elastic sheath with infoldings that invaginate the fiber interior. Each muscle fiber is composed of numerous delicate strands—myofibrils, the contractile elements of muscle. **C,** Myofibrils consist of smaller filaments that form a repeating banding pattern along the length of the myofibril. One unit of this serially repeating pattern is called a sarcomere. The sarcomere is the functional unit of the contractile system of muscle. **D,** The banding pattern of the sarcomere is formed by the organization of thick and thin filaments, composed of the proteins myosin and actin, respectively. The actin filaments are attached at one end but are free along their length to interdigitate with the myosin filaments. The thick filaments are arranged in a hexagonal fashion. A cross-section through the area of overlap shows the thick filaments surrounded by six equally spaced thin filaments. **E,** The lollipop-shaped molecules of each myosin filament are arranged so that the long tails form a sheaf with the heads, or cross-bridges, projecting from it. The cross-bridges point in one direction along half of the filament and in the other direction along the other half. Only a portion of one half of a filament is shown here. The cross-bridges are an essential element in the mechanism of muscle contraction, extending outward to interdigitate with receptor sites on the actin filaments. Each actin filament is a double helix, appearing as two strands of beads spiraling around each other. Two additional proteins, tropomyosin and troponin, are associated with the actin helix and play an important role in regulating the interdigitation of the actin and myosin filaments. Tropomyosin is a long polypeptide chain that lies in the grooves between the helices of actin. Troponin is a globular molecule attached at regular intervals to the tropomyosin. *Adapted from Williams, P. & Warwick, R. (1980). Gray's Anatomy (36th ed., pp. 506–515). Edinburgh: Churchill Livingstone.*

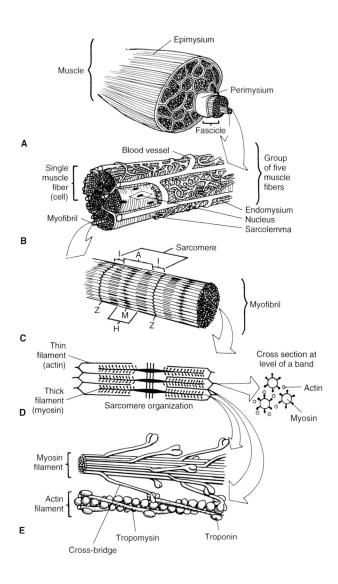

Each sarcomere is composed of the following:

1. The thin filaments (approximately 5 nm in diameter) composed of the protein actin
2. The thick filaments (approximately 15 nm in diameter) composed of the protein myosin (Fig. 6-l, D & E)
3. The elastic filaments composed of the protein titin (Fig. 6-2)
4. The inelastic filaments composed of the proteins nebulin and titin

Actin, the chief component of the thin filament, has the shape of a double helix and appears as two strands of beads spiraling around each other. Two additional proteins, troponin and tropomyosin, are important constituents of the actin helix because they appear to regulate the making and breaking of contacts between the actin and myosin filaments during contraction. Tropomyosin is a long polypeptide chain that lies in the grooves between the helices of actin. Troponin is a globular molecule attached at regular intervals to the tropomyosin (Fig. 6-1, *D & E*).

The thick filaments are located in the central region of the sarcomere, where their orderly, parallel arrangement gives rise to dark bands known as A bands because they are strongly anisotropic. The thin filaments are attached at either end of the sarcomere to a structure known as the Z line, which consists of short elements that link the thin filaments of adjacent sarcomeres, defining the limits of each sarcomere. The thin filaments extend from the Z line toward the center of the sarcomere, where they overlap with the thick filaments. Recently it was shown that there is a third set of myofibril filaments in the vertebrate striated muscles. This connecting filament, named titin, links the thick filaments with the Z line (elastic I band region of titin) and is part of the thick filaments (A band region of titin). This filament maintains the central position of the A band throughout contraction and relaxation and might act as a template during myosin assembly.

Myosin, the thicker filament, is composed of individual molecules, each of which resembles a lollipop with a globular "head" projecting from a long shaft or "tail." Several hundred such molecules are packed tail to tail in a sheaf with their heads pointed in one direction along half of the filament and in the opposite direction along the other half, leaving a head-free region (the H zone) in between. The globular heads spiral about the myosin filament in the region where actin and myosin overlap (the A band) and extend as cross-bridges to interdigitate with sites on the actin filaments, thus forming the structural and functional link between the two filament types.

The intramyofibrillar cytoskeleton includes inelastic nebulin filaments, which span from the Z line to the actin filaments. Nebulin might also act as a template for the thin filament assembly.

Titin is 1 μm long. It is the largest polypeptide and spans from the Z line to the M line. Titin is an elastic filament. The part between the Z line and myosin has a string-like appearance. Titin has been suggested to contribute greatly to the passive force development of muscle during stretch (Fig. 6-2). It also might act as a template for the thick filament assembly (Linke et al., 1998; Squire et al., 1997; Stromer et al., 1998).

The I band is bisected by the Z lines, which contain the portion of the thin filaments that does not overlap with the thick filaments and the elastic part of titin. In the center of the A band, in the gap between the ends of the thin filaments, is the H zone, a light band containing only thick filaments and that part of titin that is integrated in the thick filaments. A narrow, dark area in the center of the H zone is the M line, pro-

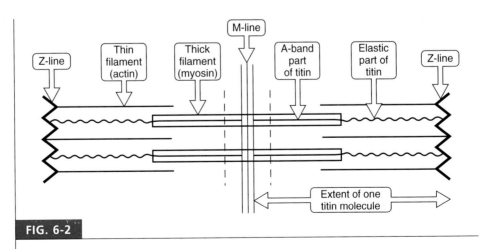

FIG. 6-2

The arrangement of titin molecules within the sarcomere. *Adapted from Craig, R.(1994). The structure of the contract filaments. In A.G. Engel & Franzini-Armstrong (eds.), Myology (2nd ed., p. 150). New York: McGraw-Hill, Inc.*

duced by transversely and longitudinally oriented proteins that link adjacent thick filaments, maintaining their parallel arrangement. The various areas of the banding pattern are apparent in the photomicrograph of human skeletal muscle shown in Figure 6-3.

Closely correlated with the repeating pattern of the sarcomeres is an organized network of tubules and sacs known as the sarcoplasmic reticulum. The tubules of the sarcoplasmic reticulum lie par-

allel to the myofibrils and tend to enlarge and fuse at the level of the junctions between the A and I bands, forming transverse sacs, or the terminal cisternae, that surround the individual myofibril completely.

The terminal cisternae enclose a smaller tubule that is separated from them by its own membrane. The smaller tubule and the terminal cisternae above and below it are known as a triad. The enclosed

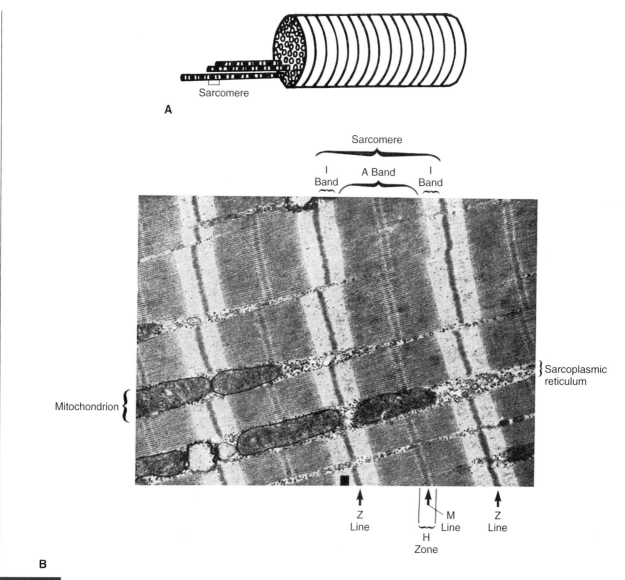

FIG. 6-3

A, Single muscle fiber with three protruding myofibrils. **B,** Electron photomicrograph of a cross-section of human skeletal muscle. The sarcomeres are apparent along the myofibrils. Characteristic regions of the sarcomere are indicated.

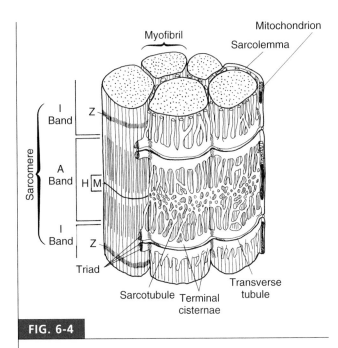

Myofibril

Mitochondrion

Sarcolemma

I Band

Z

Sarcomere

A Band

H M

I Band

Z

Triad

Sarcotubule Terminal cisternae

Transverse tubule

Diagram of a portion of a skeletal muscle fiber illustrating the sarcoplasmic reticulum that surrounds each myofibril. The various regions of the sarcomere are indicated on the left myofibril to show the correlation of these regions with the sarcoplasmic reticulum, shown surrounding the middle and right myofibrils. The transverse tubules represent an infolding of the sarcolemma, the plasma membrane that encompasses the entire muscle fiber. Two transverse tubules supply each sarcomere at the level of the junctions of the A band and I bands. Terminal cisternae are located on each side of the transverse tubule, and together these structures constitute a triad. The terminal cisternae connect with a longitudinal network of sarcotubules spanning the region of the A band. *Adapted from Ham, A.W. & Cormack, D.H. (1979). Histology (8th ed.). Philadelphia: J.B. Lippincott.*

tubule is part of the transverse tubule system, or T system, which are invaginations of the surface membrane of the fiber. This membrane, the sarcolemma, is a plasma membrane that invests every striated muscle (Fig. 6-4).

Molecular Basis of Muscle Contraction

The most widely held theory of muscle contraction is the sliding filament theory, proposed simultaneously by A.F. Huxley and H.E. Huxley in 1964 and subsequently refined (Huxley, 1974). According to this theory, active shortening of the sarcomere, and

hence of the muscle, results from the relative movement of the actin and myosin filaments past one another while each retains its original length. The force of contraction is developed by the myosin heads, or cross-bridges, in the region of overlap between actin and myosin (the A band). These cross-bridges swivel in an arc around their fixed positions on the surface of the myosin filament, much like the oars of a boat. This movement of the cross-bridges in contact with the actin filaments produces the sliding of the actin filaments toward the center of the sarcomere. A muscle fiber contracts when all sarcomere shorten simultaneously in an all-or-nothing fashion, which is called a twitch.

Because a single movement of a cross-bridge produces only a small displacement of the actin filament relative to the myosin filament, each individual cross-bridge detaches itself from one receptor site on the actin filament and reattaches itself to another site further along, repeating the process five or six times, "with an action similar to a man pulling on a rope hand over hand" (Wilkie, 1968). The cross-bridges do not act in a synchronized manner; each acts independently. Thus, at any given moment only approximately half of the cross-bridges actively generate force and displacement, and when these detach, others take up the task so that shortening is maintained. The shortening is reflected in the sarcomere as a decrease in the I band and a decrease in the H zone as the Z lines move closer together; the width of the A band remains constant.

A key to the sliding mechanism is the calcium ion (Ca^{2+}), which turns the contractile activity on and off. Muscle contraction is initiated when calcium is made available to the contractile elements and ceases when calcium is removed. The mechanisms that regulate the availability of calcium ions to the contractile machinery are coupled to electric events occurring in the muscle membrane (sarcolemma). An action potential in the sarcolemma provides the electric signal for the initiation of contractile activity. The mechanism by which the electric signal triggers the chemical events of contraction is known as excitation-contraction coupling.

When the motor neuron stimulates the muscle at the neuromuscular junction (Fig. 6-5A) and the propagated action potential depolarizes the muscle cell membrane (sarcolemma), there is an inward spread of the action potential along the T system. (Details of this process are given in Figure 6-5, A–C and in Box 6-1, which summarizes the events during the excitation, contraction, and relaxation of muscle. Figure 6-5D shows the struc-

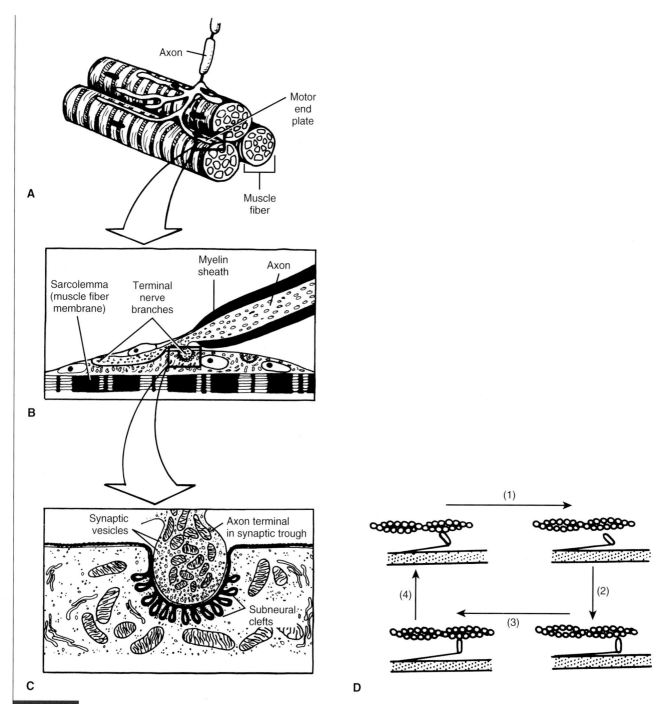

FIG. 6-5

Schematic representation of the innervation of muscle fibers. **A,** An axon of a motor neuron (originating from the cell body in the anterior horn of the spinal cord) branches near its end to innervate several skeletal muscle fibers, forming a neuromuscular junction with each fiber. The region of the muscle membrane (sarcolemma) lying directly under the terminal branches of the axon has special properties and is known as the motor end plate, or motor end plate membrane. The rectangular area is shown in detail in **B. B,** The fine terminal branches of the nerve (axon terminals), devoid of myelin sheaths, lie in grooves on the sarcolemma. The rectangular area in this section is shown in detail in **C. C,** Ultrastructure of the junction of an axon terminal and the sarcolemma. The invagination of the sarcolemma forms the synaptic trough into which the axon terminal protrudes. The invaginated sarcolemma has many folds, or subneural clefts, which greatly increase its surface area. Acetylcholine is stored in synaptic vesicles in the axon terminal. **B** and **C,** *adapted from Brobeck, J.R. (Ed.) (1979). Best and Taylor's Physiological Basis of Medical Practice (10th ed., pp. 59–113). Baltimore: Williams & Wilkins.* **D,** Cross-bridge cycle of muscle contraction.

BOX 6-1   Events During Excitation, Contraction, and Relaxation of Muscle Fiber

1. An action potential is initiated and propagated in a motor axon.
2. This action potential causes the release of acetylcholine from the axon terminals at the neuromuscular junction.
3. Acetylcholine is bound to receptor sites on the motor end plate membrane.
4. Acetylcholine increases the permeability of the motor end plate to sodium and potassium ions, producing an end-plate potential.
5. The end-plate potential depolarizes the muscle membrane (sarcolemma), generating a muscle action potential that is propagated over the membrane surface.
6. Acetylcholine is rapidly destroyed by acetylcholinesterase on the end plate membrane.
7. The muscle action potential depolarizes the transverse tubules.
8. Depolarization of the transverse tubules leads to the release of calcium ions from the terminal cisternae of the sarcoplasmic reticulum surrounding the myofibrils. These ions are released into the sarcoplasm in the direct vicinity of the regulatory proteins tropomyosin and troponin.
9. Calcium ions bind to troponin, allowing movement of the tropomyosin molecule away from the myosin receptor sites on the actin filament that it had been blocking and releasing the inhibition that had prevented actin from combining with myosin.
10. Actin (A) combines with myosin ATP (M-ATP). In this state, ATP has been hydrolyzed to ADP and phosphate but the products are still attached to myosin (receptor sites on the myosin cross-bridges bind to receptor sites on the actin chain):

$$A + M \cdot ATP \rightarrow A \cdot M \cdot ATP$$

11. Actin activates the myosin ATPase found on the myosin cross-bridge, enabling ATP to be split (hydrolyzed.) This process releases energy used to produce movement of the myosin cross-bridges:

$$A \cdot M \cdot ATP \rightarrow A \cdot M + ADP + P_1$$

12. Oar-like movements of the cross-bridges produce relative sliding of the thick and thin filaments past each other.
13. Fresh ATP binds to the myosin cross-bridge, breaking the actin-myosin bond and allowing the cross-bridge to dissociate from actin:

$$A \cdot M + ATP \rightarrow A + M \cdot ATP$$

14. The ATPase hydrolyzes the myosin ATP complex to the M · ATP complex, which represents the relaxed state of the sarcomere:

$$M \cdot ATP \rightarrow M \cdot ATP$$

15. Cycles of binding and unbinding of actin with the myosin cross-bridges at successive sites along the actin filament (steps 11, 12, 13, and 14) continue as long as the concentration of calcium remains high enough to inhibit the action of the troponin-tropomyosin system.
16. Concentration of calcium ions falls as they are pumped into the terminal cisternae of the sarcoplasmic reticulum by an energy-requiring process that splits ATP.
17. Calcium dissociates from troponin, restoring the inhibitory action of troponin-tropomyosin. The actin filament slides back and the muscle lengthens. In the presence of ATP, actin and myosin remain in the dissociated, relaxed state.

(Modified from Luciano et al. (1978). In Human Function and Structure *(Fig 5.5D). New York: McGraw-Hill; and adapted from Craig, R. (1994).* Myology *(2nd ed., p. 162). New York: McGraw-Hill.)*

tural features between actin and the cross-bridges of myosin.)

THE MOTOR UNIT

The functional unit of skeletal muscle is the motor unit, which includes a single motor neuron and all of the muscle fibers innervated by it. This unit is the smallest part of the muscle that can be made to con- tract independently. When stimulated, all muscle fibers in the motor unit respond as one. The fibers of a motor unit are said to show an all-or-none response to stimulation: they contract either maximally or not at all.

The number of muscle fibers forming a motor unit is closely related to the degree of control required of the muscle. In small muscles that perform very fine movements, such as the extraocular muscles, each motor unit may contain less than a dozen muscle fibers; in large muscles that perform coarse movements, such as the gastrocnemius, the motor unit may contain 1,000 to 2,000 muscle fibers.

The fibers of each motor unit are not contiguous but dispersed throughout the muscle with fibers of other units. Thus, if a single motor unit is stimulated, a large portion of the muscle appears to contract. If additional motor units of the nerve innervating the muscle are stimulated, the muscle contracts with greater force. The calling in of additional motor units in response to greater stimulation of the motor nerve is called recruitment.

THE MUSCULOTENDINOUS UNIT

The tendons and the connective tissues in and around the muscle belly are viscoelastic structures that help determine the mechanical characteristics of whole muscle during contraction and passive extension. Hill (1970) showed that the tendons represent a spring-like elastic component located in series with the contractile component (the contractile proteins of the myofibril, actin, and myosin), while the epimysium, perimysium, endomysium, and sarcolemma represent a second elastic component located in parallel with the contractile component (Fig. 6-6).

When the parallel and series elastic components stretch during active contraction or passive extension of a muscle, tension is produced and energy is stored; when they recoil with muscle relaxation, this energy is released. The series elastic fibers are more important in the production of tension than are the parallel elastic fibers (Wilkie, 1956). Several investigators have suggested that the cross-bridges of the myosin filaments have a spring-like property and also contribute to the elastic properties of muscle (Hill, 1968).

The distensibility and elasticity of the elastic components are valuable to the muscle in several ways:

1. They tend to keep the muscle in readiness for contraction and assure that muscle tension is produced and transmitted smoothly during contraction.
2. They assure that the contractile elements return to their original (resting) positions when contraction is terminated.
3. They may help prevent the passive overstretch of the contractile elements when these elements are relaxed, thereby lessening the danger of muscle injury.

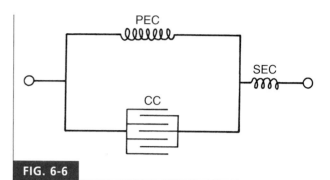

FIG. 6-6

The musculotendinous unit may be depicted as consisting of a contractile component (*CC*) in parallel with an elastic component (*PEC*) and in series with another elastic component (*SEC*). The contractile component is represented by the contractile proteins of the myofibril, actin, and myosin. (The myosin cross-bridges may also exhibit some elasticity.) The parallel elastic component comprises the connective tissue surrounding the muscle fibers (the epimysium, perimysium, and endomysium) and the sarcolemma. The series elastic component is represented by the tendons. *Adapted from Keele, C.A., Neil, E., & Joels, N. (1982). Muscle and the nervous system. In Samson Wright's Applied Physiology (13th ed., pp. 248–259). Oxford: Oxford University Press.*

4. The viscous property of the series and parallel elastic components allows them to absorb energy proportional to the rate of force application and to dissipate energy in a time-dependent manner. (For a discussion of viscoelasticity, see Chapter 4.)

This viscous property, combined with the elastic properties of the musculotendinous unit, is demonstrated in everyday activities. For example, when a person attempts to stretch and touch the toes, the stretch is initially elastic. As the stretch is held, however, further elongation of the muscle results from the viscosity of the muscle-tendon structure, and the fingers slowly reach closer to the floor.

Mechanics of Muscle Contraction

Electromyography provides a mechanism for evaluating and comparing neural effects on muscle and the contractile activity of the muscle itself in vivo and in vitro. Much has been learned by using electromyography to study various aspects of the contractile process, particularly the time relationship between the onset of electrical activity in the muscle and actual contraction of the muscle or muscle fiber. The following sections discuss the mechanical response of a muscle to electrical (neural) stimulation and the various ways in which the muscle contracts to move a joint, control its motion, or maintain its position.

SUMMATION AND TETANIC CONTRACTION

The mechanical response of a muscle to a single stimulus of its motor nerve is known as a twitch, which is the fundamental unit of recordable muscle activity. Following stimulation there is an interval of a few milliseconds known as the latency period before the tension in the muscle fibers begins to rise. This period represents the time required for the "slack" in the elastic components to be taken up. The time from the start of tension development to peak tension is the contraction time, and the time from peak tension until the tension drops to zero is the relaxation time. The contraction time and relaxation time vary among muscles, depending largely on the muscle fiber makeup (described below). Some muscle fibers contract with a speed of only 10 msec; others may take 100 msec or longer.

An action potential lasts only approximately 1 to 2 msec. This is a small fraction of the time taken for the subsequent mechanical response, or twitch, even in muscles that contract quickly; thus it is possible for a series of action potentials to be initiated before the first twitch is completed if the activity of the motor axon is maintained. When mechanical responses to successive stimuli are added to an initial response, the result is known as summation (Fig. 6-7). If a second stimulus occurs during the latency period of the first muscle twitch, it produces no additional response and the muscle is said to be completely refractory.

The frequency of stimulation is variable and is modulated by individual motor units. The greater the frequency of stimulation of the muscle fibers, the greater the tension produced in the muscle as a whole. However, a maximal frequency will be reached beyond which the tension of the muscle no longer increases. When this maximal tension is sustained as a result of summation, the muscle is said to contract tetanically. In this case, the rapidity of stimulation outstrips the contraction-relaxation

time of the muscle so that little or no relaxation can occur before the next contraction is initiated (Fig. 6-8).

The considerable gradation of contraction exhibited by whole muscles is achieved by the differential

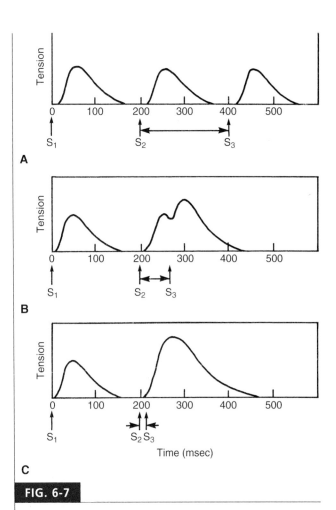

FIG. 6-7

Summation of contractions in a muscle held at a constant length. **A,** An initial stimulus (S_1) is applied to the muscle, and the resulting twitch lasts 150 msec. The second (S_2) and third (S_3) stimuli are applied to the muscle after 200-msec intervals when the muscle has relaxed completely, thus no summation occurs. **B,** S_1 is applied 60 msec after S_2, when the mechanical response from S_2 is beginning to decrease. The resulting peak tension is greater than that of the single twitch. **C,** The interval between S_2 and S_3 is further reduced to 10 msec. The resulting peak tension is even greater than in B, and the increase in tension produces a smooth curve. The mechanical response evoked by S_3 appears as a continuation of that evoked by S_2. *Adapted from Luciano, D.S., Vander, A.J., & Sherman, J.H. (1978).* Human Function and Structure *(pp. 113–136). New York: McGraw-Hill.*

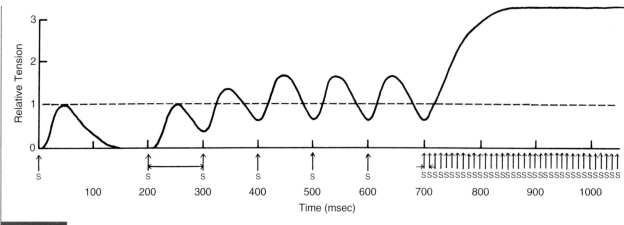

FIG. 6-8

Generation of muscle tetanus. As the frequency of stimulation (*S*) increases (i.e., the intervals shorten from 200 to 100 msec), the muscle tension rises as a result of summation. When the frequency is increased to 100/second, summation becomes *maximal* and the muscle contracts tetanically, exerting sustained peak tension. *Adapted from Luciano, D.S., Vander, A.J., & Sherman, J.H. (1978).* Human Function and Structure *(pp. 113–136). New York: McGraw-Hill.*

activity of their motor units, in both stimulation frequency and the number of units activated. The repetitive twitching of all recruited motor units of a muscle in an asynchronous manner results in brief summations or more prolonged subtetanic or tetanic contractions of the muscle as a whole and is a principal factor responsible for the smooth movements produced by the skeletal muscles.

TYPES OF MUSCLE CONTRACTION

During contraction, the force exerted by a contracting muscle on the bony lever(s) to which it is attached is known as the muscle tension, and the external force exerted on the muscle is known as the resistance, or load. As the muscle exerts its force, it generates a turning effect, or moment (torque), on the involved joint because the line of application of the muscle force usually lies at a distance from the center of motion of the joint. The moment is calculated as the product of the muscle force and the perpendicular distance between its point of application and the center of motion (this distance is known as the lever arm, or moment arm, of the force).

Muscle contractions and the resulting muscle work can be classified according to the relationship between either the muscle tension and the resistance to be overcome or the muscle moment generated and the resistance to be overcome, as shown in Box 6-2 (Kroemer et al., 1990).

Although no motion is accomplished and no mechanical work is performed during an isometric contraction, muscle work (physiological work) is performed: energy is expended and is mostly dissipated as heat, which is also called the isometric heat production. All dynamic contractions involve what may be considered an initial static (isometric) phase as the muscle first develops tension equal to the load it is expected to overcome.

The tension in a muscle varies with the type of contraction. Isometric contractions produce greater tension than do concentric contractions. Studies suggest that the tension developed in an eccentric contraction may even exceed that developed during an isometric contraction. These differences are thought to be due in large part to the varying amounts of supplemental tension produced in the series elastic component of the muscle and to differences in contraction time. The longer contraction time of the isometric and eccentric contractions allows greater cross-bridge formation by the contractile components, thus permitting greater tension to be generated (Kroll, 1987). More time is also available for this tension to be transmitted to the series elastic component as the muscle-tendon unit is stretched. The longer contraction time allows the recruitment of additional motor units.

Komi (1986) has pointed out that concentric, isometric, and eccentric muscle contractions seldom

BOX 6-2	Types of Muscle Work and Contraction

Dynamic work: Mechanical work is performed and joint motion is produced through the following forms of muscle contraction:

1. Concentric (*con,* together; *centrum,* center) contraction: When muscles develop sufficient tension to overcome the resistance of the body segment, the muscles shorten and cause joint movement. The net moment generated by the muscle is in the same direction as the change in joint angle. An example of a concentric contraction is the action of the quadriceps in extending the knee when ascending stairs.

2. Eccentric (e.g., out of-, centrum, center) contraction: When a muscle cannot develop sufficient tension and is overcome by the external load, it progressively lengthens instead of shortening. The net muscle moment is in the opposite direction from the change in joint angle. One purpose of eccentric contraction is to decelerate the motion of a joint. For example, when one descends stairs, the quadriceps works eccentrically to decelerate flexion of the knee, thus decelerating the limb. The tension that it applies is less than the force of gravity pulling the body downward, but it is sufficient to allow controlled lowering of the body.

3. Isokinetic (*iso,* constant; *kinetic,* motion) contraction: This is a type of dynamic muscle work in which movement of the joint is kept at a constant velocity, and hence the velocity of shortening or lengthening of the muscle is constant. Because velocity is held constant, muscle energy cannot be dissipated through acceleration of the body part and is entirely converted to a resisting moment. The muscle force varies with changes in its lever arm throughout the range of joint motion (Hislop & Perrine, 1967). The muscle contracts concentrically and eccentrically with different directions of joint motion. For example, the flexor muscles of a joint contract concentrically during flexion and eccentrically during extension, acting as decelerators during the latter.

4. Isoinertial (*iso,* constant; *inertial,* resistance) contraction: This is a type of dynamic muscle work wherein the resistance against which the muscle must contract remains constant. If the moment (torque) produced by the muscle is equal to or less than the resistance to be overcome, the muscle length remains unchanged and the muscle contracts isometrically. If the moment is greater than the resistance, the muscle shortens (contracts concentrically) and causes acceleration of the body part. Isoinertial contraction occurs, for example, when a constant external load is lifted. At the extremes of motion, the inertia of the load must be overcome; the involved muscles contract isometrically and muscle torque is maximal. In the midrange of the motion, with the inertia overcome, the muscles contract concentrically and the torque is submaximal.

5. Isotonic (*iso,* constant; *tonic,* force) contraction: This term is commonly used to define muscle contraction in which the tension is constant throughout a range of joint motion. This term does not take into account the leverage effects at the joint. However, because the muscle force moment arm changes throughout the range of joint motion, the muscle tension must also change. Thus, isotonic muscle contraction in the truest sense does not exist in the production of joint motion (Kroll, 1987).

Static work: No mechanical work is performed and posture or joint position is maintained through the following form of muscle contraction:

1. Isometric (*iso,* constant; *metric,* length) contraction: Muscles are not always directly involved in the production of joint movements. They may exercise either a restraining or a holding action, such as that needed to maintain the body in an upright position in opposing the force of gravity. In this case the muscle attempts to shorten (i.e., the myofibrils shorten and in doing so stretch the series elastic component, thereby producing tension), but it does not overcome the load and cause movement; instead, it produces a moment that supports the load in a fixed position (e.g., maintains posture) because no change takes place in the distance between the muscle's points of attachment.

occur alone in normal human movement. Instead, one type of contraction or load is preceded by a different type. An example is the eccentric loading prior to the concentric contraction that occurs at the ankle from midstance to toe-off during gait.

Because muscles normally shorten or lengthen at varying velocities and with varying amounts of tension, performance and measurement of isokinetic work require the use of an isokinetic dynamometer. This device provides constant velocity of joint motion and maximum external resistance throughout the range of motion of the involved joint, thereby requiring maximal muscle torque. The use of the isokinetic dynamometer provides a method of selective training and measurement, but physiological movement is not simulated.

Force Production in Muscle

The total force that a muscle can produce is influenced by its mechanical properties, which can be described by examining the length-tension, load-velocity, and force-time relationships of the muscle and the skeletal muscle architecture. Other principal factors in force production are muscle temperature, muscle fatigue, and prestretching.

LENGTH-TENSION RELATIONSHIP

The force, or tension, that a muscle exerts varies with the length at which it is held when stimulated. This relationship can be observed in a single fiber contracting isometrically and tetanically, as illustrated by the length-tension curve in Figure 6-9. Maximal tension is produced when the muscle fiber is approximately at its "slack," or resting, length. If the fiber is held at shorter lengths, the tension falls off slowly at first and then rapidly. If the fiber is lengthened beyond the resting length, tension progressively decreases.

The changes in tension when the fiber is stretched or shortened primarily are caused by structural alterations in the sarcomere. Maximal isometric tension can be exerted when the sarcomeres are at their resting length (2.0–2.25 μm), because the actin and myosin filaments overlap along their entire length and the number of cross-bridges is maximal. If the sarcomeres are lengthened, there are fewer junctions between the filaments and the active tension decreases. At a sarcomere length of approximately 3.6 μm, there is no overlap and hence no active tension. Sarcomere shortening to less than its resting length decreases the active ten-

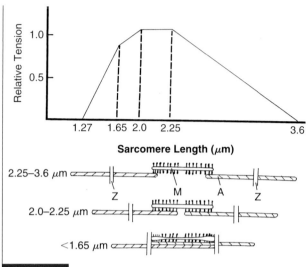

FIG. 6-9

Tension-length curve from part of an isolated muscle fiber stimulated at different lengths. The isometric tetanic tension is closely related to the number of cross-bridges on the myosin filament overlapped by the actin filament. The tension is maximal at the slack length, or resting length, of the sarcomere (2 μm), where overlap is greatest, and falls to zero at the length where overlap no longer occurs (3.6 μm). The tension also decreases when the sarcomere length is reduced below the resting length, falling sharply at 1.65 μm and reaching zero at 1.27 μm as the extensive overlap interferes with cross-bridge formation. The structural relationship of the actin and myosin filaments at various stages of sarcomere shortening and lengthening is portrayed below the curve. *A*, actin filaments; *M*, myosin filaments; *Z*, Z lines. *Adapted from Crawford, C.N.C. & James, N.T. (1980). The design of muscles. In R. Owen, J. Goodfellow, & P. Bullough (Eds.),* Scientific Foundations of Orthopaedics and Traumatology *(pp. 67–74). London: William Heinemann; as modified from Gordon, A.M., Huxley, A.F.I., & Julian, F.J. (1966). The variation in isometric tension with sarcomere length in vertebrate muscle fibers.* J Physiol, 184, 170.

sion because it allows overlapping of the thin filaments at opposite ends of the sarcomere, which are functionally polarized in opposite directions. At a sarcomere length of less than 1.65 μm, the thick filaments on the Z line and the tension diminish sharply.

The length-tension relationship illustrated in Figure 6-9 is for an individual muscle fiber. If this relationship is measured in a whole muscle contracting isometrically and tetanically, the tension produced by both active components and passive components must be taken into account (Fig. 6-10).

The curve labeled "active tension" in Figure 6-10 represents the tension developed by the contractile elements of the muscle, and it resembles the curve for the individual fiber. The curve labeled "passive tension" reflects the tension developed when the muscle surpasses its resting length and the noncontractile muscle belly is stretched. This passive tension is mainly developed in the parallel and series elastic components (Fig. 6-6). When the belly contracts, the combined active and passive tensions produce the total tension exerted. The curve demonstrates that as a muscle is progressively stretched beyond its resting length, the passive tension rises and the active tension decreases.

Most muscles that cross only one joint normally are not stretched enough for the passive tension to play an important role, but the case is different for two-joint muscles, in which the extremes of the

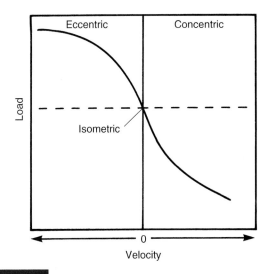

FIG. 6-11

Load-velocity curve generated by plotting the velocity of motion of the muscle lever arm against the external load. When the external load imposed on the muscle is negligible, the muscle contracts concentrically with maximal speed. With increasing loads the muscle shortens more slowly. When the external load equals the maximum force that the muscle can exert, the muscle fails to shorten (i,e., has zero velocity) and contracts isometrically. When the load is increased further, the muscle lengthens eccentrically. This lengthening is more rapid with greater load.

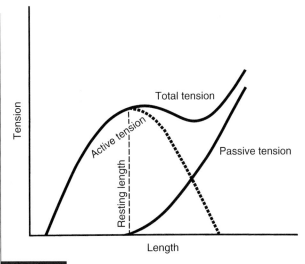

FIG. 6-10

The active and passive tension exerted by a whole muscle contracting isometrically and tetanically is plotted against the muscle's length. The active tension is produced by the contractile muscle components and the passive tension by the series and parallel elastic components, which develop stress when the muscle is stretched beyond its resting length. The greater the amount of stretching, the larger the contribution of the elastic component to the total tension. The shape of the active curve is generally the same in different muscles, but the passive curve, and hence the total curve, varies depending on how much connective tissue (elastic component) the muscle contains. *Adapted from Crawford, C.N.C. & James, N.T. (1980). The design of muscles. In R. Owen, J. Goodfellow, & P. Bullough (Eds.), Scientific Foundations of Orthopaedics and Traumatology (pp. 67–74). London: William Heinemann.*

length-tension relationship may be functioning (Crawford & James, 1980). For example, the hamstrings shorten so much when the knee is fully flexed that the tension they can exert decreases considerably. Conversely, when the hip is flexed and the knee extended, the muscles are so stretched that it is the magnitude of their passive tension that prevents further elongation and causes the knee to flex if hip flexion is increased.

LOAD-VELOCITY RELATIONSHIP

The relationship between the velocity of shortening or eccentric lengthening of a muscle and different constant loads can be determined by plotting the velocity of motion of the muscle lever arm at various external loads, thereby generating a load-velocity curve (Fig. 6-11). The velocity of shortening of a muscle contracting concentrically is inversely related to the external load applied (Guyton, 1986). The velocity of shortening is greatest when the ex-

Gastrocnemius Muscle Tear

A 22-year-old male professional athlete tears his gastrocnemius during a race (Fig. cs6-1-1). The tensile overload that happens during strenuous eccentric and concentric contractions increases the risk of injury, especially when the forces involve bi-articular muscles such as the gastrocnemius. This indirect trauma is associated with high tensile forces during rapid contraction (high velocity) and continued changes in muscle length. The status of muscle contraction at the time of overload is usually eccentric, and failure most often occurs at or near the myotendinous junction unless the muscle has been previously injured (Kasser, 1996). Swelling from hemorrhage occurs initially in the inflammatory phase. The cellular response is more rapid and repair is more complete if the vascular channels are not disrupted and the nutrition of the tissue is not disturbed. The degree of injury from a tensile overload will dictate the potential host response and the time needed for repair.

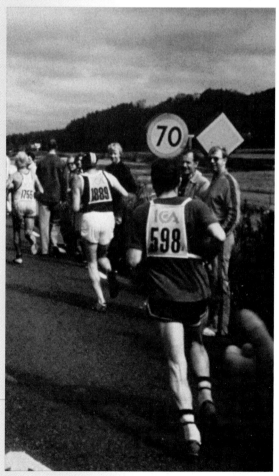

Case Study Figure 6-1-1.

ternal load is zero, but as the load increases the muscle shortens more and more slowly. When the external load equals the maximal force that the muscle can exert, the velocity of shortening becomes zero and the muscle contracts isometrically. When the load is increased still further, the muscle contracts eccentrically: it elongates during contraction. The load-velocity relationship is reversed from that of the concentri-cally contracting muscle; the muscle eccentrically lengthens more quickly with increasing load (Kroll, 1987) (Case Study 6-1).

FORCE-TIME RELATIONSHIP

The force, or tension, generated by a muscle is proportional to the contraction time: the longer the contraction time, the greater is the force developed, up to the point of maximum tension. In Figure 6-12, this relationship is illustrated by a force-time curve for a whole muscle contracting isometrically. Slower contraction leads to greater force production because time is allowed for the tension produced by the contractile elements to be transmitted through the parallel elastic components to the tendon. Although tension production in the contractile component can reach a maximum in as little as 10 msec, up to 300 msec may be needed for that tension to be transferred to the elastic components. The tension in the tendon will reach the maximum tension developed by the contractile element only if the active contraction process is of sufficient duration (Ottoson, 1983).

EFFECT OF SKELETAL MUSCLE ARCHITECTURE

The muscles consist of the contractile component, the sarcomere, which produces active tension. The arrangement of the contractile components affects the contractile properties of the muscle dramatically. The more sarcomere lie in series, the longer the myofibril will be; the more sarcomere lie parallel, the larger the cross-sectional area of the myofibril will be. These two basic architectural patterns of myofibrils (long or thick) affect the contractile properties of the muscles in the following ways:

1. The force the muscle can produce is proportional to the cross-section of the myofibril (Fig. 6-13A).
2. The velocity and the excursion (working range) that the muscle can produce are proportional to the length of the myofibril (Fig. 6-13B).

Muscles with shorter fibers and a larger cross-sectional area are designed to produce force, whereas muscles with long fibers are designed for excursion and velocity. The quadriceps muscle contains shorter myofibrils and appears to be specialized for force production. The sartorius muscle has longer fibers and a smaller cross-sectional area and is better suited for high excursion (Baratta et al., 1998; Lieber & Bodine-Fowler, 1993).

EFFECT OF PRESTRETCHING

It has been demonstrated in amphibians and in humans (Cuillo & Zarins, 1983) that a muscle performs more work when it shortens immediately after being stretched in the concentrically contracted state than when it shortens from a state of isometric contraction. This phenomenon is not entirely accounted for by the elastic energy stored in the series elastic component during stretching but must also be caused by energy stored in the contractile com-

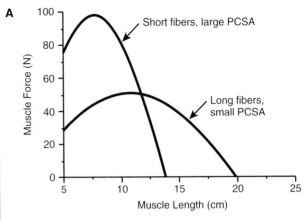

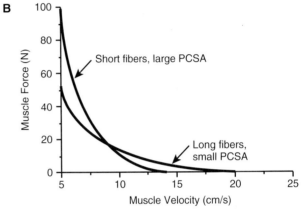

FIG. 6-13

Isometric and isotonic properties of muscles with different architecture. **A,** Force-length relationship. **B,** Force-velocity relationship. *PSCA,* physiological cross-sectional area.
Reprinted with permission of the American Physical Therapy Association, from Lieber, R.L. (1993). Skeletal muscle mechanics: Implications for rehabilitation. Physical Therapy, 73(12), 852.

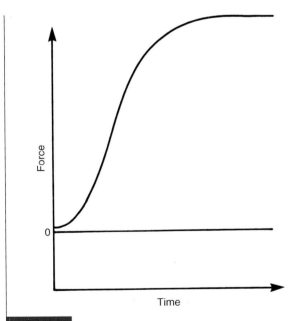

FIG. 6-12

Force-time curve for a whole muscle contracting isometrically. The force exerted by the muscle is greater when the contraction time is longer because time is required for the tension created by the contractile components to be transferred to the parallel elastic component and then to series elastic component as the musculotendinous unit is stretched.

ponent. It has been suggested that changes in the intrinsic mechanical properties of myofibrils are important in the stretch-induced enhancement of work production (Takarada et al., 1997).

EFFECT OF TEMPERATURE

A rise in muscle temperature causes an increase in conduction velocity across the sarcolemma (Phillips & Petrofsky, 1983), increasing the frequency of stimulation and hence the production of muscle force. Rising of the muscle temperature from 6 to 34°C results in an almost linear increase of the tension/stiffness ratio (Galler et al., 1998).

A rise in temperature also causes greater enzymatic activity of muscle metabolism, thus increasing the efficiency of muscle contraction. A further effect of a rise in temperature is the increased elasticity of the collagen in the series and parallel elastic components, which enhances the extensibility of the muscle-tendon unit. This increased prestretch increases the force production of the muscle.

Muscle temperature increases by means of two mechanisms:

1. Increase in blood flow, which occurs when an athlete "warms up" his or her muscles
2. Production of the heat of reaction generated by metabolism, by the release of the energy of contraction, and by friction as the contractile components slide over each other

However, at low temperature (10°C), it has been shown that the maximum shortening velocity and the isometric tension are inhibited significantly. This is caused by decreased pH (acidosis) in the muscle. The pH plays a much less important role at temperatures close to the physiological level (Pate et al., 1995).

EFFECT OF FATIGUE

The ability of a muscle to contract and relax is dependent on the availability of adenosine triphosphate (ATP) (Box 6-1). If a muscle has an adequate supply of oxygen and nutrients that can be broken down to provide ATP, it can sustain a series of low-frequency twitch responses for a long time. The frequency must be low enough to allow the muscle to synthesize ATP at a rate sufficient to keep up with the rate of ATP breakdown during contraction. If the frequency of stimulation increases and outstrips the rate of replacement of ATP, the twitch responses soon grow progressively weaker and eventually fall to zero (Fig. 6-14). This drop in tension following prolonged stimulation is muscle fatigue. If the frequency is high enough to produce tetanic contractions, fatigue occurs even sooner. If a period of rest is allowed before stimulation is continued, the ATP concentration rises and the muscle briefly recovers its contractile ability before again undergoing fatigue.

Three sources supply ATP in muscle: creatine phosphate, oxidative phosphorylation in the mitochondria, and substrate phosphorylation during anaerobic glycolysis. When contraction begins, the

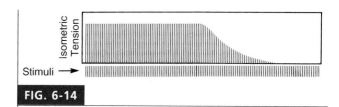

FIG. 6-14

Fatigue in a muscle contracting isometrically. Prolonged stimulation occurs at a frequency that outstrips the muscle's ability to produce sufficient ATP for contraction. As a result, tension production declines and eventually ceases. *Adapted from Luciano, D.S., Vander, A.J., & Sherman, J.H. (1978).* Human Function and Structure *(pp. 113–136). New York: McGraw-Hill.*

myosin ATPase rapidly breaks down ATP. The increase in adenosine diphosphate (ADP) and phosphate (Pi) concentrations resulting from this breakdown ultimately leads to increased rates of oxidative phosphorylation and glycolysis. After a short lapse, however, these metabolic pathways begin to deliver ATP at a high rate. During this interval, the energy for ATP formation is provided by creatine phosphate, which offers the most rapid means of forming ATP in the muscle cell.

At moderate rates of muscle activity, most of the required ATP can be formed by the process of oxidative phosphorylation. During intense exercise, when ATP is being broken down rapidly, the cell's ability to replace ATP by oxidative phosphorylation may be limited, primarily by inadequate delivery of oxygen to the muscle by the circulatory system.

Even when oxygen delivery is adequate, the rate at which oxidative phosphorylation can produce ATP may be insufficient to sustain intense exercise because the enzymatic machinery of this pathway is relatively slow. Anaerobic glycolysis then begins to contribute an increasing portion of the ATP. The glycolytic pathway, although it produces much smaller amounts of ATP from the breakdown of glucose, operates at a much faster rate. It can also proceed in the absence of oxygen, with the formation of lactic acid as its end product. Thus, during intense exercise, anaerobic glycolysis becomes an additional source for rapidly supplying the muscle with ATP.

The glycolytic pathway has the disadvantage of requiring large amounts of glucose for the production of small amounts of ATP. Thus, even though muscle stores glucose in the form of glycogen, existing glycogen supplies may be depleted quickly when muscle activity is intense. Finally, myosin ATPase may break down ATP faster than even glycolysis can replace it, and fatigue occurs rapidly as ATP concentrations drop.

After a period of intense exercise, creatine phosphate levels have become low and much of the muscle glycogen may have been converted to lactic acid. For the muscle to be returned to its original state, creatine phosphate must be resynthesized and the glycogen stores must be replaced. Because both processes require energy, the muscle will continue to consume oxygen at a rapid rate even though it has stopped contracting. This sustained high oxygen uptake is demonstrated by the fact that a person continues to breathe heavily and rapidly after a period of strenuous exercise.

When the energy necessary to return glycogen and creatine phosphate to their original levels is taken into account, the efficiency with which muscle converts chemical energy to work (movement) is usually no more than 20 to 25%, the majority of the energy being dissipated as heat. Even when muscle is operating in its most efficient state, a maximum of only approximately 45% of the energy is used for contraction (Arvidson et al., 1984; Guyton, 1986).

In growth biomechanics, muscle fatigue is first observed by the lack of coordination of movement and its effect in the increasing of loads in tissue. Researchers including Bates et al. (1977) have indicated that the skill of the person in performing a given action is affected by fatigue. They studied the fatigue effect on runners and observed that runners decrease their knee extension when fatigue occurs (Bates et al., 1977). Parnianpour (1988) studied the motion coupling of the spine at exhaustive extension flexion. This study showed that when an individual became fatigued, the coupled motion increased and therefore the spinal torque increased. The most deleterious component of the neuromuscular adaptation to the fatigue state was the reduction in accuracy control and speed of contraction, which may predispose an individual to injury if muscle fatigue occurs.

Muscle Fiber Differentiation

In the preceding section, we described the major factors that determine the total tension developed by the whole muscle when it contracts. Individual muscle fibers also display distinct differences in their rates of contraction, development of tension, and susceptibility to fatigue.

Many methods of classifying muscle fibers have been devised. As early as 1678, Lorenzini observed anatomically the gross difference between red and white muscle, and in 1873 Ranvier typed muscle on the basis of speed of contractility and fatigability. Although considerable confusion has existed concerning the method and terminology for classifying skeletal muscle, recent histological and histochemical observations have led to the identification of three distinct types of muscle fibers on the basis of differing contractile and metabolic properties (Brandstater & Lambert, 1969; Buchtahl & Sohmalburch, 1980) (Table 6-1).

The fiber types are distinguished mainly by the metabolic pathways by which they can generate ATP and the rate at which its energy is made available to the contractile system of the sarcomere, which determines the speed of contraction. The three fiber types are termed type I, slow-twitch oxidative (SO) fibers; type IIA, fast-twitch oxidative-glycolytic (FOG) fibers; and type IIB, fast-twitch glycolytic (FG) fibers.

Type I (SO) fibers are characterized by a low activity of myosin ATPase in the muscle fiber and, therefore, a relatively slow contraction time. The glycolytic (anaerobic) activity is low in this fiber type, but a high content of mitochondria produces a high potential for oxidative (aerobic) activity. Type I fibers are difficult to fatigue because the high rate of blood flow to these fibers delivers oxygen and nutrients at a sufficient rate to keep up with the relatively slow rate of ATP breakdown by myosin ATPase. Thus, the fibers are well suited for prolonged, low-intensity work. These fibers are relatively small in diameter and so produce relatively little tension. The high myoglobin content of type I fibers gives the muscle a red color.

Type II muscle fibers are divided into two main subgroups, IIA and IIB, on the basis of differing susceptibility to treatment with different buffers prior to incubation (Brooke & Kaiser, 1970). A third subgroup, the type IIC fibers, are rare, undifferentiated fibers, which are usually seen before the 30th week of gestation. This fiber type is infrequent in human muscle (Banker, 1994). Type IIA and IIB fibers are characterized by a high activity of myosin ATPase, which results in relatively fast contraction.

Type IIA (FOG) fibers are considered intermediate between type I and type IIB because their fast contraction time is combined with a moderately well-developed capacity for both aerobic (oxidative) and anaerobic (glycolytic) activity. These

TABLE 6-1

Properties of Three Types of Skeletal Muscle Fibers

	TYPE 1 Slow-Twitch Oxidative (SO)	TYPE IIA Fast-Twitch Oxidative-Glycolytic (FOG)	TYPE IIB Fast-Twitch Glycolytic (FG)
Speed of contraction	Slow	Fast	Fast
Primary source of ATP production	Oxidative phosphorylation	Oxidative phosphorylation	Anaerobic glycolysis
Glycolytic enzyme activity	Low	Intermediate	High
Capillaries	Many	Many	Few
Myoglobin content	High	High	Low
Glycogen content	Low	Intermediate	High
Fiber diameter	Small	Intermediate	Large
Rate of fatigue	Slow	Intermediate	Fast

fibers also have a well-developed blood supply. They can maintain their contractile activity for relatively long periods; however, at high rates of activity, the high rate of ATP splitting exceeds the capacity of both oxidative phosphorylation and glycolysis to supply ATP, and these fibers thus eventually fatigue. Because the myoglobin content of this muscle type is high, the muscle is often categorized as red muscle.

Type IIB (FG) fibers rely primarily on glycolytic (anaerobic) activity for ATP production. Few capillaries are found in the vicinity of these fibers and because they contain little myoglobin they are often referred to as white muscle. Although type IIB fibers are able to produce ATP rapidly, they fatigue easily because their high rate of ATP splitting quickly depletes the glycogen needed for glycolysis. These fibers generally are of large diameter and are thus able to produce great tension, but only for short periods before they fatigue.

It has been well demonstrated that the nerve innervating the muscle fiber determines its type (Burke et al., 1971); thus, the muscle fibers of each motor unit are of a single type. In humans and other species, electrical stimulation was found to change the fiber type (Munsat, McNeal, & Waters, 1976). In animal studies, transecting the nerves that innervate slow-twitch and fast-twitch muscle fibers and then crossing these nerves was noted to reverse the fiber types. After recovery from the cross-innervation, the slow-twitch fibers became fast in their con-

tractile and histochemical properties and the fast-twitch fibers became slow.

The fiber composition of a given muscle depends on the function of that muscle. Some muscles perform predominantly one form of contractile activity and are often composed mostly of one muscle fiber type. An example is the soleus muscle in the calf, which primarily maintains posture and is composed of a high percentage of type *I* fibers. More commonly, however, a muscle is required to perform endurance-type activity under some circumstances and high-intensity strength activity under others. These muscles generally contain a mixture of the three muscle fiber types.

In a typical mixed muscle exerting low tension, some of the small motor units, composed of type I fibers, contract. As the muscle force increases, more motor units are recruited and their frequency of stimulation increases. As the frequency becomes maximal, greater muscle force is achieved by recruitment of larger motor units composed of type IIA (FOG) fibers and eventually type IIB (FG) fibers. As the peak muscle force decreases, the larger units are the first to cease activity (Guyton, 1986; Luciano, Vander, & Sherman, 1978).

It is generally, but not universally, accepted that fiber types are genetically determined (Costill et al., 1976; Gollnick, 1982). In the average population, approximately 50 to 55% of muscle fibers are type I, approximately 30 to 35% are type IIA, and approximately 15% are type IIB, but these percentages vary greatly among individuals.

In elite athletes, the relative percentage of fiber types differs from that in the general population and appears to depend on whether the athlete's principal activity requires a short, explosive, maximal effort or involves submaximal endurance. Sprinters and shot putters, for example, have a high percentage of type II fibers, whereas distance runners and cross-country skiers have a higher percentage of type I fibers. Endurance athletes may have as many as 80% type I fibers, and those engaged in short, explosive efforts as few as 30% of these fibers (Saltin et al., 1977).

The genetically determined fiber typing may be responsible for the natural selective process by which athletes are drawn to the type of sport for which they are most suited. Because fiber types are determined by the nerve that innervates the muscle fiber, there may be some cortical control of this innervation that influences an athlete to choose the sport in which he or she is genetically able to excel.

Muscle Injuries

Muscle injuries comprise contusion, laceration, ruptures, ischemia, compartment syndromes, and denervation. These injuries weaken the muscles and can cause significant disability. Blunt trauma can diminish muscle strength, limit joint motion, and finally lead to myositis ossificans. Muscle laceration, surgical incisions, and traumatic lesion to muscle tissue and denervation weaken the muscles, sometimes significantly. Ruptures in muscles also can cause weakness. Like the other injuries, they may result from direct trauma, but muscle contractions against resistance also can lead to tears in muscle tissue.

Acute muscle ischemia and compartment syndromes can cause extensive muscle necrosis. The many potential causes of compartment syndrome all result in increased pressure within a confined muscle compartment. In this case, failure to relieve the pressure rapidly may cause complications that range from weakness and decreased motion to loss of an entire limb.

Studies have shown that healthy skeletal muscle has a substantial capacity to repair itself. This repair process following a specific injury is inferred by the prior innovation pattern, vascularization,

physical constraint of the surrounding tissues, the extent and condition of extracellular matrices, and the development of repair cells. Muscle injuries are important but the topic is not within the scope of this chapter. Injuries should be investigated carefully if suspicion arises that a patient has muscle damage.

Muscle Remodeling

The remodeling of muscle tissue is similar to that of other skeletal tissues such as bone, articular cartilage, and ligaments. As in these other tissues, muscle atrophies in response to disuse and immobilization and hypertrophies when subjected to greater use than usual.

EFFECTS OF DISUSE AND IMMOBILIZATION

Disuse and immobilization have detrimental effects on muscle fibers. These effects include loss of endurance and strength and muscle atrophies on a microstructural and macrostructural level, such as decreased numbers and size of fiber. Biochemical changes occur and affect aerobic and anaerobic energy production. These effects are dependent on fiber type and muscle length during immobilization. Immobilization in a lengthened position has a less deleterious effect (Appell, 1997; Kasser, 1996; Ohira et al., 1997; Sandmann, et al., 1998).

Clinical and laboratory studies of human and animal muscle tissue suggest that a program of immediate or early motion may prevent muscle atrophy after injury or surgery. In a study of crush injuries to rat muscle, the effect of immobilization of the crushed limb was compared with that of immediate motion. The muscle fibers were found to regenerate in a more parallel orientation in the mobilized animal than in the immobilized animal, capillarization occurred more rapidly, and tensile strength returned more quickly. Similar results were found in a later study on the effect of immobilization on the morphology of rat calf muscles (Kannus et al., 1998a).

It has been found clinically that atrophy of the quadriceps muscle that develops while the limb is immobilized in a rigid plaster cast cannot be reversed through the use of isometric exercises. Atrophy may be limited by allowing early motion such as that permitted by a partly mobile cast brace. In this case, dynamic exercises can be performed.

Human muscle biopsy studies have shown that it is mainly the type I fibers that atrophy with immobilization; their cross-sectional area decreases and their potential for oxidative enzyme activity is reduced (Kannus et al., 1998b). Early motion may prevent this atrophy. It appears that if the muscle is placed under tension when the body segment moves, afferent (sensory) impulses from the intrafusal muscle spindles will increase, leading to increased stimulation of the type I fiber. Although intermittent isometric exercise may be sufficient to maintain the metabolic capacity of the type II fiber, the type I fiber (the postural fiber) requires a more continuous impulse. Evidence also suggests that electric stimulation may prevent the decrease in type I fiber size and the decline in its oxidative enzyme activity caused by immobilization (Eriksson et al., 1981).

In elite athletes, inactivity following injury, surgery, or immobilization rapidly decreases the size and aerobic capability of muscle fibers, particularly in the fiber type affected by the chosen sport. In endurance athletes, type I fibers are affected, while in athletes engaged in an explosive activity such as sprinting, type II fibers are affected.

EFFECTS OF PHYSICAL TRAINING

Physical training increases the cross-sectional area of all muscle fibers, accounting for the increase in muscle bulk and strength. Some evidence suggests that the relative percentage of fiber types composing a person's muscles may also change with physical training (Arvidson, Eriksson, & Pitman, 1984). The cross-sectional area of the fibers affected by the athlete's principal activity increases. For example, in endurance athletes, the area of muscle taken up by type I and type IIA fibers increases at the expense of the total area of type IIB fibers (Case Study 6-2).

Stretching increases muscle flexibility, maintains and augments the range of joint motion, and increases the elasticity and length of the musculotendinous unit (Brobeck, 1979; Cuillo & Zarins, 1983). It also permits the musculotendinous unit to store more energy in its viscoelastic and contractile components.

The events that take place during muscle stretching are complex and incompletely under-

stood (Gollnick, 1982; Guyton, 1986). It appears that these events are controlled or modified by both the intrafusal muscle spindles, located in parallel with the extrafusal fibers of the muscle belly, and the Golgi tendon organs, located in series with

---

CASE STUDY 6-2

Ruptured Left Anterior Cruciate Ligament

A 25-year-old male, status postsurgical repair of the ruptured left anterior cruciate ligament, had torque measurements taken from the involved and uninvolved limb 10 weeks after the surgical procedure (Fig. cs6-2-1*A*) and repeated 6 weeks after the training began (Fig. cs6-2-1*B*). An increase of muscle torque is shown in the repeated isokinetic test. The initial deficit of the involved side was approximately 63% when compared with the uninvolved side. After 6 weeks of training, the deficit of the involved side compared with the uninvolved side decreased to 43%.

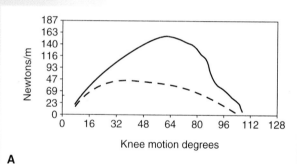

A

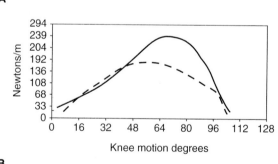

B

Case Study Figure 6-2-1 Isokinetic test at 180°/sec. **A,** Measurement of the quadriceps femoris torque production at 10 weeks postsurgical procedure. The *dashed line* represents torque output by the involved limb. The *solid line* represents torque output by the noninvolved limb. **B,** Measurements of the quadriceps femoris torque production at 16 weeks postsurgical procedure and 6 weeks after training sessions. The *dashed line* represents torque output by the involved limb. The *solid line* represents torque output by the noninvolved limb.

these fibers. The spindles respond to an increase in muscle length and the Golgi apparatus to an increase in muscle tension. The resulting spindle reflex increases muscle contraction, while the Golgi reflex inhibits contraction and enhances muscle relaxation.

The intrafusal muscle spindles are of two types: primary and secondary. The primary spindles respond to changes in the rate of muscle lengthening (dynamic response) and the actual amount of lengthening. The secondary spindles respond only to the actual length change (static response). The static response is weak and the dynamic response is strong; therefore, keeping the rate of stretch low may allow the dynamic response to be bypassed, essentially negating the effect of the spindles. Conversely, the increase in muscle tension during stretching may activate the relaxing effect of the Golgi apparatus and thus enhance further stretching. The various methods and theories of stretching all have as a common goal inhibition of the spindle effect and enhancement of the Golgi effect to relax the muscle and promote further lengthening.

Summary

1 The structural unit of skeletal muscle is the fiber, which is encompassed by the endomysium and organized into fascicles encased in the perimysium. The epimysium surrounds the entire muscle.

2 The fibers are composed of myofibrils, aligned so as to create a band pattern. Each repeat of this pattern is a sarcomere, the functional unit of the contractile system.

3 The myofibrils are composed of thin filaments of the protein actin and thick filaments of the protein myosin, and the intramyofibrillar cytoskeleton is composed of the elastic filaments titin and the inelastic filaments nebulin.

4 According to the sliding filament theory, active shortening of the muscle results from the relative movement of the actin and myosin filaments past one another. The force of contraction is developed by movement of the myosin heads, or cross-bridges, in contact with the actin filaments. Troponin and tropomyosin, two proteins in the actin helix, regulate the making and breaking of the contacts between filaments.

5 A key to the sliding mechanism is the calcium ion, which turns the contractile activity on and off.

6 The motor unit, a single motor neuron and all muscle fibers innervated by it, is the smallest part of the muscle that can contract independently. The calling in of additional motor units in response to greater stimulation of the motor nerve is known as recruitment.

7 The tendons and the endomysium, perimysium, sarcolemma, and epimysium represent parallel and series elastic components that stretch with active contraction or passive muscle extension and recoil with muscle relaxation.

8 Summation occurs when mechanical responses of the muscle to successive stimuli are added to an initial response. When maximal tension is sustained as a result of summation, the muscle contracts tetanically. The muscle fiber contracts in an all-or-nothing fashion.

9 Muscles may contract concentrically, eccentrically, or isometrically depending on the relationship between the muscle tension and the resistance to be overcome. Concentric and eccentric contractions involve dynamic work, in which the muscle moves a joint or controls its movement.

10 Force production in muscle is influenced by the length-tension, load-velocity, and force-time relationships of the muscle. The length-tension relationship in a whole muscle is influenced by both active (contractile) and passive (series and parallel elastic) components.

11 Two other factors that increase force production are prestretching of the muscle and a rise in muscle temperature.

12 The energy for muscle contraction and its release is provided by the hydrolytic splitting of ATP. Muscle fatigue occurs when the ability of the muscle to synthesize ATP is insufficient to keep up with the rate of ATP breakdown during contraction.

13 Three main fiber types have been identified: type I, slow-twitch oxidative; type IIA, fast-twitch oxidative-glycolytic; and type IIB, fast-twitch glycolytic fibers. Most muscles contain a mixture of these types.

14 Muscle atrophies occur under disuse and immobilization; muscle trophism can be restored through early and active remobilization.

REFERENCES

Appell, H.J. (1997). The muscle in the rehabilitation process. *Orthopade, 26*(11), 930–934.

Arvidson, I., Eriksson, E., & Pitman, M. (1984). Neuromuscular basis of rehabilitation. In E. Hunter & J. Funk (Eds.), *Rehabilitation of the Injured Knee* (pp. 210–234). St. Louis: C. V. Mosby.

Banker, B.Q. (1994). Basic reaction of muscle. In A.G. Engel & C. Franzini-Armstrong (Eds.), *Myology* (2nd ed.). New York: McGraw-Hill, Inc.

Baratta R.V., Solomonow, M., Zhou, B.H. (1998). Frequency domain-based models of skeletal muscle. *J Electromyogr Kinesiol, 8*(2), 79-91.

Bates, B.T., Osterning, L.R., James, S.L. (1977). Fatigue effects in running. *J Motor Behav, 9*, 203–207.

Brobeck, J. R. (Ed.) (1979). *Best and Taylor's Physiological Basis of Medical Practice* (10th ed., pp. 59–113). Baltimore: Williams & Wilkins.

Brooke, M.H. & Kaiser, K.K. (1970). Three myosin adenosine triphosphatase systems: The nature of their pH liability and sulfhydryl dependence. *J Histochem Cytochem, 18*, 670.

Buchtahl, F. & Sohmalburch, H. (1980). Motor units of mammalian muscle. *Physiol Rev, 60*, 90.

Burke, R.E., Levine, D.N., Zajac, F.E. (1971). Mammalian motor units: Physiological histochemical correlation in three types of motor units in cat gastrocnemius. *Science, 174*, 709.

Costill, D.L., Coyle, E.F., Fink, W.F., Lesmes, G.R., Wilzmann, F.A. (1979). Adaptation in skeletal muscles following strength training. *J Appl Physiol, 46*,96-9.

Craig, R. (1994). The structure of the contract filaments. In A.G. Engel & C. Franzini-Armstrong (Eds.), *Myology* (2nd ed.). New York: McGraw-Hill, Inc.

Crawford, C.N.C. & James, N.T. (1980). The design of muscles. In R. Owen, J. Goodfellow, & P. Bullough (Eds.) *Scientific Foundations of Orthopaedics and Traumatology* (pp. 67–74). London: William Heinemann.

Cuillo, J.V. & Zarins, B. (1983). Biomechanics of the musculotendinous unit: Relation to athletic performance and injury. *Clin Sports Med, 2*, 71.

Eriksson, E., Haggmark, T., Kiessling, K.H., et al. (1981). Effect of electrical stimulation on human skeletal muscle. *Int Sports Med, 2*, 18.

Galler, S., Hilber, K. (1998). Tension/stiffness ratio of skinned rat skeletal muscle fibre types at various temperatures. *Act Physiol Scand, 162*(2), 119–126.

Gollnick, P.D. (1982). Relationship of strength and endurance with skeletal muscle structure and metabolic potential. *Int J Sports Med [Suppl], 3*, 26.

Gordon, A.M., Huxley, A.F.I., & Julian, F.J. (1966). The variation in isometric tension with sarcomere length in vertebrate muscle fibers. *J Physiol, 184*, 170.

Guyton, A.C. (1986). *Textbook of Medical Physiology* (7th ed.). Philadelphia: W.B. Saunders.

Ham, A.W. & Cormack, D.H. (1979). *Histology* (8th ed.). Philadelphia: J.B. Lippincott.

Hill, A.V. (1970). *First and Last Experiments in Muscle Mechanics*. Cambridge: Cambridge University Press.

Hill, D.K. (1968). Tension due to interaction between the sliding filaments of resting striated muscle. The effect of stimulation. *Physiol [Lond], 199*, 637.

Hislop, H.J. & Perrine, J. (1967). The isokinetic concept of exercise. *Phys Ther, 47*, 114.

Huxley, A.F. (1974). Muscular contraction. *J Physiol, 243*, 1.

Huxley, A.F. & Huxley, H.E. (1964). Organizers of a discussion of the physical and chemical basis of muscular contraction. *Proc R Sec, B160*, 433.

Kannus, P., Jozsa, L., Kvist, M., Jarvinen, T., Jarvinen, M. (1998a). Effects of immobilization and subsequent low- and high-intensity exercise on morphology of rat calf muscles. *Scand J Med Sci Sports, 8*(3), 160–171.

Kannus, P., Jozsa, L., Jarvinen, T.L., Kvist, M., Vieno, T., Jarvinen, M. (1998b). Free mobilization and low- to high-intensity exercise in immobilization-induced muscle atrophy. *J Appl Physiol, 84*(4), 1418–1424.

Kasser, J.R. (1996). General Knowledge. In J.R. Kasser (Ed.) *Orthopaedic Knowledge Update 5: Home Study Syllabus.* Illinois: American Academy of Orthopaedic Surgeons.

Keele, C.A., Neil, E., & Joels, N. (1982). Muscle and the nervous system. In *Samson Wright's Applied Physiology* (13th ed., pp. 248–259). Oxford: Oxford University Press.

Komi, P.V. (1986). The stretch-shortening cycle and human power output. In N.L. Jones, N. McCartney, & A.J. McConas (Eds.) *Human Muscle Power* (pp. 27–39). Champaign, IL: Human Kinetics Publishers.

Kroemer, K.H.E., Marras, W.M., McGlothlin, J.D., et al. (1990). On the measurement of human strength. *Int J Indust Ergonomics, 6*, 199–210.

Kroll, P.G. (1987). *The effect of previous contraction condition on subsequent eccentric power production in elbow flexor muscles.* Unpublished doctoral dissertation, New York University, New York.

Lieber, RL. & Bodine-Fowler, S.C. (1993). Skeletal muscle mechanics. Implications for rehabilitation. *Phys Ther, 73*(12), 844–856.

Linke, W.A., Ivemeyer, M., Mundel, P., Stockmeier, M.R., Kolmerer, B. (1998). Nature of PEVK-titin elasticity in skeletal muscle. *Proc Natl Acad Sci USA, 95*(14), 8052–8057.

Luciano, D.S., Vander, A.J., & Sherman, J.H. (1978). *Human Function and Structure* (pp. 113–136). New York: McGraw-Hill.

Munsat, T.L., NcNeal, D., & Waters, R. (1976). Effects of nerve stimulation on human muscle. *Arch Neurol, 33*, 608.

Ohira, Y., Yasui, W., Roy, R.R., Edgerton, V.R. (1997). Effects of muscle length on the response to unloading. *Acta Anat (Basel), 159*(2–3), 90–98.

Ottoson, D. (1983). *Physiology of the Nervous System* (pp. 78–116). New York: Oxford University Press.

Parnianpour, M., Nordin, M., Kahanovitz, N., et al. (1988). The triaxial coupling torque generation of trunk muscles during isometric exertions and the effect of fatiguing isoinertial movements on the motor output and movement patterns. *Spine, 13*(9).

Pate, E., Bhimani, M., Franks-Skiba, K., Cook, R. (1995). Reduced effect of pH on skinned rabbit psoas muscle mechanics at high temperatures: Implications for fatigue. *J Physiol (Lond), 486*(Pt 3), 689–694.

Phillips, C.A. & Petrofsky, J.S. (1983). *Mechanics of Skeletal and Cardiac Muscle*. Springfield: Charles C. Thomas.

Saltin, B., et al. (1977). Fiber types and metabolic potentials of skeletal muscles in sedentary man and endurance runners. *Ann NY Acad Sci, 301*, 3.

Sandmann, M.E., Shoemann, J.A., Thompson, L.V. (1998). The fiber-type-specific effect of inactivity and intermittent weight-bearing on the gastrocnemius of 30-month-old rats. *Arch Phys Med Rehabil, 79*(6), 658–662.

Squire, J.M. (1997). Architecture and function in the muscle sarcomere. *Curr Opin Struct Biol, 7*(2), 247–257.

Stromer, M.H. (1998). The cytoskeleton in skeletal, cardiac and smooth muscle cells. *Histol Histopathol, 13*(1), 283–291.

Takarada, Y., Iwamoto, H., Sugi, H., Hirano, Y., Ishii, N. (1997). Stretch-induced enhancement of mechanical work production in long frog single fibers and human muscle. *J Appl Physiol, 83*(5), 1741–1748.

Wilkie, D.R. (1956). The mechanical properties of muscle. *Br Med Bull, 12,* 177.

Wilkie, D.R. (1968). *Muscle.* London: Edward Arnold.

Williams, P. & Warwick, R. (1980). *Gray's Anatomy* (36th ed., pp. 506–515). Edinburgh: Churchill Livingstone.

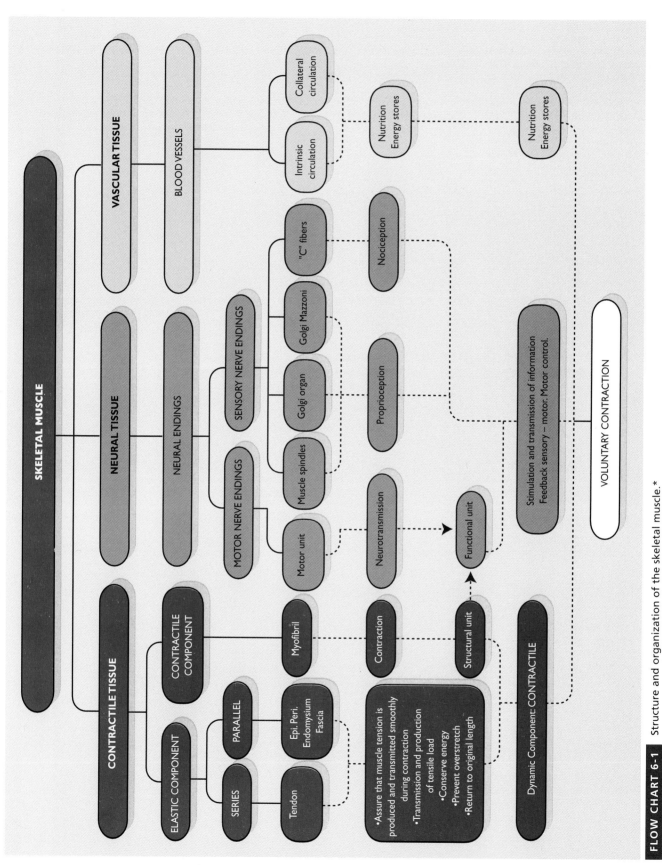

FLOW CHART 6-1 Structure and organization of the skeletal muscle. *

*This flow chart is designed for classroom or group discussion. Flow chart is not meant to be exhaustive.

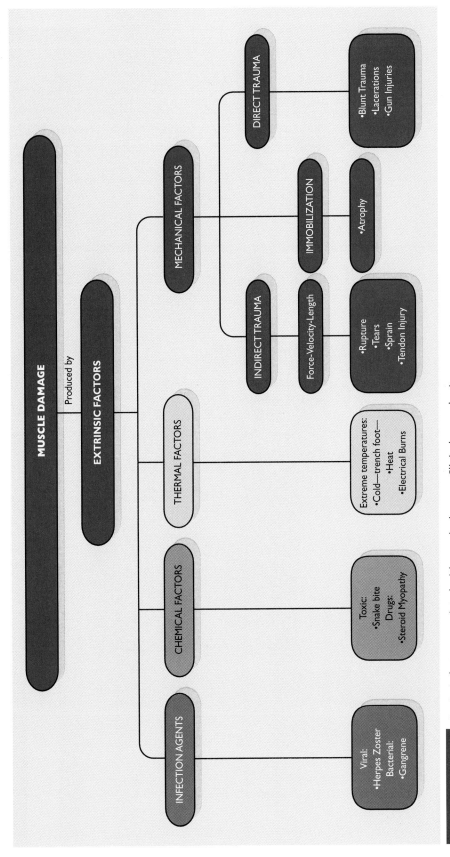

FLOW CHART 6-2   Extrinsic factors associated with muscle damage. Clinical examples.*

*This flow chart is designed for classroom or group discussion. Flow chart is not meant to be exhaustive.

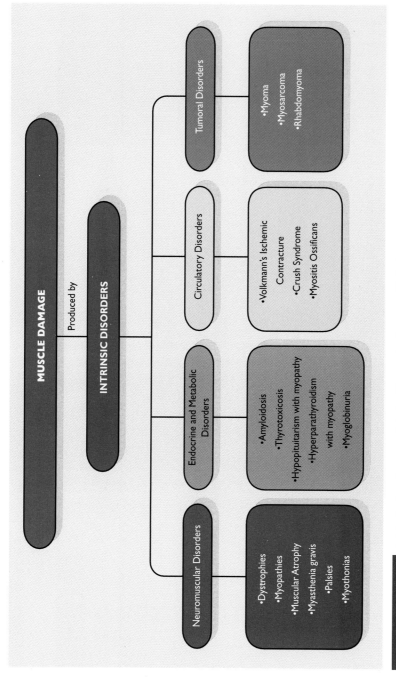

FLOW CHART 6-3   Intrinsic disorders associated with muscle damage. Clinical examples.*

*This flow chart is designed for classroom or group discussion. Flow chart is not meant to be exhaustive.

PART II

Biomechanics of Joints

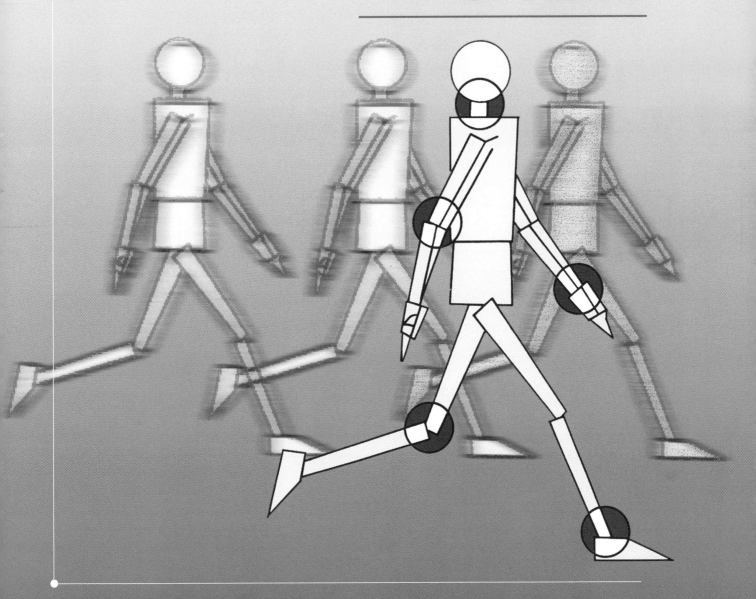

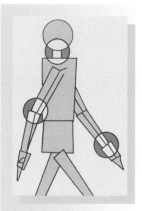

CHAPTER 7

Biomechanics
of the Knee

Margareta Nordin, Victor H. Frankel

Introduction

The knee transmits loads, participates in motion, aids in conservation of momentum, and provides a force couple for activities involving the leg. The human knee, the largest and perhaps most complex joint in the body, is a two-joint structure composed of the tibiofemoral joint and the patellofemoral joint (Fig. 7-1). The knee sustains high forces and moments and is situated between the body's two longest lever arms (the femur and the tibia), making it particularly susceptible to injury. This chapter utilizes the knee to introduce the basic terms, explain the methods, and demonstrate the calculations necessary for analyzing joint motion and the forces and moments acting on a joint. This information is applied to other joints in subsequent chapters.

The knee is particularly well suited for demonstrating biomechanical analyses of joints because these analyses can be simplified in the knee and still yield useful data. Although knee motion occurs simultaneously in three planes, the motion in one plane is so great that it accounts for nearly all of the motion. Also, although many muscles produce forces on the knee, at any particular instant one muscle group predominates, generating a force so great that it accounts for most of the muscle force acting on the knee. Thus, basic biomechanical analyses can be limited to motion in one plane and to the force produced by a single muscle group and still give an understanding of knee motion and an estimation of the magnitude of the principal forces and moments on the knee. Advanced biomechanical dynamic analyses of the knee joint that include all

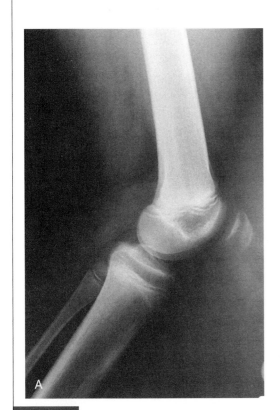

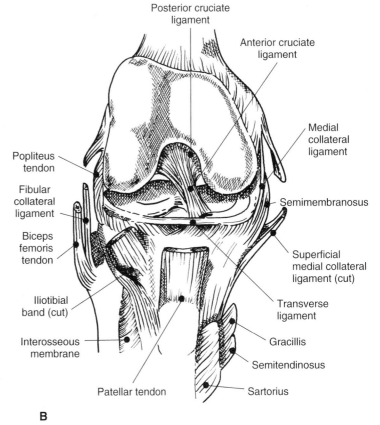

FIG. 7-1

Two-joint structure of the knee. **A,** Lateral view of a knee joint with open growth plates.
B, Anterior view without patella.

soft tissue structures are complex and still under investigation.

Analysis of motion in any joint requires the use of kinematic data. Kinematics is the branch of mechanics that deals with motion of a body without reference to force or mass. Analysis of the forces and moments acting on a joint necessitates the use of both kinematic and kinetic data. Kinetics is the branch of mechanics that deals with the motion of a body under the action of given forces and/or moments.

Kinematics

Kinematics defines the range of motion and describes the surface motion of a joint in three planes: frontal (coronal or longitudinal), sagittal, and transverse (horizontal) (Fig. 7-2, *A & B*). Clinical measurements of joint range of motion define the anatomical position as a zero position for measurement. This taxonomy will be used for joint motion throughout this book. Other taxonomies and reference systems exist (Andriacchi et al., 1979; Grood &

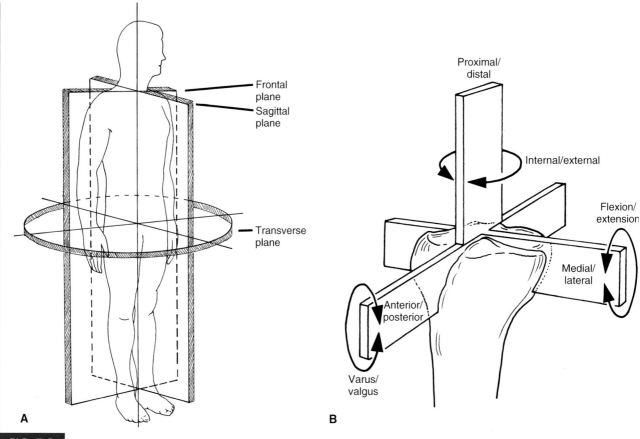

FIG. 7-2

A, Frontal (coronal or longitudinal), sagittal, and transverse (horizontal) planes in the human body performed easily for both the tibiofemoral and the patellofemoral joint. **B,** Depiction and nomenclature of the six degrees of freedom of knee motion: anterior posterior translation, medial/lateral translation and proximal distal translation, flexion-extension rotation, internal-external rotation, varus-valgus rotation.
Adapted from Wilson, S.A., Vigorita, V.J., & Scott, W.N. (1994). *Anatomy. In N. Scott (Ed.), The Knee (p. 17). Philadelphia: Mosby-Year Book.*

Suntay 1983; Kroemer et al., 1990; Özkaya & Nordin, 1999), but the anatomical reference system by far is the most commonly used among clinicians. Of the two joints composing the knee, the tibiofemoral joint lends itself particularly well to an analysis of range of joint motion. Analysis of surface joint motion can be performed easily for both the tibiofemoral and the patellofemoral joint. Any impediment of range of motion or surface joint motion will disturb the normal loading pattern of a joint and bear consequences.

RANGE OF MOTION

The range of motion of any joint can be measured in any plane. Gross measurements can be made with a goniometer, but more specific measurements require the use of more precise methods such as electrogoniometry, roentgenography, stereophotogrammetry, or photographic and video techniques using skeletal pins.

In the tibiofemoral joint, motion takes place in all three planes, but the range of motion is greatest by far in the sagittal plane. Motion in this plane from full extension to full flexion of the knee is from 0° to approximately 140°.

Motion in the transverse plane, internal and external rotation, is influenced by the position of the joint in the sagittal plane. With the knee in full extension, rotation is almost completely restricted by the interlocking of the femoral and tibial condyles, which occurs mainly because the medial femoral condyle is longer than the lateral condyle. The range of rotation increases as the knee is flexed, reaching a maximum at 90° of flexion; with the knee in this position, external rotation ranges from 0° to approximately 45° and internal rotation ranges from 0° to approximately 30°. Beyond 90° of flexion, the range of internal and external rotation decreases, primarily because the soft tissues restrict rotation.

Motion in the frontal plane, abduction and adduction, is similarly affected by the amount of joint flexion. Full extension of the knee precludes almost all motion in the frontal plane. Passive abduction and adduction increase with knee flexion up to 30°, but each reaches a maximum of only a few degrees. With the knee flexed beyond 30°, motion in the frontal plane again decreases because of the limiting function of the soft tissues.

The range of tibiofemoral joint motion required for the performance of various physical activities can be determined from kinematic analysis. Motion

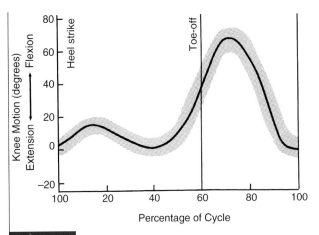

FIG. 7-3

Range of motion of the tibiofemoral joint in the sagittal plane during level walking in one gait cycle. The *shaded area* indicates variation among 60 subjects (age range 20 to 65 years). *Adapted from Murray, M.P., Drought, A.B., Kory, R.C. (1964). Walking patterns of normal men.* J Bone Joint Surg, 46A, *335.*

in this joint during walking has been measured in all planes. The range of motion in the sagittal plane during level walking was measured with an electrogoniometer by Lamoreaux (1971) and Murray et al. (1964). Full or nearly full extension was noted at the beginning of the stance phase (0% of cycle) at heel strike, and at the end of the stance phase before toe-off (around 60% of cycle) (Fig. 7-3). Maximum flexion (approximately 60°) was observed during the middle of the swing phase (see Chapter 18, Biomechanics of Gait, for more detailed information). These measurements are velocity-dependent and must be interpreted with caution.

Motion in the transverse plane during walking has been measured by several investigators. Using a photographic technique involving the placement of skeletal pins through the femur and tibia, Levens and associates (1948) found that total rotation of the tibia with respect to the femur ranged from approximately 4 to 13° in 12 subjects (mean 8.6°). Greater rotation (mean 13.3°) was noted by Kettelkamp and coworkers (1970), who used electrogoniometry on 22 subjects. In both studies, external rotation began during knee extension in the stance phase and reached a peak value at the end of the swing phase just before heel strike. Internal rotation was noted during flexion in the swing phase.

TABLE 7-1

Range of Tibiofemoral Joint Motion in the Sagittal Plane During Common Activities

Activity	Range of Motion from Knee Extension to Knee Flexion (Degrees)
Walking	0–67[a]
Climbing stairs	0–83[b]
Descending stairs	0–90
Sitting down	0–93
Tying a shoe	0–106
Lifting an object	0–117

[a]Data from Kettelkamp et al. (1970). Mean for 22 subjects. A slight difference was found between right and left knees (mean for right knee 68.1°, mean for left knee 66.7°).

[b]These and subsequent data from Laubenthal et al. (1972). Mean for 30 subjects.

Kettelkamp's group (1970) also measured motion in the frontal plane during walking. In nearly all of the 22 subjects, maximal abduction of the tibia was observed during extension at heel strike and at the beginning of the stance phase; maximal adduction occurred as the knee was flexed during the swing phase. The total amount of abduction and adduction averaged 11°.

Values for the range of motion of the tibiofemoral joint in the sagittal plane during several common activities are presented in Table 7-1. Maximal knee flexion occurs during lifting. A range of motion from full extension to at least 117° of flexion appears to be required for an individual to carry out the activities of daily living in a normal manner. Any restriction of knee motion can be compensated for by increased motion in other joints. In studying the range of tibiofemoral joint motion during various activities, researchers found that an increased speed of movement requires a greater range of motion in the tibiofemoral joint (Holden et al., 1997; Perry et al., 1977). As the pace accelerates from walking slowly to running, progressively more knee flexion is needed during the stance phase (Table 7-2).

SURFACE JOINT MOTION

Surface joint motion, which is the motion between the articulating surfaces of a joint, can be described for any joint in any plane with the use of stereophotogrammetric methods (Selvik, 1978, 1983). Be-

cause these methods are highly technical and complex, a simpler method evolved in the nineteenth century is still used (Reuleaux, 1876). This method, called the instant center technique, allows surface joint motion to be analyzed in the sagittal and frontal planes but not in the transverse plane. The instant center technique provides a description of the relative uniplanar motion of two adjacent segments of a body and the direction of displacement of the contact points between these segments.

The skeletal portion of a body segment is called a link. As one link rotates about the other, at any instant there is a point that does not move, that is, a point that has zero velocity. This point constitutes an instantaneous center of motion, or instant center. The instant center is found by identifying the displacement of two points on a link as the link moves from one position to another in relation to an adjacent link, which is considered to be stationary. The points on the moving link in its original position and in its displaced position are designated on a graph and lines are drawn connecting the two sets of points. The perpendicular bisectors of these two lines are then drawn. The intersection of the perpendicular bisectors is the instant center.

Clinically, a pathway of the instant center for a joint can be determined by taking successive roentgenograms of the joint in different positions (usually 10° apart) throughout the range of motion in one plane and applying the Reuleaux method for locating the instant center for each interval of motion.

When the instant center pathway has been determined for joint motion in one plane, the surface joint motion can be described. For each interval of motion, the point at which the joint surfaces make contact is located on the roentgenograms used for the instant center analysis, and a line is drawn from

TABLE 7-2

Amount of Knee Flexion During Stance Phase of Walking and Running

Activity	Range in Amount of Knee Flexion During Stance Phase (Degrees)
Walking	
Slow	0–6
Free	6–12
Fast	12–18
Running	18–30

Data from Perry et al. (1977). Range for seven subjects.

the instant center to the contact point. A second line drawn at right angles to this line indicates the direction of displacement of the contact points. The direction of displacement of these points throughout the range of motion describes the surface motion in the joint. In most joints, the instant centers lie at a distance from the joint surface, and the line indicating the direction of displacement of the contact points is tangential to the load-bearing surface, demonstrating that one joint surface is gliding on the other (load-bearing) surface. In the case in which the instant center is found on the surface, the joint has a rolling motion and there is no gliding function. Because the instant center technique allows a description of motion in one plane only, it is not useful for describing the surface joint motion if more than 15° of motion takes place in any plane other than the one being measured.

In the knee, surface joint motion occurs between the tibial and femoral condyles and between the femoral condyles and the patella. In the tibiofemoral joint, surface motion takes place in all three planes simultaneously but is considerably less in the transverse and frontal planes. Surface motion in the patellofemoral joint takes place in two planes simultaneously, the frontal and transverse, but is far greater in the frontal plane.

Tibiofemoral Joint

An example will illustrate the use of the instant center technique to describe the surface motion of the tibiofemoral joint in the sagittal plane. To determine the pathway of the instant center of this joint during flexion, a lateral roentgenogram is taken of the knee in full extension and successive films are taken at 10° intervals of increased flexion. Care is taken to keep the tibia parallel to the x-ray table and to prevent rotation about the femur. When a patient has limited knee motion, the knee is flexed or extended only as far as the patient can tolerate.

Two points on the femur that are easily identified on all roentgenograms are selected and desig-

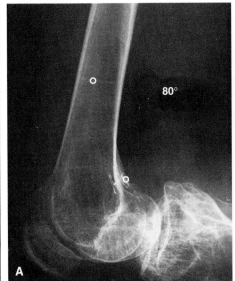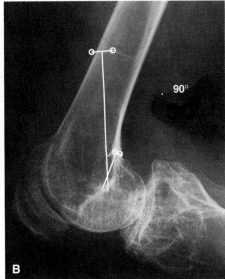

FIG. 7-4

Locating the instant center. **A,** Two easily identifiable points on the femur are designated on a roentgenogram of a knee flexed 80°. **B,** This roentgenogram is compared with a roentgenogram of the knee flexed 90°, on which the same two points have been indicated. The images of the tibiae are superimposed, and lines are drawn connecting each set of points. The perpendicular bisectors of these two lines are then drawn. The point at which these perpendicular bisectors intersect is the instant center of the tibiofemoral joint for the motion between 80 and 90° of flexion. *Courtesy of Ian Goldie, M.D. University of Gothenburg, Gothenburg, Sweden.*

nated on each roentgenogram (Fig. 7-4A). The films are then compared in pairs, with the images of the tibiae superimposed on each other. Roentgenograms with marked differences in tibial alignment are not used. Lines are drawn between the points on the femur in the two positions, and the perpendicular bisectors of these lines are then drawn. The point at which these perpendicular bisectors intersect is the instant center of the tibiofemoral joint for each 10° interval of motion (Fig. 7-4B). The instant center pathway throughout the entire range of knee flexion and extension can then be plotted. In a normal knee, the instant center pathway for the tibiofemoral joint is semicircular (Fig. 7-5).

After the instant center pathway has been determined for the tibiofemoral joint, the surface motion can be described. On each set of superimposed roent-genograms the point of contact of the tibiofemoral joint surfaces (the narrowest point in the joint space) is determined and a line is drawn connecting this point with the instant center. A second line drawn at right angles to this line indicates the direction of displacement of the contact points. In a normal knee, this line is tangential to the surface of the tibia for each interval of motion from full extension to full flexion, demonstrating that the femur is gliding on the tibial condyles (Frankel et al., 1971) (Fig. 7-6). During normal knee motion in the sagittal plane from full extension to full flexion, the instant center pathway moves posteriorly, forcing a combination of rolling and sliding to occur between the articular surface (Fig 7-6, A & B). The unique mechanism prevents the femur from rolling off the posterior aspect of the tibia plateau as the knee goes into increased flexion (Draganich et al., 1987; Fu et al., 1994; Kapandji, 1970). The mechanism that prevents this roll-off is the link formed between the tibial and femoral attachment sites of the anterior and posterior cruciate ligaments and the osseous geometry of the femoral condyles (Fu et al., 1994) (Fig. 7-6, B–D).

Frankel and associates (1971) determined the instant center pathway and analyzed the surface motion of the tibiofemoral joint from 90° of flexion to full extension in 25 normal knees; tangential gliding was noted in all cases. They also determined the instant center pathway for the tibiofemoral joint in 30 knees with internal derangement and found that, in all cases, the instant center was displaced from the normal position during some portion of the motion examined. The abnormal instant cen-

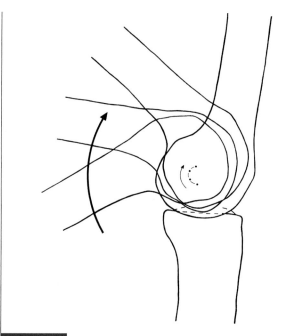

FIG. 7-5

Semicircular instant center pathway for the tibiofemoral joint in a 19-year-old man with a normal knee.

ter pathway for one subject, a 35-year-old man with a bucket-handle derangement, is shown in Figure 7-7.

If the knee is extended and flexed about an abnormal instant center pathway, the tibiofemoral joint surfaces do not glide tangentially throughout the range of motion but become either distracted or compressed (Fig. 7-8). Such a knee is analogous to a door with a bent hinge that no longer fits into the door jamb. If the knee is continually forced to move about a displaced instant center, a gradual adjustment to the situation will be reflected either by stretching of the ligaments and other supporting soft tissues or by the imposition of abnormally high pressure on the articular surfaces.

Internal derangements of the tibiofemoral joint may interfere with the so-called screw-home mechanism, which is external rotation during extension of the tibia (Fig. 7-9). The tibiofemoral joint is not a simple hinge joint; it has a spiral, or helicoid, motion. The spiral motion of the tibia about the femur during flexion and extension results from the anatomical configuration of the

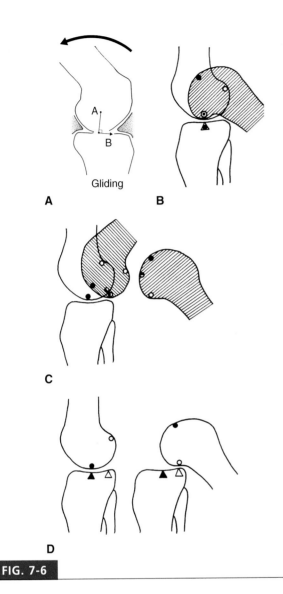

Gliding

A   B

C

D

FIG. 7-6

A, In a normal knee, a line drawn from the instant center of the tibiofemoral joint to the tibiofemoral contact point (*line A*) forms a right angle with a line tangential to the tibial surface (*line B*). The *arrow* indicates the direction of displacement of the contact points. Line B is tangential to the tibial surface, indicating that the femur glides on the tibial condyles during the measured interval of motion. **B,** Pure sliding of the femur on the tibia with knee extension. Note that the contact point of the tibia does not change as the femur slides over it. Eventually impingement would occur if all surface motion was restricted to sliding. Round points delineate contact points at the femur and triangles delineate contact points at the tibia. **C,** Pure rolling of the femur on the tibia with knee flexion. Note that both the tibia and the femoral contact points change as the femur rolls on the tibia. Also note that with moderate flexion, the femur will begin to roll off the tibia if surface motion was restricted to rolling. **D,** Actual knee motion including both sliding and rolling.

medial femoral condyle; in a normal knee, this condyle is approximately 1.7 cm longer than the lateral condyle. As the tibia moves on the femur from the fully flexed to the fully extended position, it descends and then ascends the curves of the medial femoral condyle and simultaneously rotates externally. This motion is reversed as the tibia moves back into the fully flexed position. This screw-home mechanism (rotation around the longitudinal axis of the tibia) provides more stability to the knee in any position than would a simple hinge configuration of the tibiofemoral joint.

Matsumoto et al. (2000) investigated the axis of tibia axial rotation and its change with knee flexion angle in 24 fresh-frozen normal knee cadaver specimens ranging in age from 22 to 67 years. The magnitude and location of the longitudinal axis of tibia rotation were measured at 15° increments between 0 and 90° of knee flexion. The magnitude of tibia rotation was 8° at 0°

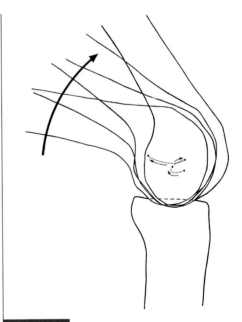

FIG. 7-7

Abnormal instant center pathway for a 35-year-old man with a bucket-handle derangement. The instant center jumps at full extension of the knee. *Adapted from Frankel, V.H., Burstein, A.H., & Brooks, D.B. (1971). Biomechanics of internal derangement of the knee. Pathomechanics as determined by analysis of the instant centers of motion. J Bone Joint Surg, 53A, 945.*

of knee flexion. The tibial rotation increased rapidly as the knee flexion angle increased and reached a maximum of 31° at 30° of knee flexion. It then decreased again with additional flexion (Fig 7-10). The location of the longitudinal rotational axis was close to the insertion of the anterior cruciate ligament (ACL) at 0° of flexion. At continuous flexion up to 60°, the rotational axis moved toward the insertion of the posterior cruciate ligament. Between 60 and 90° of flexion, the rotational axis moved anteriorly again (Fig 7-11). This study showed that the rotational axis remains approximately in the area between the two cruciate ligaments. Any change of direction and tension of the cruciate ligaments and surrounding soft tissue may affect the movement and the location of the longitudinal tibia axis of rotation and thereby affect joint load distribution.

A clinical test, the Helfet test, is often used to determine whether external rotation of the tibio-

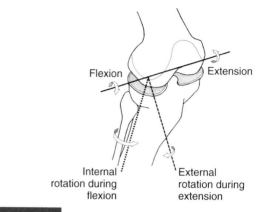

FIG. 7-9

Screw-home mechanism of the tibiofemoral joint. During knee extension, the tibia rotates externally. This motion is reversed as the knee is flexed. **A,** Oblique view of the femur and tibia. The *shaded area* indicates the tibial plateau. **B,** Top view showing the position of the tibial plateau on the femoral condyles in knee flexion (top) and extension (bottom). The *solid outlines* represent the femoral condyles; the *broken lines* represent the tibial plateau. *Adapted from Helfet, A.J. (1974). Anatomy and mechanics of movement of the knee joint. In A. Helfet (Ed.),* Disorders of the Knee *(pp. 1–17). Philadelphia: J.B. Lippincott.*

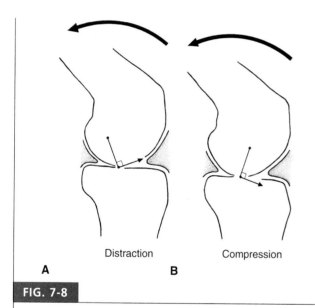

FIG. 7-8

Surface motion in two tibiofemoral joints with displaced instant centers. In both joints, the *arrowed line* at right angles to the line between the instant center and the tibiofemoral contact point indicates the direction of displacement of the contact points. **A,** The *small arrow* indicates that with further flexion, the tibiofemoral joint will be distracted. **B,** With increased flexion, this joint will be compressed.

femoral joint takes place during knee extension, thereby indicating whether the screw-home mechanism is intact. This clinical test is performed with the patient sitting with the knee and hip flexed 90° and the leg hanging free. The medial and lateral borders of the patella are marked on the skin. The tibial tuberosity and the midline of the patella are then designated, and the alignment of the tibial tuberosity with the patella is checked. In a normal knee flexed 90°, the tibial tuberosity aligns with the medial half of the patella (Fig. 7-12*A*). The knee is then extended fully and the movement of the tibial tuberosity is observed. In a normal knee, the tibial tuberosity moves laterally during extension and aligns with the lateral half of the patella at full extension (Fig. 7-12*B*). Rotatory motion in a normal knee may be as great as half the width of the patella. In a deranged knee, the tibia may not rotate externally during extension. Because of the altered surface motion in such a knee, the tibiofemoral joint will be abnormally compressed if the knee is forced into extension, and the joint surfaces may be damaged.

Patellofemoral Joint

The surface motion of the patellofemoral joint in the frontal plane may also be described by means of the instant center technique. This joint is shown to have a gliding motion (Fig. 7-13). From full extension to full flexion of the knee, the patella glides caudally approximately 7 cm on the femoral condyles. Both the medial and lateral facets of the femur articulate with the patella from full extension to 140° of flexion (Hehne, 1990) (Fig. 7-14). Beyond 90° of flexion, the patella rotates externally, and only the medial femoral facet articulates with the patella (Fig. 7-14B). At full flexion, the patella sinks into the intercondylar groove (Goodfellow et al., 1976). The contact area of the lateral facet joint of the patella is larger than the medial contact areas and ranges from 0.5 to 2.5 cm² and less than 0.5 to 2 cm², respectively. Contact areas increase with an increased amount of flexion of the knee joint and increased pulling force of the quadriceps muscle (Hehne, 1990).

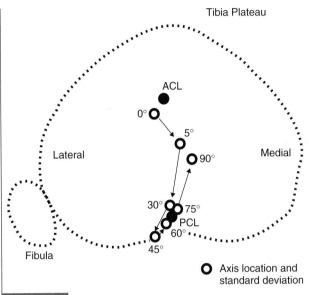

FIG. 7-11

Location of the axis of tibia axial rotation. The location of the axis was close to the tibial insertion of the anterior cruciate ligament (ACL) at 0° of flexion and gradually moved toward that of the posterior cruciate ligament at 45 and 90° of knee flexion. The axis then moved anterior again and was approximately at equal distance from the two insertions of the cruciate ligaments at 90° of knee flexion. ACL, insertion of the anterior cruciate ligament; PCL, tibial insertion of the posterior cruciate ligament. *Reprinted with permission from Matsumoto, H., Seedhom, B.B., Suda, Y., et al. (2000). Axis of tibial rotation and its change with flexion angle. Clin Orthop, 371, 178–182.*

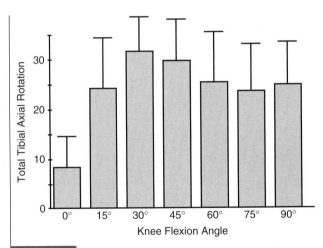

FIG. 7-10

The total tibial axial rotation (y-axis) plotted against the magnitude of knee flexion (x-axis) in fresh-frozen specimens tested under unloaded axial conditions. The magnitude of tibial rotation was below 9° at 0° of knee flexion. Maximum rotation (31.7°) was measured between 30 to 45° of knee flexion. *Reprinted with permission from Matsumoto, H., Seedhom, B.B., Suda, Y., et al. (2000). Axis of tibial rotation and its change with flexion angle. Clin Orthop, 371, 178–182.*

Kinetics

Kinetics involves both static and dynamic analysis of the forces and moments acting on a joint. Statics is the study of the forces and moments acting on a body in equilibrium (a body at rest or moving at a constant speed). For a body to be in equilibrium, two equilibrium conditions must be met: force (translatory) equilibrium, in which the sum of the forces is zero, and moment (rotatory) equilibrium, in which the sum of the moments is zero. Dynamics is the study of the moments and forces acting on a body in motion (an accelerating or decelerating body). In this case, the forces do not add up to zero, and the body displaces and/or the moments do not add up to zero and the body

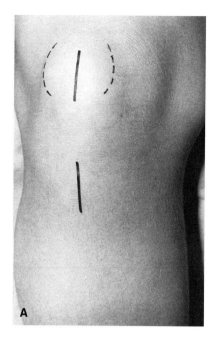 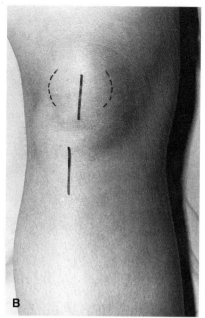

Knee flexed 90°   Knee fully extended

FIG. 7-12

Helfet test. **A,** In a normal knee flexed 90°, the tibial tuberosity aligns with the medial half of the patella. **B,** When the knee is fully extended, the tibial tuberosity aligns with the lateral half of the patella.

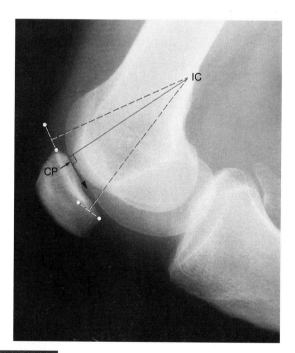

FIG. 7-13

After the instant center (*IC*) is determined for the patellofemoral joint for the motion from 75 to 90° of knee flexion, a line is drawn from the instant center to the contact point (*CP*) between the patella and the femoral condyle. A line drawn at right angles to this line is tangential to the surface of the patella, indicating gliding.

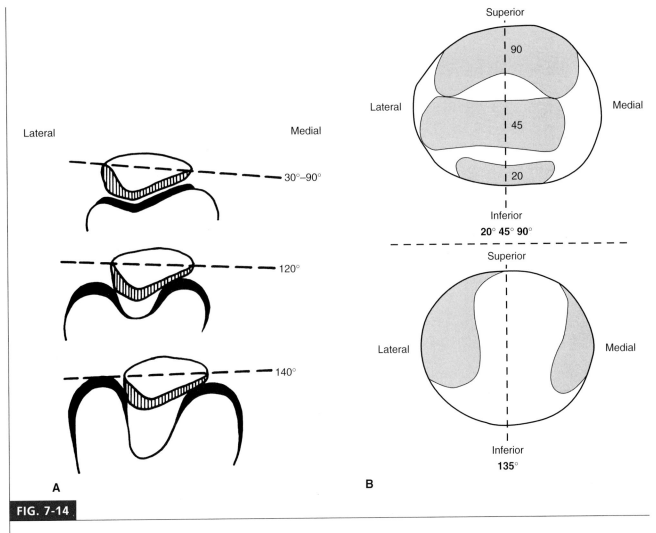

FIG. 7-14

A, The position of the patella at different ranges of knee flexion motion. **B,** Contact areas during different degrees of flexion. Beyond 90° of flexion, the patella rotates slightly outwards. *Adapted from Goodfellow, J., Hungerford, D.S., & Zindel, M. (1976). Patellofemoral joint mechanics and pathology. 1.*

Functional anatomy of the patellofemoral joint. J Bone Joint Surg, 58B, 287; and from Hehne, H.J. (1990). Biomechanics of the patellofemoral joint and its clinical relevance. Clin Orthop, 258, 73–85.

rotates around an axis perpendicular to the plane of the forces producing the moments. Kinetic analysis allows one to determine the magnitude of the moments and forces on a joint produced by body weight, muscle action, soft tissue resistance, and externally applied loads in any situation, either static or dynamic, and to identify those situations that produce excessively high moments or forces.

In this and subsequent chapters, the discussion of statics and dynamics of the joints of the skeletal system concerns the magnitude of the forces and moments acting to move a joint about an axis or to maintain its position. It does not take into account the deforming effect of these forces and moments on the joint structures. This effect is indeed present, but the discussion is not within the scope of this text.

STATICS OF THE TIBIOFEMORAL JOINT

Static analysis may be used to determine the forces and moments acting on a joint when no motion takes place or at one instant in time during a dynamic activity such as walking, running, or lifting an object. It can be performed for any joint in any position and under any loading configuration. In such analyses, either graphic or mathematical methods may be used to solve for the unknown forces or moments.

A complete static analysis involving all moments and all forces imposed on a joint in three dimensions is complicated. For this reason, a simplified technique is often used. The technique utilizes a free-body diagram and limits the analysis to one plane, to the three main coplanar forces acting on the free-body, and to the main moments acting about the joint under consideration. The minimum magnitudes of the forces and moments are obtained.

When the simplified free-body technique is used to analyze coplanar forces, one portion of the body is considered as distinct from the entire body, and all forces acting on this free-body are identified. A diagram is drawn of the free-body in the loading situation to be analyzed. The three principal coplanar forces acting on the free-body are identified and designated on the free-body diagram.

These forces are designated as vectors if four characteristics are known: magnitude, sense, line of application, and point of application. (The term "direction" includes line of application and sense.) If the points of application for all three forces and the directions for two forces are known, all remaining characteristics can be obtained for a force equilibrium situation. When the free-body is in equilibrium, the three principal coplanar forces are concurrent; that is, they intersect at a common point. In other words, these forces form a closed system with no resultant (i.e., their vector sum is zero). For this reason, the line of application for one force can be determined if the lines of application for the other two forces are known. Once the lines of application for all three forces are known, a triangle of forces can be constructed and the magnitudes of all three forces can be scaled from this triangle.

An example will illustrate the application of the simplified free-body technique for coplanar forces to the knee. In this case, the technique is used to estimate the minimum magnitude of the joint reaction force acting on the tibiofemoral joint of the weight-bearing leg when the other leg is lifted during stair climbing. The lower leg is considered as a free-body,

distinct from the rest of the body, and a diagram of this free-body in the stair-climbing situation is drawn (Calculation Box 7-1). From all forces acting on the free-body, the three main coplanar forces are identified as the ground reaction force (equal to body weight[1]), the tensile force through the patellar tendon exerted by the quadriceps muscle, and the joint reaction force on the tibial plateau. The ground reaction force (W) has a known magnitude (equal to body weight), sense, line of application, and point of application (point of contact between the foot and the ground). The patellar tendon force (P) has a known sense (away from the knee joint), line of application (along the patellar tendon), and point of application (point of insertion of the patellar tendon on the tibial tuberosity), but an unknown magnitude. The joint reaction force (J) has a known point of application on the surface of the tibia (the contact point of the joint surfaces between the tibial and femoral condyles, estimated from a roentgenogram of the joint in the proper loading configuration), but an unknown magnitude, sense, and line of application. Using vectors calculations and triangles laws the joint reaction force (J) and the patellar tendon force (P) can be calculated (Calculation Box 7-1)

It can be seen that the main muscle force has a much greater influence on the magnitude of the joint reaction force than does the ground reaction force produced by body weight. Note that, in this example (Calculation Box 7-1), only the minimum magnitude of the joint reaction force has been calculated. If other muscle forces are considered, such as the force produced by the contraction of the hamstring muscles in stabilizing the knee, the joint reaction force increases.

The next step in the static analysis is analysis of the moments acting around the center of motion of the tibiofemoral joint with the knee in the same position and the loading configuration shown in Calculation Box Figure 7-1-1. The moment analysis is used to estimate the minimum magnitude of the moment produced through the patellar tendon, which counterbalances the moment on the lower leg produced by the weight of the body as the subject ascends stairs (Calculation Box 7-2).

---

[1]In this case, the ground reaction force is actually equal to body weight minus the weight of the lower leg. Because the weight of the lower leg is minimal (less than one tenth of the body), it can be disregarded, and the figure for total body weight can be utilized in the calculation.

Free-Body Diagram of the Knee Joint

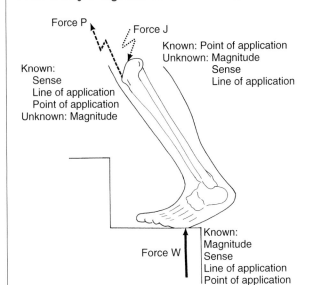

The three main coplanar forces acting on the lower leg: Ground reaction force (W), patellar tendon force (P), and joint reaction force (J) are designated on a free-body diagram of the lower leg while climbing stairs (Calculation Box Fig 7-1-1).

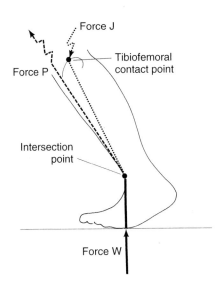

Because the lower leg is in equilibrium, the lines of application for all three forces intersect at one point. Because the lines of application for two forces (W and P) are known, the line of application for the third force (J) can be determined. The lines of application for forces W and P are extended until they intersect. The line of application for J can then be drawn from its point of application on the tibial surface through the intersection point (Calculation Box Fig. 7-1-2).

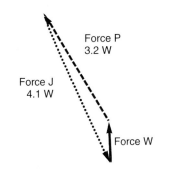

Now that the line of application for J has been determined, it is possible to construct a triangle of forces (Calculation Box Fig. 7-1-3). First, a vector representing W is drawn. Next, P is drawn from the head of vector W. Then, to close the triangle, force J is drawn from the head of vector W. The point at which forces P and J intersect defines the length of these vectors. Now that the length of all three vectors is known, the magnitude of forces P and J can be scaled from force W, which is equal to body weight. It is determining the number of times the length of force W can be aligned along the force P and J, respectively. In this case, force P is 3.2 times body weight, and force J is 4.1 times body weight.

CALCULATION BOX 7-2

Free-Body Diagram of the Lower Leg During Stair Climbing

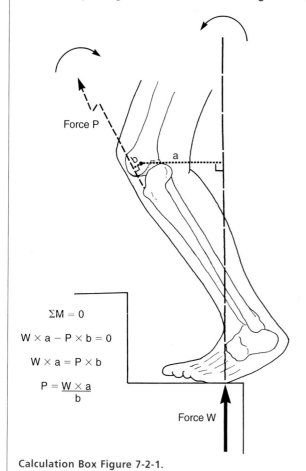

Force P

$\Sigma M = 0$

$W \times a - P \times b = 0$

$W \times a = P \times b$

$P = \dfrac{W \times a}{b}$

Force W

Calculation Box Figure 7-2-1.

The two main moments acting around the center of motion of the tibiofemoral joint (solid dot) are designated on the free-body diagram of the lower leg during stair climbing (Calculation Box Fig. 7-2-1).

The flexing moment on the lower leg is the product of the weight of the body[2] (W, the ground reaction force) and its lever arm (a), which is the perpendicular distance of the force W to the center of motion of the tibiofemoral joint. The counterbalancing extending moment is the product of the quadriceps muscle force through the patellar tendon (P) and its lever arm (b). Because the lower leg is in equilibrium, the sum of these two moments must equal zero ($\Sigma M = 0$).

In this example, the counterclockwise moment is arbitrarily designated as positive ($W \times a - P \times b = 0$). Values for lever arms a and b can be measured from anatomical specimens or on soft tissue imaging or fluoroscopy (Kellis & Baltzopoulos, 1999; Wretenberg et al., 1996), and the magnitude of W can be determined from the body weight of the individual. The magnitude of P can then be found from the moment equilibrium equation:

$$P = \frac{W \times a}{b}$$

[2]Again the weight of the lower leg is disregarded because it is less than one tenth of body weight.

DYNAMICS OF THE TIBIOFEMORAL JOINT

Although estimations of the magnitude of the forces and moments imposed on a joint in static situations are useful, most of our activities are of a dynamic nature. Analysis of the forces and moments acting on a joint during motion requires the use of a different technique for solving dynamic problems.

As in static analysis, the main forces considered in dynamic analysis are those produced by body weight, muscles, other soft tissues, and externally applied loads. Friction forces are negligible in a normal joint and thus not considered here. In dynamic analysis, two factors in addition to those in static analysis must be taken into account: the acceleration of the body part under consideration and the mass moment of inertia of the body part. (The mass moment of inertia is the unit used to express the amount of torque needed to accelerate a body and depends on the shape of the body.) (For more in-depth studies of dynamics, see Özkaya & Nordin, 1999.)

The steps for calculating the minimum magnitudes of the forces acting on a joint at a particular instant in time during a dynamic activity are as follows:

1. The anatomical structures are identified: definitions of structures, anatomical landmarks, point of contact of articular surface, and lever

arms involved in the production of forces for the biomechanical analyses.

2. The angular acceleration of the moving body part is determined.
3. The mass moment of inertia of the moving body part is determined.
4. The torque (moment) acting about the joint is calculated.
5. The magnitude of the main muscle force accelerating the body part is calculated.
6. The magnitude of the joint reaction force at a particular instant in time is calculated by static analysis.

In the first step, the structures of the body involved in producing forces on the joint are identified. These are the moving body part and the main muscles in that body part that are involved in the production of the motion. Great care must be taken in applying this first step. For example, the lever arms for all major knee muscles change according to the degree of knee flexion and gender (Wretenberg et al., 1996).

In joints of the extremities, acceleration of the body part involves a change in joint angle. To determine this angular acceleration of the moving body part, the entire movement of the body part is recorded photographically. Recording can be done with a stroboscopic light and movie camera, with video photogrammetry, with Selspot systems, with stereophotogrammetry, or with other methods (Gardner et al., 1994; Ramsey & Wretenberg, 1999; Winter, 1990). The maximal angular acceleration for a particular motion is calculated.

Next, the mass moment of inertia for the moving body part is determined. Anthropometric data on the body part can be used for this determination. As calculating these data is a complicated procedure, tables are commonly used (Drillis et al., 1964).

The torque about the joint can now be calculated using Newton's second law of motion, which states that when motion is angular, the torque is a product of the mass moment of inertia of the body part and the angular acceleration of that part:

$$T = I\alpha \, ,$$

where

T   is the torque expressed in newton meters (Nm)
I   is the mass moment of inertia expressed in newton meters $\times$ seconds squared (Nm sec^2)
α is the angular acceleration expressed in radians per second squared (r/sec^2).

The torque is not only a product of the mass moment of inertia and the angular acceleration of the body part but also a product of the main muscle force accelerating the body part and the perpendicular distance of the force from the center of motion of the joint (lever arm). Thus,

$$T = Fd$$

where

F   is the force expressed in newtons (N)
d   is the perpendicular distance expressed in meters (m).

Because T is known and d can be measured on the body part from the line of application of the force to the center of motion of the joint, the equation can be solved for F. When F has been calculated, the remaining problem can be solved like a static problem using the simplified free-body technique to determine the minimum magnitude of the joint reaction force acting on the joint at a certain instant in time.

A classic example will illustrate the use of dynamic analysis in calculating the joint reaction force on the tibiofemoral joint at a particular instant during a dynamic activity (e.g., kicking a football) (Frankel & Burstein, 1970). A stroboscopic film of the knee and lower leg was taken, and the angular acceleration was found to be maximal at the instant the foot struck the ball; the lower leg was almost vertical at this instant. From the film, the maximal angular acceleration was computed to be 453 r/sec^2. From anthropometric data tables (Drillis et al., 1964), the mass moment of inertia for the lower leg was determined to be 0.35 Nm sec^2. The torque about the tibiofemoral joint was calculated according to the equation; torque equals mass moment of inertia times angular acceleration (T = Iα),

$$0.35 \text{ Nm sec}^2 \times 453 \text{ r/sec}^2 = 158.5 \text{ Nm}$$

After the torque had been determined to be 158.5 Nm and the perpendicular distance from the subject's patellar tendon to the instant center for the tibiofemoral joint had been found to be 0.05 m, the muscle force acting on the joint through the patellar tendon was calculated using the equation torque equals force times distance (T = Fd),

$$158.5 \text{ Nm} = F \times 0.05 \text{ m}$$

$$F = \frac{158.5 \text{ Nm}}{0.05 \text{ m}}$$

$$F = 3170 \text{ N}$$

Thus, 3,170 N was the maximal force exerted by the quadriceps muscle during the kicking motion.

Static analysis can now be performed to determine the minimum magnitude of the joint reaction force on the tibiofemoral joint. The main forces on this joint are identified as the patellar tendon force (P), the gravitational force of the lower leg (T), and the joint reaction force (J). P and T are known vectors. J has an unknown magnitude, sense, and line of application. The free-body technique for three coplanar forces is used to solve for J, which is found to be only slightly lower than P.

As is evident from the calculations, the two main factors that influence the magnitude of the forces on a joint in dynamic situations are the acceleration of the body part and its mass moment of inertia. An increase in angular acceleration of the body part will produce a proportional increase in the torque about the joint. Although in the body the mass moment of inertia is anatomically set, it can be manipulated externally. For example, it is increased when a weight boot is applied to the foot during rehabilitative exercises of the extensor muscles of the knee. Normally, a joint reaction force of approximately 50% of body weight results when the knee is slowly (with no acceleration forces) extended from 90° of flexion to full extension. In a person weighing 70 kg, this force is approximately 350 N. If a 10-kg weight boot is placed on the foot, it will exert a gravitational force of 100 N. This will increase the joint reaction force by 1,000 N, making this force almost four times greater than it would be without the boot.

Dynamic analysis has been used to investigate the peak magnitudes of the joint reaction forces, muscle forces, and ligament forces on the tibiofemoral joint during walking. Morrison (1970) calculated the magnitude of the joint reaction force transmitted through the tibial plateau in male and female subjects during level walking. He simultaneously recorded muscle activity electromyographically to determine which muscles produced the peak magnitudes of this force on the tibial plateau during various stages of the gait cycle (Fig. 7-15).

Just after heel strike, the joint reaction force ranged from two to three times body weight and was associated with contraction of the hamstring muscles, which have a decelerating and stabilizing effect on the knee. During knee flexion in the beginning of the stance phase, the joint reaction force was approximately two times body weight and was associated with the contraction of the quadriceps muscle, which acts to prevent buckling of the knee. The peak joint reaction force occurred during the late stance phase just before toe-off. This force ranged from two to four times body weight, varying among the subjects tested, and was associated with contraction of the gastrocnemius muscle. In the late swing phase, contraction of the hamstring muscles resulted in a joint reaction force approximately equal to body weight. No significant difference was found between the joint reaction force magnitudes for men and women when the values were normalized by dividing them by body weight.

Andriacchi & Strickland (1985) studied the normal moment patterns around the knee joint during level walking for 29 healthy volunteers (15 women and 14 men with an average age of 39 years). Figure 7-16 depicts the flexion-extension, abduction-adduction, and internal-external moments during the stance and swing phase of level walking. The moments are normalized to the individual's body weight and height and are presented as a percentage. The flexion-

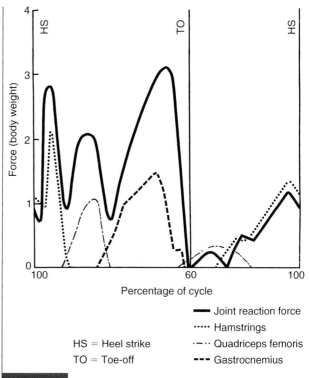

HS = Heel strike
TO = Toe-off

Joint reaction force
Hamstrings
Quadriceps femoris
Gastrocnemius

FIG. 7-15

Joint reaction forces expressed as body weight transmitted through the tibial plateau during walking, one gait cycle (12 subjects). The muscle forces producing the peak magnitudes of this force are also designated. *Adapted from Morrison, J.B. (1970). The mechanics of the knee joint in relation to normal walking.* J Biomech, 3, 51.

extension moments during the stance phase are approximately 20 to 30 times larger than the moment produced in the frontal (abduction-adduction) and transverse (internal-external) planes.

An increase in knee joint flexion-extension moment amplitude has been reported at increased walking speeds (Andriacchi & Strickland, 1985; Holden et al., 1997). An increase in the production of adduction knee joint moment during stair climbing compared with level walking was reported by Yu et al. (1997).

During the gait cycle, the joint reaction force shifts from the medial to the lateral tibial plateau. In the stance phase, when the force reaches its peak value, it is sustained mainly by the medial plateau (adduction moment); in the swing phase, when the force is minimal, it is sustained primarily by the lateral plateau. The contact area of the medial tibial plateau is approximately 50% larger than that of the lateral tibial plateau (Kettelkamp & Jacobs, 1972). Also, the cartilage on this plateau is approximately three times thicker than that on the lateral plateau. The larger surface area and the greater thickness of the medial plateau allow it to more easily sustain the higher forces imposed on it.

In a normal knee, joint reaction forces are sustained by the menisci as well as by the articular cartilage. The function of the menisci was investigated by Seedhom and coworkers (1974), who examined the distribution of stresses in knees of human autopsy subjects with and without menisci. Their results suggest that in load-bearing situations, the magnitude of the stresses on the tibiofemoral joint when the menisci have been removed may be as much as three times greater than when these structures are intact. Fukuda et al. (2000) studied in vitro the load-compressive transmission of the knee joint and the role of menisci and articular cartilage. The load simulated was static and dynamic impact loading. The testing was done in neutral, varus, and valgus alignment of the knee joints in 40 fresh-frozen pig knee specimens. The compressive stress on the medial subchondral bone was up to five times higher with the menisci removed. This study points to the importance of the menisci as a structure to absorb load and protect the cartilage and subchondral bone under dynamic conditions.

In a normal human knee, stresses are distributed over a wide area of the tibial plateau. If the menisci are removed, the stresses are no longer distributed over such a wide area but instead are limited to a contact area in the center of the plateau (Fig. 7-17). Thus, removal of the menisci not only increases the

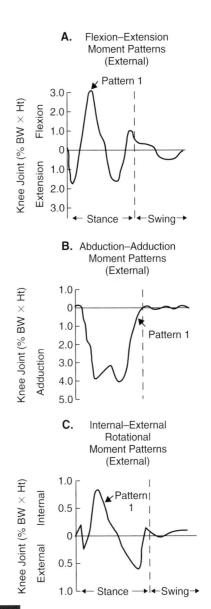

FIG. 7-16

Flexion-extension (**A**), abduction-adduction (**B**), and internal-external rotation (**C**) moments produced during one gait cycle in normal subjects. The moments are normalized to each individual body weight X height and expressed as a percentage. *Reprinted with permission from Andriacchi, T.P. & Strickland, A.B. (1985). Gait analysis as a tool to assess joint kinetics. In N. Berme, A.E. Engin, D.A. Correis, et al. (Eds.), Biomechanics of Normal and Pathological Human Articulating Joints. (NATO ASI series, Vol 93, pp. 83–102). Drodrecht, Netherlands: Martinus Nijhoff.*

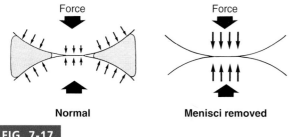

FIG. 7-17

Stress distribution in a normal knee and in a knee with the menisci removed. Removal of the menisci increases the magnitude of stresses on the cartilage of the tibial plateau and changes the size and location of the tibiofemoral contact area. With the menisci intact, the contact area encompasses nearly the entire surface of the tibial plateau. With the menisci removed, the contact area is limited to the center of the tibial plateau.

magnitude of the stresses on the cartilage and subchondral bone at the center of the tibial plateau but also diminishes the size and changes the location of the contact area. Over the long term, the high stresses placed on this smaller contact area may be harmful to the exposed cartilage, which is usually soft and fibrillated in that area. The menisci are

thought to carry up to 70% of the load across the knee. Movement during knee flexion of the menisci would therefore protect the articulating surfaces while avoiding injury to it.

Vedi et al. (1999) studied menisci movement in 16 young football players with normal knees with MRI. The knee flexion movement was scanned from full knee extension to 90° of knee flexion. The imaging technique allowed for both standing (weight-bearing) and sitting (non–weight-bearing) and was performed simultaneously in the sagittal and transverse plane. Figure 7-18 shows the movements in the transverse plane of the medial and lateral menisci expressed in millimeters (mean) from full extension to 90° flexion of knee joint motion. Movement was significantly greater in weight-bearing than in non–weight-bearing for both lateral and medial menisci. The contributions of the menisci are therefore not only to protect the articular cartilage and subchondral bone but also to contribute actively to knee joint stability.

STABILITY OF THE KNEE JOINT

The key to a healthy knee joint is joint stability. The osseous configuration, the menisci, the ligaments, the capsule, and the muscles surrounding the knee joint produce joint stability (Fig. 7-1, *A & B*). If any

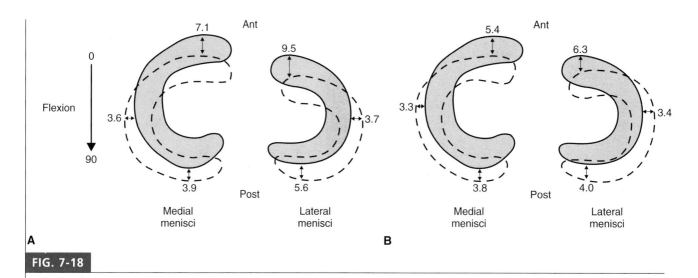

FIG. 7-18

Simplified diagrams showing the mean movements of the medial and lateral menisci from full knee extension to 90° knee flexion during two conditions. **A,** Erect and weight-bearing. **B,** Sitting, relaxed, and bearing no weight. *Adapted with permission from Vedi, V., Williams, A., Tennant, S.J., et al. (1999). Meniscal movement. An in-vivo study using dynamic MRI. J Bone Joint Surg, 81B(1), 37–41.*

ACL Injury

A 30-year-old male suffered an external rotation trauma in his right knee while downhill skiing. Following the trauma, he experienced sharp pain, progressive joint effusion, and subjective instability. During careful examination by a specialist, an anterior positive drawer test was diagnosed, and the Lachman test and pivot shift test were found positive. An MRI confirmed the ACL rupture (Case Study Fig 7-1-1).

The rupture of the primary stabilizer of the knee joint (ACL) leads to a progressive structural alteration of the knee. A primary objective of the treatment is the prevention of re-injury of the knee in the hope of preventing additional ligamentous injuries, meniscal injuries, and possible cartilage degeneration. In this case, the patient first completed a course of conservative treatment with physical therapy. After 6 months, the subjective instability was present during sports and daily activities such as gait and stair climbing. To compensate for the ACL deficiency, the patient altered his gait patterns, presenting quadriceps avoidance gait to prevent the anterior translation of the tibia when the quadriceps contracts at the midstance phase of the gait (Andriacchi & Birac, 1993; Berchuck et al., 1990).

The patient went for surgical treatment. The MRI below (Case Study Fig. 7-1-2) shows the ACL status after patella bone-tendon-bone autograft was performed 10 months post-trauma.

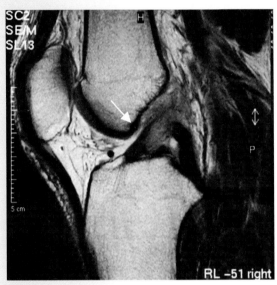

Case Study Figure 7-1-1.

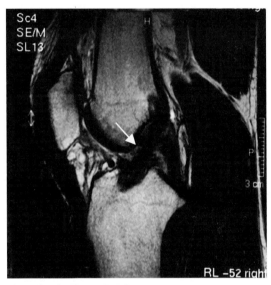

Case Study Figure 7-1-2.

of these structures are malfunctioning or disturbed, knee joint instability will occur. The ligaments are the primary stabilizer for anterior and posterior translation, varus and valgus angulation, and internal and external rotation of the knee joint (Case Study 7-1).

Fu et al. (1994) summarized the functions of the knee ligaments. The ACL is the predominant restraint to anterior tibial displacement. The ligament accepts 75% of the anterior force at full extension and an additional 10% (up to 90°) of knee flexion. The posterior cruciate ligament is the primary restraint to posterior tibial translation; it sustains 85 to 100% of the posterior force at both 30 and 90° of knee flexion. The lateral collateral ligament is the primary restraint to varus angulation and it resists approximately 55% of the applied load at full extension. The role of the lateral collateral ligament increases with joint flexion as the posterior structures become lax. The medial collateral ligament (superficial portion) is the primary restraint to valgus (adduction) angulation and resists 50% of the external valgus load. The capsule, the anterior and posterior cruciate ligaments, share the remaining valgus load. Internal rotational laxity seen in the 20 to 40° range of knee flexion is restrained by the medial collateral ligament and the ACL. Finally, external rotation laxity seen in the 30 to 40° range of knee flexion is restrained by the posterior cruciate ligament at 90° of knee flexion.

In vivo measurement of the normal ACL has been performed by Beynnon et al. (1992). They placed a strain transducer arthroscopically in the ACL. The results showed that strain in the ACL was related to knee flexion (with the most strain occurring near full extension) and increased with quadriceps contraction. Less strain occurred with co-contractions of both the quadriceps and the hamstring muscle groups and at greater degrees of knee flexion. This indicates that muscle contraction and co-contraction contribute to the stability of the knee joint by increasing the stiffness of the joint. Kwak et al. (2000) studied in vitro the effect of hamstrings and iliotibial band forces on the kinematics of the knee. At various knee flexion angles, human knee specimens were tested with different muscle-loading patterns. The quadriceps muscle force was always present, and the test was performed with and without hamstring muscle force and with and without iliotibial band force. With loading of simultaneous quadriceps and hamstring muscle force, the tibia translated posteriorly and rotated externally. The effect was similar for the iliotibial band simulated forces but the effect was smaller.

Many in vitro studies suggest that the hamstrings are important anterior and rotational stabilizers of the tibia. In vivo studies have shown that co-contractions of the quadriceps and hamstring muscles are highly present in normal knee joints and daily activities (Baratta et al., 1988; Solomonow & D'Ambrosia, 1994). The co-contraction mechanisms also increase the knee joint stability in vivo (Åagaard et al., 2000; Markholf et al., 1978; Solomonow & D'Ambrosia, 1994). However, the complex mechanism in vivo of muscle activity as a knee stabilizer, the extent of protection, and the biomechanical and clinical importance needs further research (Grabiner & Weiker, 1993).

FUNCTION OF THE PATELLA

The patella serves two important biomechanical functions in the knee. First, it aids knee extension by producing anterior displacement of the quadriceps tendon throughout the entire range of motion, thereby lengthening the lever arm of the quadriceps muscle force. Second, it allows a wider distribution of compressive stress on the femur by increasing the area of contact between the patellar tendon and the femur. The contribution of the patella to the length of the quadriceps muscle force lever arm varies from full flexion to full extension of the knee (Lindahl & Movin, 1967; Smidt, 1973). At full flexion, when the patella is in the intercondylar groove, it produces little anterior displacement of the quadriceps

tendon and it contributes the least to the length of the quadriceps muscle force lever arm (approximately 10% of the total length). As the knee is extended, the patella rises from the intercondylar groove, producing significant anterior displacement of the tendon. The length of the quadriceps force lever arm rapidly increases with extension up to 45°, at which point the patella lengthens the lever arm by approximately 30%.

With knee extension beyond 45°, the length of the lever arm is diminished slightly. With this decrease in its lever arm, the quadriceps muscle force must increase for the torque about the knee to remain the same. In an in vitro study of normal knees, Lieb and Perry (1968) showed that the quadriceps muscle force required to extend the knee the last 15° increased by approximately 60% (Fig. 7-19).

If the patella is removed from a knee, the patellar tendon lies closer to the center of motion of the tibiofemoral joint (Fig. 7-20). Acting with a shorter lever arm, the quadriceps muscle must produce even more force than is normally required for a certain torque about the knee to be maintained during

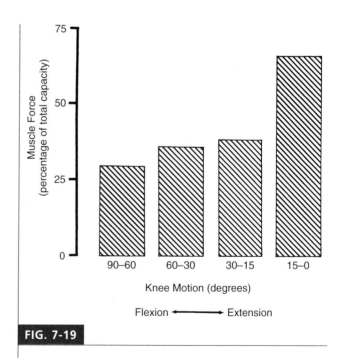

FIG. 7-19

Quadriceps muscle force required during knee motion from 90° of flexion to full extension. *Adapted from Lieb, F.J. & Perry, J. (1968). Quadriceps function. An anatomical and mechanical study using amputated limbs.* J Bone Joint Surg, 50A, *1535.*

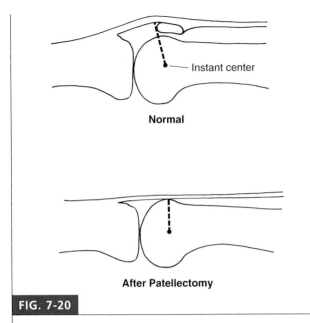

Normal

After Patellectomy

FIG. 7-20

Quadriceps muscle lever arm (represented by the *broken line*) in a normal knee and in a knee in which the patella has been removed. The lever arm is the perpendicular distance between the force exerted by the quadriceps muscle through the patellar tendon and the instant center of the tibiofemoral joint for the last two degrees of extension. The patellar tendon lies closer to the instant center in the knee without a patella. *Adapted from Kaufer, H. (1971). Mechanical function of the patella.* J Bone Joint Surg, 53A, *1551.*

the last 45° of extension. Full active extension of such a knee may require as much as 30% more quadriceps force than is normally required (Kaufer, 1971). This increase in force may be beyond the capacity of the quadriceps muscle in some patients, particularly those who have intra-articular disease or are advanced in age.

STATICS AND DYNAMICS OF THE PATELLOFEMORAL JOINT

During dynamic activities, the magnitude of the muscle forces acting on a joint directly affects the magnitude of the joint reaction force. In general, the greater the muscle forces, the greater the joint reaction force.

In the patellofemoral joint, the quadriceps muscle force increases with knee flexion. During relaxed upright standing, minimal quadriceps muscle forces are required to counterbalance the small flexion moments about the patellofemoral joint because the center of gravity of the body above the

knee is almost directly above the center of rotation of the patellofemoral joint. As knee flexion increases, the center of gravity shifts further away from the center of rotation, thereby greatly increasing the flexion moments to be counterbalanced by the quadriceps muscle force. As the quadriceps muscle force rises, so does the patellofemoral joint reaction force (Hungerford & Barry, 1979; Reilly & Martens, 1972).

Knee flexion also influences the patellofemoral joint reaction force by affecting the angle between the patellar tendon force and the quadriceps tendon force. The angle of these two force components becomes more acute with knee flexion, increasing the magnitude of the patellofemoral joint reaction force (Calculation Box 7-3). Reilly and Martens (1972) determined the magnitude of the patellofemoral joint reaction force during several dynamic activities involving varying amounts of knee flexion. During level walking, which requires relatively little knee flexion, the reaction force was low. The peak value, in the middle of the stance phase when flexion was greatest, was one-half body weight.

The joint reaction force was much greater during activities that require greater flexion. During knee bends to 90°, this force reached 2.5 to 3 times body weight with the knee flexed 90° (Fig. 7-21). Through-

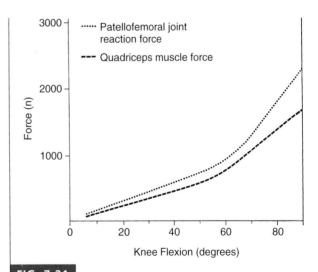

FIG. 7-21

Patellofemoral joint reaction force and quadriceps muscle force during knee bend to 90° (three subjects). *Adapted from Reilly, D.T. & Martens, M. (1972). Experimental analysis of the quadriceps muscle force and patellofemoral joint reaction force for various activities.* Acta Orthop Scand, 43, *126*

CALCULATION BOX 7-3

Joint Reaction Forces at the Knee in Flexion

Knee flexion influences the patellofemoral joint reaction force by changing the angle between the patellar tendon and the quadriceps tendon (Calculation Box Fig. 7-3-1, A & B).

The angle between the patellar tendon (P) and the quadriceps tendon (Q) is 35° with the knee flexed 5° (left top) and 80° with the knee flexed 90° (left bottom). Values for the tendon angles are from Matthews and Associates (1977), who determined the angle roentgenographically after placing two metal wires along each of these tendons.

The patellofemoral joint reaction force with the knee in 5 and 90° of flexion is obtained by constructing a parallelogram of forces for each situation and using trigonometric calculations. The patellofemoral joint reaction force (J) is the resultant of the two equal force components through the patellar tendon (P) and the quadriceps tendon (Q). As the angle between these force components becomes more acute with greater knee flexion, the resultant joint reaction force (J) becomes larger. *Adapted from Wiktorin, C.v.H. & Nordin, M. (1986).* Introduction to Problem Solving in Biomechanics *(pp. 87–129). Philadelphia: Lea & Febiger.*

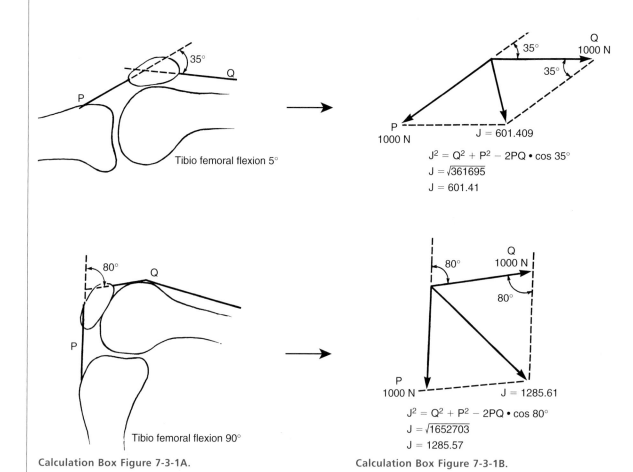

$$J^2 = Q^2 + P^2 - 2PQ \cdot \cos 35°$$
$$J = \sqrt{361695}$$
$$J = 601.41$$

$$J^2 = Q^2 + P^2 - 2PQ \cdot \cos 80°$$
$$J = \sqrt{1652703}$$
$$J = 1285.57$$

Calculation Box Figure 7-3-1A.

Calculation Box Figure 7-3-1B.

CASE STUDY 7-2

Extensor Mechanism Injury

A 30-year-old basketball player had a forceful knee flexion while coming down from a jump. A strong eccentric contraction of the quadriceps produced abnormally high tensile loads in the patella, leading to a fracture at the inferior pole. In this case, the patella fracture occurred because the muscle forces of the quadriceps overcame the osseous strength of the patella. The weakest link was the patella.

The picture shows a fracture at the patella accompanied by a significant fracture separation that resulted from the quadriceps traction force.

Because of the fracture, the extensor mechanism is unable to function and extend the knee. It will directly affect the stability of the patellofemoral joint and the distribution of the compressive stresses on the femur. At the same time, the impaired function of the quadriceps decreases the dynamic stability at the knee joint (patellofemoral and tibiofemoral joints) that is necessary for daily activities such as gait and stair climbing.

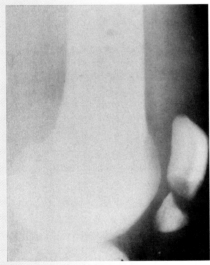

Case Study Figure 7-2-1.

out knee bend, the patellofemoral joint reaction force remained higher than the quadriceps muscle force. During stair climbing and descent, at the point when knee flexion reached a maximum of approximately 60°, the peak value equaled 3.3 times body weight.

When the knee is extended, the lower part of the patella rests against the femur. As the knee is flexed to 90°, the contact surface between the patella and femur shifts cranially in vivo and under weight-bearing conditions (Komistek et al., 2000). The

contact surface area increases in size somewhat (Goodfellow et al., 1976). To some extent, this increase in the contact surface with knee flexion compensates for the larger patellofemoral joint reaction force. If a tight iliotibial band is present, the patellofemoral joint force may shift laterally, causing abnormal patellar kinematics and load-bearing (Kwak et al., 2000).

The quadriceps muscle force and the torque around the patellofemoral joint can be extremely high under certain circumstances, particularly when the knee is flexed—for instance, when a basketball player suffers a patella fracture as a result of indirect forces played by an eccentric contraction of the quadriceps (Case Study 7-2). Another extreme situation was observed during a study of the external torque on the knee produced by weight lifting: one subject ruptured his patellar tendon when he lifted a barbell weighing 175 kg (Zernicke et al., 1977). At the instant of tendon rupture, the knee was flexed 90°; the torque on the knee joint was 550 Nm and the quadriceps muscle force was approximately 10,330 N.

Because of the high magnitude of quadriceps muscle force and joint reaction force during activities requiring a large amount of knee flexion, patients with patellofemoral joint derangements experience increased pain when performing these activities. An effective mechanism for reducing these forces is to limit the amount of knee flexion.

Summary

1 The knee is a two-joint structure that is composed of the tibiofemoral joint and the patellofemoral joint.

2 In the tibiofemoral joint, surface motion occurs in three planes simultaneously but is greatest by far in the sagittal plane. In the patellofemoral joint, surface motion occurs simultaneously in two planes, the frontal and the transverse, and is greater in the frontal plane.

3 The surface joint motion can be described with the use of an instant center technique. When performed on a normal knee, the technique reveals the following: the instant center for successive intervals of motion of the tibiofemoral joint in the sagittal plane follows a semicircular pathway, and the direction of displacement of the tibiofemoral contact points is tangential to the surface of the tibia, indicating gliding throughout the range of motion.

4 The screw-home mechanism of the tibiofemoral joint adds stability to the joint in full extension. Additional passive stability to the knee is given by the ligamentous structure and menisci and the dynamic stability by the muscles around the knee.

5 The tibiofemoral and patellofemoral joints are subjected to great forces. Muscle forces have the greatest influence on the magnitude of the joint reaction force, which can reach several times body weight in both joints. In the patellofemoral joint, knee flexion also affects the joint reaction force, with greater knee flexion resulting in a higher joint reaction force.

6 Although the tibial plateaus are the main load-bearing structures in the knee, the cartilage, menisci, and ligaments also bear loads. The menisci aid in distributing the stresses and reducing the load imposed on the tibial plateaus.

7 The patella aids knee extension by lengthening the lever arm of the quadriceps muscle force throughout the entire range of motion and allows a wider distribution of compressive stress on the femur.

REFERENCES

Åagaard, P., Simonsen, E.B., Andersen, J.L., et al. (2000). Antagonist muscle co-activation during isokinetic extension. *Scan J Med Sci Sports, 10*(2), 58–67.

Andriacchi, T. P. & Birac, D. (1993). Functional ligament testing in the anterior cruciate ligament deficient knee. *Clin Orthop Rel Res, 288 (March),* 40–47.

Andriacchi, T.P., Kramer, G. M., & Landon, G. C. (1979). Three-dimensional coordinate data processing in human motion analysis. *J Biomech Eng, 101,* 279–283.

Andriacchi, T.P. & Strickland, A.B. (1985). Gait analysis as a tool to assess joint kinetics. In N. Berme, A.E. Engin, D.A. Correis, et al. (Eds.). *Biomechanics of Normal and Pathological Human Articulating Joints* (NATO ASI series, Vol 93, pp. 83–102). Drodrecht, Netherlands: Martinus Nijhoff.

Baratta, R., Solomonow, M., Zhou, B.H., Letson, D., Chuinard, R., D'Ambrosia, R. (1988). Muscular co-activation: The role of the antagonist musculature in maintaining knee stability. *Am J Sports Med, 16,* 113–122.

Berchuck M., Andriacchi, T.P., Bach, B.R., Reider, B. (1990) Gait adaptions by patients who have a deficient anterior cruciate ligament. *J Bone Joint Surg, 72A,* 871–877.

Beynnon, B., Howe, J.G., & Pope, M.H. (1992). The measurements of anterior cruciate ligament strain in vivo. *Int Orthop, 16,* 1–12.

Draganich, L.D., Andriacchi, T.P., & Andersson, G.B.J. (1987). Interaction between intrinsic knee mechanism and the knee extensor mechanism. *J Orthop Res, 5,* 539–547.

Drillis, R., Contini, R., & Bluestein, M. (1964). Body segment parameters. A survey of measurement techniques. *Artif Limbs, 8,* 44.

Frankel, V.H. & Burstein, A.H. (1970). *Orthopaedic Biomechanics.* Philadelphia: Lea & Febiger.

Frankel, V.H., Burstein, A.H., & Brooks, D.B. (1971). Biomechanics of internal derangement of the knee. Pathomechanics as determined by analysis of the instant centers of motion. *J Bone Joint Surg, 53A,* 945.

Fu, F.H., Harner, C.D., Johnson, D.L., et al. (1994). Biomechanics of the knee ligaments: Basic concepts and clinical application. *Instr Course Lecture, 43,* 137–148.

Fukuda, Y., Takai, S., Yoshino, N., et al. (2000). Impact load transmission of the knee joint—influence of leg alignment and the role of meniscus and articular cartilage. *Clinical Biomech, 15,* 516–521.

Gardner, T.R., Ateshian, G.A., Grelsamer, R.P., et al. (1994). A 6 DOF knee testing device to determine patellar tracking and patellofemoral joint contact area via stereophotogrammetry. *Adv Bioeng ASME BED, 28,* 279–280

Goodfellow, J., Hungerford, D.S., & Zindel, M. (1976). Patellofemoral joint mechanics and pathology. 1. Functional anatomy of the patellofemoral joint. *J Bone Joint Surg, 58B,* 287.

Grabiner, M.D. & Weiker, G.G. (1993). Anterior cruciate ligament injury and hamstring co-activation. *Clinical Biomech, 8,* 216–219.

Grood, E.S. & Suntay, W.J. (1983). A coordinate system for clinical description of three dimensional motion: Application to the knee. *J Biomech Eng, 105,* 136–144.

Hehne, H.J. (1990). Biomechanics of the patellofemoral joint and its clinical relevance. *Clin Orthop, 258,* 73–85.

Helfet, A.J. (1974). Anatomy and mechanics of movement of the knee joint. In A. Helfet (Ed.), *Disorders of the Knee* (pp. 1–17). Philadelphia: J.B. Lippincott.

Holden, J.P., Chou, G., & Stanhope, S.J. (1997). Changes in knee joint function over a wide range of walking speeds. *Clinical Biomech, 12*(6), 375–382.

Hungerford, D.S. & Barry, M. (1979). Biomechanics of the patellofemoral joint. *Clin Orthop, 144,* 9–15.

Kapandji, I.A. (1970). The knee. In I.A. Kapandjii (Ed.), *The Physiology of the Joints* (Vol 2, pp. 72–135). Paris: Editions Maloine.

Kaufer, H. (1971). Mechanical function of the patella. *J Bone Joint Surg, 53A,* 1551.

Kellis, E. & Baltzopoulus, V. (1999). In vivo determination of the patella and hamstrings moment arms in adult males using videofluoroscopy during submaximal knee extension and flexion. *Clinical Biomech, 14,* 118–124.

Kettelkamp, D.B., Johnson, R.J., Smidt, G.L., Chao, E.Y., Walker, M. (1970). An electrogoniometric study of knee motion in normal gait. *J Bone Joint Surg, 52A,* 775.

Kettelkamp, D.B. & Jacobs, A.W. (1972). Tibiofemoral contact area—determination and implications. *J Bone Joint Surg, 54A,* 349.

Komistek, R.D., Dennis, D.A., Mabe, J.A., et al. (2000). An in vivo determination of patellofemoral contact positions. *Clinical Biomech, 15,* 29–36.

Kroemer, K.H., Marras, W.S., McGlothin, J.D., et al. (1990). On the measurements of human strength. *Int J Industrial Ergonomics, 6,* 199–210.

Kwak, S.D., Ahmad, C.S., Gardner, T.R., et al. (2000). Hamstrings and iliotibial forces affect knee ligaments and contact pattern. *J Orthop Res,18,* 101–108.

Lamoreaux, L. (1971). Kinematic measurements in the study of human walking. Biomechanics Lab, University of California, San Francisco. *Bull Prosthetic Res, Sp 1971,* 10–15.

Laubenthal, K.N., Smidt, G.L., & Kettelkamp, D.B. (1972). A quantitative analysis of knee motion during activities of daily living. *Phys Ther, 52,* 34.

Levens, A.S., Inman, V.T., & Blosser, J.A. (1948). Transverse rotation of the segments of the lower extremity in locomotion. *J Bone Joint Surg, 3OA,* 859.

Lieb, F.J. & Perry, J. (1968). Quadriceps function. An anatomical and mechanical study using amputated limbs. *J Bone Joint Surg, 50A,* 1535.

Lindahl, O. & Movin, A. (1967). The mechanics of extension of the knee joint. *Acta Orthop Scand, 38,* 226.

Markholf, K., Graff-Radford, A., & Amstutz, H. (1978). In vivo knee stability. *J Bone Joint Surg, 60A,* 664–674.

Matsumoto, H., Seedhom, B.B., Suda, Y., et al. (2000). Axis of tibial rotation and its change with flexion angle. *Clin Orthop, 371,* 178–182.

Matthews, L.S., Sonstegard, D.A., & Henke, J.A. (1977). Load bearing characteristics of the patellofemoral joint. *Acta Orthop Scand, 48,*511.

Morrison, J.B. (1970). The mechanics of the knee joint in relation to normal walking. *J Biomech, 3,* 51.

Murray, M.P., Drought, A.B., Kory, R.C. (1964). Walking patterns of normal men. *J Bone Joint Surg, 46A,* 335.

Özkaya, N. & Nordin, M. (1999). *Fundamentals of Biomechanics: Equilibrium, Motion, and Deformation* (2nd ed.). New York: Springer-Verlag.

Perry, J., Norwood, L., & House, K. (1977). Knee posture and biceps and semimembranosus muscle action in running and cutting (an EMG study). *Trans Orthop Res Soc, 2,* 258.

Ramsey, D.K. & Wretenberg, P.F. (1999). Biomechanics of the knee: Methodological considerations in the in vivo kinematic analysis of the tibiofemoral and patellofemoral joint. Review paper. *Clinical Biomech, 14,* 595–611.

Reilly, D.T. & Martens, M. (1972). Experimental analysis of the quadriceps muscle force and patellofemoral joint reaction force for various activities. *Acta Orthop Scand, 43,* 126.

Reuleaux, F. (1876). In *The Kinematics of Machinery: Outline of a Theory of Machines.* London: Macmillan.

Seedhom, B.B., Dowson, D., & Wright, V. (1974). The load-bearing function of the menisci: A preliminary study. In O.S. Ingwersen, et al. (Eds.), *The Knee Joint: Recent Advances in Basic Research and Clinical Aspects* (pp. 37–42). Amsterdam: Excerpta Medica.

Selvik, G. (1978). Roentgen stereophotogrammetry in Lund, Sweden. In A.M. Coblenz & R.E. Herron (Eds.), *Applications of Human Biostereometrics. Proc. SPIE (166)* (pp. 184–189).

Selvik, G. (1983). Roentgen stereophotogrammetry in orthopaedics. In R.E. Herron (Ed.), *Biostereometrics '82. Proc SPIE (361)* (pp. 178–185).

Smidt, G.L. (1973). Biomechanical analysis of knee flexion and extension. *J Biomech, 6,* 79.

Solomonow, M. & D'Ambrosia, R. (1994). Neural reflex arcs and muscle control of knee stability and motion. In W.N. Scott (Ed.), *The Knee* (pp. 107–120). New York: Mosby.

Vedi, V., Williams, A., Tennant, S.J., et al. (1999). Meniscal movement. An in-vivo study using dynamic MRI. *J Bone Joint Surg, 81B*(1), 37–41.

Winter, D.A. (1990). In *Biomechanics and Motor Control of Human Behaviour* (2nd ed.). New York: John Wiley & Sons.

Wiktorin, C.v.H. & Nordin, M. (1986). *Introduction to Problem Solving in Biomechanics* (pp. 87–129). Philadelphia: Lea & Febiger.

Wilson, S.A., Vigorita, V.J., & Scott, W.N. (1994). Anatomy. In N. Scott (Ed.), *The Knee* (p. 17). Philadelphia: Mosby.

Wretenberg, P., Németh, G., Lamontagne, M., et al. (1996). Passive knee muscle moment arms measured in vivo with MRI. *Clinical Biomech, 11*(8), 439–446.

Yu, B., Stuart, M.J., Kienbarcher, T., et al. (1997). Valgus-varus motion of the knee in normal level walking and stair climbing. *Clinical Biomech, 12*(5), 286–293.

Zernicke, R.F., Garhammer, J., & Jobe, F.W. (1977). Human patellar tendon rupture. *J Bone Joint Surg, 59A,* 179–183.

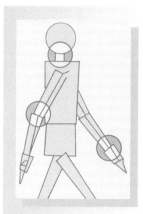

CHAPTER 8

Biomechanics
of the Hip

Margareta Nordin, Victor H. Frankel

Introduction

The hip joint is one of the largest and most stable joints in the body. In contrast to the knee, the hip joint has intrinsic stability provided by its relatively rigid ball-and-socket configuration. It also has a great deal of mobility, which allows normal locomotion in the performance of daily activities. Derangements of the hip can produce altered stress distributions in the joint cartilage and bone, leading to degenerative arthritis. Such damage is further potentiated by the large forces borne by the joint.

Anatomical Considerations

The hip joint is composed of the head of the femur and the acetabulum of the pelvis (Fig. 8-1). This articulation has a loose joint capsule and is surrounded by large, strong muscles. The construction of this stable joint allows for the wide range of motion required for normal daily activities such as walking, sitting, and squatting. Such a joint must be precisely aligned and controlled.

THE ACETABULUM

The acetabulum is the concave component of the ball-and-socket configuration of the hip joint. The acetabular surface is covered with articular cartilage that thickens peripherally (Kempson et al., 1971) and predominantly laterally (Rushfeld et al., 1979). The cavity of the acetabulum faces obliquely forward, outward, and downward. The osseous acetabulum in the hip is deep and provides substantial static stability to the hip. A plane through the circumference of the acetabulum at its opening would intersect with the sagittal plane at an angle of 40° opening posteriorly and with the transverse plane at an angle of 60° opening laterally. The acetabular cavity is deepened by the labrum, a flat rim of fibrocartilage, and the transverse acetabular ligament (Fig. 8-2). The labrum contains free nerve endings and sensory end organs in its superficial layer, which may participate in nociceptive and proprioceptive mechanisms (Kim & Azuma, 1995).

The unloaded acetabulum has a smaller diameter than the femoral head (Greenwald & Haynes, 1972) (Fig. 8-3). The acetabulum deforms about the femoral head when the hip joint is loaded. It undergoes elastic deformation to become congruous with the femoral head, and contact is made about the periphery of the anterior, superior, and posterior

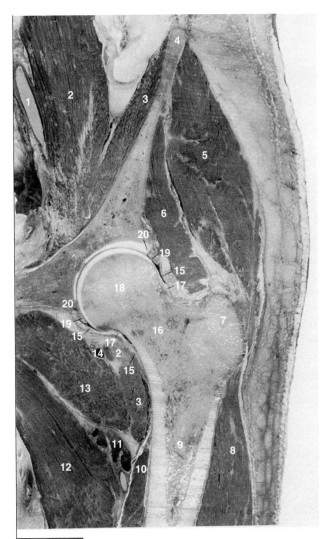

FIG. 8-1

The hip joint (front view) 1. External iliac artery. 2. Psoas major muscle. 3. Iliacus muscle. 4. Iliac crest. 5. Gluteus medius muscle. 6. Gluteus minimus muscle. 7. Greater trochanter. 8. Vastus lateralis muscle. 9. Shaft of femur. 10. Vastus medialis muscle. 11. Profunda femoris vessels. 12. Adductor longus muscle. 13. Pectineus muscle. 14. Medial circumflex femoral vessels. 15. Capsule of the hip joint. 16. Neck of femur. 17. Zona orbicularis of capsule. 18. Head of femur. 19. Acetabular labrum. 20. Rim of acetabulum. *Reprinted with permission from McMinn, R.H. & Huchings, R.H.R. (1988). Color Atlas of Human Anatomy (2nd ed., p. 302). Chicago: Year Book Medical Publishers, Inc.*

articular surface of the acetabulum (Konrath et al., 1998). Load distribution of the acetabulum was studied in vitro in human specimens (Greenwald & Haynes, 1972; Konrath et al., 1998). Joint reaction forces were simulated to physiological levels. The loading pattern of the acetabulum is shown in Figure 8-3. Removal of the transverse acetabular ligament and labrum sequentially did not affect the loading pattern of the acetabulum significantly (Konrath et al., 1998).

THE FEMORAL HEAD

The femoral head is the convex component of the ball-and-socket configuration of the hip joint and forms two-thirds of a sphere. The articular cartilage covering the femoral head is thickest on the medial-central surface and thinnest toward the periphery. The variations in the cartilage thickness result in a different strength and stiffness in various regions of the femoral head (Kempson et al.,

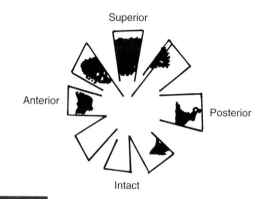

FIG. 8-3

Loading pattern of a human acetabulum in vitro with intact labrum and transverse acetabular ligament. Note: This pattern was grossly unchanged after removal of the transverse acetabular ligament, or the labrum, or both, and therefore those patterns are not displayed. *Adapted from Konrath, G.A., Hamel, A.J., Olson, S.A., et al. (1998). The role of the acetabular labrum and the transverse acetabular ligament in load transmission of the hip. J Bone Joint Surg, 80A(12), 1781–1788.*

1971). Rydell (1965) suggested that most load was transmitted in the femoral head through the superior quadrant. Von Eisenhart-Rothe et al. (1997) demonstrated in an in vitro study that the magnitude of load influenced the loading pattern on the femoral head. At smaller loads, the load-bearing area was concentrated at the periphery of the lunate surface of the femoral head, and at higher loads to the center of the lunate and the anterior and posterior horns. It is still not known exactly how the stresses in vivo on the normal femoral head are distributed, but indications from in vivo measurements with an instrumented prosthetic head show that the anterior and medial lunate is transmitting most of the load during daily activities (Bergmann et al., 1993, 1995).

THE FEMORAL NECK

The femoral neck has two angular relationships with the femoral shaft that are important to hip joint function: the angle of inclination of the neck to the shaft in the frontal plane (the neck-to-shaft angle) and the angle of inclination in the transverse plane (the angle of anteversion). Freedom of motion of the hip joint is facilitated by the neck-to-shaft angle, which offsets the femoral shaft from the pelvis laterally. In most adults, this angle is approximately

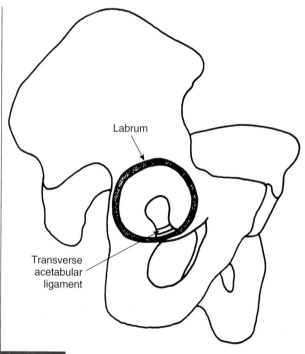

FIG. 8-2

Schematic drawing showing the lateral view of the acetabulum with the labrum and the transverse acetabular ligament intact. *Adapted from Konrath, G.A., Hamel, A.J., Olson, S.A., et al. (1998). The role of the acetabular labrum and the transverse acetabular ligament in load transmission of the hip. J Bone Joint Surg, 80A(12), 1781–1788.*

125°, but it can vary from 90 to 135°. An angle exceeding 125° produces a condition known as coxa valga; an angle less than 125° results in coxa vara (Fig. 8-4). Deviation of the femoral shaft in either way alters the force relationships about the hip joint and has a nontrivial effect on the lever arms to muscle force and line of gravity.

The angle of anteversion is formed as a projection of the long axis of the femoral head and the transverse axis of the femoral condyles (Fig. 8-5). In adults, this angle averages approximately 12°, but it varies a great deal. Anteversion of more than 12° causes a portion of the femoral head to be uncovered and creates a tendency toward internal rotation of the leg during gait to keep the femoral head in the acetabular cavity. An angle of less than 12° (retroversion) produces a tendency toward external rotation of the leg during gait. Both anteversion and retroversion are fairly common in children but are usually outgrown.

The interior of the femoral neck is composed of cancellous bone with trabeculae organized into medial and lateral trabecular systems (Fig. 8-1, 8-6). The fact that the joint reaction force on the femoral head parallels the trabeculae of the medial

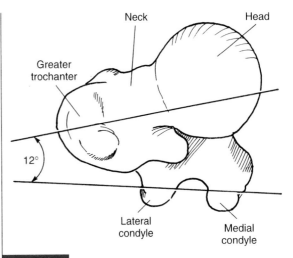

FIG. 8-5

Top view of the proximal end of the left femur showing the angle of anteversion, formed by the intersection of the long axis of the femoral head and the transverse axis of the femoral condyles. This angle averages approximately 12° in adults.

system (Frankel, 1960) indicates the importance of the system for supporting this force. The epiphyseal plates are at right angles to the trabeculae of the medial system and are thought to be perpendicular to the joint reaction force on the femoral head (Inman, 1947). It is likely that the lateral trabecular system resists the compressive force on the femoral head produced by contraction of the abductor muscles—the gluteus medius, the gluteus minimus, and the tensor fasciae latae. The thin shell of cortical bone around the superior femoral neck progressively thickens in the inferior region.

With aging, the femoral neck gradually undergoes degenerative changes: the cortical bone is thinned and cancellated and the trabeculae are gradually resorbed (see Fig. 2-50). These changes may predispose the femoral neck to fracture. It is noteworthy that the femoral neck is the most common fracture site in elderly persons (Case Study 8-1).

Kinematics

In considering the kinematics of the hip joint, it is useful to view the joint as a stable ball-and-socket configuration wherein the femoral head and acetabulum can move in all directions.

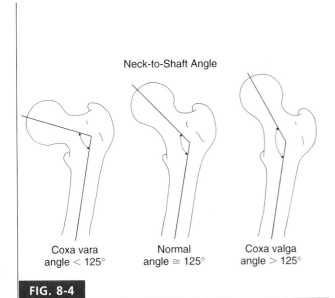

FIG. 8-4

The normal neck-to-shaft angle (angle of inclination of the femoral neck to the shaft in the frontal plane) is approximately 125°. The condition in which this angle is less than 125° is called coxa vara. If the angle is greater than 125°, the condition is called coxa valga.

three planes. Measurements in the sagittal plane during level walking (Murray, 1967) showed that the joint was maximally flexed during the late swing phase of gait, as the limb moved forward for heel strike. The joint extended as the body moved forward at the beginning of stance phase. Maximum extension was reached at heel-off. The joint reversed into flexion during swing phase and again reached maximal flexion, 35 to 40°, prior to heel strike. Figure 8-8A shows the pattern of hip joint motion in the sagittal plane during a gait cycle and

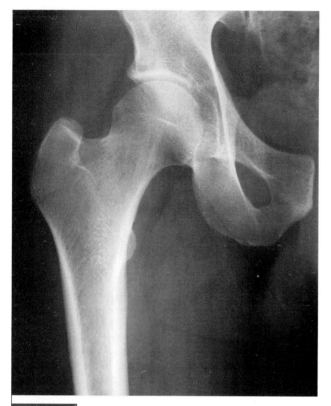

FIG. 8-6

Roentgenogram of a femoral neck showing the medial and lateral trabecular systems. The thin shell of cortical bone around the superior femoral neck progressively thickens in the inferior region.

RANGE OF MOTION

Hip motion takes place in all three planes: sagittal (flexion-extension), frontal (abduction-adduction), and transverse (internal-external rotation) (Fig. 8-7). Motion is greatest in the sagittal plane, where the range of flexion is from 0 to approximately 140° and the range of extension is from 0 to 15°. The range of abduction is from 0 to 30°, whereas that of adduction is somewhat less, from 0 to 25°. External rotation ranges from 0 to 90° degrees and internal rotation from 0 to 70° when the hip joint is flexed. Less rotation occurs when the hip joint is extended because of the restricting function of the soft tissues.

The range of motion of the hip joint during gait has been measured electrogoniometrically in all

CASE STUDY 8-1

Femoral Intertrochanteric Fractures

An 80-year-old woman falls from her own height after losing her balance. She presented with sharp pain in her hip and an inability to stand and walk by herself. She is transported to the E.R. and after a careful examination and x-ray evaluation, a right intertrochanteric fracture is diagnosed.

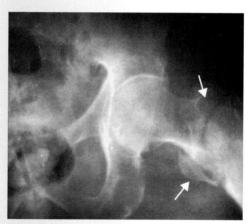

Case Study Figure 8-1-1.

The radiograph illustrates a right femoral intertrochanteric unstable fracture with separation of the lesser trochanter. The image shows osteoporotic changes characteristic of the aging process. The decrease in the bone mass at the femoral neck leads to reduced bone strength and stiffness as a result of diminution in the amount of cancellous bone and thinning of cortical bone. It increases the likelihood of a fracture at the weakest level.

During the fall, the magnitude of the compressive forces at the femoral neck overcame its stiffness and strength. In addition, the tensile forces produced by protective contraction of muscles such as the iliopsoas generated a traction fracture at the lesser trochanter level.

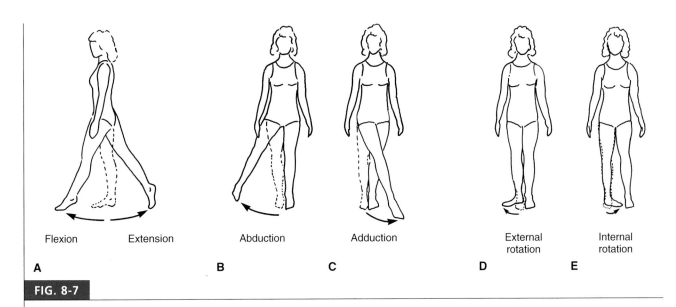

Flexion   Extension   Abduction   Adduction   External   Internal
                                                                rotation   rotation

A   **B**   **C**   **D**   **E**

FIG. 8-7

Movements of the hip joint. **A,** Flexion-extension. **B,** Abduction. **C,** Adduction. **D,** External
rotation. **E,** Internal rotation.

allows a comparison of this motion with that of the knee and ankle.

Motion in the frontal plane (abduction-adduction) and transverse plane (internal-external rotation) during gait (Johnston & Smidt, 1969) is illustrated in Figure 8-8B. Abduction occurred during swing phase, reaching its maximum just after toe-off; at heel strike, the hip joint reversed into adduction, which continued until late stance phase. The hip joint was externally rotated throughout the swing phase, rotating internally just before heel strike. The joint remained internally rotated until late stance phase, when it again rotated externally. The average ranges of motion recorded for the 33 normal men in this study were 12° for the frontal plane and 13° for the transverse plane.

As people age, they use a progressively smaller portion of the range of motion of the lower extremity joints during ambulation. Murray and coworkers (1969) studied the walking patterns of 67 normal men of similar weight and height ranging in age from 20 to 87 years and compared the gait patterns of older and younger men. The differences in the sagittal body positions of the two groups at the instant of heel strike are illustrated in Figure 8-9. The older men had shorter strides, a decreased range of hip flexion and extension, decreased plantar flexion of the ankle, and a decreased heel-to-floor angle of the tracking limb; they also showed reduced dorsiflexion of the ankle and diminished elevation of the toe of the forward limb.

The range of motion in three planes during common daily activities such as tying a shoe, sitting down on a chair, rising from it, picking up an object from the floor, and climbing stairs was measured electrogoniometrically in 33 normal men by Johnston and Smidt (1970). The mean motion during these activities is shown in Table 8-1. Maximal motion in the sagittal plane (hip flexion) was needed for tying the shoe and bending down to squat to pick up an object from the floor. The greatest motion in the frontal and transverse planes was recorded during squatting and during shoe tying with the foot across the opposite thigh. The values obtained for these common activities indicate that hip flexion of at least 120° abduction and external rotation of at least 20° are necessary for carrying out daily activities in a normal manner.

SURFACE JOINT MOTION

Surface motion in the hip joint can be considered as gliding of the femoral head on the acetabulum. The pivoting of the ball and socket in three planes around the center of rotation in the femoral head (estimated at the center of the femoral head) produces this glid-

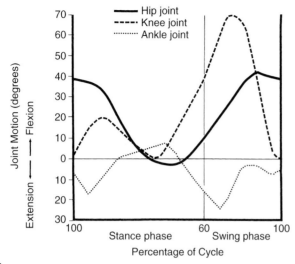

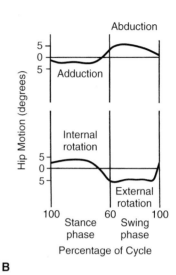

FIG. 8-8

A, Range of hip joint motion in the sagittal plane for 30 normal men during level walking, one gait cycle. The ranges of motion for the knee and ankle joints are shown for comparison. *Adapted from Murray, M.P. (1967). Gait as a total pattern of movement. Am J Phys Med, 46, 290.* **B,** A typical pattern for range of motion in the frontal plane (*top*) and transverse plane (*bottom*) during level walking, one gait cycle. *Adapted from Johnston, R.C. & Smidt, G.L. (1969). Measurement of hip-joint motion during walking. Evaluation of an electrogoniometric method. J Bone Joint Surg, 51A, 1083.*

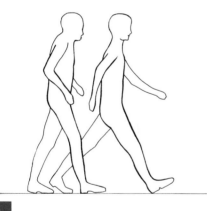

FIG. 8-9

Differences in the sagittal body positions of older men (*left*) and younger men (*right*) at the instant of heel strike. The older men showed shorter strides, a decreased range of hip flexion and extension, decreased plantar flexion of the ankle, and a decreased heel-to-floor angle of the tracking limb; they also showed less dorsiflexion of the ankle and less elevation of the toe of the forward limb. *Reprinted with permission from Murray, M.P., Kory, R.C., & Clarkson, B.H. (1969). Walking patterns in healthy old men. J Gerontol, 24, 169–178.*

ing of the joint surfaces. If incongruity is present in the femoral head, gliding may not be parallel or tangential to the joint surface and the articular cartilage may be abnormally compressed or distracted. Instant center analysis by means of the Reuleaux method cannot be performed accurately in the hip joint because motion takes place in three planes simultaneously. Locating the center of rotation of the hip joint is essential for prosthetic surgery of the hip to reconstruct an optimal lever arm of the gluteus medius muscle (Fessy et al., 1999).

Kinetics

Kinetic studies have demonstrated that substantial forces act on the hip joint during simple activities (Hurwitz & Andriacchi, 1997, 1998). The factors involved in producing these forces must be understood if rational rehabilitation programs are to be

TABLE 8-1

Mean Values for Maximum Hip Motion in Three Planes During Common Activities

Activity	Plane of Motion	Recorded Value (Degrees)
Tying shoe with foot on floor	Sagittal	124
	Frontal	19
	Transverse	15
Tying shoe with foot across opposite thigh	Sagittal	110
	Frontal	23
	Transverse	33
Sitting down on chair and rising from sitting	Sagittal	104
	Frontal	20
	Transverse	17
Stooping to obtain object from floor	Sagittal	117
	Frontal	21
	Transverse	18
Squatting	Sagittal	122
	Frontal	28
	Transverse	26
Ascending stairs	Sagittal	67
	Frontal	16
	Transverse	18
Descending stairs	Sagittal	36

Mean for 33 normal men. Data from Johnston, R.C. & Smidt, G.L. (1970). Hip motion measurements for selected activities of daily living. *Clin Orthop, 72,* 205.

developed for patients with pathological conditions of the hip. The abductor muscle group (the gluteus medius and minimus muscles) is the main stabilizer during one-legged stance (Kumagai et al., 1997; University of California, 1953)

STATICS

During a two-leg stance, the line of gravity of the superincumbent body passes posterior to the pubic symphysis, and, because the hip joint is stable, an erect stance can be achieved without muscle contraction through the stabilizing effect of the joint capsule and capsular ligaments. With no muscle activity to produce moments around the hip joint, calculation of the joint reaction force becomes simple: the magnitude of this force on each femoral head during upright two-legged stance is one half the weight of the superincumbent body. Because each lower extremity is one sixth of body

weight, the reaction force on each hip joint will be one half of the remaining two thirds, or one third of body weight; however, if the muscles surrounding the hip joint contract to prevent swaying and to maintain an upright position of the body (e.g., during prolonged standing), this force increases in proportion to the amount of muscle activity.

When a person changes from a two-leg to a single-leg stance, the line of gravity of the superincumbent body shifts in all three planes, producing moments around the hip joint that must be counteracted by muscle forces and thus increasing the joint reaction force. The magnitude of the moments, and hence the magnitude of the joint reaction force, depends on the posture of the spine, the position of the non–weight-bearing leg and upper extremities, and the inclination of the pelvis (McLeish & Charnley, 1970). Figure 8-10 demonstrates how the line of gravity in the frontal plane shifts with four different positions of the upper body and inclinations of the pelvis: standing with the pelvis in a neutral position, standing with a maximum tilt of the upper body over the supporting hip joint, standing with the upper body tilting away from the supporting hip joint, and standing with the pelvis sagging away from the supporting hip joint (Trendelenburg's test). The shift in the gravity line, and hence in the length of the lever arm of the gravitational force (the perpendicular distance between the gravity line and the center of rotation in the femoral head), influences the magnitude of the moments about the hip joint and, consequently, the joint reaction force. The gravitational force lever arm and the joint reaction force are minimized when the trunk is tilted over the hip joint (Fig. 8-10B).

Two methods are used for deriving the magnitude of the joint reaction force acting on the femoral head: the simplified free-body technique for coplanar forces and a mathematical method utilizing equilibrium equations. The simplified free-body technique for coplanar forces was described in detail in Chapter 7, in Calculation Box 7.1. This technique is used in the hip to estimate the joint reaction force in the frontal plane acting on the femoral head during a single-leg stance with the pelvis in a neutral position (Calculation Box 8-1). The second method is a mathematical calculation of the joint reaction force on the femoral head using equilibrium equations for a single-leg stance with the pelvis level (Calculation Box 8-2).

To understand and solve the equations it is necessary to indicate first the location of the external forces acting on the body during the single-leg

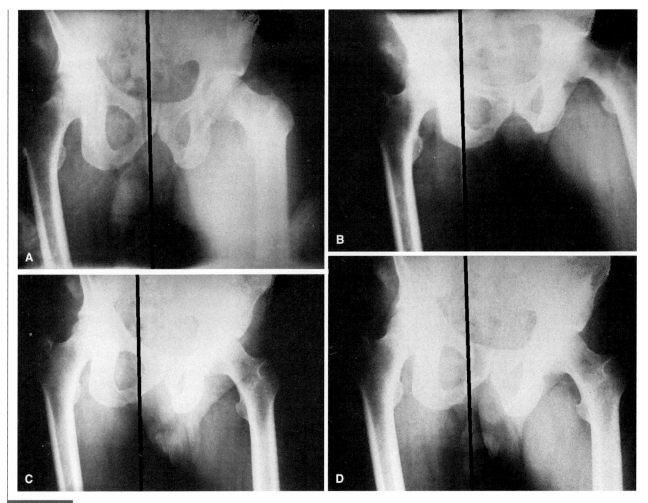

FIG. 8-10

Roentgenograms utilizing a plumb line (*black line*) show that the line of gravity shifts in the frontal plane with different positions of the upper body and inclinations of the pelvis. **A,** The pelvis is in a neutral position. The gravity line falls approximately through the pubic symphysis. The lever arm for the force produced by body weight (the perpendicular distance between the gravity line and the center of rotation in the femoral head) influences the moment about the hip joint and hence the joint reaction force. **B,** The shoulders are maximally tilted over the supporting hip joint. The gravity line has shifted and is now nearest the supporting hip. Because this shift minimizes the lever arm, the moment about the hip joint and the joint reaction force are also minimized. **C,** The shoulders are maximally tilted away from the supporting hip joint. Again the gravity line has shifted toward the supporting hip, thus decreasing the joint reaction force. **D,** The pelvis sags away from the supporting hip joint (Trendelenburg's test). The shift in the gravity line is similar to that in **C.** *(Courtesy of John C. Baker, M.D., Case Western Reserve University, Cleveland, Ohio)* Note: In **B,** the antalgic gait is illustrated, which lowers the load on the head of the femur but alters the load line to a more vertical position. Following arthroplasty for arthritis, the abductor muscles are weak and atrophic as a result of the disease process and the surgery. External support such as a cane should be used until the abductor muscles are rehabilitated. The best indication for a rehabilitated abductor muscle is the lack of limping.

stance on a free-body diagram (Calculation Box Fig. 8-2-1). Because the body is in equilibrium (i.e., the sum of the moments and the sum of the forces both equal zero), the ground reaction force is equal to the gravitational force of the body, which can be divided into two components, the gravitational force of the stance leg (equal to one-sixth body weight) and the remaining force (equal to five-sixths body weight).

Next, the body is divided at the hip joint into two free-bodies. The main coplanar forces and moments acting on these free-bodies must be determined. The upper free-body is considered first (Calculation Box Fig. 8-2-2). In this free-body, two moments are

required for stability. The moment arising from the superincumbent body weight (equal to $5/6$ W) must be balanced by a moment arising from the force of the abductor muscles. The force produced by the superincumbent body weight ($5/6$ W) acts at a distance of b from the center of rotation of the hip (Q), thus producing a moment of $5/6$ W times b. The force produced by the principal abductor, the gluteus medius, designated as A, acts at a distance of c from the center of rotation, producing a counterbalancing moment of A times c. For the body to remain in moment equilibrium, the sum of the moments must equal zero. In this example, the moments acting

---

CALCULATION BOX 8-1

Simplified Free-Body Technique for Coplanar Forces

The stance limb is considered as a free-body, and a free-body diagram is drawn. From all of the forces acting on the free-body, the three main coplanar forces are identified as the force of gravity against the foot (the ground reaction force), which is transmitted through the tibia to the femoral condyles; the force produced by contraction of the abductor muscles; and the joint reaction force on the femoral head. The ground reaction force (W) has a known magnitude equal to five-sixths of body weight and a known sense, line of application, and point of application. The abductor muscle force (A) has a known sense, a known line of application, and point of application estimated from the muscle origin and insertion on a roentgenogram but an unknown magnitude. Because several muscles are involved in the action of hip abduc-

tion, simplifying assumptions are made in determining the direction of this force (McLeish & Charnley, 1970). Furthermore, forces produced by other muscles active in stabilizing the hip joint are not taken into account. The joint reaction force (J) has a known point of application on the surface (lunate) of the femoral head but an unknown magnitude, sense, and line of application.

The magnitudes of the abductor muscle force and the joint reaction force can be derived by designating all three forces on the free-body diagram (Calculation Box Fig. 8-1-1) and constructing a triangle of forces (Calculation Box Fig. 8-1-2). The muscle force is found to be approximately two times body weight, whereas the joint reaction force is somewhat greater.

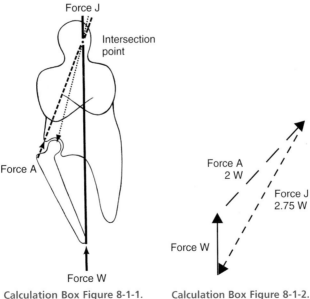

Calculation Box Figure 8-1-1.

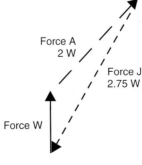

Calculation Box Figure 8-1-2.

CALCULATION BOX 8-2

External Forces Acting on the Body in Equilibrium During a Single-Leg Stance

Calculation Box Figure 8-2-1 shows external forces acting on the body in equilibrium during a single-leg stance. The ground reaction force is equal to body weight (W). The gravitational force of the stance leg is equal to one-sixth of body weight; the remaining force is equal to five-sixths of body weight.

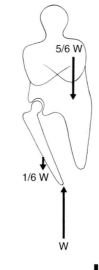

Calculation Box Figure 8-2-1.

The internal forces acting on the hip joint are found by separating the joint into an upper and lower free-body; the upper free-body is considered first. In this free-body, two moments are required for stability. Moment equilibrium is attained by the production of two equal moments. A moment arising from the force of the abductor muscle (A) times abductor force lever arm (c) counterbalances the moment arising from the gravitational force of the superincumbent body (5/6 W) times gravitational force lever arm (b), which tends to tilt the pelvis away from the supporting lower extremity. Q, center of rotation of the hip joint.

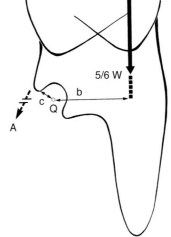

Calculation Box Figure 8-2-2.

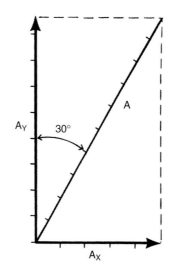

$$A = 2\,W$$
$$A_X = A \cdot \sin 30°$$
$$A_X = 0.5\,A = W$$

$$A_Y = A \cdot \cos 30°$$
$$A_Y = 0.8\,A = 1.7\,W$$

Calculation Box Figure 8-2-3.

Force A is equal to two times body weight and has a direction of 30° from the vertical. The magnitudes of its horizontal (A_x) and vertical (A_y) components are found by vector analysis. Perpendiculars are drawn from the tail of A to a horizontal and a vertical line representing A_x and A_y, respectively. A_x and A_y can then be scaled off. Alternatively, trigonometry is used to find the magnitudes of the components.

clockwise are arbitrarily considered to be positive and the counterclockwise moments are considered to be negative. Thus,

$$(\tfrac{5}{6}W \times b) - (A \times c) = 0$$

$$A = \frac{\tfrac{5}{6}W \times b}{c}$$

To solve for A it is necessary to find the values of b and c. The gravitational force lever arm (b) is found roentgenographically. Because the center of gravity must lie over the base of support, a plumb line intersecting the heel can be extended upward; a perpendicular line drawn from the center of rotation in the femoral head (Q) to the line represents distance b. The muscle force lever arm (c) is similarly found by identifying the gluteus medius muscle on a roentgenogram (Nemeth & Ohlsen, 1985, 1989) and drawing a perpendicular line from the center of rotation of the femoral head to a line approximating the gluteus medius muscle tendon.

In this example, a value for A of two times body weight was derived from the static free-body diagram and confirmed by instrumented in vivo measurements (English & Kilvington, 1979; Rydell, 1966). The direction of force A is found from a roentgenogram to be 30° from the vertical. The horizontal and vertical components of this force are found by vector analysis (Calculation Box Fig. 8-2-3). The horizontal component (A_x) is equal to body weight; the vertical component (A_Y) is approximately 1.7 times body weight.

Attention is then directed to the lower free-body (Calculation Box Fig 8-3-1). The gravitational forces (W and $\tfrac{1}{6}$ W) are known. The joint reaction force (force J) has an unknown magnitude and direction but originates from the most narrow joint space in the radiograph and must pass through the estimated center of rotation in the femoral head. The magnitude of force J is determined by finding the horizontal and vertical force components and adding them (Calculation Box Fig. 8-3-2).

The value of J is found by vector addition (Calculation Box Fig. 8-3-3), and its direction is measured on the parallelogram of forces. The joint reaction force on the femoral head in a single-leg stance with the pelvis leveled in the horizontal plane is found to be approximately 2.7 times body weight, and its direction is 69° from the horizontal (Calculation Box Fig. 8-3-4).

A key factor influencing the magnitude of the joint reaction force on the femoral head is the ratio of the abductor muscle force lever arm (c) to the gravitational force lever arm (b) (Calculation Box

Fig. 8-2-2). This is particularly important in prosthetic replacements of the hip joint (Delp & Maloney, 1993; Free & Delp, 1996; Lim et al., 1999; Sutherland et al., 1999; Vasavada et al., 1994). The center of motion can be altered by the prosthetic design and the lever arm for the abductor muscles can be slightly changed by surgery techniques. A change of the center of location of the hip joint can decrease the abduction force by more than 40% and thereby the generated abductor moment by almost 50% (Delp & Maloney, 1993). Figure 8-11 illustrates the relationship of this ratio to the joint reaction force. A low ratio (i.e., a small muscle force lever arm and a large gravitational force lever arm) yields a greater joint reaction force than does a high ratio.

A short lever arm of the abductor muscle force, as in coxa valga (Fig. 8-4), results in a small ratio and thus a somewhat elevated joint reaction force. Moving the greater trochanter laterally during total hip replacement lowers the joint reaction force, as it increases the lever arm ratio by increasing the muscle force lever arm (Free & Delp, 1996). Inserting a prosthetic cup deeper in the acetabulum reduces the gravitational force lever arm, thereby increasing the ratio and decreasing the joint reaction force. It is difficult, however, to change the lever arm ratio in such a way as to reduce the joint reaction force significantly because the curve formed from plotting the ratios becomes asymptotic when the ratio of c to b approaches 0.8 (Fig. 8-11).

DYNAMICS

The loads on the hip joint during dynamic activities have been studied by several investigators (Andriacchi et al., 1980; Draganich et al., 1980; English & Kilvington, 1979: Rydell, 1966). Using a force plate system and kinematic data for the normal hip, J. P. Paul, 1967, (Forces at the human hip joint. Unpublished doctoral theses, University of Chicago) examined the joint reaction force on the femoral head in normal men and women during gait and correlated the peak magnitudes with specific muscle activity recorded electromyographically. In the men, two peak forces were produced during the stance phase when the abductor muscles contracted to stabilize the pelvis. One peak of approximately four times body weight occurred just after heel strike, and a large peak of approximately seven times body weight was reached just before toe-off (Fig. 8-12A). During foot flat, the joint reaction force decreased to approximately

CALCULATION BOX 8-3

Free-Body Diagram of the Lower Extremity

In Calculation Box Figure 8-3-1, the supporting lower extremity is considered as a free-body, and the forces acting on the free-body are identified. A, abductor muscle force; J, joint reaction force; 1/6 W, gravitational force of the limb; W, ground reaction force; Q, center of rotation of the hip joint.

In Calculation Box Figure 8-3-2, the forces acting on the lower free-body are divided into horizontal and vertical components. Because the body is in force equilibrium, the sum of the forces in the horizontal direction must equal zero and so must the forces in the vertical direction. The horizontal and vertical forces are added and the magnitudes of J_x and J_y are found from force equilibrium equations:

$A_x - J_x = 0$

$A_x = J_x$

$A_x = W$

$J_x = W$

From the Calculation Box 8.2 $A_y = 1.7W$

$A_y - J_y - \frac{1}{6}W + W = 0$

$1.7W - J_y - \frac{1}{6}W + W = 0$

$J_y \approx 1.7W - \frac{1}{6}W + W$

$J_y \approx 1.7W + \frac{5}{6}W$

$J_y \cong 2.5W$

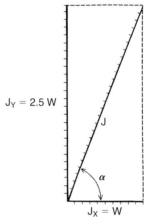

$J_Y = 2.5\ W$

$\tan \alpha = \dfrac{J_Y}{J_X}$

$\tan \alpha = 2.5$

$\alpha = 69°$

$J_X = W$

Calculation Box Figure 8-3-3.

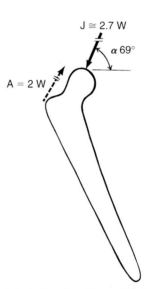

$J \cong 2.7\ W$

$\alpha\ 69°$

$A = 2\ W$

Calculation Box Figure 8-3-4.

Addition of the horizontal and vertical components J_x and J_y is performed graphically in Figure 8-3-3, and the joint reaction force (J) is scaled off. A parallelogram is constructed and the diagonal of the parallelogram indicates the inclination of the force J. Its inclination in relation to the horizontal plane is measured (α) on the parallelogram. Alternately, trigonometry is used to find the direction of J using tangent equations (Fig. 8-3-4).

The joint reaction force has a magnitude of approximately 2.7 times body weight and acts at an angle 69° from the horizontal.

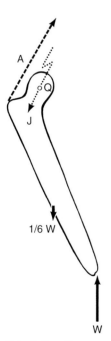

Calculation Box Figure 8-3-1.

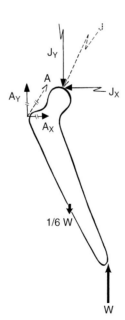

Calculation Box Figure 8-3-2.

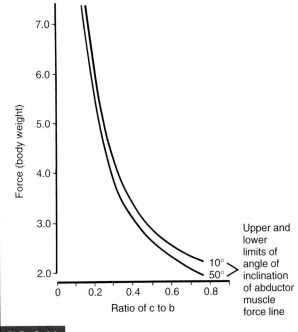

FIG. 8-11

The value of the ratio of the abductor muscle force lever arm (*c*) to the gravitational force lever arm (*b*) is plotted against the joint reaction force on the femoral head in units of body weight. Because the line of application of the abductor muscle force (its angle of inclination in the frontal plane) has finite upper and lower limits (10 and 50°), the force envelope is plotted. The curve can be utilized to determine the minimal force acting on the femoral head during a one-leg stance if the ratio of c to b is known. *Adapted from Frankel, V.H. (1960). In* The Femoral Neck: Function, Fracture Mechanisms, Internal Fixation. *Springfield: Charles C. Thomas.*

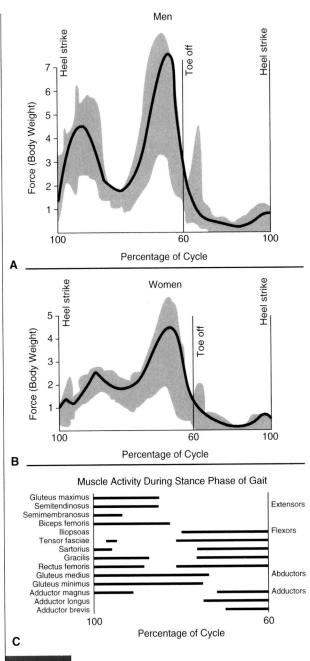

FIG. 8-12

Hip joint reaction force in units of body weight during walking, one gait cycle. The *shaded area* indicates variations among subjects. **A,** Force pattern for normal men. **B,** Force pattern for normal women. *Adapted from Paul, J.P. (1967).* Forces at the human hip joint. *Unpublished doctoral thesis, University of Chicago.* **C,** Muscle activity during stance phase of gait. The first peak corresponds mainly for the extensor and abductor muscles. The last peak is for the flexors and adductor muscles. *Adapted from the University of California. (1953). The pattern of muscular activity in the lower extremity during walking.* Univ Cal Prosthet Dev Res Rep, 2(25), 1–41.

body weight because of the rapid deceleration of the body's center of gravity. During the swing phase, the joint reaction force was influenced by contraction of the extensor muscles in decelerating the thigh, and the magnitude remained relatively low, approximately equal to body weight.

In the women, the force pattern was the same but the magnitude was somewhat lower, reaching a maximum of only approximately four times body weight at late stance phase (Fig. 8-12*B*). The lower magnitude of the joint reaction force in the women may have been the result of several factors: a wider female pelvis, a difference in the inclination of the femoral neck-to-shaft angle, a difference in footwear, and differences in the general pattern of gait.

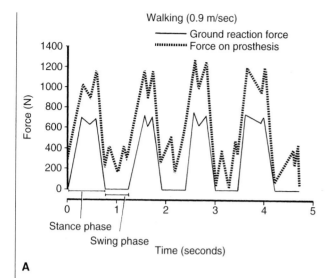

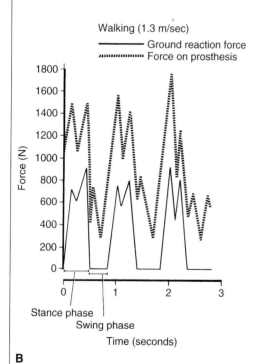

A, Walking speed 0.9 m per second.

B, Walking speed 1.3 m per second.

FIG. 8-13

Forces on an instrumented hip prosthesis during walking. The *broken line* represents the force on the prosthesis, and the *solid line* represents the ground reaction force. **A,** Walking speed 0.9 m per second. **B,** Walking speed 1.3 m per second. An increase in muscle activity at the faster cadence resulted in higher forces on the prosthesis. *Adapted from Rydell, N. (1965). Forces in the hip-joint. Part II: Intravital measurements. In R.M. Kenedi (Ed.), Biomechanics and Related Bio-Engineering Topics (pp. 351–357). Oxford: Pergamon Press.*

In vivo measurements of the forces acting on an instrumented hip joint prosthesis demonstrate the lower joint reaction force of the femoral head during the stance phase of gait compared with external measurements and calculations (Rydell, 1965) (Fig. 8-13*A*). At a faster cadence, the forces acting on the prosthesis greatly increased because of an increase in muscle activity (Fig. 8-13*B*). At both cadences, the magnitude of the forces during swing phase was approximately half that during stance phase.

Table 8-2 summarizes the typical peak joint forces on the hip joint load expressed as body weight from different studies and with different methods. The pattern of loading for walking is similar for all studies, but the magnitude of joint peak load differs. External measurements generally yield higher calculated peak force on the hip joint while instrumented implant in vivo measurements yield lower peak forces. There are many reasons for the difference, for example, the method and instrumentation, the normal hip versus the "abnormal" instrumented implant, the gait velocity, and age. Activities other than walking, such as stair ascending/descending, yield loads of around 2.6 to 5.5 body weight measured

TABLE 8-2

Range of Typical Reported Peak Hip Joint Forces From Selected Studies

Activity	Reported Peak Force BW	Instrumentation	Reference
Walking	2.7–4.3	Instrumented implants	Bergmann et al., 1993, 1995
	2.7–3.6	Instrumented implants	Kotzar et al., 1991
	2.7	Instrumented implants	English et al., 1979
	1.8–3.3	Instrumented implants	Rydell et al., 1966
Walking	4.9–7.0	EMG /force plate	Paul, 1967
	4.5–7.5	EMG /force plate	Crowninshield et al., 1978
	5.0–8.0	EMG /force plate	Rohrle et al., 1984
	2.2–2.8	accelerometers	van den Bogert et al., 1999

BW, body weight; EMG, electromyography

CASE STUDY 8-2

Fatigue Fracture of the Hip

A 64-year-old, very active retired man experienced a femoral neck fracture after changing his training regime to prepare for a marathon. The fracture was classified as a fatigue fracture caused by overload of the hip joint.

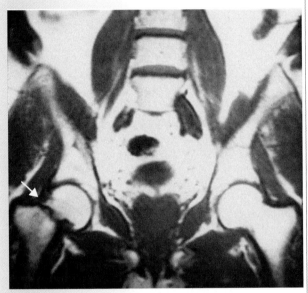

Case Study Figure 8-2-1.

The figure shows an MRI (frontal view) of the pelvis and both hip joints. The fracture is seen in the left femoral neck distal to the femoral head. The fracture is believed to have occurred during running and after an extensive change of training program. Because of the high repetitive loading, muscle fatigue, and the change in the load pattern on the hip joint and femoral neck, the bone fractured.

with an instrumented hip implant (Bergmann et al., 1995; Kotzar et al., 1991). The highest magnitudes of load during daily activities are measured during stair climbing and getting up from a low chair when the hip is flexed more than 100° (Catani et al., 1995; Johnston et al., 1979). Co-contraction of the biarticular muscles was evident during these activities. Running and skiing using accelerometers yielded calculated forces up to eight times body weight in middle-aged and older people (van den Bogert et al., 1999) (Case Study 8-2).

Insertion of an instrumented nail plate in the proximal femur after osteotomy or during fixation of a femoral neck fracture allowed a subsequent determination of the forces acting on the implant during activities of daily living (Fig. 8-14) (Frankel et al., 1971). Although the device measured forces on the implant and not on the hip joint, it was possible to determine the proportion of the load transmitted through the device and to calculate the total load acting on the hip joint by means of static analysis. In the case illustrated in Figure 8-14, the nail plate transmitted one fourth of the total load.

Strong forces acting on the nail plate were encountered during such diverse activities as moving onto a bedpan, transferring to a wheelchair, and walking. The magnitude of the forces was greatly modified by skillful assistance from the nurse or therapist to control the patient's movement. Forces of up to four times body weight acted on the hip joint when the patient used the elbows and heels to elevate the hips while being placed on a bedpan (Fig. 8-15), but these forces were greatly reduced through the use of a trapeze and assistance from an attendant (Fig. 8-15B). A 5-kg extension traction on the hip had little effect in modifying the forces acting on the hip joint. Exercises of the foot and ankle increased these forces.

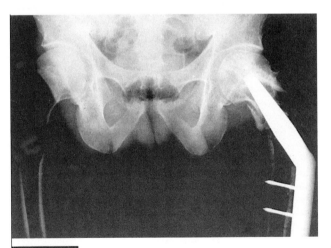

FIG. 8-14

An instrumented nail plate in the proximal end of the femur was used to determine the forces acting on the implant during the activities of daily living following fracture of the femoral neck. In this case, the nail plate was found to transmit one fourth of the total load on the hip joint.

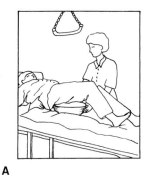
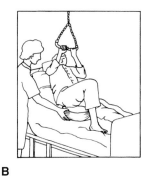

A　　　　　　　**B**

A, When the patient used elbows and heels to elevate the hips while being placed on a bedpan, the force on the tip of the instrumented nail was 670 N. With a spica cast, the force on the tip of the nail was 190 N. **B,** The use of a trapeze and assistance from an attendant reduced the force to 190 N without a cast and to 70 N with a spica cast. *Reprinted with permission from Frankel, V.H. (1973). Biomechanics of the hip. In R.G. Tronzo (Ed.), Surgery of the Hip Joint (pp. 105–125). Philadelphia: Lea & Febiger.*

Use of the instrumented nail plate demonstrated that, for a bedridden patient with a fractured femoral neck, the forces on the femoral head during activities of daily living approached those during walking with external supports. These studies support clinical protocols for early mobilization of patients and decreased bed rest for patients with hip fractures. The magnitude (approximately 8 Nm) of the moments acting on the nail-plate junction in the transverse plane (i.e., during internal and external rotation) was only approximately one half the magnitude (18 Nm) of the moments acting in the frontal plane (i.e., during abduction) for many activities.

EFFECT OF EXTERNAL SUPPORT ON THE HIP JOINT REACTION FORCE

Static analysis of the joint reaction force on the femoral head during walking with a cane demonstrates that the cane should be used on the side opposite the painful or operated hip. Neumann (1998)

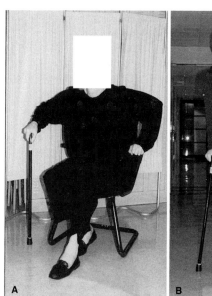
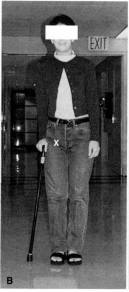
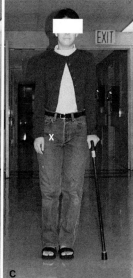

A　　　　　　　**B**　　　　　　　**C**

High and low load on the hip joint during daily activities. Raising from a low chair produces approximately 8 times body weight (**A**). Walking with a cane on the ipsilateral side of the affected hip produces approximately 3.4 times body weight (**B**), and walking with a cane on the contralateral side of the affected hip reduces hip joint load substantially to 2.2 times body weight (**C**). This figure illustrates how load on the hip joint can be manipulated by simple means (**X** denotes affected hip).

CALCULATION BOX 8-4

Effect of External Support on the Hip Joint Reaction Force

Kinematic data were used to determine the joint reaction force acting on the femoral head in the late swing phase of the gait cycle for an 8-year-old boy weighing 24 kg and wearing a long-leg brace. The main muscle force was produced by contraction of the gluteus maximus muscle and identified through electromyography. The torque about the hip joint was calculated according to the formula

$$T = I\alpha,$$

where

T   is the torque expressed in newton meters (Nm)

I   is the mass moment of inertia expressed in newton meters times seconds squared (Nm sec²)

a   is the angular acceleration in late swing phase, expressed in radians per second squared (r/sec²).

In the case of the braced side, $I = I_L + I_B$ where

I_L is the mass moment of inertia of the leg

I_B is the mass moment of inertia of the brace.

On the normal side,
I = 0.45 Nm sec²
α = 24 r/sec².

On the braced side,
I = 0.45 Nm sec² + 0.35 Nm sec²
α = 24 r/sec²

Thus,
I = 0.45 Nm sec²
   × 24 r/sec²
T = 10.8 Nm.

Thus,
T = (.45 Nm sec² + .35 Nm sec²)
   × 24 r/sec²
T = 19.2 Nm.

The extensor muscle force (E) was then found from the moment relationship

$$T = Fd,$$

where F is the extensor muscle force and d is the perpendicular distance from the center of rotation of the femur to the middle of the gluteus maximus muscle. Distance d was measured from a roentgenogram and found to be 3.2 cm. From the equation E = T/d, the muscle force on the normal side was calculated to be 338 N, and on the braced side, 600 N. The joint reaction force on the femoral head (J) is equal to the muscle force (E) minus the gravitational force produced by the weight of the limb (W_L). In this example, W_L was estimated to be 40 N.

On the normal side,
J = E – W_L
J = 338 N – 40 N
J = 298 N.

On the braced side,
J = E – W_L
J = 600 N – 40 N
J = 560 N.

Thus, the joint reaction force on the femoral head in the braced limb was over 80% higher than the force in the non-braced limb, reaching more than two times body weight.

---

studied the effects of cane use in 24 subjects with a mean age of 63 years. During walking, the electromyographic activity of the hip abductor muscles was measured. Neumann found that use of a cane on the contralateral side of the affected hip joint, with careful instructions to use with near maximal effort, could reduce the muscle activity by 42% (Fig. 8-16). This calculates to a reduction of approximately one times body weight from 2.2 body weight with a cane, compared with 3.4 body weight without a cane. These studies give important information to the clinician about ways to moderate the load for the patient with hip problems.

Such use reduces the force on the femoral head of the painful joint without necessitating an antalgic body position. A cane used on the side of the painful hip works through a shorter lever arm and thus an even greater push on the cane is needed to decrease the joint reaction force. For the older patient, such

a large push may not be possible because of a lack of strength in the upper extremities.

The use of a brace on the leg may alter the forces on the hip joint but may not always reduce the joint reaction force on the femoral head. An ischial long-leg brace used in the treatment of Perthes' disease raises the joint reaction force during late swing phase because the large mass moment of inertia of the brace results in a higher extensor muscle force during this part of the gait cycle (Calculation Box 8-4).

Summary

1 The hip joint is a ball-and-socket joint composed of the acetabulum and femoral head.

2 The thickness and mechanical properties of the cartilage on the femoral head and acetabulum vary from point to point.

3 Hip flexion of at least 120°, abduction of at least 20°, and external rotation of at least 20° are necessary for carrying out daily activities in a normal manner.

4 A joint reaction force of approximately three times body weight acts on the hip joint during a single-leg stance with the pelvis in a neutral position; its magnitude varies as the position of the upper body changes.

5 The magnitude of the hip joint reaction force is influenced by the ratio of the abductor muscle force and gravitational force lever arms. A low ratio yields a greater joint reaction force than does a high ratio.

6 The hip joint reaction force during gait reaches levels of three to six times body weight or more in stance phase and is approximately equal to body weight during swing phase.

7 An increase in gait velocity increases the magnitude of the hip joint reaction force in both swing and stance phase.

8 The forces acting on an internal fixation device during the activities of daily living vary greatly depending on the nursing care and the therapeutic activities undertaken by the patient.

9 The use of a cane or a brace on the leg can alter the magnitude of the hip joint reaction force.

REFERENCES

Andriacchi, T.P., Andersson, G.B., Fermier, R.W., Stern, D., Galanie, J.O. (1980). A study of lower-limb mechanics during stair-climbing. *J Bone Joint Surg, 62A*, 749.

Bergmann, G., Graichen, F., & Rohlmann, A. (1993). Hip joint loading during walking and running measured in two patients. *J Biomech, 26*(8), 969–990.

Bergmann, G., Graichen, F., & Rohlmann, A. (1995). Is staircase walking a risk for the fixation of hip implants? *J Biomech, 28*(5), 535–553.

Catani, F., Hodge, A., Mann, R.W., et al. (1995). The role of muscular co-contraction of the hip during movement. *Chir Organi Mov, 80*(2), 227–236.

Crowninshield, R.D., Johnston, R.C., Brand, R.A. (1978). The effects of walking velocity and age on hip kinematics and kinetics. *Clin Orthop Rel Res, 132,*140–144.

Delp, S.L. & Maloney, W. (1993). Effects of hip center location on the moment-generating capacity of the muscles. *J Biomech, 26*(5), 485–499.

Draganich, L.F., Andriacchi, T.P., Strongwater, A.M., et al. (1980). Electronic measurement of instantaneous foot-floor contact patterns during gait. *J Biomech, 13*, 875.

English, T.A. & Kilvington, M. (1979). In vivo records of hip loads using a femoral implant with telemetric output (a preliminary report). *J Biomed Eng, 1*(2), 111.

Fessy, M.H., N'Diaye, A., Carret, J.P., et al. (1999). Locating the center of rotation of the hip. *Surg Radiol Anat, 21*(4), 247–250.

Frankel, V.H. (1973). Biomechanics of the hip. In R.G. Tronzo (Ed.), *Surgery of the Hip Joint* (pp. 105–125). Philadelphia: Lea & Febiger.

Frankel, V.H. (1960). In *The Femoral Neck: Function, Fracture Mechanisms, Internal Fixation.* Springfield: Charles C. Thomas.

Frankel, V.H., Burstein, A.H., Lygre, L., et al. (1971). The telltale nail. *J Bone Joint Surg, 53A*, 1232.

Free, S.A. & Delp, S.L. (1996). Trochanteric transfer in total hip replacement: Effects on the moment arms and force-generating capacities of the hip abductors. *J Orthop Res, 14*(2), 245–250.

Greenwald, A.S. & Haynes, D.W. (1972). Weight-bearing areas in the human hip joint. *J Bone Joint Surg, 54B*(1), 157–163.

Hurwitz, D.E. & Andriacchi, T.P. (1998). Biomechanics of the hip. In J.J. Callaghan, A.G. Rosenberg, & H.E. Rubash (Eds.), *The Adult Hip* (pp. 75–85). Philadelphia: Lippincott-Raven Publishers.

Hurwitz, D.E. & Andriacchi, T.P. (1997). Biomechanics of the hip and the knee. In M. Nordin, G.B.J. Andersson, & M.H. Pope (Eds.), *Musculoskeletal Disorders in the Workplace. Principles and Practice* (pp. 486–496). Philadelphia: Mosby-Year Book.

Inman, V.T. (1947). Functional aspects of the abductor muscles of the hip. *J Bone Joint Surg, 29A*, 607.

Johnston, R.C., Brand, R.A., & Crowninshield, R.D. (1979). Reconstruction of the hip. *J Bone Joint Surg, 61A*(5), 646–652.

Johnston, R.C. & Smidt, G.L. (1969). Measurement of hip-joint motion during walking. Evaluation of an electrogoniometric method. *J Bone Joint Surg, 51A*, 1083.

Johnston, R.C. & Smidt, G.L. (1970). Hip motion measurements for selected activities of daily living. *Clin Orthop, 72*, 205.

Kempson, G.E., Spivey, C.J., Swanson, S.A.V., et al. (1971). Patterns of cartilage stiffness on normal and degenerate human femoral heads. *J Biomech, 4*, 597.

Kim, Y.T. & Azuma, H. (1995). The nerve endings of the acetabular labrum. *Clin Orthop, 320*, 176–181.

Konrath, G.A., Hamel, A.J., Olson, S.A., et al. (1998). The role of the acetabular labrum and the transverse acetabular ligament in load transmission of the hip. *J Bone Joint Surg, 80A*(12), 1781–1788.

Kotzar, G.M., Davy, D.T., Goldberg, V.M., et al. (1991). Telemitrized in vivo hip joint force data. A report on two patients after total hip surgery. *J Orthop Res, 9*, 621–633.

Kumagai, M., Shiba, N., Higuchi, F., et al. (1997). Functional evaluation of hip abductor muscles with use of magnetic resonance imaging. *J Orthop Res, 15*(6), 888–893.

Lim, L.A., Carmichael, S.W., & Cabanela, M.E. (1999). Biomechanics of total hip arthroplasty. *Anat Rec, 257*(3), 110–116.

McLeish, R.D. & Charnley, J. (1970). Abduction forces in the one-legged stance. *J Biomech, 3*, 191.

McMinn, R.H. & Huchings, R.H.R. (1988). In *Color Atlas of Human Anatomy* (2nd ed., p. 302). Chicago: Year Book Medical Publishers, Inc.

Murray, M.P. (1967). Gait as a total pattern of movement. *Am J Phys Med, 46*, 290.

Murray, M.P., Kory, R.C., & Clarkson, B.H. (1969). Walking patterns in healthy old men. *J Gerontol, 24,* 169–178.

Nemeth, G. & Ohlsen, H. (1985). In vivo moment arm lengths for hip extensor muscles at different angles of hip flexion. *J Biomech, 18,* 129–149.

Nemeth, G. & Ohlsen, H. (1989). Moment arms of hip abductor and adductor muscles in vivo by computed tomography. *Clin Biomech, 4,* 133–136.

Neumann, D.A. (1998). Hip abductor muscle activity as subjects with hip prostheses walk with different methods of using a cane. *Phys Ther, 78*(5), 490–501.

Röhrle, H., Scholten R., Sigolotto, C., et al. (1984). Joint forces in the human pelvis-leg skeleton during walking. *J Biomech, 17,* 409–424.

Rushfeld, P.D., Mann, R.W., & Harris, W.H. (1979). Influence of cartilage geometry on the pressure distribution in the human hip joint. *Science, April 27, 204*(4391), 413–415.

Rydell, N.W. (1966). Forces acting on the femoral head prosthesis: A study on strain gauge supplied prostheses in living persons. *Acta Orthop Scand, Suppl 88,* 1–132.

Rydell, N. (1965). Forces in the hip-joint. Part II: Intravital measurements. In R.M. Kenedi (Ed.), *Biomechanics and Related Bio-Engineering Topics* (pp. 351–357). Oxford: Pergamon Press.

Sutherland, A.G., D'Arcy, S., Smart, D., et al. (1999). Abductor muscle weakness and stress around acetabular components of total hip arthroplasty: A finite element analysis. *Int Orthop, 23*(5), 275–278.

University of California. (1953). The pattern of muscular activity in the lower extremity during walking. *Univ Cal Prosthet Dev Res Rep, 2*(25), 1–41.

van den Bogert, A.J., Read, L., & Nigg, B.M. (1999). An analysis of hip joint loading during walking, running and skiing. *Med Sci Sports, 31*(1), 131–142.

Vasavada, A.N., Delp, S.L., Maloney, W.J., et al. (1994). Compensating for changes in muscle length in total hip arthroplasty. Effects on the moment generating capacity of the muscles. *Clin Orthop, 302,* 121–133.

Von Eisenhart-Rothe, R., Eckstein, F., Muller-Gerbl, M., et al. (1997). Direct comparison of contact areas, contact stress and subchondral mineralization in human hip joint specimens. *Anat Embryol (Berl), 195*(3), 279–288.

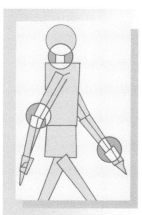

CHAPTER 9

Biomechanics of the Foot and Ankle

G. James Sammarco, Ross Todd Hockenbury

Introduction

The biomechanics of the foot and ankle are complex and intricately associated with each other. The foot is an integral mechanical part of the lower extremity necessary for a smooth and stable gait. The ankle transfers load from the lower extremity to the foot and closely influences foot orientation with the ground.

The foot is comprised of 28 bones (including sesamoids) whose motions are closely interrelated (Fig. 9-1). Besides acting as a structural supporting platform capable of withstanding repetitive loads of multiples of body weight, the foot/ankle complex also must be able to adjust to different ground surfaces and varying speeds of locomotion. The unique qualities of the foot allow it to be rigid when necessary, as in ballet dancing on point, or quite flexible, as in walking barefoot on the sand. The transition from shock-absorbing platform to rigid lever capable of forward propulsion occurs with each step of the gait cycle.

The ankle is comprised of three bones that form the ankle mortise. This joint complex consists of the tibiotalar, fibulotalar, and tibiofibular joints (Fig. 9-2). The ankle is a hinge joint whose stability depends on joint congruency and the medial, lateral, and syndesmotic ligaments.

This chapter discusses the motions that occur in the foot and ankle during the various phases of gait as well as during extremes of motion. The close interplay between lower extremity rotation and forefoot orientation is explained. The ground (foot-to-floor) reaction force and distribution of forces on the plantar aspect of the foot are explored. The location of forces as they pass from the tibiofibular complex into the dome of the talus and then into the foot is discussed. We also discuss the roles of ligaments and muscles in the support of the medial longitudinal arch. Finally, ankle motion and ligamentous stability is outlined.

A discussion of sophisticated electromyographic activity during walking is not within the scope of this chapter; however, the activity of certain extrinsic and intrinsic muscles is by necessity presented to allow a better understanding of foot and ankle control during gait. The moments produced about joints by muscle action and resultant effects on foot and ankle position are detailed. Joint axes and instant centers of joint motion are described. Refer to Chapter 18 for information about the application of biomechanics to gait.

Any pathological change in foot or ankle structure or motion, however subtle, may have a profound impact on the foot and ankle's shock-absorbing, propulsive, and stabilizing roles. Clinical correlation of alterations in biomechanical function is presented in case studies. Footwear in Western society may vary from a rigid ski boot to a soft moccasin. These externally restrictive materials may alter normal foot and ankle biomechanics and ultimately influence the development of some pathological conditions, such as hallux valgus.

Growth of the Foot

The foot is formed when the limb buds develop during the eighth week of gestation. Foot length and width increases linearly from age 3 to 12 in girls and age 3 to 15 in boys at an average of 8 to 10 mm per year, followed by a plateau in growth (Cheng et al., 1997). Blais and associates (1956) showed that the foot appears to be closer to the adult size at all times during normal development of the child than are other parts of the limb. On average, at age 1 year in girls and 18 months in boys, the length of the foot is one half the length of the respective adult foot (Fig. 9-3). This situation contrasts with that in the femur and tibia, which do not attain their mature length until 3 years later in both boys and girls. The relatively large size of the foot, then, is important for providing a broad base on which the child's body is supported, and this base may at times compensate for the child's lack of muscle strength and coordination.

Kinematics of the Foot

Gross motion of the foot is complex and occurs around three axes and on three planes (Fig. 9-4). Flexion-extension occurs in the sagittal plane, abduction-adduction occurs in the horizontal or transverse plane, and inversion-eversion occurs in the coronal or frontal plane. Supination and pronation are terms commonly used to describe positioning of the plantar surface of the foot and occur primarily at the subtalar (talocalcaneal) joint. During supination the sole faces medially, and during pronation the sole faces laterally. Supination is a combination of inversion, flexion, and adduction. Pronation is a combination of eversion, extension, and abduction (Fig. 9-5). Toe motion includes flexion, extension, adduction, and abduction.

For practical purposes, foot motion can be considered to be of two distinct types: non–weight-

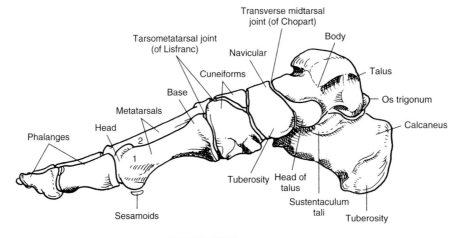

MEDIAL VIEW

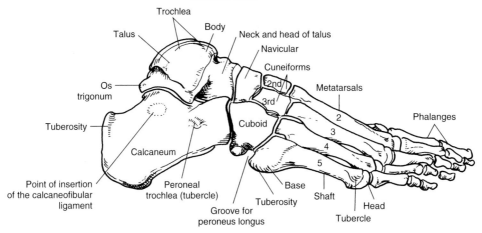

LATERAL VIEW

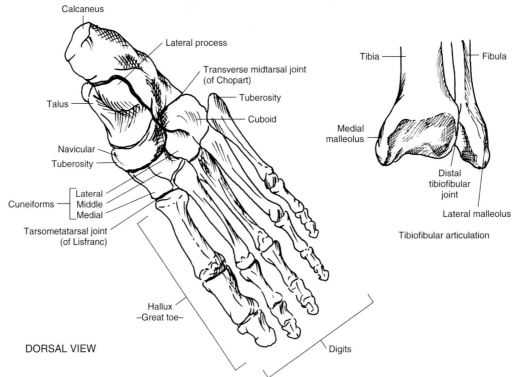

DORSAL VIEW

Tibiofibular articulation

FIG. 9-1

Top, View of the medial aspect of the foot. *Middle,* View of the lateral aspect of the foot.
Bottom left, Superior view of the foot. *Bottom right,* Anterior view of the ankle mortise.

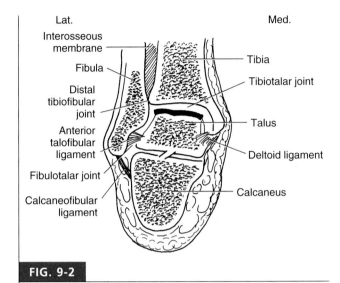

Lat.   Med.

Interosseous membrane

Fibula

Distal tibiofibular joint

Anterior talofibular ligament

Fibulotalar joint

Calcaneofibular ligament

Tibia

Tibiotalar joint

Talus

Deltoid ligament

Calcaneus

FIG. 9-2

Ankle joint complex composed of the tibiotalar, fibulotalar, and distal tibiofibular joints.

bearing and weight-bearing. Passive, non–weight-bearing motion may be tested with the patient seated and the foot and ankle hanging free. Subtalar motion is evaluated by grasping the tibia with one hand and inverting and everting the heel with the other hand. Abduction and adduction of the fore-foot can be tested if the heel is held immobile. Supination and pronation of the forefoot may also be tested with the heel fixed, as may flexion and extension of the tarsometatarsal joints and toes.

Active, weight-bearing motion of the foot differs from passive motion because the forces produced by body weight and by muscle contraction act to stabilize the joints. Generally, functional active foot motion during gait tends to be less than passive foot motion. Active subtalar inversion can be demonstrated by viewing heel orientation from behind while asking the patient to raise up on his or her toes. External rotation of the leg while bearing weight on the foot causes the heel to invert and the forefoot to pronate, therefore raising the arch. Rotating the leg internally has the opposite effect: it lowers the arch.

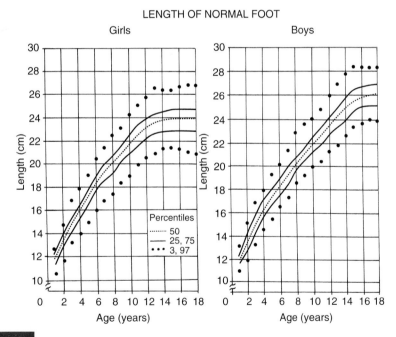

LENGTH OF NORMAL FOOT

Girls   Boys

Percentiles
.... 50
—— 25, 75
••• 3, 97

FIG. 9-3

Lengths of normal girls' and boys' feet derived from serial measures of 512 children aged 1 to 18 years. *Left,* Foot length versus age in girls. Note plateau in growth after age 12. *Right,* Foot length versus age in boys. Note plateau in growth after age 15 . *Adapted with permission from Blais, M.M., Green, W.T., & Anderson, M. (1956). Lengths of the growing foot. J Bone Joint Surg, 38A, 988.*

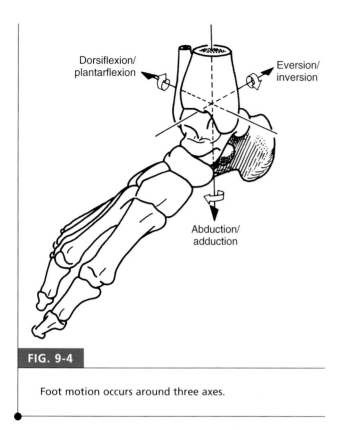

FIG. 9-4

Foot motion occurs around three axes.

FOOT AND ANKLE MOTION DURING GAIT

The gait cycle consists of a stance phase and a swing phase. The stance phase encompasses 62% of the gait cycle and the swing phase makes up the remaining 38%. The stance phase is subdivided into heel strike, foot flat, heel rise, push-off, and toe-off. Swing phase is divided into acceleration, toe clearance, and deceleration phases (Fig. 9-6). The part of stance phase spent with both feet on the ground is termed double limb support and occurs through the first and last 12% of stance phase (Fig. 9-7). Normal men have an average gait velocity of 82 m/min and 58 heel strikes/min (Waters et al., 1978). Running is defined as a gait speed past 201 m/min. At this speed, double stance disappears and a float phase develops in which both feet are off of the ground (Fig. 9-8).

During normal walking, the entire lower extremity (including the pelvis, femur, and tibia) rotates internally through the first 15% of stance phase. From heel strike through foot flat the subtalar joint everts, the foot pronates, and the forefoot becomes flexible to absorb shock and adapt to irregularities in the ground floor surface. The subtalar joint everts in part because the point of contact of the heel is lateral to the center of the ankle joint, thus producing a valgus

thrust on the subtalar joint. In the middle of stance phase and at push-off, the entire lower extremity begins to reverse and rotate externally as the subtalar joint simultaneously inverts (Fig. 9-9). With inversion of the subtalar joint and supination of the foot, the foot is transformed into a rigid structure capable of propulsion. Olerud and Rosendahl (1987) and Lundberg et al. (1989a–d) have experimentally measured the coupling of tibial rotation to subtalar motion. They have shown that the foot supinates 1° for every 0.2 to 0.44° of tibial external rotation.

Causes of Leg Rotation During the Gait Cycle

Mann (1993) has described the coordination of ankle and subtalar motion in an elegant model called a mitered hinge (Fig. 9-10). As the tibia internally rotates, the subtalar joint everts (pronates). Conversely, external rotation of the tibia causes inversion (supination) of the subtalar joint. He attributes the internal rotation of the lower extremity in early stance to the obliquity of a general ankle joint axis (see Ankle Joint Motion). According to the "single" axis model of the ankle joint, the ankle joint axis is angled downward and posteriorly from medial to lateral (Fig. 9-11). Because of the obliquity of the ankle

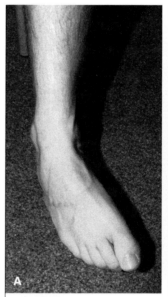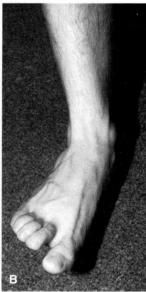

FIG. 9-5

A, During foot supination the sole faces medially. **B,** During foot pronation the sole faces laterally.

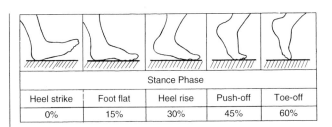

Stance Phase				
Heel strike	Foot flat	Heel rise	Push-off	Toe-off
0%	15%	30%	45%	60%

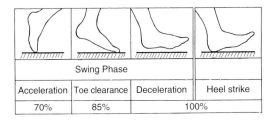

Swing Phase			
Acceleration	Toe clearance	Deceleration	Heel strike
70%	85%	100%	

FIG. 9-6

62% of the normal gait cycle is spent in stance phase and 38% is spent in swing phase.

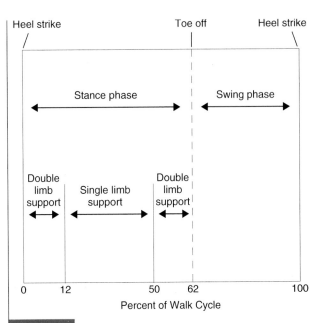

FIG. 9-7

Stance phase consists of two periods of double limb support and one period of single limb support.

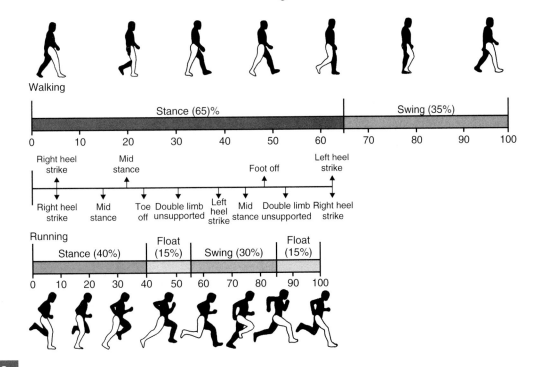

FIG. 9-8

Comparison of walking and running cycles. In the running cycle, stance phase decreases, swing phase increases, double limb support disappears, and a double limb unsupported or float phase develops.

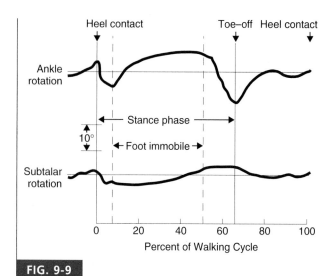

FIG. 9-9

Ankle motion and subtalar rotation during normal walking. Maximal subtalar eversion occurs at foot flat in early stance phase. Maximum subtalar inversion occurs at toe-off.

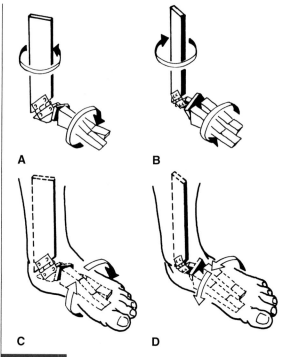

FIG. 9-10

Mitered hinge model of leg, ankle, and subtalar motion. **A,** Outward rotation of the upper stick causes inward rotation of the lower stick. **B,** Inward rotation of the upper stick causes outward rotation of the lower stick. **C,** External tibial rotation causes supination of the foot. **D,** Internal tibial rotation causes pronation of the foot.

joint axis, the leg internally rotates with ankle dorsiflexion and externally rotates with ankle plantarflexion. Additional mechanisms by which leg external rotation occurs during late stance include the swing of the opposite leg that causes external rotation of the planted leg and the obliquity of the metatarsal break (Fig. 9-12). The metatarsal break is an oblique axis of 50 to 70° with respect to the long axis of the foot formed by the centers of rotation of the metatarsophalangeal joints. With push-off, the foot and lower extremity externally rotate with respect to the sagittal plane because of this oblique axis.

MUSCLE ACTION DURING GAIT

Although the motions of the foot and ankle during the walking cycle occur primarily as a result of the passive constraints of joints and ligaments, electromyography has shown that muscle activity does occur during normal gait (Fig. 9-13). At heel strike, the pretibial musculature fires eccentrically to slow down the descent of the forefoot and prevent a foot slap. At midstance, the calf musculature contracts to slow down the forward movement of the body over the foot and prevent a crouch gait. The intrinsics also contract during midstance to toe-off to aid in rigidity of the forefoot. Toe-off is primarily a passive event. The pretibial musculature again contracts during swing phase to ensure that the foot clears the floor during swing-through.

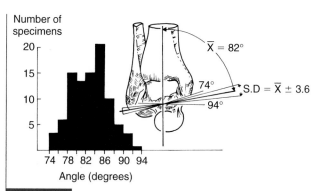

FIG. 9-11

Variations in the angle between the midline of the tibia and the empirical axis of the ankle. The axis is angled obliquely and inferolaterally 82°. The histogram shows variability among specimens.

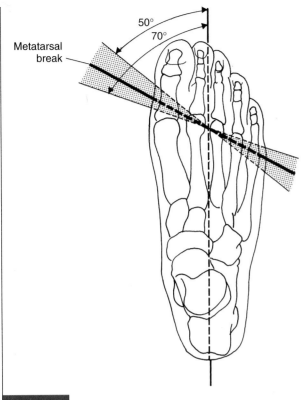

FIG. 9-12

The metatarsal break (*top view*), a generalization of the instant centers of rotation of all five metatarsophalangeal joints, may vary among individuals from 50 to 70° in its orientation to the long axis of the foot. *Adapted with permission from Mann, R.A. (1975). Biomechanics of the foot. In AAOS Atlas of Orthotics: Biomechanical Principles and Application (pp. 257–266). St. Louis: C.V. Mosby Co.*

The muscles of the lower extremity are more active during running. The gluteus maximus and hamstrings are active in midstance through toe-off and increase their activity 30 to 50% to decelerate the stance phase limb. Dorsiflexors of the foot and ankle are active in 70% of the running cycle. The intrinsics, plantar flexors, and peroneals are important stabilizers of the plantar surface and hindfoot during the foot flat phase (Adelaar, 1986).

MOTION OF THE TARSAL BONES

Subtalar Joint Motion

The joint between the talus and calcaneus is termed the subtalar joint. Its complex motion in three planes produces the motions of supination and pronation, clinically referred to as subtalar in-

version and eversion. The subtalar joint is responsible along with the transverse tarsal joint (consisting of the talonavicular and calcaneocuboid joints) for transforming tibial rotation into forefoot supination and pronation. Because the ankle joint is to some degree a single-axis joint, subtalar motion reduces the rotatory stresses to the ankle joint. Congenitally blocked motion of the subtalar joint may result in the formation of a ball-and-socket ankle as a result of the increased rotatory stress to the joint. Manter (1941) determined the subtalar axis of rotation to be oriented upward at an angle of 42° from the horizontal and medially 16° from the midline (Fig. 9-14). The subtalar facets resemble segments of a "spiral of Archimedes," a right-handed screw in the right foot, so that the calcaneus actually translates anteriorly along the subtalar axis as it rotates clockwise during the motion of subtalar inversion (Fig. 9-15). Average subtalar motion is 20 to 30° inversion and 5 to 10° eversion. Functional subtalar joint motion during gait is 10 to 15°. During the gait cycle, the heel strikes the ground in slight inversion, followed by rapid eversion to a maximum of 5 to 10° at 10% of the gait cycle (Fig. 9-9) (Sarrafian, 1993a,b).

Transverse Tarsal Joint Motion

The transverse tarsal joint, Chopart's joint, consists of the talonavicular joint and calcaneocuboid joint. Manter (1941) described two axes of motion in the

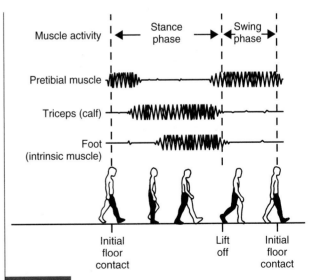

FIG. 9-13

Schematic phasic activity of leg and foot muscles during normal gait.

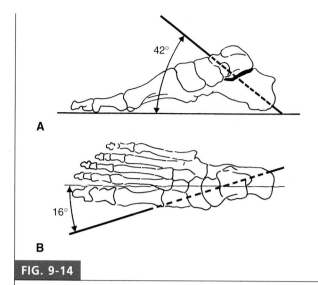

FIG. 9-14

Subtalar joint axis. **A**, Sagittal plane (lateral view). The axis rises up at a 42° angle from the plantar surface. **B**, Transverse plane (top view). The axis is oriented 16° medial to the midline of the foot. *Reprinted with permission from Manter, J.T. (1941). Movements of the subtalar and transverse tarsal joints.* Anat Rec, 80, 397.

transverse tarsal joint: a longitudinal axis and an oblique axis. The longitudinal axis is oriented 15° upward from the horizontal and 9° medially from the longitudinal axis of the foot. Inversion and eversion occur about the longitudinal axis (Fig. 9-16). The oblique axis is oriented 52° upward from the horizontal and 57° anteromedially. Flexion and extension occur primarily about this axis (Fig. 9-17). Ouzonian and Shereff (1989) determined in vitro talonavicular motion to be 7° in flexion-extension and 17° in pronation-supination. Calcaneocuboid motion is 2° flexion-extension and 7° pronation-supination.

The motions of the subtalar joint and transverse tarsal joint interrelate to produce either foot flexibility or rigidity. Elftman (1960) showed that the major axes of the calcaneocuboid joint and talonavicular joint are in parallel when the subtalar joint is everted, thus allowing motion of the transverse tarsal joint. As the subtalar joint inverts, the axes of these joints are convergent, thus locking the transverse tarsal joint and providing rigidity to the midfoot (Fig. 9-18). During the period of midstance to toe-off, the foot therefore becomes a rigid lever through inversion of the subtalar joint and locking of the transverse tarsal joint.

Astion (1997) showed the close interplay between the subtalar, talonavicular, and calcaneocuboid joints

in a study entailing experimental selective fusion of these joints. Subtalar joint arthrodesis reduced talonavicular motion to 26% of its normal motion and reduced calcaneocuboid motion to 56% normal. Calcaneocuboid arthrodesis reduced subtalar motion to 92% normal and talonavicular motion to 67% normal. Selective fusion of the talonavicular joint had the most profound effect on the remaining joints, reducing their remaining motion to only 2° each. Beaudoin (1991) showed that experimental subtalar fusion resulted in significant reduction in talonavicular joint contact and also reduced ankle joint contact.

Tarsometatarsal and Intertarsal Motion

The joints between the three cuneiforms, cuboid, and five metatarsals produce little motion. The intertarsal joints are closely congruent and exhibit minimal gliding motion between one another. The tarsometatarsal joints, known as Lisfranc's joint,

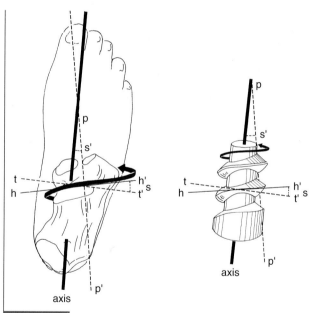

FIG. 9-15

Comparison of the posterior calcaneal facet of the right subtalar joint with a right-handed screw. The *arrow* represents the path of the body following the screw. The horizontal plane in which motion is occurring is hh′; tt′ is a plane perpendicular to the axis of the screw; s is the helix angle of the screw, equal to s′, which is obtained by dropping a perpendicular (pp′) from the axis. As the calcaneus inverts, it rotates clockwise and translates forward along the axis.
Reprinted with permission from Manter, J.T. (1941). Movements of the subtalar and transverse tarsal joints. Anat Rec, 80, 397.

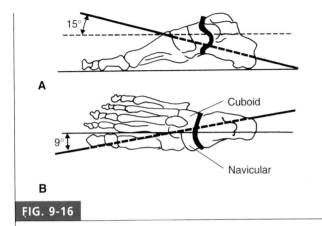

FIG. 9-16

Longitudinal axis of the transverse tarsal joint. Inversion and eversion occur about this axis. **A,** Lateral view. **B,** Top view. *Reprinted with permission from Manter, J.T. (1941). Movements of the subtalar and transverse tarsal joints. Anat Rec, 80, 397.*

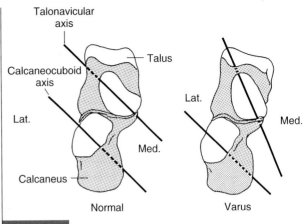

FIG. 9-18

Anteroposterior view of the transverse tarsal joint of the right foot. The anterior articulations of the talar head and calcaneus are shown. The major axes of the talonavicular and calcaneocuboid joints are shown in the neutral position (parallel) and with the heel in varus (convergent).

are intrinsically stable because of their arch-like configuration best seen in cross-section. The second metatarsal base is recessed into the midfoot, forming a key-like configuration with the intermediate cuneiform (Fig. 9-19). A strong ligament

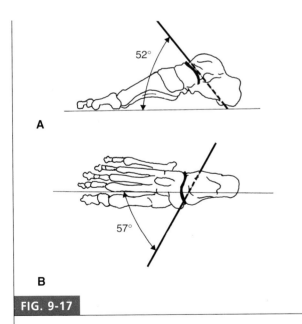

FIG. 9-17

Oblique axis of the transverse tarsal joint. Flexion and extension occur about this axis. **A,** Lateral view. **B,** Top view. *Reprinted with permission from Manter, J.T. (1941). Movements of the subtalar and transverse tarsal joints. Anat Rec, 80, 397.*

known as the Lisfranc's ligament connects the second metatarsal base to the medial cuneiform. The motion of the first three metatarsocuneiform joints is minimal compared with the fourth and fifth metatarsocuboid joints. Ouzonian and Shereff determined the first metatarsal-medial cuneiform motion to be 3.5° flexion-extension and 1.5° pronation-supination, while the fourth and fifth metatarsotarsocuboid joints were 9 to 10° flexion-extension and 9 to 11° pronation-supination. An in vivo study of first metatarsocuneiform motion found a mean sagittal motion of 4.4° (Fritz & Prieskorn, 1995). An in vitro study of first metatarsocuneiform motion showed that only 11% of 100 specimens demonstrated any adduction-abduction (Wanivenhaus & Pretterklieber, 1989). There has been recent concern that hypermobility of the first metatarsocuneiform joint may lead to offloading of the first ray and subsequent hallux valgus deformity (Klaue, Hansen, & Masquelet, 1994). Mizel (1993) described the plantar first metatarsocuneiform ligament as the major restraint to dorsal angulation and subsequent dorsal displacement of the distal first metatarsal head.

Motion of the Hallux

The hallux must accommodate a wide range of motion of the foot to perform a great variety of tasks.

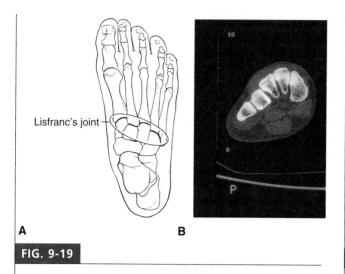

FIG. 9-19

A, Top view of the tarsometatarsal joints, known as Lisfranc's joint. Note the recessed second metatarsal base. **B,** Cross-sectional view of Lisfranc's joint seen on computed tomography scan. Note the arch-like structure.

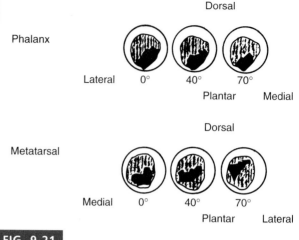

FIG. 9-21

Contact distribution of the first metatarsophalangeal joint in 0° (neutral), 40° of extension, and 70° of extension. *Top,* Joint contact of the proximal phalanx. *Bottom,* Joint contact of the metatarsal head. With increasing extension, joint surface contacts shift dorsally on the metatarsal head.

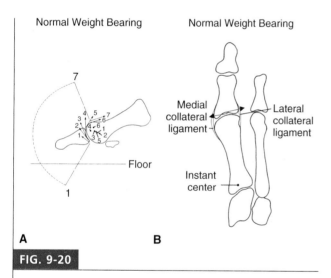

FIG. 9-20

A, Instant center and surface motion analysis of the metatarsophalangeal joint of the hallux in the sagittal plane. Each *arrow* denoting direction of displacement of the contact points corresponds to the similarly numbered instant center. Gliding takes place throughout most of the motion except at the limit of extension, which occurs at toe-off in the gait cycle and with squatting. At full extension, joint compression takes place. The range of motion of the hallux is indicated by the arc. **B,** Instant center analysis of the metatarsophalangeal joint of the hallux in the transverse plane during normal weight-bearing. Gliding (denoted by *arrows*) occurs at the joint surface even though the range of motion is small.

One need only consider the dorsiflexed position of the great toe of a baseball catcher crouching behind home plate to appreciate the degree of motion possible in the great toe. The first metatarsophalangeal joint has a range of motion from 30° plantarflexion to 90° dorsiflexion with respect to the long axis of the first metatarsal shaft. The first metatarsal is inclined 20° with respect to the floor; therefore, range of motion of the hallux is 50° plantarflexion to 70° dorsiflexion referenced to the floor surface. During the toe-off phase of normal walking, maximum dorsiflexion of the first metatarsophalangeal joint is required.

Analysis of motion of the hallux in the sagittal plane reveals that instant centers of motion often fall within the center of the metatarsal head, with minimal scatter (Fig. 9-20). The surface motion of the first metatarsophalangeal joint is characterized as tangential sliding from maximum plantarflexion to moderate dorsiflexion, with some joint compression at maximum dorsiflexion (Sammarco, 1980; Shereff, Bejahi, & Kummer, 1986). Ahn et al. (1997) determined the first metatarsal head surface contact area to be 0.38 cm^2 in the neutral position, which decreases to 0.04 cm^2 in full dorsiflexion (Fig. 9-21). The metatarsal head surface contact area shifts dorsally with full extension and is associated with joint compression. This explains the characteristic formation of dorsal osteophytes and limited dorsiflexion of the proximal phalanx in cases of hallux rigidus (Fig. 9-22).

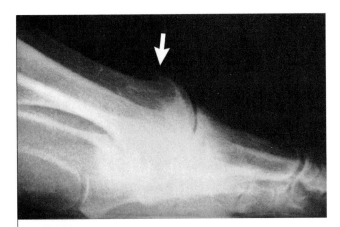

FIG. 9-22

Lateral view of hallux rigidus. Note osteophytes on the dorsal aspect of the metatarsal head, which limit joint extension.

The great toe provides stability to the medial aspect of the foot through the windlass mechanism of the plantar aponeurosis (see The Medial Longitudinal Arch). As the body passes over the foot in toe-off, the proximal phalanx passes over the metatarsal head and depresses it. This has been confirmed by force plate analysis in the late stance phase, which shows that pressure under the first metatarsal head increases in this phase of gait (Clark, 1980). In hallux valgus, the proximal phalanx shifts laterally and pronates on the first metatarsal head. This abnormal position of the proximal phalanx decreases its ability to depress the metatarsal head during toe-off. Any clinical situation that affects the normal depression of the metatarsal head may transfer plantar forces laterally to the second and third metatarsal heads and result in the formation of painful plantar calluses called transfer lesions (Case Study 9-1 and Figs. 9-23 and 9-24).

Motion of the Lesser Toes

The lateral four toes are analogous to the digits of the hand. The lesser toes have three phalanges, the motion of each being controlled by extrinsic muscles, which originate within the leg, and intrinsic muscles, which originate within the foot. Normal motion of the metatarsophalangeal joint is approximately 90° extension to 50° flexion. The extrinsic and intrinsic muscles contribute to the toe extensor hood, which controls motion of the metatarsophalangeal and interphalangeal joints

CASE STUDY 9-1

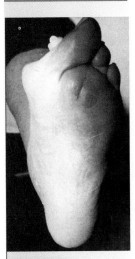

A 50-year-old woman who has been wearing shoes with a narrow toebox for almost 35 years. By compressing the forefoot medially and laterally, these abnormal forces can lead to a hallux valgus deformation. In this way, the proximal phalanx shifts laterally and pronates on the first metatarsal head. This abnormal position of the proximal phalanx decreases its ability to depress the metatarsal head during toe-off (Fig. 9-23).

FIG. 9-23

A view of the plantar surface of the foot of a patient with severe hallux valgus. Note calluses underlying the second and third metatarsal heads (transfer lesions), which indicate a transfer of plantar forces away from the first metatarsal head to the lesser metatarsal heads.

The altered joint mechanics produced by hallux valgus is evident in analysis of instant centers of rotation, which demonstrate joint distraction and jamming where gliding normally occurs (Fig. 9-24).

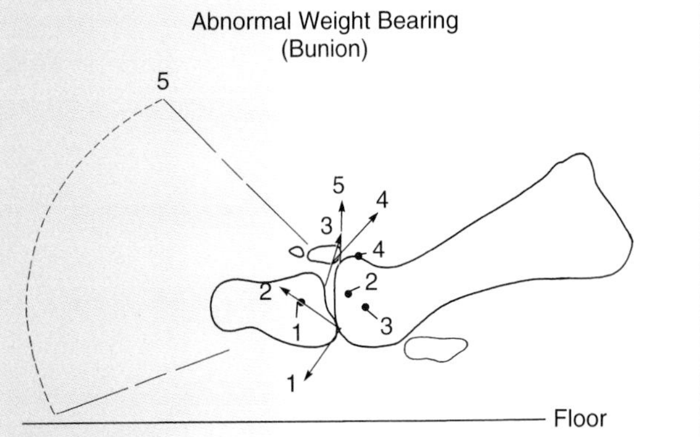

Abnormal Weight Bearing
(Bunion)

Floor

FIG. 9-24

Altered instant centers caused by the presence of a bunion, seen through analysis of motion of the metatarsophalangeal joint of the hallux in the sagittal plane. Each *arrow* denoting direction of displacement of the contact points corresponds to a similarly numbered instant center. The arc indicates the range of motion of the hallux, which is more limited than that in a normal foot.

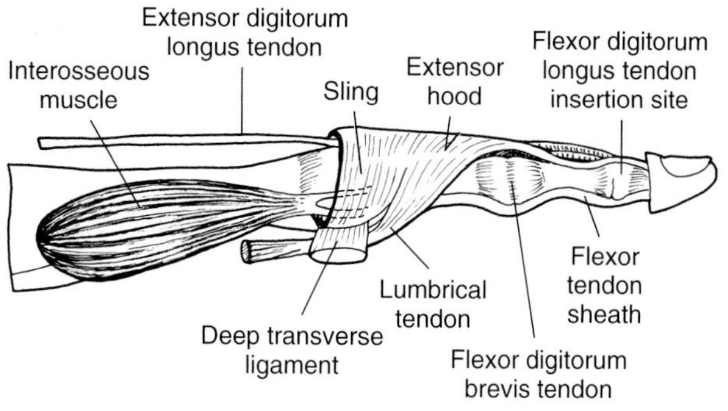

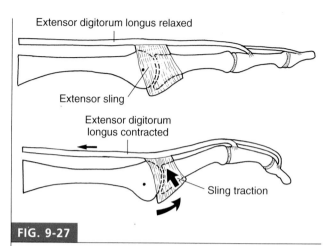

FIG. 9-25

Lateral view of the lesser toe illustrating the extensor hood with contributing muscles and ligaments.

FIG. 9-27

Lateral diagram showing the action of the extensor sling. When the extensor digitorum longus contracts (**bottom**), the proximal phalanx is lifted into extension through the sagittal bands.

(Fig. 9-25). The extrinsics consist of the long toe flexors and extensors. The lumbricals and interossei are the main intrinsic contributors to the extensor hood. The intrinsics act to flex the metatarsophalangeal joints and extend the interphalangeal joints (Fig. 9-26). The long toe extensors extend the metatarsophalangeal joint through the action of the sagittal bands by lifting the proximal phalanges into extension (Fig. 9-27). The flexor digitorum brevis is the primary flexor of the proximal interphalangeal joint. The flexor digitorum longus is the primary flexor of the distal interphalangeal joint.

Neurological conditions, such as diabetic neuropathy or Charcot-Marie-Tooth disease, initially affect the intrinsic muscles of the foot and result in an intrinsic minus condition. The extrinsic muscles overpower the intrinsics and a claw toe deformity is produced with extension of the metatarsophalangeal joint and flexion of the interphalangeal joints (Fig. 9-28).

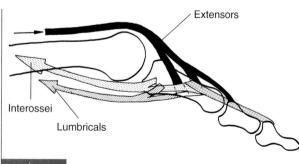

FIG. 9-26

The intrinsic muscles (interossei and lumbricals) act to flex the metatarsophalangeal joint and extend the interphalangeal joints.

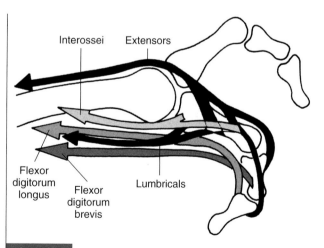

FIG. 9-28

A claw toe deformity is produced by an imbalance of the extrinsic and intrinsic muscles. Relative weakness of the interossei and lumbricals with overpull of the extrinsic toe extensors and flexors produces an intrinsic minus deformity of metatarsophalangeal extension and interphalangeal joint flexion.

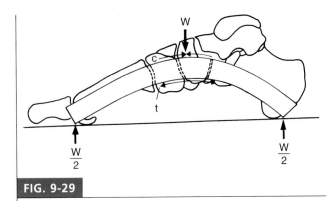

FIG. 9-29

The beam model of the longitudinal arch. The arch is a curved beam consisting of interconnecting joints and supporting plantar ligaments. Tensile forces are concentrated on the inferior beam surface; compressive forces are generated at the superior surface.

THE MEDIAL LONGITUDINAL ARCH

Two models exist to describe the medial longitudinal arch of the foot: the beam model and the truss model (Sarrafian, 1987). The beam model states that the arch is a curved beam made up of interconnecting joints whose structure is dependent on joint and ligamentous interconnections for stability. Tensile forces are produced on the inferior surface of the beam and compressive forces are concentrated on the superior surface of the beam (Fig. 9-29). The truss model states that the arch has a triangular structure with two struts connected at the base by a

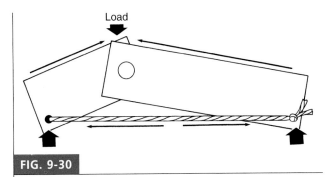

FIG. 9-30

The truss model of the longitudinal arch. The two wooden members, or struts, are connected at the base by a rope, or tie rod. The struts are analogous to bony structures of the foot and the tie rod is analogous to the plantar fascia. The shorter the tie rod, the higher the arch is raised.

tie rod. The struts are under compression and the tie rod is under tension (Fig. 9-30). Both models have validity and can be demonstrated clinically.

The structure analogous to the tie rod in the truss model is the plantar fascia. The plantar fascia originates on the medial tuberosity of the calcaneus and spans the transverse tarsal, tarsometatarsal, and metatarsophalangeal joints to insert on the metatarsophalangeal plantar plates and collateral ligaments as well as the hallucal sesamoids. Dorsiflexion of the metatarsophalangeal joints places traction on the plantar fascia and causes elevation of the arch through a mechanism known as the "windlass effect" (Hicks, 1954) (Fig. 9-31). During toe-off in the gait cycle, the toes are dorsiflexed passively as the body passes over the foot and the plantar fascia tightens and acts to shorten the distance between the metatarsal heads and the heel, thus elevating the arch. The traction on the plantar fascia also assists in inverting the calcaneus through its attachment on the medial plantar aspect of the calcaneus.

The arch has both passive and active support. Huang et al. (1993) performed an in vitro study of the loaded foot and found that division of the plantar fascia resulted in a 25% decrease in arch stiffness. They found the three most important static contributors to arch stability in order of impor-

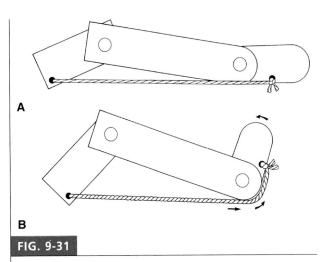

FIG. 9-31

A, Schematic of a truss. The far left wooden segment represents the hindfoot, the middle wooden segment represents the forefoot, and the far right wooden segment is the proximal phalanx. The rope is the plantar fascia. **B,** Dorsiflexion of the proximal phalanx raises the arch through traction on the plantar fascia.

tance were the plantar fascia, the long and short plantar ligaments, and the spring ligament (calcaneonavicular ligament). The spring ligament forms a sling for the talar head, which prevents medial and plantar migration of the talar head, and therefore provides static arch support (Davis et al., 1996). Basmajian (1963) demonstrated electromyographi-cally that the muscles of the calf did not contribute to support of the medial longitudinal arch when a load was applied to the leg of a seated individual; however, his experimental model did not simulate normal walking or running, when arch integrity is under greater challenge. Thordarson et al. (1995) performed a dynamic study of arch support by simulating stance phase of gait by applying proportional loads to tendons while the foot was loaded. In this study, the plantar fascia contributed the most to arch stability through toe dorsiflexion. The posterior tibialis contributed the most to dynamic arch support. In a similar cadaveric study, Kitaoka et al. (1997) demonstrated a 0.5 mm decrease in arch height and an angular change in the bones of the arch when tension on the posterior tibial tendon was released during simulated stance. A clinical study of 14 feet postplantar fasciotomy at greater than 4 years follow-up showed a decrease in arch height of 4.1 mm, thus supporting the truss model of arch stability (Daly et al., 1992).

Neuropathic joint changes or trauma may disrupt the bone and joint support of the arch, leading to arch collapse and a resultant rocker bottom foot deformity (Fig. 9-32). This sequela of joint destruction lends credence to the beam model of arch stability.

MUSCLE CONTROL OF THE FOOT

Twelve of the thirteen extrinsic and nineteen intrinsic muscles control the foot and ankle. The plantaris muscle is an extrinsic muscle that generally has no contribution to muscle control of the foot or ankle. The extrinsic muscles are the strongest and most important in providing active control during gait. According to Fick's principle (1911), the strength of a muscle is proportional to its cross-sectional area. Accordingly, Silver et al. (1985) have weighed and measured muscle fiber length to determine the relative strengths of muscles acting on the foot and ankle (Table 9-1).

The muscles of the leg fire in a pattern during normal gait to ensure an efficient transfer of muscle force to the floor and smooth progression of

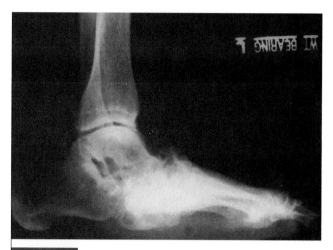

FIG. 9-32

A lateral radiograph of a rocker bottom foot, demonstrating loss of the bony and ligamentous support of the arch.

body weight forward along the axis of progression (Fig. 9-33). The moment produced by each muscle tendon unit can be predicted by their relationship to the ankle and subtalar axes (Fig. 9-34).

The soleus and gastrocnemius combine to form the Achilles tendon, which inserts onto the calcaneus and is the strongest flexor of the ankle. A mathematical model has predicted peak Achilles tendon forces to be 5.3 to 10 times body weight during running (Burdett, 1982). Firing of the ankle plantarflexors during midstance acts to slow the forward motion of the tibia over the foot.

TABLE 9-1

The Relative Strengths of Muscles Acting on the Foot and Ankle

Plantarflexor Strength Percentage	Dorsiflexor Strength Percentage
Soleus 29.9	Tibialis anterior 5.6
Gastrocnemius 19.2	Extensor digitorum longus 1.7
Flexor hallucis longus 3.6	Extensor hallucis longus 1.2
Flexor digitorum longus 1.8	Peroneus tertius 0.9
Inverters	**Everters**
Tibialis posterior 6.4	Peroneus longus 5.5
	Peroneus brevis 2.6

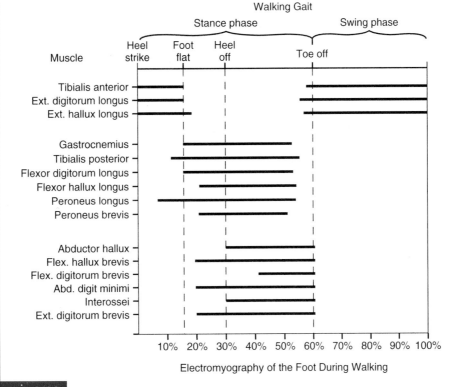

FIG. 9-33

Electromyography of the musculature of the foot and ankle during one normal gait cycle (heel strike to heel strike).

The strongest extensor of the ankle is the tibialis anterior, which is most active during stance phase from heel strike to foot flat. The ankle and toe extensors fire eccentrically to slow the descent of the foot and prevent foot slap. They also are necessary to allow foot clearance from the floor during the swing phase.

The strongest inverter of the foot and ankle is the posterior tibialis muscle. The posterior tibialis is a dynamic supporter of the medial longitudinal arch. It functions to invert the subtalar joint during mid- and late stance, thereby locking the transverse tarsal joint and ensuring rigidity of the foot during toe-off. Loss of this muscle results in acquired pes planus with flattening of the arch, abduction of the forefoot, and eversion of the heel (Fig. 9-35). Patients with posterior tibialis tendon dysfunction usually are unable to actively invert their heel while attempting a single toe rise. They have difficulty performing a single toe rise because of their inability to form a rigid platform on which to support their weight.

The primary everters of the foot and ankle are the peroneals. The peroneus longus inserts on the base of the first metatarsal and medial cuneiform and acts to depress the metatarsal head. Injury or paralysis of this muscle may allow elevation of the first metatarsal head and decrease loads borne by the first metatarsals and can result in the development of a dorsal bunion. The peroneus brevis stabilizes the forefoot laterally by resisting inversion and was found by Hintermann and associates (1994) to be the strongest everter of the foot. Loss of peroneal muscle strength can result in varus of the hindfoot (Sammarco, 1995).

The interosseus muscles are active during late stance and are thought to aid in stabilizing the forefoot during toe-off. An imbalance between the intrinsics and extrinsics will lead to toe deformities such as hammer toes, claw toes, or mallet toes.

Both intrinsic and extrinsic muscles mediate the positional control of the great toe. A cross-section of the proximal phalanx shows the relative position of

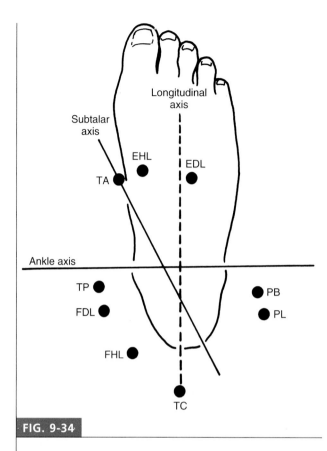

FIG. 9-34

Subtalar and ankle axes in relationship to extrinsic muscles. *EDL,* extensor digitorum longus; *EHL,* extensor hallucis longus; *FDL,* flexor digitorum longus; *FHL,* flexor hallucis longus; *PB,* peroneus brevis; *PL,* peroneus longus; *TA,* tibialis anterior; *TC,* tendon calcaneus; *TP,* tibialis posterior.

the flexors, extensors, abductors, and adductors (Fig. 9-36). The tibial and fibular sesamoids lie within the toe tendons of the flexor hallucis brevis muscle, beneath the head of the first metatarsal. Similar to the patella, they increase the lever arm distance of the pull of the flexor hallucis brevis muscle and enable greater flexion torque to be generated at the metatarsophalangeal joint. They also act to transfer loads from the ground to the first metatarsal head.

Kinetics of the Foot

The magnitude of loads experienced by the foot is astounding. Peak vertical forces reach 120% body weight during walking, and they approach 275% during running. It is estimated that an average 150-lb

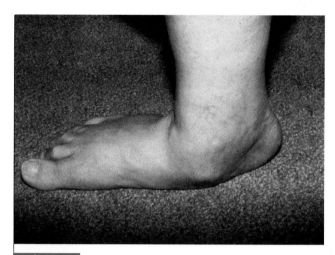

FIG. 9-35

Loss of the medial longitudinal arch in an acquired adult flatfoot secondary to posterior tibial tendon deficiency.

man absorbs 63.5 tons on each foot while walking. Running one mile would produce 110 tons per foot in that same 150-lb man (Mann, 1982).

Manter measured the compressive loads under static loading in cadaveric feet to determine the distribution of forces through the joints of the foot (Fig. 9-37). The highest part of the longitudinal arch, the talonavicular and naviculocuneiform

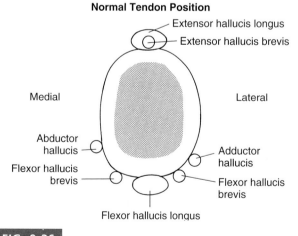

FIG. 9-36

Diagrammatic cross-section of the proximal phalanx of the hallux showing normal positions of the various tendons in relation to the bone.

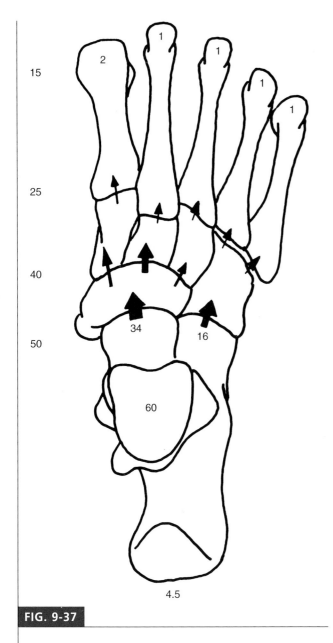

FIG. 9-37

Compressive forces of the foot after a 60-lb load is applied to the talus. The majority of the force passes through the talonavicular joint and into the first through third metatarsals.

The distribution of loads under the foot during stance has been the subject of intense investigation for the last half century. Initially, the concept of a "transverse metatarsal arch" was promoted, in which loads were borne primarily by the heel, first, and fifth metatarsal, as if the foot were a tripod. This concept was disputed by Morton (1935), who thought the forefoot had six contact points that shared equally in weight distribution, namely, the two sesamoids and the four lesser metatarsal heads. Recent plantar pressure studies by Cavanaugh et al. (1987) of subjects standing barefoot have determined that the distribution of load in the foot is as follows: heel 60%, midfoot 8%, forefoot 28%, and toes 4% (Fig. 9-38). Peak pressures under the heel are 2.6 times greater than forefoot pressures (Fig. 9-39). Forefoot peak pressures occur under the second metatarsal head (Fig. 9-40).

Static foot radiographic measurements fail to predict 65% of the variance found among dynamic pressures measured in various subjects. Therefore, the dynamics of gait exert the primary influence on plantar pressure during walking (Cavanagh et al., 1997). Hutton et al. (1973) studied the progression of the center of pressure across the sole of the foot during gait (Fig. 9-41). During barefoot walking, the center of pressure is initially located in the central heel and accelerates rapidly across the midfoot to reach the forefoot, where the velocity decreases. Peak forefoot pressures are reached at 80% stance phase and are centered under the second metatarsal.

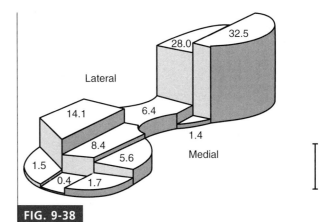

FIG. 9-38

Mean regional weight distribution expressed as a percentage of total load carried by the foot in barefoot standing. Over 60% of the weight is distributed in the rearfoot, 8% in the midfoot, and 28% in the forefoot. The toes have little involvement in the weight-bearing process.

joints bear the majority of the load through the tarsal joints. The medial column of the foot, consisting of the talus, navicular, cuneiforms, and first through third metatarsals, bears the majority of the load. The lateral column, made up of the calcaneocuboid joint and lateral two metatarsals, transmits the lesser load.

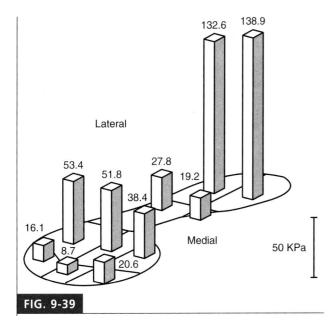

FIG. 9-39

Mean regional peak pressures during standing measured in kilopascals (kPa). The ratio of peak rearfoot to peak forefoot pressures is approximately 2.6:1.

At toe-off, the center of pressure is located under the hallux. The metatarsal heads are in contact with the floor at least 50% of stance phase. Soames (1985) determined that the highest peak pressure and greatest foot-floor impulse during barefoot walking was under the third metatarsal head instead of the second.

The distribution of plantar pressures changes with shoewear. Shoewear reduces peak heel pressure by producing a more even distribution of pressure under the heel. With shoes, forefoot load distribution shifts medially with maximum pressure under the first and second metatarsal heads. The pressures under the toes also increase with shoewear (Soames, 1985).

The distribution of plantar pressure during running has identified two types of runners characterized by their first point of contact with the ground: rearfoot strikers and midfoot strikers (Fig. 9-42). Rearfoot strikers make initial ground contact with the posterior third of the shoe. The initial contact for the midfoot strikers is in the middle third of the shoe. In both groups, first contact occurs along the lateral border of the foot. Peak pressure does not differ between runner types. The center of pressure is in the distal-most 20 to 40% of the shoe in both contact groups for most of contact time, indicating most time is spent on the forefoot (Cavanagh et al., 1987).

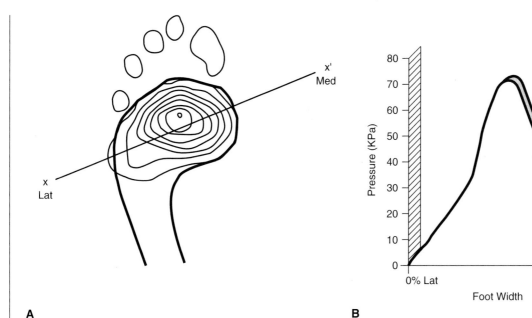

A **B**

FIG. 9-40

Metatarsal head pressure distribution during standing. **A,** A line (XX') drawn in the contour plot between the approximate locations of the first and fifth metatarsal heads. **B,**

The distribution of pressure along the metatarsal head line (XX') indicating maximum pressure under the second metatarsal head.

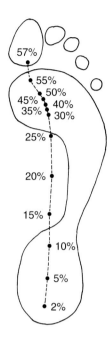

FIG. 9-41

The progression of the center of pressure along the sole of the foot during normal walking is expressed as a *broken line*. Each point on the sole corresponds to a percentage of the gait cycle. Note the rapid progression across the heel and midfoot to reach the forefoot, where most of stance phase is spent. It then progresses rapidly along the plantar aspect of the hallux.

During walking and running, several forces are acting between the foot and the ground: vertical force, fore and aft shear (anteroposterior shear), medial and lateral shear, and rotational torque (Fig. 9-43). The vertical ground reaction force exhibits a double peak following the initial heel strike spike. The first peak follows heel strike in early stance and the second peak occurs in late stance prior to toe-off. The fore and aft shear forces demonstrate initial braking by the foot as the foot places a forward shear force on the ground, followed by a backward shear on the ground as it pushes off in late stance. Most of the medial-lateral shear is directed laterally because the body's center of gravity is oriented medially over the foot. Medial (internal rotation) torque is generated early in stance as the tibia internally rotates and the foot pronates, followed by lateral (external rotation) torque as the leg externally rotates and the foot supinates.

SOFT TISSUES OF THE FOOT

The soft tissues of the foot are modified to provide traction, cushioning, and protection to the underlying structures. The dorsal skin of the foot is loosely at-

tached as is evident by the sometimes dramatic dorsal foot swelling found during trauma or infection of the foot or ankle. The plantar skin is firmly attached to the underlying bones, joints, and tendon sheaths of the heel and forefoot by specialized extensions of the plantar fascia. This function of the plantar fascia is essential for traction between the floor and the foot's weight-bearing skeletal structures to occur. During extension of the metatarsophalangeal joints, these plantar fascial ligaments restrict the movement of skin of the forefoot and plantar metatarsal fat pad (Bojsen-Moller & Lamoreux, 1979).

The heel pad is a highly specialized structure designed to absorb shock. The average heel pad area is 23 cm². For the average 70-kg man, the heel loading pressure is 3.3 kg/cm², which increases to 6 kg/cm² with running. At a repetition rate of 1,160 heel impacts per mile, the cumulative effect of running is impressive. These cumulative forces would normally result in tissue necrosis in other parts of the body (Perry, 1983). The heel pad consists of comma-shaped or U-shaped fat-filled columns arrayed vertically. The septae are reinforced internally with elas-

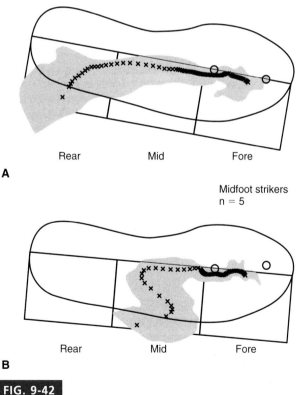

FIG. 9-42

Two types of runners characterized by initial ground contact. **A,** Rearfoot strikers. **B,** Midfoot strikers.

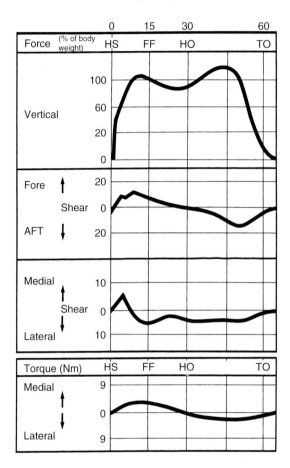

FIG. 9-43

Ground reactive forces acting on the foot during the gait cycle. *HS,* heel strike; *FF,* foot flat; *HO,* heel-off; *TO,* toe-off. *Reprinted with permission from Mann, R.A. (1982). Biomechanics of running. In AAOS Symposium on the Foot and Leg in Running Sports (pp.30–44). St. Louis: C.V. Mosby Co.*

tic transverse and diagonal fibers to produce a spiral honeycomb effect (Fig. 9-44). The multiple small closed cells are arranged to most effectively absorb and dissipate force. With age, septal degeneration and fat atrophy occur, which predispose the calcaneus and foot to injury (Jahss et al., 1992a,b).

Ankle Joint Biomechanics

KINEMATICS

The ankle mortise forms a simple hinge consisting of the talus, medial malleolus, tibial plafond, and lateral malleolus. The talus is shaped like a truncated cone, or frustum, with the apex directed medially (Inman, 1976). The talus is 4.2 mm wider

anteriorly than posteriorly (Sarrafian, 1993a,b). A single ankle joint axis has been described as passing just distal to the medial malleolus and just distal and anterior to the lateral malleolus (Inman, 1976). This empirical "general" ankle axis can be estimated by palpating the tips of the malleoli (Fig. 9-45). The single ankle axis is angulated posterolaterally in the transverse plane and inferolaterally in the coronal plane. Several authors have disputed the theory of a single axis of ankle motion and have described multiple axes of motion as the ankle moves from dorsiflexion to plantarflexion (Barnett & Napier, 1952; Hicks, 1953; Hintermann & Nigg, 1995; Lundberg et al., 1989a–d; Sammarco et al., 1973). Barnett and Napier (1952) describe a dorsiflexion axis inclined downward

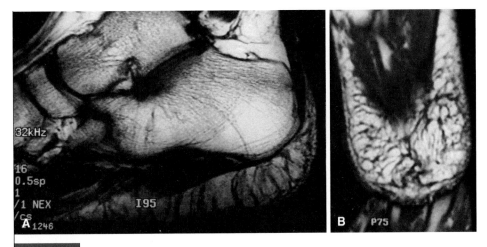

FIG. 9-44

Structure of a normal heel pad as seen on magnetic resonance imaging (MRI). **A,** Lateral view. Note vertically oriented fat-filled columns. **B,** Top view of the heel pad demonstrating the spiral structure of the septae, which separate the fat-filled cells.

and laterally and a plantarflexion axis angled downward and medially (Fig. 9-46). The ankle joint axes for dorsiflexion and plantarflexion differ by 20 to 30° in the coronal plane but remain parallel in the transverse plane.

A small amount of talar rotation occurs during ankle motion, which varies with axial load. Lundberg

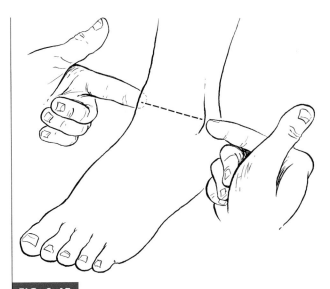

FIG. 9-45

The empirical axis of the ankle joint estimated through palpation of the malleoli. The axis angles downward and posteriorly, moving from medial to lateral.

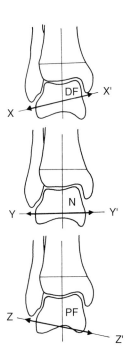

FIG. 9-46

Ankle joint axis variation. *Top,* In dorsiflexion (DF) the axis of motion XX' is inclined downward and laterally. *Middle,* In neutral the axis of motion YY' is almost horizontal. *Bottom,* In plantarflexion the axis ZZ' is inclined downward and medially.

et al. (1989a–d) used stereophotogrammetry to measure talar rotation during motion of the weight-bearing ankle in normal volunteers. The talus externally rotated 9° from neutral to 30° dorsiflexion. From 0 to 10° plantarflexion, the talus internally rotated 1.4°, followed by external rotation of 0.6° at 30° plantarflexion (Fig. 9-47). An in vitro study of loaded ankles demonstrated 2.5° external rotation in 25° dorsiflexion, and <1° internal rotation at 35° plantarflexion (Michelson & Helgemo, 1995.)

RANGE OF MOTION

Ankle motion occurs primarily in the sagittal plane and is described as plantarflexion (flexion) and dorsiflexion (extension). A wide range of normal motion for the ankle has been reported and depends on whether the motion is measured clinically with a goniometer or whether it is measured radiographically. Goniometric measurements yield a normal motion of 10 to 20° dorsiflexion and 40 to 55° plantarflexion. Lundberg et al. (1989a–d) found that the joints of the midfoot contribute 10 to 41% of clinical plantarflexion from neutral to 30° plantarflexion. Therefore, what appears to be clinical

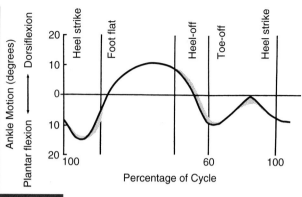

FIG. 9-48

Range of ankle joint motion in the sagittal plane during level walking in one gait cycle. The *shaded area* indicates variation among 60 subjects (age 20 to 65 years). *Reprinted with permission from Stauffer, R.N., Chao, E.Y.S., & Brewster, R.L. (1977). Force and motion analysis of the normal, diseased and prosthetic ankle joints.* Clin Orthop, 127, 189.

ankle plantarflexion is actually occurring distal to the ankle itself. This midfoot motion explains the apparent ability of the foot to dorsiflex and plantarflex following ankle fusion. It also explains the ability of dancers and gymnasts to align the foot with the long axis of the leg during toe point. Sammarco and associates (1973) found average non–weight-bearing ankle motion measured radiographically to be 24° dorsiflexion and 24° plantarflexion.

The normal pattern of ankle motion has been studied extensively (Lamoreaux, 1971; Murray et al., 1964; Stauffer et al., 1977; Wright et al., 1964). At heel strike, the ankle is in slight plantarflexion. Plantarflexion increases until foot flat, but the motion rapidly reverses to dorsiflexion during midstance as the body passes over the foot. The motion then returns to plantarflexion at toe-off. The ankle again dorsiflexes in the middle of swing phase and changes to slight plantarflexion at heel strike (Figs. 9-9 and 9-48). Ankle motion during normal walking averages 10.2° dorsiflexion and 14.2° plantarflexion, with a total motion of 25°. Maximum dorsiflexion occurs at 70% stance phase and maximum plantarflexion occurs at toe-off (Stauffer et al., 1977).

SURFACE JOINT MOTION

Sammarco et al. (1973) performed analyses of instant centers of rotation and surface velocities in both normal and diseased ankles. They found that

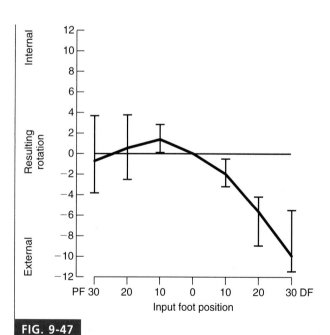

FIG. 9-47

Horizontal rotation of the talus around the vertical axis at different positions of ankle dorsiflexion-plantarflexion. Moving from plantarflexion to dorsiflexion, the talus initially internally rotates slightly, then externally rotates markedly.

the instant centers of rotation fell within the tali of normal ankles but that their positions changed with ankle motion (Fig. 9-49). This confirms that the ankle axis of rotation does not remain constant with motion. Surface motion from full plantarflexion to full dorsiflexion was also determined. Beginning in full plantarflexion, the ankle joint showed early distraction as dorsiflexion began. Joint gliding then took place until full dorsiflexion was reached and jamming of the joint occurred. It is possible that distraction and jamming of the tibiotalar joint play a role in lubrication of the joint. In arthritic ankles the direction of displacement of the contact points showed no consistent pattern. The tibiotalar joint surfaces distracted in an unpredictable manner, and they jammed when the joint was in neutral position rather than at the end of dorsiflexion (Fig. 9-50).

ANKLE JOINT STABILITY

Stability of the talocrural joint depends on both joint congruency and supporting ligamentous structures. The lateral ankle ligaments responsible for resistance to inversion and internal rotation are the anterior talofibular ligament, the calcaneofibular

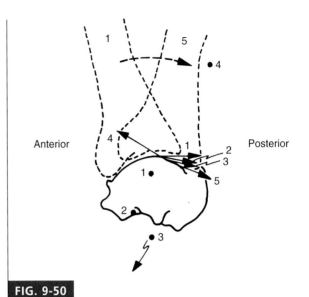

FIG. 9-50

Instant center and surface velocity analysis in an arthritic ankle. The instant centers vary considerably. Joint compression occurs early in motion and distraction occurs in dorsiflexion (velocity 4).

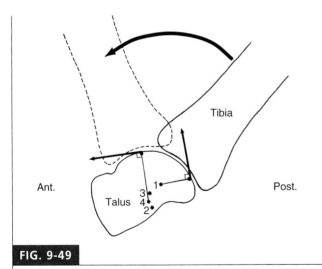

FIG. 9-49

Instant center pathway for surface joint motion at the tibiotalar joint in a normal ankle from full plantarflexion to full dorsiflexion. All instant centers fall within the talus. The direction of displacement of the contact points shows distraction of the joint surfaces at the beginning of motion (points 1 and 2) and gliding thereafter (points 3 and 4). *Reprinted with permission from Sammarco, G.J., Burnstein, A.H., & Frankel, V.H. (1973). Biomechanics of the ankle: A kinematic study. Orthop Clin North Am, 4, 75.*

ligament, and the posterior talofibular ligament (Fig. 9-51). The superficial and deep deltoid ligaments are responsible for resistance to eversion and external rotation stress. The ligaments responsible for maintaining stability between the distal fibula and tibia are the syndesmotic ligaments. The syndesmotic ligaments consist of the anterior tibiofibular ligament, the posterior tibiofibular ligament, the transverse tibiofibular ligament (also referred to as a deep portion of the posterior tibiofibular), and the interosseous ligament (Fig. 9-52).

The lateral ankle ligaments are the most commonly injured and therefore the most frequently studied. The anterior talofibular and calcaneofibular ligaments form a 105° angle with one another (Fig. 9-53). They act synergistically to resist ankle inversion forces. The anterior talofibular ligament is under greatest tension in plantarflexion and the calcaneofibular ligament is under greatest tension in ankle dorsiflexion (Cawley & France, 1991; Inman,1976; Nigg et al., 1990; Renstrom et al.,1988). The anterior talofibular ligament therefore resists ankle inversion in plantarflexion and the calcaneofibular ligament resists ankle inversion during ankle dorsiflexion. The accessory functions of the anterior talofibular ligament are resistance to anterior talar displacement

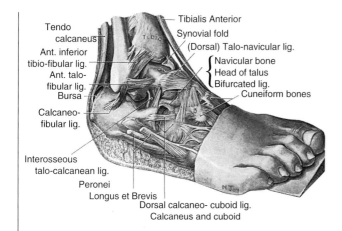

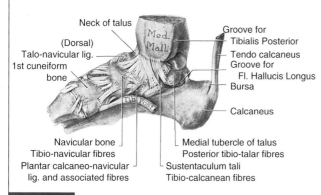

FIG. 9-51

Top, Lateral side of the foot and ankle. *Bottom,* Medial side of the foot and ankle. *From Anderson, J. (Ed.) (1978).* Grant's Atlas of Anatomy. *Baltimore, MD. Lippincott, Williams & Wilkins.*

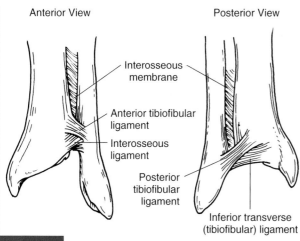

FIG. 9-52

Components of the ankle syndesmosis.

from the mortise, clinically referred to as anterior drawer, and resistance to internal rotation of the talus within the mortise (Fig. 9-54). The calcaneofibular ligament spans both the lateral ankle joint and lateral subtalar joint, thus contributing to subtalar joint stability (Stephens & Sammarco, 1992). The posterior talofibular ligament is under greatest strain in ankle dorsiflexion and acts to limit posterior talar displacement within the mortise as well as limit talar external rotation (Fig. 9-55) (Sarrafian, 1993a). In vitro testing of unloaded ankles subjected to anterior drawer testing demonstrated that the anterior talofibular ligament was most important in plantarflexion and that the calcaneofibular and posterior talofibular ligaments were most important in ankle dorsiflexion (Bulucu et al., 1991).

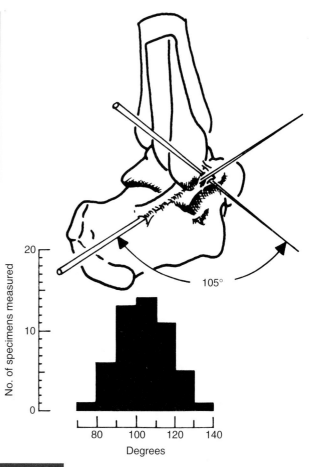

FIG. 9-53

Average angle between the calcaneofibular and talofibular ligaments in the sagittal plane. The average angle is 105° with considerable variation from 70 to 140° among measured subjects.

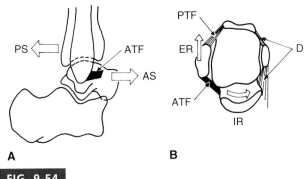

FIG. 9-54

Function of the anterior talofibular ligament (ATF). **A,** The ATF limits anterior shift (AS) of the talus or posterior shift (PS) of the tibia-fibula. **B,** The ATF limits internal rotation (IR) of the talus or external rotation (ER) of the fibula. *PTF,* posterior talofibular ligament; *D,* deltoid ligament.

Clinically, the most commonly sprained ankle ligament is the anterior talofibular ligament, followed by the calcaneofibular ligament. These injuries most commonly occur as a result of landing or falling on a plantarflexed and inverted ankle (Case Study 9-2). During periods of ankle unloading, the ankle rests in a position of plantarflexion and inversion. If the ground is met unexpectedly, lateral ligament injury occurs. Ataarian et al. (1985) tested the strength of the ankle ligaments by loading cadaver ligaments to failure and found the strength of the various ligaments from weakest to strongest to be anterior

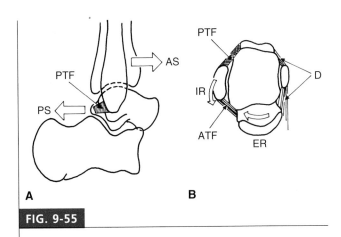

FIG. 9-55

Function of the posterior talofibular ligament (PTF). **A,** The PTF limits posterior shift (PS) of the talus or anterior shift (AS) of the tibia-fibula. **B,** The PTF limits external rotation (ER) of the talus or internal rotation (IR) of the fibula. *ATF,* anterior talofibular ligament; *D,* deltoid ligament.

Sprain Injury

A basketball player with an injury that results from a fall on a plantarflexed and inverted ankle position during a game (Case Study Fig. 9-2-1).

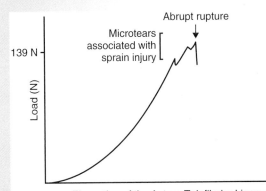

Case Study Figure 9-2-1.

An abnormally high load in conjunction with the loading rate produces the injury (Case Study Fig. 9-2-2). The sprain inversion injury produced by high stress (load per unit of area) in the plantarflexion and inversion direction will most commonly affect the antero talofibular ligament (failure load ~139N). This produces lateral instability in the ankle joint an abnormal anterior talar displacement from the mortise, decreasing the resistance to internal rotation of the talus within the mortise.

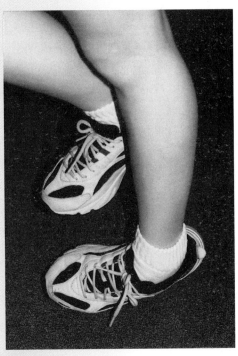

Case Study Figure 9-2-2.

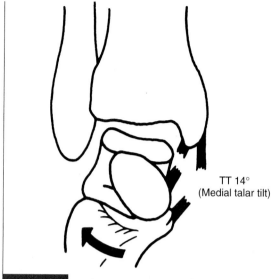

FIG. 9-56

Transection of both superficial and deep components of the deltoid ligament resulted in an average 14° of valgus talar tilt (TT) among 24 cadaver specimens.

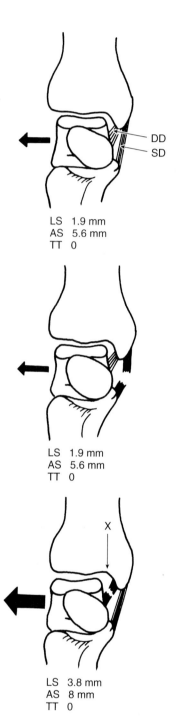

FIG. 9-57

The lateral malleolus is excised to simulate a fibular fracture or distal syndesmotic ligament injury. A laterally directed load is applied to the talus in an unloaded ankle model. The talar lateral shift (LS), anterior shift (AS), and valgus talar tilt (TT) are measured. Sectioning of the deep deltoid (DD) doubled the lateral talar shift from 1.9 to 3.8 mm. *SD*, superficial deltoid.

talofibular 139 N, posterior talofibular 261 N, calcaneofibular 346 N, and deltoid 714 N. Therefore, incidence of ankle ligamentous injury tends to match both mechanism of injury and ligamentous strength.

The deltoid ligament acts to resist eversion, external rotation, and plantarflexion of the ankle joint (Fig. 9-56) (Harper, 1987; Kjaersgaard-Andersen et al., 1989; Nigg et al., 1990). It also resists lateral talar shift within the mortise when the mortise is widened by distal syndesmotic ligamentous injury or distal fibular fracture (Fig. 9-57) (Michelson, Clark, & Jinnah, 1990; Harper, 1987).

Under physiological load, the ankle articular surface congruency takes on more importance (Cawley & France, 1991; Stiehl et al., 1993; Stormont et al., 1985). Stormont et al. found that in a loaded state the ankle articular surfaces provided 30% of rotational stability and 100% of resistance to inversion/eversion. They hypothesized that during weight-bearing, the ankle ligaments do not contribute to ankle versional stability, although rotational instability may still occur. Cawley and France showed that the force to cause ankle inversion and eversion increased by 91% and 80%, respectively, with loading. Stiehl et al. (1993) found that loading of the ankle resulted in decreased range of motion (especially plantarflexion), decreased anteroposterior drawer, as well as increased stability against version and rotation. Cass and Settles (1994) performed CT scans of loaded cadaveric ankles in an apparatus that did not constrain rotation and demonstrated that talar tilt of an average 20° still occurred in loaded ankles after sectioning both anterior talofibular and calcaneofibular ligaments. They did not feel that the articular surfaces prevented inversion instability during ankle loading. Most studies agree that loading of the ankle results in increased stability as a result of articular surface congruency, especially in ankle dorsiflexion.

Syndesmotic stability is dependent on the integrity of both malleoli, the syndesmotic ligaments, and the deltoid ligamentous complex. During ankle dorsiflexion, there is approximately 1 mm of mortise widening and 2° of external rotation of the fibula (Close, 1956). The normal distal fibular migration with loading is 1 mm (Wang et al., 1996). This distal fibular migration serves to deepen the ankle mortise for added bony stability (Scranton, McMaster, & Kelly, 1976). With disruption of the mortise in an external rotation injury, the syndesmotic ligaments and deltoid ligaments are torn, the distal fibula fractures, and the talus displaces laterally. A study of cadaveric ankles by Olgivie-Harris et al. (1994) defined the contribution to resistance to lateral talar displacement by the syndesmotic ligaments to be 35% for the anterior tibiofibular ligament, 40% for the posterior tibiofibular ligament, 22% for the interosseous ligament, and less than 10% for the interosseous membrane.

The deltoid ligament appears to be key in preventing lateral talar shift. Burns et al. (1993) found only minimal talar shift in a loaded cadaveric ankle study with sectioning of the syndesmotic ligaments until the deltoid ligament was sectioned. Michelson and colleagues (1990) simulated 4 mm of lateral fibular displacement in a cadaver study and placed the ankle under a 100-lb load. Lateral talar shift doubled from 1 to 2 mm following sectioning of the deltoid ligament. Pereira et al. (1996) simulated a laterally displaced fibular fracture of 4 mm and placed cadaveric ankles under a 500-N load in various static positions of ankle dorsiflexion and plantarflexion. Cutting the deltoid ligament in this study did not result in significant lateral talar shift or alteration in joint contact area or pressure. They hypothesized that under static loading the talus moves to a position of maximum congruence within the mortise rather than displacing laterally with the distal fibula. Most studies agree that the deltoid ligament and medial malleolus are most important in resisting talar external rotation and lateral talar shift.

Subtalar joint and ankle joint inversion are often difficult to separate clinically. The calcaneofibular ligament provides stability to inversion and torsional stresses to both the ankle and subtalar joints. Stephens and Sammarco (1992) provided an inversion stress to cadaveric ankles and sequentially sectioned the anterior talofibular and calcaneofibular ligaments. They found that up to 50% of the inversion observed clinically was coming from the subtalar joint. The structures that contribute to stability of the subtalar joint are the calcaneofibular ligament, the cervical ligament, the interosseous ligament, the lateral talocalcaneal ligament, the ligament of Rouviere, and the extensor retinaculum (Harper, 1991) (Fig. 9-58).

Kinetics of the Ankle Joint

The reaction forces on the ankle joint during gait are equal to or greater than the hip and knee joints, respectively. The following static and dynamic analyses give an estimate of the magnitude of the reaction forces acting on the ankle joint during standing, walking, and running.

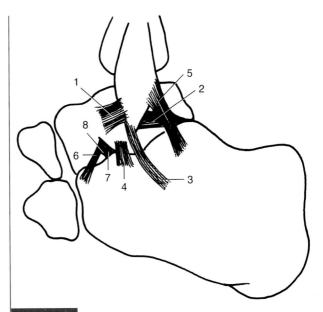

FIG. 9-58

Ligaments of the lateral ankle and subtalar joints: 1, anterior talofibular ligament; 2, posterior talofibular ligament; 3, calcaneofibular ligament; 4, lateral talocalcaneal ligament; 5, fibulotalocalcaneal ligament, or ligament of Rouviere; 6, cervical ligament; 7, ligament of the anterior capsule of the posterior talocalcaneal joint; 8, interosseous ligament.

STATICS

In a static analysis of the forces acting on the ankle joint, the magnitude of the force produced by contraction of the gastrocnemius and the soleus muscles through the Achilles tendon, and consequently the magnitude of the joint reaction force, can be calculated through use of a free-body diagram. In the following example, the muscle force transmitted through the Achilles tendon and the reaction force on the ankle joint are calculated for a subject standing on tiptoe on one leg. In this example, the foot is considered a free-body with three main coplanar forces acting on it: the ground reaction force (W), the muscle force through the Achilles tendon (A), and the joint reaction force on the dome of the talus (J) (Calculation Box 9-1).

The ground reaction force (equaling body weight) is applied under the forefoot and is directed upward vertically. The Achilles force has an unknown magnitude but a known point of application (point of insertion on the calcaneus) and a known direction (along the Achilles tendon). The talar dome joint reactive force has a known point of application on the dome of the talus, but the magnitude and line of direction are unknown. The magnitude of A and J can be derived by designating the forces on a free-body diagram and constructing a triangle of forces. Not surprisingly, these forces are found to be quite large. The joint reactive force is approximately 2.1 times body weight, and the Achilles tendon force reaches approximately 1.2 times body weight. The great force required for rising up on tiptoe explains why the patient with weak gastrocnemius and soleus muscles has difficulty performing the exercise 10 times in rapid succession. The magnitude of the ankle joint reaction force explains why a patient with degenerative arthritis of the ankle has pain while rising on tiptoe.

An in vitro study by Wang et al. (1996) found that the fibula transmits 17% of the load in the lower extremity. With the ankle positioned in varus or plantarflexion, the fibular load decreased. During ankle valgus or dorsiflexion, fibular load transmission increased. Cutting the distal syndesmotic ligaments decreased fibular load transmission and increased distal fibular migration. Cutting the interosseous membrane had no effect on fibular load transmission. The distal syndesmotic ligaments are therefore important for preventing distal migration of the fibula and maintaining fibular load.

The Free-Body Diagram of the Foot

A, On a free-body diagram of the foot, including the talus, the lines of application for W and A are extended until they intersect (intersection point). The line of application for J (dotted line) is then determined by connecting its point of application, the tibiotalar contact point, with the intersection point for W and A (Calculation Box Fig. 9-1-1). **B,** A triangle of forces is constructed. Force A is 1.2 times body weight and force J is 2.1 times body weight (Calculation Box Fig. 9-1-2).

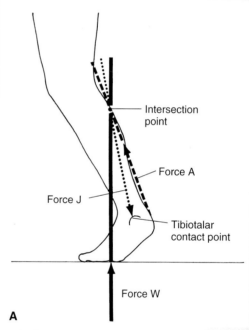

Calculation Box Figure 9-1-1.

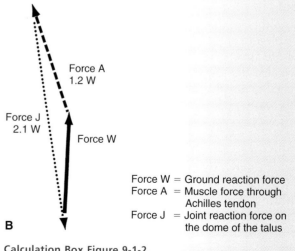

Force W = Ground reaction force
Force A = Muscle force through Achilles tendon
Force J = Joint reaction force on the dome of the talus

Calculation Box Figure 9-1-2.

ANKLE LOAD DISTRIBUTION

The ankle has a relatively large load-bearing surface area of 11 to 13 cm², resulting in lower stresses across this joint than in the knee or hip (Greenwald, 1977). The load distribution on the talus is determined by ankle position and ligamentous integrity. During weight-bearing, 77 to 90% of the load is transmitted through the tibial plafond to the talar dome, with the remainder on the medial and lateral talar facets (Calhoun et al., 1994). As the loaded ankle moves into inversion, the medial talar facet is loaded more. Ankle eversion increases the load on the lateral talar facet. The centroid of contact area moves from posterior to anterior, from plantarflexion to dorsiflexion, and from medial to lateral during the motion from inversion to eversion. The total talar contact was greatest and the average high pressure was lowest in ankle dorsiflexion (Calhoun et al., 1994) (Fig. 9-59).

Talar load distribution is also determined by ligamentous forces. Sectioning of the tibiocalcaneal fascicle of the superficial deltoid ligament in a loaded cadaver model resulted in a 43% decrease in talar contact area, a 30% increase in peak pressures, and a 4 mm lateral shift of the centroid (Earll et al., 1996).

DYNAMICS

Dynamic studies of the ankle joint are needed to appreciate the forces that act on the normal ankle during walking and running. Stauffer et al. (1977) used force plate, high-speed photography, radiographs, and free-body calculations to determine ankle joint compressive and shear forces. The main compressive force across the normal ankle during gait is produced by contraction of the gastrocnemius and soleus muscles. The pretibial musculature produces mild compressive forces in early stance of <20% body weight. A compressive force of five times body weight was produced in late stance by contraction of the posterior calf musculature (Fig. 9-60A). The shear force reached a maximum value of 0.8 times body weight during heel-off (Fig. 9-60B). Proctor and Paul (1982) also measured ankle compressive forces during gait and found peak compressive forces of four times body weight. In contrast to work by Stauffer et al. (1977), they found substantial compressive forces equal to body weight produced by contraction of the anterior tibial muscle group.

The pattern of ankle joint reactive force during gait differs with different walking cadences (Fig. 9-61). In a faster cadence, the pattern showed two

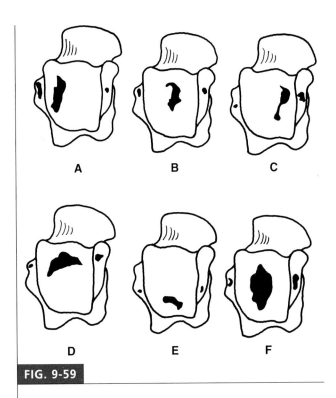

FIG. 9-59

Schematic demonstration of prints on pressure-sensitive film representing high pressure contact areas on the left talus. **A,** 490-N load in eversion; note lateral shift of talar contact area. **B,** 490-N load in neutral version. **C,** 490-N load in inversion; note medial shift of talar contact area. **D,** 490-N load in 10° dorsiflexion; note anterior shift of talar contact area and an increase in contact area. **E,** 490-N load in 30° plantarflexion; note posterior shift of talar contact area. **F,** 980-N load in neutral; note increase in talar contact area with increased load.

peak forces of three to five times body weight, one in early stance phase and the other in late stance phase. In the slower cadence, only one peak force of approximately five times body weight was reached during late stance phase (Stauffer et al., 1977). During running, localized ankle forces may be as high as 13 times body weight (Burdett, 1982).

Effects of Shoewear on Foot/Ankle Biomechanics

Western society places great importance on the appearance of footwear, especially among women. Women's footwear is designed to make the foot appear smaller and the leg appear longer by narrowing the toebox and elevating the heel. A narrow toebox compresses the forefoot medially and laterally, thus contributing to the development of hallux valgus, hammer toes, and bunionettes. A study of 356 women by Frey et al. (1993) found that 88% of women with foot pain wore shoes that were on average 1.2 cm narrower than their foot. Women who wore shoes on average 0.5 cm wider than the foot had no symptoms and less deformity. Shoes with elevated heels increase forefoot pressure compared with standing barefoot (Snow, Williams, & Holmes, 1992). A 1.9 cm heel increased forefoot pressure by 22%, a 5 cm heel increased peak pressure by 57%, and an 8.3 cm heel increased peak pressure by 76%. An elevated heel can cause pain

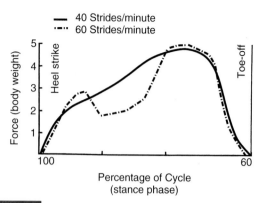

FIG. 9-61

Ankle joint reaction force expressed in multiples of body weight in a normal ankle during the stance phase of gait at two velocities. In the faster cadence, there were two peaks of three to five times body weight, one in early stance and one in late stance phase. In the slower cadence, only one peak force of approximately five times body weight was reached during late stance phase. *Reprinted with permission from Stauffer, R.N., Chao, E.Y.S., & Brewster, R.L. (1977). Force and motion analysis of the normal, diseased and prosthetic ankle joints.* Clin Orthop, 127, *189.*

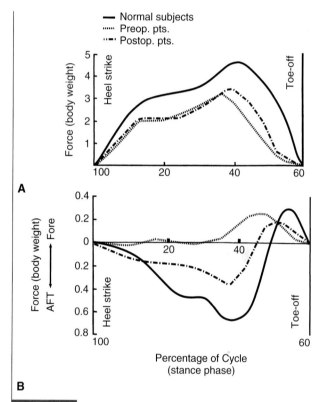

FIG. 9-60

A, The compressive component of the ankle joint reaction force expressed in multiples of body weight during the stance phase of normal walking for five normal subjects and nine patients with joint disease before and after prosthetic ankle replacement. **B,** The fore-aft shear component produced in the ankle during the stance phase of walking for the same subjects. *Reprinted with permission from Stauffer, R.N., Chao, E.Y.S., & Brewster, R.L. (1977). Force and motion analysis of the normal, diseased and prosthetic ankle joints.* Clin Orthop, 127, *189.*

under the metatarsal heads and may also contribute to interdigital neuroma formation. Elevation of the heel also may over time result in Achilles contracture, limited ankle dorsiflexion, and an altered gait. The amount of ankle joint motion in the gait cycle decreases as heel height increases (Murray et al., 1970).

Summary

1. The foot alternates in form and function between shock-absorbing flexible platform and rigid propulsive lever during different phases of the gait cycle.

2. The ankle and subtalar joint act like a mitered hinge. Ankle dorsiflexion and tibial internal rotation are associated with subtalar eversion (pronation); ankle plantarflexion and tibial external rotation are associated with subtalar inversion (supination).

3. Subtalar motion is screw-like and influences the flexibility of the transverse tarsal joint. Subtalar inversion locks the transverse joint and causes the foot to become rigid; subtalar eversion unlocks the transverse tarsal joint and allows foot flexibility.

4 The Lisfranc's joint (tarsometatarsal joints) is intrinsically stable and relatively immobile as a result of its arch-like configuration and the key-like structure of the second tarsometatarsal joint.

5 The first metatarsophalangeal joint exhibits a wide range of motion, with gliding throughout most of its range and jamming at full extension.

6 The medial longitudinal arch acts like both a beam and a truss. The arch is elevated through the windlass mechanism of the plantar fascia. The posterior tibial tendon provides dynamic support to the arch.

7 Foot muscle action during standing is relatively silent, but sequential firing of both extrinsic and intrinsic muscles is necessary to produce a normal gait pattern. The anterior tibial musculature fires during early stance to slow foot plantarflexion and prevent foot slap. The posterior calf musculature fires during mid- and late stance to control progression of the body over the foot.

8 During barefoot standing, the heel bears 60% of the load and the forefoot bears 28%. Forefoot peak pressures occur under the second metatarsal head.

9 During walking, the center of pressure moves from the posterolateral heel rapidly across the midfoot to the forefoot with peak pressures under the second or third metatarsal head. At toe-off, the hallux bears the most pressure.

10 The heel fat pad is specifically designed to absorb shock during heel strike. The plantar fascia attaches the skin of the heel and forefoot to the underlying bony and ligamentous structures.

11 The ankle joint has multiple axes that change during motion. Minimal talar rotation occurs during dorsiflexion and plantarflexion.

12 Ankle joint instant centers of rotation fall within the talus during range of motion. In movement from plantarflexion to dorsiflexion, joint surfaces first distract, then glide and eventually jam at the end of dorsiflexion.

13 Ankle joint stability is determined by joint congruency and ligamentous integrity. Ankle stability increases and depends more on articular surface congruency during weight-bearing.

14 The anterior talofibular and calcaneofibular ligaments synergistically provide stability against inversion during ankle motion.

15 The deltoid ligament prevents ankle eversion, external rotation, and lateral talar shift. It is key in maintaining the integrity of the syndesmosis.

16 The fibula bears approximately one sixth of the force exerted through the lower extremity.

17 The distal syndesmotic ligaments prevent separation of the distal fibula and tibia and help transmit force through the distal fibula on weight-bearing.

18 Ankle joint centroid (center of pressure) position changes with ankle flexion-extension and inversion-eversion. Talar surface contact is maximized and joint pressure is minimized in dorsiflexion.

19 The forces acting on the ankle can rise to levels exceeding five times body weight during walking and thirteen times body weight during running.

20 Narrow shoes and high heels can adversely affect foot mechanics, leading to forefoot deformities, heel pain, and Achilles contracture.

REFERENCES

Adelaar, R.S. (1986). The practical biomechanics of running. *Am J Sports Med, 14,* 497.

Ahn, T.K., Kitaoka, H.B., Luo, Z.P., et al. (1997). Kinematics and contact characteristics of the first metatarsophalangeal joint. *Foot Ankle Int, 18,* 170.

Astion, D.J., Deland, J.T., Otis, J.C., et al. (1997). Motion of the hindfoot after simulated arthrodesis. *J Bone Joint Surg, 79A,* 241.

Ataarian, D.E., McCrackin, H.J., Devito, D.P., et al. (1985). Biomechanical characteristics of human ankle ligaments. *Foot Ankle, 6,* 54.

Barnett, C.J. & Napier, J.R. (1952). The axis of rotation at the ankle joint in man. Its influence upon the form of the talus and the mobility of the fibula. *J Anat, 86,* 1.

Basmajian, J.V. & Stecko, G. (1963). The role of muscles in arch support of the foot. *J Bone Joint Surg, 45A,* 1184.

Beaudoin, A.J., Fiore, S.M., Krause, W.R., et al. (1991) Effect of isolated talocalcaneal fusion on contact in the ankle and talonavicular joints. *Foot Ankle, 12,* 19.

Blais, M.M., Green, W.T., & Anderson, M. (1956). Lengths of the growing foot. *J Bone Joint Surg, 38A,* 988.

Bojsen-Moller, F. & Lamoreux, L. (1979). Significance of free dorsiflexion of the toes in walking. *Acta Orthop Scand, 50,* 471.

Bulucu, C., Thomas, K.A., Halvorson, T.L., et al. (1991). Biomechanical evaluation of the anterior drawer test: The contribution of the lateral ankle ligaments. *Foot Ankle, 11,* 389.

Burdett, R.G. (1982). Forces predicted at the ankle during running. *Med Sci Sports Exerc, 14,* 308–316.

Burns, W.C. II, Prakash, K., Adelaar, R., et al. (1993). Tibiotalar joint dynamics: Indications for the syndesmotic screw—A cadaver study. *Foot Ankle, 14,* 153–158.

Calhoun, J.H., Eng, M., Li, F., et al. (1994). A comprehensive study of pressure distribution in the ankle joint with inversion and eversion. *Foot Ankle Int, 15,* 125–133.

Cass, J.R. & Settles, H. (1994). Ankle in stability: In vitro kinematics in response to axial load. *Foot Ankle Int, 15(3),* 134–140.

Cavanagh, P.R., Morag, E., Boulton, A.J.M., et al. (1997). The relationship of static foot structure to dynamic foot function. *J Biomechanics, 30,* 243–250.

Cavanagh, P.R., Rodgers, M.M., & Iiboshi, A. (1987). Pressure distribution under symptom-free feet during barefoot standing. *Foot Ankle, 7,* 262.

Cawley, P.W. & France, E.P. (1991). Biomechanics of the lateral ligaments of the ankle: An evaluation of the effects of axial load and single plane motion on ligament strain patterns. *Foot Ankle, 12,* 92.

Cheng, J.C.Y., Leung, S.S.F., Leung, A.K.L., et al. (1997). Change of foot size with weightbearing. A study of 2829 children 3 to 18 years of age. *Clin Orthop, 342,* 123.

Clark, T.E. (1980). *The Pressure Distribution Under the Foot During Barefoot Walking.* University Park, Pennsylvania: Penn State University.

Close, J.R. (1956). Some applications of the functional anatomy of the ankle joint. *J Bone Joint Surg, 386,* 761.

Daly, P.J., Kitaoka, H.B., & Chao, E.Y.S. (1992). Plantar fasciotomy for intractable plantar fasciitis: Clinical results and biomechanical evaluation. *Foot Ankle, 13,* 188.

Davis, W.H., Sobel, M., Diarlo, E.F., et al. (1996). Gross, histological, and microvascular anatomy and biomechanical testing of the spring ligament complex. *Foot Ankle Int, 17,* 95.

Earll, M., Wayne, J., Brodrick, C., et al. (1996). Contribution of the deltoid ligament to ankle joint contact characteristics: A cadaver study. *Foot Ankle Int, 17,* 317.

Elftman, H. (1960). The transverse tarsal joint and its control. *Clin Orthop, 16,* 41.

Fick, R. (1911). *Handbuch der Anatomie und Mechanik der Gelenke.* Jena Fischer.

Frey, C., Thompson, F., Smith, J., et al. (1993). American Orthopaedic Foot and Ankle Society women's shoe survey. *Foot Ankle, 14,* 78–81.

Fritz, G.R. & Prieskorn, D. (1995). First metatarsocuneiform motion: A radiographic and statistical analysis. *Foot Ankle Int, 16,* 117.

Greenwald, S. (1977). Unpublished data cited in R.N. Stauffer, E.Y.S. Chao, and C. Brewster. Force and motion analysis of the normal, diseased, and prosthetic ankle joint. *Clin Orthop, 127,* 189.

Harper, M. (1987). Deltoid ligament: An experimental evaluation of function. *Foot Ankle, 8,* 19.

Harper, M. (1991). The lateral ligamentous support of the subtalar joint. *Foot Ankle, 11,* 354.

Hicks, J.H. (1954). The mechanics of the foot II: The plantar aponeurosis and the arch. *J Anat, 88,* 25.

Hintermann, B. & Nigg, B.M. (1995). In vitro kinematics of the axially loaded ankle complex in response to dorsiflexion and plantarflexion. *Foot Ankle Int, 16,* 514.

Huang, C.K., Kitaoka, H.B., An, K.N., et al. (1993). Biomechanical evaluation of longitudinal arch stability. *Foot Ankle, 14,* 353.

Hutton, W.C., Scott, J.R.R., & Stokes, I.A.F. (1973) The mechanics of the foot. In L. Klenerman (Ed.). *The Foot and Its Disorders* (p. 41). Oxford: Blackwell Scientific Publications.

Inman, V.T. (1976). *The Joints of the Ankle.* Baltimore: Williams & Wilkins.

Jahss, M.H., Kummer, F., & Michelson, J.D. (1992a). Investigation into the fat pads of the sole of the foot: Heel pressure studies. *Foot Ankle, 13,* 227.

Jahss, M.H., Michelson, J.D., Desai, P., et al. (1992b). Investigations into the fat pads of the sole of the foot: Anatomy and histology. *Foot Ankle, 13,* 233.

Kitaoka, H.B., Luo, Z.P., & An, K.N. (1997). Effect of posterior tibial tendon on the arch of the foot during simulated weightbearing: Biomechanical analysis. *Foot Ankle Int, 18,* 43.

Kjaersgaard-Andersen, P., Wethelund, J.O., Helmig, P., et al. (1989). Stabilizing effect of the tibiocalcaneal fascicle of the deltoid on hindfoot joint movements: An experimental study. *Foot Ankle, 10,* 30.

Klaue, K., Hansen, S.T., & Masquelet, A.C. (1994). Clinical, quantitative assessment of first tarsometatarsal mobility on the sagittal plane and its relation to hallux valgus deformity. *Foot Ankle Int, 15(1),* 9–13.

Lamoreaux, L.W. (1971). Kinematic measurements in the study of human walking. *Bull Prosthet Res, 10,* 1.

Lundberg, A., Goldie, I., Kalin, B., et al. (1989a). Kinematics of the ankle/foot complex: Plantarflexion and dorsiflexion. *Foot Ankle, 9,* 194–200.

Lundberg, A., Svensson, O.K., Bylund, C., et al. (1989b). Kinematics of the ankle/foot complex—Part 2: Pronation and supination. *Foot Ankle, 9,* 248.

Lundberg, A., Svenson, O.K., Nemeth, G., et al. (1989c). Kinematics of the ankle/foot complex—Part 3: Influence of leg rotation. *Foot Ankle, 9,* 304.

Lundberg, A., Svenson, O.K., Nemeth, G., et al. (1989d). The axis of rotation of the ankle joint. *J Bone Joint Surg, 71B,* 94–99.

Mann, R.A. (1982). Biomechanics of running. In *AAOS Symposium on the Foot and Leg in Running Sports* (pp. 30–44). St. Louis: CV Mosby Co.

Mann, R.A. (1975). Biomechanics of the foot. In *AAOS Atlas of Orthotics: Biomechanical Principles and Application* (pp. 257–266). St. Louis: C.V. Mosby Co.

Mann, R.A. (1993). Biomechanics of the foot and ankle. In *Surgery of the Foot and Ankle* (pp. 3–43). St. Louis: C.V. Mosby Co.

Manter, J.T. (1941). Movements of the subtalar and transverse tarsal joints. *Anat Rec, 80,* 397.

Michelson, J.D., Clarke, H.J., & Jinnah, R.H. (1990). The effect of loading on tibiotalar alignment in cadaver ankles. *Foot Ankle, 10,* 280.

Michelson, J.D. & Helgemo, S.L. Jr. (1995). Kinematics of the axially loaded ankle. *Foot Ankle Int, 16,* 577.

Mizel, M.S. (1993). The role of the plantar first metatarsal cuneiform ligament in weightbearing on the first metatarsal. *Foot Ankle, 14,* 82.

Morton, D.J. (1935). *The Human Foot. Its Evolution, Physiology and Functional Disorders.* New York: Columbia University Press.

Murray, M.P., Drought, A.B., & Kory, R.C. (1964). Walking patterns in normal men. *J Bone Joint Surg, 46A,* 335–360.

Murray, M.P., Kory, R.C., & Sepic, S.B. (1970). Walking patterns of normal women. *Arch Phys Med Rehabil, 51,* 637.

Nigg, B.M., Skorvan, G., Frank, C.B., et al. (1990). Elongation and forces of ankle ligaments in a physiological range of motion. *Foot Ankle, 11,* 30.

Olerud, C. & Rosendahl, Y. (1987). Torsion-transmitting properties of the hindfoot. *Clin Orthop, 214,* 285.

Olgivie-Harris, D.J., Reed, S.C., & Hedman, T.P. (1994). Disruption of the ankle syndesmosis: Biomechanical study of ligamentous restraints. *Arthroscopy, 10,* 558–560.

Ouzonian, T.J. & Shereff, M.J. (1989). In vitro determination of midfoot motion. *Foot Ankle, 10,* 140.

Pereira, D.S., Koval, K.J., Resnick, R.B., et al. (1996). Tibiotalar contact area and pressure distribution: The effect of mortise widening and syndesmosis fixation. *Foot Ankle Int, 17,* 269.

Perry, J. (1983). Anatomy and biomechanics of the hindfoot. *Clin Orthop, 177,* 9.

Proctor, P. & Paul, J.P. (1982). Ankle joint biomechanics. *J Biomech, 15,* 627.

Renstrom, P., Wertz, M., Incavo, S., et al. (1988). Strain on the lateral ligaments of the ankle. *Foot Ankle, 9,* 59.

Sammarco, G.J. (1980). Biomechanics of the foot. In V.H. Frankel & M. Nordin (Eds.), *Basic Biomechanics of the Musculoskeletal System* (2nd ed., pp. 193–219). Philadelphia: Lea & Febiger.

Sammarco, G.J. (1995). Peroneus longus tendon tears: Acute and chronic. *Foot Ankle Int, 16(5),* 245–253.

Sammarco, G.J., Burnstein, A.H., & Frankel, V.H. (1973). Biomechanics of the ankle: A kinematic study. *Orthop Clin North Am, 4,* 75.

Sarrafian, S.K. (1987). Functional characteristics of the foot and plantar aponeurosis under tibiotalar loading. *Foot Ankle, 8,* 4.

Sarrafian, S.K. (1993a). Functional anatomy of the foot and ankle. In *Anatomy of the Foot and Ankle* (pp. 474–602). Philadelphia: Lippincott.

Sarrafian, S.K. (1993b). Retaining systems and compartments. In *Anatomy of the Foot and Ankle* (pp. 137–149). Philadelphia: Lippincott.

Scranton, P.E., McMaster, J.H., & Kelly, E. (1976). Dynamic fibular function: A new concept. *Clin Orthop, 118,* 76–81.

Shereff, M.J., Bejahi, F.J., & Kummer, F.J. (1986). Kinematics of the first metatarsophalangeal joint. *J Bone Joint Surg, 68A,* 392.

Silver, R.L., de la Garza, J., & Rang, M. (1985). The myth of muscle balance: A study of relative strengths and excursions about the foot and ankle. *J Bone Joint Surg, 67B,* 432.

Snow, R.E., Williams, K.R., & Holmes, G.B. Jr (1992). The effects of wearing high heeled shoes on pedal pressures in women. *Foot Ankle, 13,* 85–92.

Soames, R.W. (1985). Foot pressures during gait. *J Biomech Eng, 7,* 120–126.

Stauffer, R.N., Chao, E.Y.S., & Brewster, R.L. (1977). Force and motion analysis of the normal, diseased and prosthetic ankle joints. *Clin Orthop, 127,* 189.

Stephens, M.M. & Sammarco, G.J. (1992). The stabilizing role of the lateral ligament complex around the ankle and subtalar joints. *Foot Ankle, 13,* 130.

Stiehl, J.B., Skrade, D.A., Needleman, R.L., et al. (1993). Effect of axial load and ankle position on ankle stability. *J Orthop Trauma, 7,* 72–77.

Stormont, D.M., Morrey, B.F., An, K.N., et al. (1985). Stability of the loaded ankle. Relation between articular restraint and primary and secondary restraints. *Am J Sports Med, 13,* 295.

Thordarson, D.B., Schmotzer, H., Chon, J., et al. (1995). Dynamic support of the human longitudinal arch. *Clin Orthop, 316,* 165.

Wang, Q.W., Whittle, M., Cunningham, J., et al. (1996). Fibula and its ligaments in load transmission and ankle joint stability. *Clin Orthop, 330,* 261.

Wanivenhaus, A. & Pretterklieber, M. (1989). First tarsometatarsal joint: Anatomical and biomechanical study. *Foot Ankle, 9,* 153.

Waters, R.L., Hislop, H.J., Perry, J., et al. (1978). Energetics: Application of the study and management of locomotor disabilities. *Orthop Clin North Am, 9,* 351.

Wright, D.G., Desai, S.M., & Henderson, W.H. (1964). Action of the subtalar and ankle joint complex during the stance phase of walking. *J Bone Joint Surg, 46A,* 361.

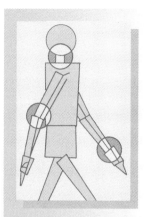

CHAPTER 10

Biomechanics of the Lumbar Spine

*Margareta Nordin, Shira Schecter Weiner adapted from
Margareta Lindh*

Introduction

The human spine is a complex structure whose principal functions are to protect the spinal cord and transfer loads from the head and trunk to the pelvis. Each of the 24 vertebrae articulates with the adjacent ones to permit motion in three planes. The spine gains stability from the intervertebral discs and from the surrounding ligaments and muscles; the discs and ligaments provide intrinsic stability and the muscles provide extrinsic support.

This chapter describes the basic characteristics of the various structures of the spine and the interaction of these structures during normal spine function. Kinematics and kinetics of the spine are also examined. The discussion of kinematics covers both the thoracic and lumbar spine, but that of kinetics involves only the lumbar spine because it is subjected to significantly greater loads than is the rest of the spine and has received more attention clinically and experimentally. The information in the chapter has been selected to provide an understanding of some fundamental aspects of lumbar spine biomechanics that can be put to practical use.

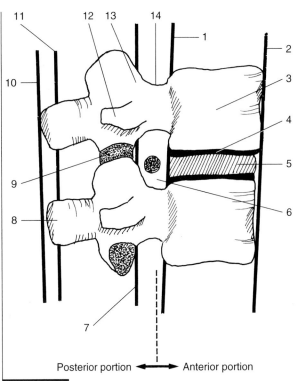

FIG. 10-2

Schematic representation of a motion segment in the lumbar spine (sagittal view). Anterior portion: 1, posterior longitudinal ligament; 2, anterior longitudinal ligament; 3, vertebral body; 4, cartilaginous end plate; 5, intervertebral disc; 6, intervertebral foramen with nerve root. Posterior portion: 7, ligamentum flavum; 8, spinous process; 9, intervertebral joint formed by the superior and inferior facets (the capsular ligament is not shown); 10, supraspinous ligament; 11, interspinous ligament; 12, transverse process (the intertransverse ligament is not shown); 13, arch; 14, vertebral canal (the spinal cord is not depicted).

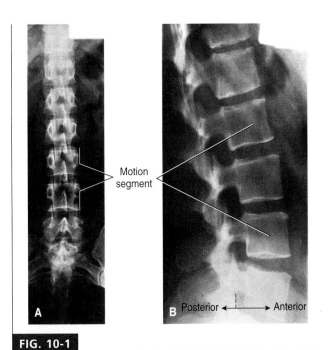

FIG. 10-1

Anteroposterior (**A**) and lateral (**B**) roentgenograms of the lumbar spine. One motion segment, the functional unit of the spine, is indicated.

The Motion Segment: The Functional Unit of the Spine

The functional unit of the spine, the motion segment, consists of two vertebrae and their intervening soft tissues (Fig. 10-1). The anterior portion of the segment is composed of two superimposed intervertebral bodies, the intervertebral disc, and the longitudinal ligaments (Fig. 10-2). The corresponding vertebral arches, the intervertebral joints formed by the facets, the transverse and spinous processes, and various ligaments make up the posterior portion. The

257

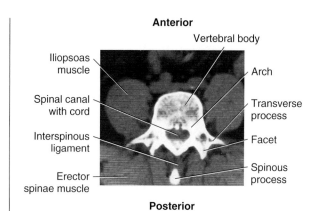

Anterior

Vertebral body

Iliopsoas muscle

Arch

Spinal canal with cord

Transverse process

Interspinous ligament

Facet

Erector spinae muscle

Spinous process

Posterior

FIG. 10-3

Transverse section of a motion segment at the L4 level viewed by computed tomography. The vertebral body, arch, spinal canal with spinal cord, and transverse processes are clearly seen. The view is taken at a level that depicts only the tip of the spinous process, with the interspinous ligament visible between the spinous process and the facets of the intervertebral joints. Directly anterior to the transverse processes and adjacent to the vertebral body are the iliopsoas muscles. Posterior to the vertebral body, the erector spinae muscles can be seen.

arches and vertebral bodies form the vertebral canal, which protects the spinal cord (Fig. 10-3).

THE ANTERIOR PORTION OF THE MOTION SEGMENT

The vertebral bodies are designed to bear mainly compressive loads and they are progressively larger caudally as the superimposed weight of the upper body increases. The vertebral bodies in the lumbar region are thicker and wider than those in the thoracic and cervical regions; their greater size allows them to sustain the larger loads to which the lumbar spine is subjected.

The intervertebral disc, which bears and distributes loads and restrains excessive motion, is of great mechanical and functional importance. It is well suited for its dual role because of its location between the vertebrae and because of the unique composition of its inner and outer structures. The inner portion of the disc, the nucleus pulposus, is a gelatinous mass. Rich in hydrophilic (water-binding) glycosaminoglycans in the young adult, it diminishes in glycosaminoglycan content with age and becomes progressively less hydrated (Urban & McMullin, 1985).

The nucleus pulposus lies directly in the center of all discs except those in the lumbar segments, where it has a slightly posterior position. This inner mass is surrounded by a tough outer covering, the annulus fibrosus, composed of fibrocartilage. The crisscross arrangement of the coarse collagen fiber bundles within the fibrocartilage allows the annulus fibrosus to withstand high bending and torsional loads (see Fig. 11-11). Discs with annular tears display increased rotational moments during loading compared with nondegenerated discs (Haughton et al., 2000). The end plate, composed of hyaline cartilage, separates the disc from the vertebral body (Fig. 10-2). The disc composition is similar to that of articular cartilage, described in detail in Chapter 3.

During daily activities, the disc is loaded in a complex manner and is usually subjected to a combination of compression, bending, and torsion. Flexion, extension, and lateral flexion of the spine produce mainly tensile and compressive stresses in the disc, whereas rotation produces mainly shear stress.

When a motion segment is transected vertically, the nucleus pulposus of the disc protrudes, indicating that it is under pressure. Measurement of the intradiscal pressure in normal and slightly degenerated cadaver lumbar nuclei pulposi has shown an intrin-

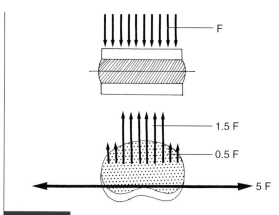

F

1.5 F

0.5 F

5 F

FIG. 10-4

Distribution of stress in a cross-section of a lumbar disc under compressive loading. The compressive stress is highest in the nucleus pulposus, 1.5 times the externally applied load (F) per unit area. By contrast, the compressive stress on the annulus fibrosus is only approximately 0.5 times the externally applied load. This part of the disc bears predominantly tensile stress, which is four to five times greater than the externally applied load per unit area. *Adapted with permission from Nachemson, A. (1975). Towards a better understanding of back pain: A review of the mechanics of the lumbar disc. Rheumatol Rehabil, 14, 129.*

sic pressure in the unloaded disc of approximately 10 N per square centimeter (Nachemson, 1960). This intrinsic pressure, or pre-stress, in the disc results from forces exerted by the longitudinal ligaments and the ligamentum flavum. During loading of the spine, the nucleus pulposus acts hydrostatically (Nachemson, 1960), allowing a uniform distribution of pressure throughout the disc; hence, the entire disc serves a hydrostatic function in the motion segment, acting as a cushion between the vertebral bodies to store energy and distribute loads.

In a disc loaded in compression, the pressure is approximately 1.5 times the externally applied load per unit area. Because the nuclear material is only slightly compressible, a compressive load makes the disc bulge laterally; circumferential tensile stress is sustained by the annular fibers. In the lumbar spine the tensile stress in the posterior part of the annulus fibrosus has been estimated to be four to five times the applied axial compressive load (Galante, 1967; Nachemson, 1960, 1963) (Fig. 10-4). The tensile stress in the annulus fibrosus in the thoracic spine is less than that in the lumbar spine because of differences in disc geometry. The higher ratio of disc diameter to height in the thoracic discs reduces the circumferential stress in these discs (Kulak et al., 1975).

Degeneration of a disc reduces its proteoglycan content and thus its hydrophilic capacity (Fig. 10-5, A–C). As the disc becomes less hydrated, its elasticity and its ability to store energy and distribute loads gradually decrease; these changes make the disc(s) more vulnerable to stresses.

THE POSTERIOR PORTION OF THE MOTION SEGMENT

The posterior portion of the motion segment guides its movement. The type of motion possible at any level of the spine is determined by the orientation of the facets of the intervertebral joints to the transverse and frontal planes. This orientation changes throughout the spine.

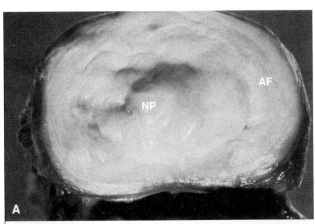

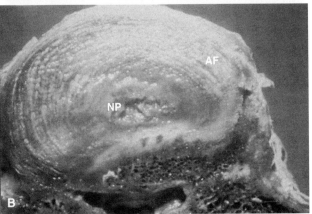

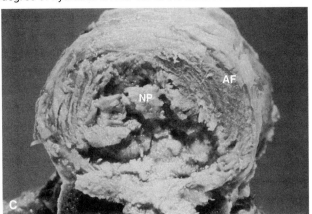

Human intervertebral disc composed of an inner gelatinous mass, the nucleus pulposus (*NP*), and a tough outer covering, the annulus fibrosus (*AF*). **A,** Normal young disc. The gelatinous nucleus pulposus is 80 to 88% water content *(reprinted with permission from Gower, W.E. & Pedrini, V. 1969. J Bone Joint Surg, 51A, 1154).* Age-related variations in protein-polysaccharides from human nucleus pulposus, annulus fibrosus, and costal cartilage are easy to distinguish from the firmer annulus fibrosus. **B,** Normal mid-age disc. The nucleus pulposus has lost water content, a normal degenerative process. The fibers on the posterior part of the annulus have sustained excessive stress. **C,** Severely degenerated disc. The nucleus pulposus has become dehydrated and has lost its gel-like character. The boundary between the nucleus and the annulus is difficult to distinguish because the degree of hydration is now about the same in both structures.

FIG. 10-5

Except for the facets of the two uppermost cervical vertebrae (Cl and C2), which are parallel to the transverse plane, the facets of the cervical intervertebral joints are oriented at a 45° angle to the transverse plane and are parallel to the frontal plane (Fig. 10-6A). This alignment of the joints of C3 to C7 allows flexion, extension, lateral flexion, and rotation. The facets of the thoracic joints are oriented at a 60° angle to the transverse plane and at a 20° angle to the frontal plane (Fig. 10-6B); this orientation allows lateral flexion, rotation, and some flexion and extension. In the lumbar region, the facets are oriented at right angles to the transverse plane and at a 45° angle to the frontal plane (Fig. 10-6C) (White & Panjabi, 1978). This alignment allows flexion, extension, and lateral flexion, but almost no rotation. The lumbosacral joints differ from the other lumbar intervertebral joints in that the oblique orientation of the facets allows appreciable rotation (Lumsden & Morris, 1968). The above-cited values for facet orientation are only approximations, as considerable variation is found within and among individuals.

The facets guide movement of the motion segment and have a load-bearing function. Load-sharing between the facets and the disc varies with the position of the spine. The loads on the facets are greatest (approximately 30% of the total load) when the spine is hyperextended (King et al., 1975). Because the facets are not the primary support structure in extension, if total compromise of these joints occurs, an alternate path of loading is established. This path involves the transfer of axial loads to the annulus and anterior longitudinal ligament as a way of supporting the spine (Haher et al., 1994). High loading of the facets is also present during forward bending, coupled with rotation (El-Bohy & King, 1986). The vertebral arches and intervertebral joints play an important role in resisting shear forces. This function is demonstrated by the fact that patients with deranged arches or defective joints (e.g., from spondylolysis and listhesis) are at increased risk for forward displacement of the vertebral body (Adams & Hutton, 1983; Miller et al., 1983) (Case Study 10-1). The transverse and spinous processes serve as sites of attachment for the spinal muscles, whose activity initiates spine motion and provides extrinsic stability.

THE LIGAMENTS OF THE SPINE

The ligamentous structures surrounding the spine contribute to its intrinsic stability (Fig. 10-2). All spine ligaments except the ligamentum flavum have a high collagen content, which limits their extensibility during spine motion. The ligamentum flavum, which connects two adjacent vertebral arches longitudinally, is an exception, having a large percentage of elastin. The elasticity of this ligament allows it to contract during extension of the spine and to elongate during flexion. Even when the spine is in a neutral position, the ligamentum flavum is under constant tension as a result of its elastic properties. Because it is located at a distance from the center of motion in the disc, it pre-stresses the disc; that is, along with the longitudinal ligaments, it creates an intradiscal pressure and thus helps provide intrinsic support to the spine (Nachemson & Evans, 1968; Rolander, 1966). Research suggests that with degenerative changes such as spondylolisthesis, traction spurs, and disc degeneration, which may lead to instability, altered mechanical stress will increasingly load the ligamentum flavum and cause hypertrophy (Fukuyama et al., 1995).

The amount of strain on the various ligaments differs with the type of motion of the spine. During flexion, the interspinous ligaments are subjected to the greatest strain, followed by the capsular ligaments and the ligamentum flavum. During extension, the anterior longitudinal ligament bears the greatest strain. During lateral flexion, the contralateral transverse ligament sustains the highest strains, followed by the ligament flavum and the capsular ligaments. The capsular ligaments of the facet joints bear the most strain during rotation (Panjabi et al., 1982).

Kinematics

Active motion of the spine as in any joint is produced by the coordinated interaction of nerves and muscles. Agonistic muscles (prime movers) initiate and carry out motion and antagonistic muscles control and modify the motion, while co-contraction of both groups stabilizes the spine. The range of motion differs at various levels of the spine and depends on the orientation of the facets of the intervertebral joints (Fig. 10-6). Motion between two vertebrae is small and does not occur independently; all spine movements involve the combined action of several motion segments. The skeletal structures that influence motion of the trunk are the rib cage, which limits thoracic motion, and the pelvis, which augments trunk movements by tilting.

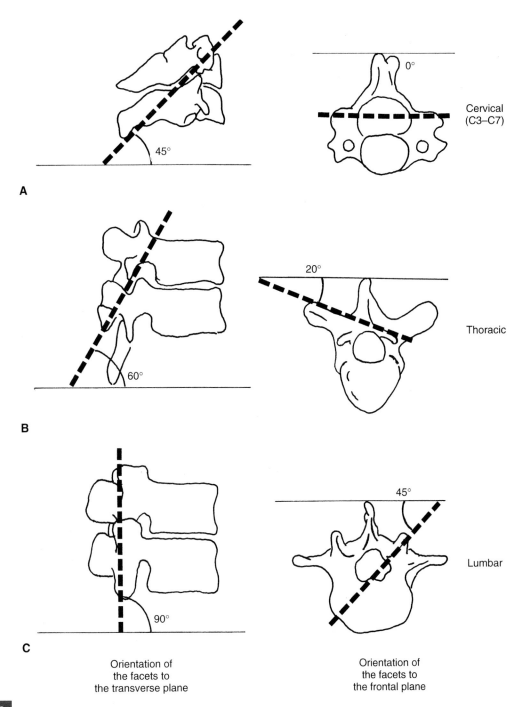

45°

Cervical
(C3–C7)

0°

A

20°

Thoracic

60°

B

45°

Lumbar

90°

C

Orientation of
the facets to
the transverse plane

Orientation of
the facets to
the frontal plane

FIG. 10-6

Orientation of the facets of the intervertebral joints (approximate values). *Reprinted with permission from White, A.A. & Panjabi, M.N. (1978).* Clinical Biomechanics of the Spine. *Philadelphia: J.B. Lippincott.* **A,** In the lower cervical spine, the facets are oriented at a 45° angle to the transverse plane and are parallel to the frontal plane. **B,** The facets of the thoracic spine are oriented at a 60° angle to the transverse plane and at a 20° angle to the frontal plane. **C,** The facets of the lumbar spine are oriented at a 90° angle to the transverse plane and at a 45° angle to the frontal plane.

Spondylolisthesis: Anterior Slippage of One Vertebra in Relation to the Vertebra Below It

A 30-year-old male gymnast complains of severe back pain with radiation to both legs. The pain is associated with periods of strenuous training and the symptoms decrease with rest or restriction of activity. After a careful examination by a specialist and MRI films, a diagnosis was made of spondylolisthesis at the level L5–S1 (Case Study Fig. 10-1-1), with concurrent bilateral pars interarticularis defects of L5 (Case Study Fig. 10-1-2).

Physiological loads during repeated flexion-extension motion of the lumbar spine caused a fatigue fracture of the pars interarticularis (aspect of the posterior arch of the vertebra that lies between the inferior and superior facets). This bilateral defect leads to an anterior displacement of the vertebra L5 onto S1. As the L5 vertebra begins to slip forward, the center of gravity of the body is displaced anteriorly. To compensate, the lumbar spine above the lesion hyperextends and the upper part of the trunk is displaced backward. Because this is a disease continuum, the abnormal forces placed on the intervertebral disc leads to herniation into the neural foramina, producing moderate stenosis of both L5–S1 nerve roots.

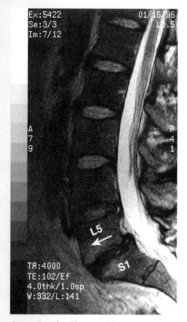

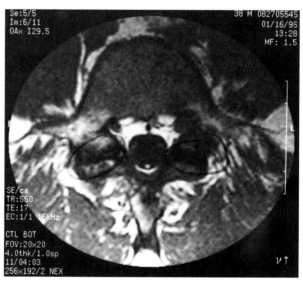

Case Study Figure 10-1-1.   **Case Study Figure 10-1-2.**

SEGMENTAL MOTION OF THE SPINE

The vertebrae have six degrees of freedom: rotation about and translation along a transverse, a sagittal, and a longitudinal axis. The motion produced during flexion, extension, lateral flexion, and axial rotation of the spine is a complex combined motion resulting from simultaneous rotation and translation.

Range of Motion

Various investigations using autopsy material or radiographic measurements in vivo have shown divergent values for the range of motion of individual motion segments, but there is agreement on the relative amount of motion at different levels of the spine. Representative values from White and Panjabi (1978) are presented in Figure 10-7 to allow a comparison of motion at various levels of the thoracic and lumbar spine. (Representative values for motion in the cervical spine are included for comparison.)

Investigations of the thoracic and lumbar spine show that the range of flexion and extension is approximately 4° in each of the upper thoracic motion segments, approximately 6° in the midthoracic region, and approximately 12° in the two lower thoracic segments. This range progressively increases in the lumbar motion segments, reaching a maximum of 20° at the lumbosacral level.

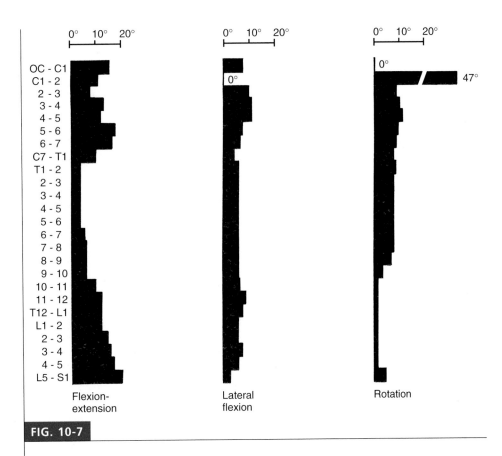

FIG. 10-7

A composite of representative values for type and range of motion at different levels of the spine. *Reprinted with permission from White, A.A. & Panjabi, M.N. (1978). Clinical Biomechanics of the Spine. Philadelphia: J.B. Lippincott.*

Lateral flexion shows the greatest range in each of the lower thoracic segments, reaching 8 to 9°. In the upper thoracic segments, the range is uniformly 6°. Six degrees of lateral flexion is also found in each of all lumbar segments except the lumbosacral segment, which demonstrates only 3° of motion.

Rotation is greatest in the upper segments of the thoracic spine, where the range is 9°. The range of rotation progressively decreases caudally, reaching 2° in the lower segments of the lumbar spine. It then increases to 5° in the lumbosacral segment.

Surface Joint Motion

Motion between the surfaces of two adjacent vertebrae during flexion-extension or lateral flexion may be analyzed by means of the instant center method of Reuleaux. The procedure is essentially the same as that described for the cervical spine in Chapter 11 (see Figs. 11-18 and 11-19). The instantaneous

center of flexion-extension and lateral flexion in a motion segment of the lumbar spine lies within the disc under normal conditions (Fig. l0-8*A*) (Cossette et al., 1971; Rolander, 1966). With abnormal conditions such as pronounced disc degeneration, the instantaneous center pathway will be altered (Fig. 10-8*B*) (Gertzbein et al., 1985; Reichmann et al., 1972).

FUNCTIONAL MOTION OF THE SPINE

Because of its complexity, the motion of a single motion segment is difficult to measure clinically. Approximate values for the normal functional range of motion of the spine can be given. Variations among individuals are large and show a Gaussian distribution in the three planes. The range of motion is strongly age-dependent, decreasing by approximately 30% from youth to old age, although with aging, loss of range of motion is noted in flexion and lateral bending while axial rotation motion is main-

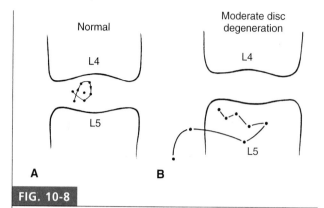

Normal

Moderate disc degeneration

L4

L4

L5

L5

A   **B**

FIG. 10-8

Instant center pathway for a normal cadaver spine (**A**) and a cadaver spine with moderate disc degeneration (**B**). Instant centers were determined for 3° intervals of motion from maximum extension to maximum flexion. In the normal spine, all instant centers fell within a small area in the disc. In the degenerated spine, the centers were displaced, and hence the surface motion was abnormal. *Reprinted with permission from Gertzbein, S.D., et al. (1985). Centrode patterns and segmental instability in degenerative disc disease. Spine, 10, 257.*

tained with evidence of increased coupled motion (McGill et al., 1999). Differences have also been noted between the sexes: men have greater mobility in flexion and extension whereas women are more mobile in lateral flexion (Biering-Sorensen, 1984; Moll & Wright, 1971). Loss of range of motion in the lumbar and/or thoracic spine is compensated for mainly by motion in the cervical spine and hips.

THE MUSCLES

The spinal muscles can be divided into flexors and extensors. The main flexors are the abdominal muscles (the rectus abdominis muscles, the internal and external oblique muscles, and the transverse abdominal muscle) and the psoas muscles. In general, muscles anterior to the vertebral column act as flexors. The main extensors are the erector spinae muscles, the multifidus muscles, and the intertransversarii muscles attached to the posterior elements. In general, the muscles posterior to the vertebral columns act as extensors (Fig. 10-9). The extensor

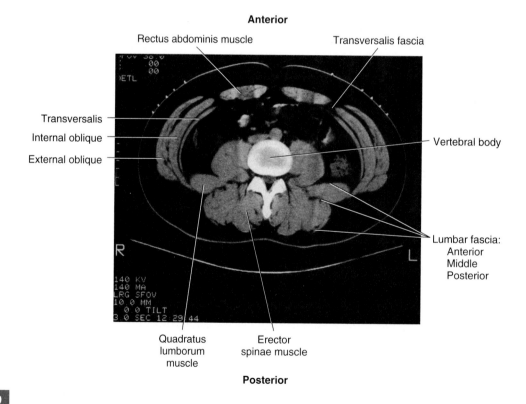

Anterior

Rectus abdominis muscle

Transversalis fascia

Transversalis

Internal oblique

External oblique

Vertebral body

Lumbar fascia:
Anterior
Middle
Posterior

R   L

Quadratus lumborum muscle

Erector spinae muscle

Posterior

FIG. 10-9

An MRI transverse cross-section of the body at the L4 level of a normal adult human spine. The major trunk muscles are shown (R, right; L, left). *By courtesy from Ali Sheikzahed, Ph.D., Hospital for Joint Diseases, Mt. Sinai, NYU Health, New York, NY, USA.*

muscles bridge between each vertebrae and motion segment as well as over several vertebrae and motion segments. When extensor muscles contract symmetrically, extension is produced. When right and left side flexors and extensor muscles contract asymmetrically, lateral bending or twisting of the spine is produced (Andersson & Lavender, 1997).

Flexion and Extension

During unloaded flexion-extension range of motion, the first 50 to 60° of spine flexion occurs in the lumbar spine, mainly in the lower motion segments (Carlsöö, 1961; Farfan, 1975). Tilting the pelvis forward allows for further flexion. During lifting and lowering a load, this rhythm occurs simultaneously, although a greater separation of these movements is noted during lifting than during lowering (Nelson et al., 1995) The thoracic spine contributes little to forward flexion of the entire spinal column because of the oblique orientation of the facets (Figs. 10-6 and 10-7), the nearly vertical orientation of the spinous processes, and the limitation of motion imposed by the rib cage.

Flexion is initiated by the abdominal muscles and the vertebral portion of the psoas muscle (Andersson & Lavender, 1997; Basmajian & DeLuca, 1985). The weight of the upper body produces further flexion, which is controlled by the gradually increasing activity of the erector spinae muscles as the forward-bending moment acting on the spine increases. The posterior hip muscles are active in controlling the forward tilting of the pelvis as the spine is flexed (Carlsöö, 1961). It has long been accepted that in full flexion, the erector spinae muscles become inactive once they are fully stretched. In this position, the forward bending moment was counteracted passively by these muscles and by the posterior ligaments, which are initially slack but become taut at this point because the spine has fully elongated (Farfan, 1975). This silencing of the erector spinae muscles is known as the flexion-relaxation phenomenon (Allen, 1948; Andersson & Lavender, 1997; Floyd & Silver, 1955; Morris et al., 1962). However, Andersson et al. (1996), using wire electrodes inserted in the trunk extensor muscles guided by ultrasound or MRI, showed that in the deep flexed position the superficial erector spinae muscles relax, while the quadratus lumborum and deep lateral lumbar erector spinae muscles become activated (Fig. 10-10). In forced flexion, the superficial extensor muscles become re-activated. From

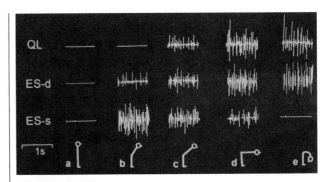

FIG. 10-10

Electromyography of the quadratus lumborum (*QL*) and erector spinae superficial (*ES-s*) and deep (*ES-d*) muscles. Wire electrodes were inserted in QL and ES-d; surface electrodes were used for ES-s. Five positions (a–e) of trunk flexion are depicted. In full nonforced trunk flexion (e), the ES-s activity is silent; however, the ES-d and QL are very active to counterbalance the trunk flexion movement. (*Courtesy of Eva Andersson, MD Ph.D, Karolinska Institute, Stockholm, Sweden.*)

full flexion to upright positioning of the trunk, the pelvis tilts backward and the spine then extends. The sequence of muscular activity is reversed. The gluteus maximus comes into action early together with the hamstrings and initiates extension by posterior rotation of the pelvis. The paraspinal muscles then become activated and increase their activity until the movement is completed (Andersson & Lavender, 1997).

Some studies have shown that the concentric exertion performed by the muscles involved in raising the trunk is greater than the eccentric exertion performed by the muscles involved in lowering the trunk (de Looze et al., 1993; Friedebold, 1958; Joseph, 1960). However, this finding has been contradicted in several studies (Reid & Costigan, 1987; Marras & Mirka, 1992). Creswell and Thortensson (1994) support the finding that less electromyographic (EMG) activity is noted during eccentric activity, as in lowering, despite high levels of force generated. The compressive load of the spine caused by the muscle exertion produced by lowering the trunk with a load or resistance can approach the spinal tolerance limits, putting the back at greater risk for injury (Davis et al., 1998).

When the trunk is hyperextended from the upright position, the extensor muscles are active during the initial phase. This initial burst of activity decreases during further extension, and the abdominal muscles become active to control and modify the motion. In extreme or forced extension, extensor activity is again required (Floyd & Silver, 1955).

Lateral Flexion and Rotation

During lateral flexion of the trunk, motion may predominate in either the thoracic or the lumbar spine. In the thoracic spine, the facet orientation allows for lateral flexion, but the rib cage restricts it (to varying degrees in different people); in the lumbar spine, the wedge-shaped spaces between the intervertebral joint surfaces show variations during this motion (Reichmann, 1971). The spinotransversal and transversospinal systems of the erector spinae muscles and the abdominal muscles are active during lateral flexion; ipsilateral contractions of these muscles initiate the motion and contralateral contractions modify it (Fig. 10-11) (Andersson & Lavender, 1997).

Significant axial rotation occurs at the thoracic and lumbosacral levels but is limited at other levels of the lumbar spine, being restricted by the vertical orientation of the facets (Fig. 10-6C). In the thoracic region, rotation is consistently associated with lateral flexion. During this coupled motion, which is most marked in the upper thoracic region, the vertebral bodies generally rotate toward the concavity of the lateral curve of the spine (White, 1969). Coupling of rotation and lateral flexion also takes place in the lumbar spine, with the vertebral bodies rotating toward the convexity of the curve (Miles & Sullivan, 1961). During axial rotation, the back and abdominal muscles are active on both sides of the spine, as both ipsilateral and contralateral muscles cooperate to produce this movement. High coactivation has been measured for axial rotation (Lavender et al., 1992; Pope et al., 1986).

Pelvic Motion

Functional trunk movements not only involve a combined motion of different parts of the spine but also require the cooperation of the pelvis because pelvic motion is essential for increasing the range of functional motion of the trunk. The relationship between pelvic movements and spinal motion is generally analyzed in terms of motion of the lumbosacral joints, the hip joints, or both (Fig. 10-12). Load transfer from the spine to the pelvis occurs through the sacroiliac (SI) joint. Biomechanical analysis of the sacroiliac joints suggests that these

joints function mainly as shock absorbers and are important in protecting the intervertebral joints (Wilder et al., 1980).

When loaded in vitro, the SI joint exhibits three-dimensional movement with joint opening rotation ranging from 0.5 to 1.2° and sacrum anterior-

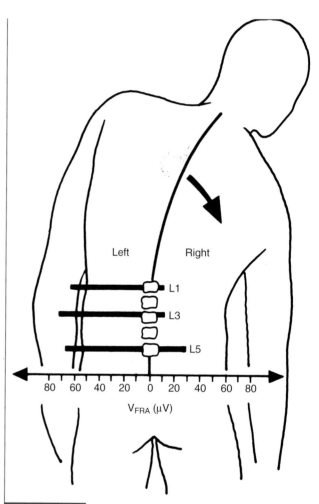

FIG. 10-11

Example of electromyographic activity of the erector spinae muscles collected with surface electrodes during side-bending of the trunk. The figure illustrates trunk bending to the right and muscle activity at the L1, L3, and L5 level of the lumbar spine. Substantial contralateral muscle activity (*left*) of the erector spinae muscles is recorded when bending to the right to maintain equilibrium. *Reproduced with permission from Andersson, G.B.J., Ortengren, R., & Nachemson, A. (1977). Intradiscal pressure, intra-abdominal pressure and myoelectric back muscle activity related to posture and loading. Clin Orthop, 129, 156.*

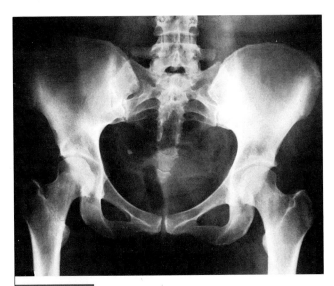

FIG. 10-12

The pelvic ring with its linkage to the spine and the lower extremities. The antero-posterior view of these structures on film gives a hint of the irregular shape of the sacroiliac joint surfaces, but an oblique projection is required for an accurate view of the joints.

posterior rotation ranging from 0.3 to 0.6°; translation ranged from 0.5 to 0.9 mm (Wang & Dumas, 1998). In vivo analysis of the SI joint utilizing roentgen stereophotogrammetry shows joint rotation mean at 2.5° and translation mean at 0.7 mm with no differences between symptomatic and asymptomatic joints (Sturesson et al., 1989).

Muscle forces acting on the SI joint have a stabilizing effect, helping to attenuate the high stress of pelvic loading (Dalstra & Huiskes, 1995).

Kinetics

Loads on the spine are produced primarily by body weight, muscle activity, pre-stress exerted by the ligaments, and externally applied loads. Simplified calculations of the loads at various levels of the spine can be made with the use of the free-body technique for coplanar forces. Direct information regarding loads on the spine at the level of individual intervertebral discs can be obtained by measuring the pressure within the discs both in vitro and in vivo. Because this method is too complex for general application, a semidirect measuring method is often

used. This involves measuring the myoelectric activity of the trunk muscles and correlating this activity with calculated values for muscle contraction forces. The values obtained correlate well with those obtained through intradiscal pressure measurement and can therefore be used to predict the loads on the spine (Andersson & Lavender, 1997; Örtengren et al., 1981; Schultz et al., 1982).

Another method is the use of a mathematical model for force estimation that allows the loads on the lumbar spine and the contraction forces in the trunk muscles to be calculated for various physical activities. The models are useful as predictors of load, for load sharing analysis under different conditions, to simulate loads, and in spine prosthetic and instrumentation design. The precision of the model depends on the assumption used for the calculations. Two categories of models currently used are the EMG-driven model based on electromyographic trunk muscle recordings and the more traditional biomechanical model based on trunk moments and forces (Chaffin & Anderson, 1991; Lavender et al., 1992; Marras & Granata, 1995; Sheikhzadeh, [1997]. *The effect of pure and combined loading on the recruitment pattern of ten selected trunk muscles.* Unpublished doctoral thesis. New York University, New York).

STATICS AND DYNAMICS

In the following section, static loads on the lumbar spine are examined for common postures such as standing and sitting and also for lifting, a common activity involving external loads. In the final section, the dynamic loads on the lumbar spine during walking and common strengthening exercises for the back and abdominal muscles are discussed.

Statics

The spine can be considered as a modified elastic rod because of the flexibility of the spinal column, the shock-absorbing behavior of the discs and vertebrae, the stabilizing function of the longitudinal ligaments, and the elasticity of the ligaments flavum. The two curvatures of the spine in the sagittal plane—kyphosis and lordosis—also contribute to the spring-like capacity of the spine and allow the vertebral column to withstand higher loads than if it were straight. A study of the capacity of cadaver thoracolumbar spines devoid of muscles to resist vertical loads showed that the critical load (the point at which buckling occurred) was approxi-

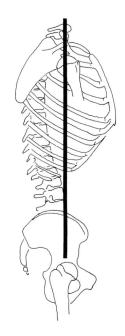

FIG. 10-13

The line of gravity for the trunk (*solid line*) is usually ventral to the transverse axis of motion of the spine and thus the spine is subjected to a constant forward-bending moment.

mately 20 to 40 N (Gregersen & Lucas, 1967; Lucas & Bresier, 1961). The critical load is much higher in vivo and varies greatly among individuals. The extrinsic support provided by the trunk muscles helps stabilize and modify the loads on the spine in both dynamic and static situations.

LOADING OF THE SPINE DURING STANDING

When a person stands, the postural muscles are constantly active. This activity is minimized when the body segments are well aligned. During standing, the line of gravity of the trunk usually passes ventral to the center of the fourth lumbar vertebral body (Asmussen & Klausen, 1962). Thus, it falls ventral to the transverse axis of motion of the spine and the motion segments are subjected to a forward-bending moment, which must be counterbalanced by ligament forces and erector spinae muscle forces (Fig. 10-13). Any displacement of the line of gravity alters the magnitude and direction of the moment on the spine. For the body to return to equilibrium, the moment must be counteracted by increased muscle activity, which causes intermittent postural sway. In addition to the erector spinae mus-

cles, the abdominal muscles are often intermittently active in maintaining the neutral upright position and stabilizing the trunk (Cholewicki et al., 1997). However, this activity is readily reduced by the command to stand relaxed (Hodges & Richardson, 1997).

The vertebral portion of the psoas muscles is also involved in producing postural sway (Basmajian, 1958; Nachemson, 1966). The level of activity in these muscles varies considerably among individuals and depends to some extent on the shape of the spine, for example, on the magnitude of habitual kyphosis and lordosis.

The pelvis also plays a role in the muscle activity and resulting loads on the spine during standing (Fig. 10-14). The base of the sacrum is inclined forward and downward. The angle of inclination, or sacral angle, is approximately 30° to the transverse plane during relaxed standing (Fig. 10-14*B*). Tilting of the pelvis about the transverse axis between the hip joints changes the angle. When the pelvis is tilted backward, the sacral angle decreases and the lumbar lordosis flattens (Fig. 10-14*A*). This flattening affects the thoracic spine, which extends slightly to adjust the center of gravity of the trunk so that the energy expenditure, in terms of muscle exertion,

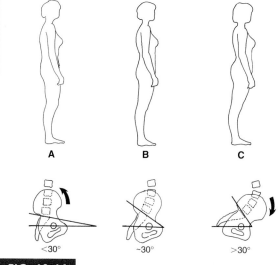

FIG. 10-14

Effect of pelvic tilting on the inclination of the base of the sacrum to the transverse plane (sacral angle) during upright standing. **A,** Tilting the pelvis backward reduces the sacral angle and flattens the lumbar spine. **B,** During relaxed standing, the sacral angle is approximately 30°. **C,** Tilting the pelvis forward increases the sacral angle and accentuates the lumbar lordosis.

is minimized. When the pelvis is tilted forward, the sacral angle increases, accentuating the lumbar lordosis and the thoracic kyphosis (Fig. 10-14C). Forward and backward tilting of the pelvis influences the activity of the postural muscles by affecting the static loads on the spine (Floyd & Silver, 1955).

COMPARATIVE LOADS ON THE LUMBAR SPINE DURING STANDING, SITTING, AND RECLINING

Body position affects the magnitude of the loads on the spine. As a result of in vivo intradiscal pressure measurement studies conducted by Nachemson (1975), it was shown that these loads are minimal during well-supported reclining, remain low during relaxed upright standing, and rise during sitting. A recent in vivo investigation of intervertebral disc pressure utilizing more sophisticated technology, and based on only one subject, suggested that in relaxed, unsupported sitting, interdiscal pressure is less than in standing (Wilke et al., 1999). Additional pertinent pressure measurements can be seen in Table 10-1. Sato et al. (1999) have verified Nachemson's (1975) findings, showing an increase in spinal load from 800 N in upright standing to 996 N in upright sitting. The relative loads on the spine during various body postures, as described by Nachemson and Wilke, are presented in Figure 10-15.

During relaxed upright standing, the load on the third and fourth lumbar disc is almost twice the weight of the body above the measured level (Nachemson & Elfström, 1970; Nachemson & Morris, 1964; Wilke et al., 1999). Trunk flexion increases the load and the forward-bending moment on the spine. During forward flexion, the annulus bulges ventrally (Klein et al., 1983) and the central portion of the disc moves posteriorly (Krag et al., 1987) (Fig. 10-16). More than trunk extension, trunk flexion stresses the posterolateral area of the annulus fibrosus. The addition of twisting motion and accompanying torsional loads further increases the stresses on the disc (Andersson et al.,1977; Shirazi-Adl, 1994; Steffen et al., 1998) (Case Study 10-2).

The loads on the lumbar spine are lower more during supported sitting than during unsupported sitting. During supported sitting, the weight of the upper body is supported by the backrest, which reduces the muscle activity, relieving intradiscal pressure (Andersson et al., 1974; Wilke et al., 1999). Backward inclination of the backrest and the use of a lumbar support further reduce the loads. The use of a support in the thoracic region, however, pushes the thoracic spine and the trunk forward and makes the lumbar spine move toward kyphosis to remain in

TABLE 10-1

Values of Intradiscal Pressure for Different Positions and Exercises As a Percentage Relative to Relaxed Standing in One Subject (Chosen Arbitrarily As 100%)

Position/Maneuver	Percentage
Lying supine	20
Side-lying	24
Lying prone	22
Lying prone, extended back, supporting elbows	50
Laughing heartily, lying laterally	30
Sneezing, lying laterally	76
Peaks by turning around	140–160
Relaxed standing	100
Standing, performing Valsalva maneuver	184
Standing, bent forward	220
Sitting relaxed, without back rest	92
Sitting actively straightening the back	110
Sitting with maximum flexion	166
Sitting bent forward with thigh supporting the elbows	86
Sitting slouched into the chair	54
Standing up from the chair	220
Walking barefoot	106–130
Walking with tennis shoes	106–130
Jogging with hard street shoes	70–190
Jogging with tennis shoes	70–170
Climbing stairs, one at a time	100–140
Climbing stairs, two at a time	60–240
Walking down stairs, one at a time	76–120
Walking down stairs, two at a time	60–180
Lifting 20 kg, bent over with round back	460
Lifting 20 kg as taught in back school	340
Holding 20 kg close to the body	220
Holding 20 kg, 60 cm away from the chest	360
Pressure increase during the night rest (over a period of 7 hours)	20–48

Adapted with permission from Wilke, H.J., Neef, P., Caimi, M., et al. (1999). New in vivo measurements of pressures in the intervertebral disc in daily life. *Spine, 24,* 755.

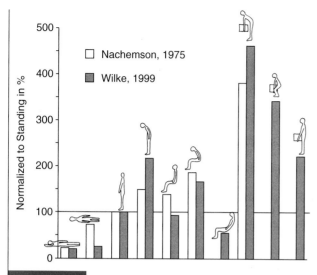

FIG. 10-15

Data from two studies using intradiscal pressure measurements. The relative loads on the third and fourth lumbar discs measured in vivo in various body positions are compared with the load during upright standing, depicted as 100%. *Adapted with permission from Nachemson, A. (1975). Towards a better understanding of back pain: A review of the mechanics of the lumbar disc. Rheumatol Rehabil, 14, 129 and from Wilke, H.J., Neef, P., Caimi, M., et al. (1999). New in vivo measurements of pressures in the intervertebral disc in daily life. Spine, 24, 755.*

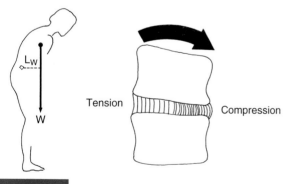

FIG. 10-16

The forward-bent position produces a bending moment on the lumbar spine. The moment is a product of the force produced by the weight of the upper body (W) and the lever arm of the force (L_W). The forward inclination of the upper body subjects the disc to increased tensile and compressive stresses. The annulus bulges on the compressive side and the nucleus is shifted posteriorly.

CASE STUDY 10-2

Nonspecific Low Back Pain

A 35-year-old male presents complaints of low back pain with radiation to the posterior aspect of the left thigh, not past the knee. His pain started 3 weeks ago, after working a 12-hour shift, when he lifted while twisting an unusually large, yet lightweight box. During the first week of pain, he visited his physician, who prescribed pain medication. Currently, he is still in pain, particularly during sitting or standing for long periods. During a follow-up physician visit, a careful examination showed the patient to be somewhat overweight, with weakness in his abdominal and back muscles and poor flexibility in his hamstrings, psoas, and back muscles. Neurological tests were normal and diagnostic x-rays were normal as well, leading to a diagnosis of nonspecific low back pain (Case Study Fig. 10-2-1).

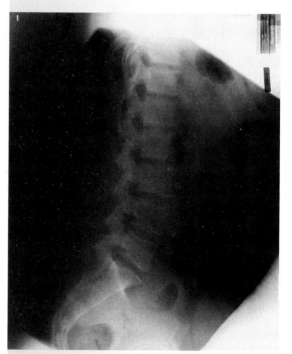

Case Study Figure 10-2-1.

Combinations of different factors have resulted in this injury. From the biomechanical point of view, although the load lifted was considered light, the vastness of the package and the resultant large lever arm (the distance from the center of gravity of the person to the package) created a larger than expected load on the lumbar spine. In addition, weakness in the abdominal and extensor muscles of the spine led to an additional mechanical disadvantage in stabilizing the lower back. Tight psoas and hamstring muscles place restrictions on the mobility of the pelvis, stressing the range of motion in the lumbar region and affecting the normal loads and motions at this level.

contact with the backrest, increasing the loads on the lumbar spine (Andersson et al., 1974) (Fig. 10-17).

Loads on the spine are minimized when an individual assumes a supine position because the loads produced by the body's weight are eliminated (Fig. 10-15). With the body supine and the knees extended, the pull of the vertebral portion of the psoas muscle produces some loads on the lumbar spine. With the hips and knees bent and supported, however, the lumbar lordosis straightens out as the psoas muscle relaxes and the loads decrease (Fig. 10-18).

STATIC LOADS ON THE LUMBAR SPINE DURING LIFTING

The highest loads on the spine are generally produced by external loads, such as lifting a heavy object. Just how much load can be sustained by the spine before damage occurs continues to be investigated. Pioneering studies by Eie (1966) of lumbar

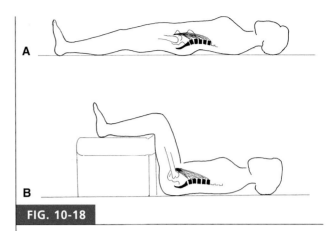

FIG. 10-18

A, When a person assumes a supine position with legs straight, the pull of the vertebral portion of the psoas muscle produces some loads on the lumbar spine. **B,** When the hips and knees are bent and supported, the psoas muscle relaxes and the loads on the lumbar spine decrease.

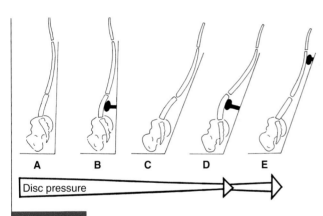

FIG. 10-17

Influence of backrest inclination and back support on loads of the lumbar spine, in terms of pressure in the third lumbar disc, during supported sitting. **A,** Backrest inclination is 90° and disc pressure is at a maximum. **B,** Addition of a lumbar support decreases the disc pressure. **C,** Backward inclination of the backrest is 110°, but with no lumbar support it produces less disc pressure. **D,** Addition of a lumbar support with this degree of backrest inclination further decreases the pressure. **E,** Shifting the support to the thoracic region pushes the upper body forward, moving the lumbar spine toward kyphosis and increasing the disc pressure. *Adapted with permission from Andersson, G.B.J., Ortengren, R., Nachemson, A., et al. (1974). Lumbar disc pressure and myoelectric back muscle activity during sitting. 1. Studies on an experimental chair.* Scand J Rehabil Med, 6, *104.*

vertebral specimens from adult humans showed that the compressive load to vertebrae failure ranged from approximately 5,000 to 8,000 N. On the whole, values reported subsequently by other authors correspond to those of Eie, although values above 10,000 N and below 5,000 N have been documented (Hutton & Adams, 1982). The application of static bending-shearing moment on lumbar motion segments revealed that bending moment of 620 Nm and shear moment of 156 Nm were tolerated before complete disruption of motion segment occurred. The flexion angle before failure was recorded as 20° with 9 mm of horizontal displacement between the two vertebrae (Osvalder et al., 1990). Both age and degree of disc degeneration influence the range preceding failure. Although the vertebral body strength is relative to the bone mass, with aging the decline in bone strength is more pronounced than is the decline in bone mass (Mosekilde, 1993).

Eie (1966) and Ranu (1990) observed that during compressive testing the fracture point was reached in the vertebral body, or end plate, before the intervertebral disc sustained damage. This finding shows that the bone is less capable of resisting compression than is an intact disc. During the testing, a yield point was reached before the vertebra or end plate fractured. When the load was removed at this point, the vertebral body recovered but was more susceptible to damage when reloaded.

Evidence exists that the spine may incur micro-damage as a result of high loads in vivo. T. Hansson (1977, *The bone mineral content and biomechanical properties of lumbar vertebrae. An in vitro study based on dual photon absorptiometry.* Unpublished thesis, University of Gothenburg, Sweden) observed microfractures in specimens from "normal" human lumbar vertebrae and interpreted this microdamage to be fatigue fractures resulting from stresses and strains on the spine in vivo. In vitro examination confirmed the existance of microdamage near the end plated with compression loading (Hasegawa et al., 1993).

Lifting and carrying an object over a horizontal distance are common situations wherein loads applied to the vertebral column may be so high as to damage the spine. Several factors influence the loads on the spine during these activities: (1) the position of the object relative to the center of motion in the spine; (2) the size, shape, weight, and density of the object; (3) the degree of flexion or rotation of the spine; and (4) the rate of loading.

Holding the object close to the body instead of away from it reduces the bending moment on the lumbar spine because the distance from the center of gravity of the object to the center of motion in the spine (the lever arm) is minimized. The shorter the lever arm is for the force produced by the weight of a given object, the lower the magnitude of the bending moment and thus the lower the loads on the lumbar spine (Andersson et al., 1976; Nachemson & Elfström, 1970; Németh, 1984; Wilke et al., 1999) (Calculation Box 10-1).

Even when identical and nonfatiguing repeated lifting tasks are performed, variability in lifting technique of the same subject has been shown in trunk kinematics, kinetics, and spinal load (Granata et al., 1999). When an individual repeatedly performs an identical lift, great variability is recorded, which indicates that the brain may have several motor strategies to do a task. It also indicates the sensitive responsiveness of the muscle system to subtle changes to maintain the performance despite fatigue.

When a person holding an object bends forward, the force produced by the weight of the object plus that produced by the weight of the upper body create a bending moment on the disc, increasing the loads on the spine. This bending moment is greater than that produced when the person stands erect while holding the object (Calculation Box 10-2).

Health professionals generally recommend that lifting be done with the knees bent and the back relatively straight to reduce the loads on the spine.

Influence of the Size of the Object on the Loads on the Lumbar Spine

The size of the object held influences the loads on the lumbar spine. If objects of the same weight, shape, and density but of different sizes are held, the lever arm for the force produced by the weight of the object is longer for the larger object, and thus the bending moment on the lumbar spine is greater (Calculation Box Fig. 10-1-1). In these two situations (Calculation Box Figs. 10-1-1 and 10-1-2), the distance from the center of motion in the disc to the front of the abdomen is 20 cm. In both cases, the object has a uniform density and weighs 20 kg. In the case of Calculation Box Figure 10-1-1, the width of the cubic object is 20 cm; in the case of Calculation Box Figure 10-1-2, the width is 40 cm. Thus, in Case 1 (Calculation Box Fig. 10-1-1), the forward-bending moment acting on the lowest lumbar disc is 60 Nm, as the force of 200 N produced by the weight of the object acts with a lever arm (L_p) of 30 cm (200 N × 0.3 m). In Case 2 (Calculation Box Fig. 10-1-2), the forward-bending moment is 80 Nm, as the lever arm (L_p) is 40 cm (200 N × 0.4 m). [Considering 1Kg ≅ 10N.]

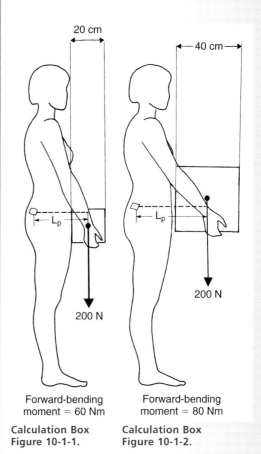

Forward-bending moment = 60 Nm

Forward-bending moment = 80 Nm

Calculation Box Figure 10-1-1.

Calculation Box Figure 10-1-2.

Influence of the Upper Body Position on the Loads at the Lumbar Spine During Lifting

In the two situations shown in Calculation Box Figures 10-2-1 and 10-2-2, an identical object weighing 20 kg is lifted. In Case 1 (Calculation Box Fig. 10-2-1) (upright standing), the lever arm of the force produced by the weight of the object (L_P) is 30 cm, creating a forward-bending moment of 60 Nm (200 N × 0.3 m). The forward-bending moment created by the upper body is 9 Nm; the length of the lever arm (LW) is estimated to be 2 cm, and the force produced by the weight of the upper body is 450 N. Thus, the total forward-bending moment in Case 1 is equal to 69 Nm (60 Nm + 9 Nm).

In Case 2 (Calculation Box Fig. 10-2-2) (upper body flexed forward), the lever arm of the force produced by the weight of the object (L_P) is increased to 40 cm, creating a forward-bending moment of 80 Nm (200 N × 0.4 m). Furthermore, the force of 450 N produced by the weight of the upper body increases in importance as it acts with a lever arm (L_W) of 25 cm, creating a forward-bending moment of 112.5 Nm (450 N × 0.25 m). Thus, the total forward-bending moment in Case 2 is 192.5 Nm (112.5 Nm + 80 Nm).

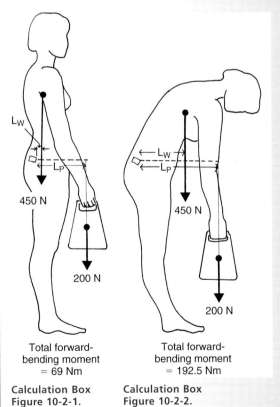

Total forward-bending moment = 69 Nm

Total forward-bending moment = 192.5 Nm

Calculation Box Figure 10-2-1.

Calculation Box Figure 10-2-2.

However, this recommendation is valid only if this technique is used correctly and optimally, with the load positioned between the feet and thereby reducing the lever arm of the external load (van Dieen et al., 1999) (Calculation Box 10-3).

A literature review revealed no significant difference in spinal compression and shear computed forces between stoop or squat lifting (van Dieene et al., 1999). However, it was suggested that loss of balance is more likely during squat lifting, which in turn may add additional stresses on the lumbar spine.

In the following example, the free-body technique for coplanar forces will be used to make a simplified calculation of the static loads on the spine as an object is lifted (Calculation Boxes 10-4*A* and 10-4*B*).

Calculations made in this way for one point in time during lifting are valuable for demonstrating how the lever arms of the forces produced by the weight of the upper body and by the weight of the object affect the loads imposed on the spine. The use of the same calculations to compute the loads produced when an 80 kg object is lifted (representing a force of 800 N) yields an approximate load of 10,000 N on the disc, which is likely to exceed the fracture point of the vertebra. Because athletes who lift weights can easily reach such calculated loads without sustaining fractures, other factors, such as intra-abdominal pressure (IAP), may be involved in reducing the loads on the spine in vivo (Krajcarski et al., 1999).

Dynamics

Almost all motion in the body increases muscle recruitment and the loads on the spine. This increase is modest during such activities as slow walking or easy twisting but becomes more marked during various exercises and the complexity of dynamic movement and dynamic loading (Nachemson & Elfström, 1970).

WALKING

In a study of normal walking at four speeds, the compressive loads at the L3–L4 motion segment ranged from 0.2 to 2.5 times body weight (Fig. 10-19) (Cappozzo, 1984). The loads were maximal around toe-off and increased approximately linearly with walking speed. Muscle action was mainly concentrated in the trunk extensors. Individual walking traits, particularly the amount of forward flexion of the trunk, influenced the loads.

CALCULATION BOX 10-3

The Technique Employed During Lifting Influences the Loads on the Lumbar Spine

In the three situations shown in Calculation Box Figures 10-3-1, 10-3-2, and 10-3-3, an identical object weighing 20 kg is lifted. Case 1 (upper body flexed forward) (Calculation Box Fig. 10-3-1) is identical to Case 2 in Calculation Box 10-2, where the total forward-bending moment is 192.5 Nm.

In Case 2 (Calculation Box Fig. 10-3-2), lifting with the knees bent and the back straight places the object closer to the trunk, decreasing the forward-bending moments. The lever arms of the forces produced by the weight of the object (L_P) and upper body (L_W) are shortened to 35 and 18 cm, respectively, at this point in the lifting process. The result is a total forward-bending moment of 151 Nm([200 N × 0.35 m] + [450 N × 0.18 m]).

Case 3 (Calculation Box Fig. 10-3-3) shows that bent knees per se do not decrease the forward-bending moments. If the object lifted is held out in front of the knees, the lever arm of the force produced by the weight of the object (L_P) increases to 50 cm, and the lever arm of the force produced by the weight of the upper body (L_W) increases to 25 cm. Thus, the total forward-bending moment created is 212.5 Nm ([200 N × 0.5 m] + [450 N × 0.25m]).

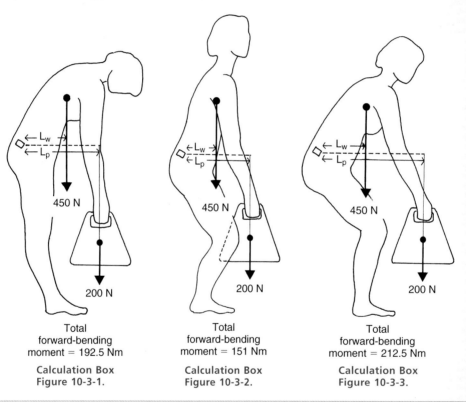

Total forward-bending moment = 192.5 Nm

Calculation Box Figure 10-3-1.

Total forward-bending moment = 151 Nm

Calculation Box Figure 10-3-2.

Total forward-bending moment = 212.5 Nm

Calculation Box Figure 10-3-3.

The greater this flexion, the larger the muscle forces and hence the compressive load. Callaghan et al. (1999) corroborated these findings and further showed that walking cadence affects lumbar loading, with increased anterior-posterior shear forces noted as speed increased. Limiting arm swing during walking resulted in increased compressive joint loading and EMG output with decreased lumbar spine motions. In conclusion, because of low tissue loading, walking is a safe and perhaps ideal therapeutic exercise for those with low back pain (Callaghan et al., 1999) while attention to speed of walking can further moderate spinal loads (Cheng et al., 1998).

Free-Body Diagram Technique for Coplanar Forces. Calculation of the Static Loads on the Spine As an Object Is Lifted

The loads on a lumbar disc will be calculated for one point in time when a person who weighs 70 kg lifts a 20 kg object The spine is flexed approximately 35°. In this example, the three principal forces acting on the lumbar spine at the lumbosacral level are: (1) the force produced by the weight of the upper body (W), calculated to be 450 N (approximately 65% of the force exerted by the total body weight); (2) the force produced by the weight of the object (P), 200 N; and (3) the force produced by contraction of the erector spinae muscles (E), which has a known direction and point of application but an unknown magnitude (Calculation Box Fig. 10-4A-1).

Because these three forces act at a distance from the center of motion in the spine, they create moments in the lumbar spine. Two forward-bending moments (WL_W and PL_P) are the products of (W) and (P) and the perpendiculars from the instant center of rotation to the lines of action of these forces (their lever arms). The lever arm (L_P) for (P) is 0.4 m and the lever arm (L_W) for (W) is 0.25 m. A counterbalancing moment (EL_E) is the product of (E) and its lever arm. The lever arm (L_E) is 0.05 m. The magnitude of (E) can be found through the use of the equilibrium equation for moments. For the body to be in moment equilibrium, the sum of the moments acting on the lumbar spine must be zero. (In this example, clockwise moments are considered to be positive and counterclockwise moments are considered to be negative.)

Thus,

$$\Sigma M = 0$$
$$(W \times L_W) + (P \times L_P) - (E \times L_E) = 0$$
$$(450\ N \times 0.25\ m) + (200\ N \times 0.4\ m) - (E \times 0.05\ m) = 0$$
$$E \times 0.05\ m = 112.5\ Nm + 80\ Nm.$$

Solving this equation for E yields 3,850 N.

The total compressive force exerted on the disc (C) can now be calculated trigonometrically (Calculation Box Fig. 10-4A-2). In the example, C is the sum of the compressive forces acting over the disc, which is inclined 35° to the transverse plane. These forces are:

1. The compressive force produced by the weight of the upper body (W), which acts on the disc inclined 35° ($W \times \cos 35°$).
2. The force produced by the weight of the object (P), which acts on the disc inclined 35° ($P \times \cos 35°$).
3. The force produced by the erector spinae muscles (E), which acts approximately at a right angle to the disc inclination.

The total compressive force acting on the disc (C) has a known sense, point of application, and line of action but an unknown magnitude. The magnitude of C can be found through the use of the equilibrium equation for forces. For the body to be in force equilibrium, the sum of the forces must be equal to zero.

Thus,

$$\Sigma \text{ forces} = 0$$
$$(W \times \cos 35°) + (P \times \cos 35°) + E - C = 0$$
$$(450\ N \times \cos 35°) + (200\ N \times \cos 35°) + 3850\ N - C = 0$$
$$C = 368.5\ N + 163.8\ N + 3850\ N.$$

Solving the equation for C yields 4,382 N.

The shear component for the reaction force on the disc (S) is found in the same way:

$$(450\ N \times \sin 35°) + (200\ N \times \sin 35°) - S = 0$$
$$S = 373\ N$$

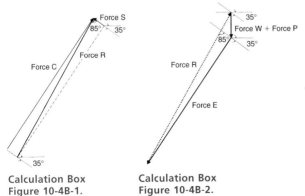

Calculation Box Figure 10-4A-1.

Calculation Box Figure 10-4A-2.

Force E (3850 N)

W·Cos 35°   W·Sin 35°

35°

Force W (450 N)

P·Cos 35°   P·Sin 35°

Force C (magnitude unknown)

Force P (200 N)

Force S (magnitude unknown)

C = 4382 N
S = 373 N

Free-Body Diagram Technique for Coplanar Forces. Calculation of the Static Loads on the Spine As an Object Is Lifted

Force S

85°   35°

Force R

Force C

35°

Calculation Box Figure 10-4B-1.

35°
Force W + Force P
85°
35°

Force R

Force E

Calculation Box Figure 10-4B-2.

Because C and S form a right angle (Calculation Box Fig. 10-4B-1), the Pythagorean theorem can be used to find the total reaction force on the disc (R):

$$(R) = \sqrt{C^2 + S^2}$$
$$R = 4398\ N$$

The direction of (R) is determined by means of a trigonometric function:

$$\sin(\alpha) = C/R$$

$(\alpha) = \arcsin(C/R) = 85°$ where (α) is the angle between the total vector force on the disc and the disc inclination.

The problem can be graphically solved by constructing a vector diagram based on the known values (Calculation Box Fig. 10-4B-2). A vertical line representing (W) + (P) is drawn first; (E) is added at a right angle to the disc inclination, and (R) closes the triangle. The direction of (R) in relation to the disc is determined.

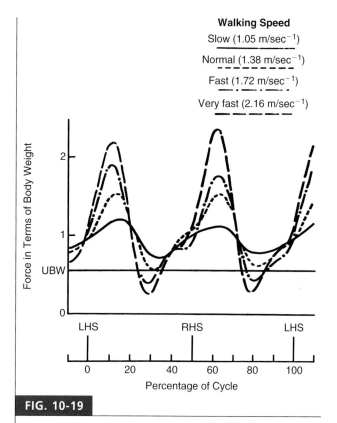

Walking Speed

Slow (1.05 m/sec^{-1})

Normal (1.38 m/sec^{-1})

Fast (1.72 m/sec^{-1})

Very fast (2.16 m/sec^{-1})

FIG. 10-19

Axial load on the L3–L4 motion segment in terms of body weight for one subject during walking at four speeds. The *horizontal line* (UBW) denotes the weight of the upper body, which represents the gravitational component of this load. Loads were predicted using experimental data from photogrammetric measurements along with a biomechanical model of the trunk. *LHS,* left heel strike; *RHS,* right heel strike. *Adapted with permission from Cappozzo, A. (1984). Compressive loads in the lumbar vertebral column during normal level walking.* J Orthop Res, 1, 292.

EXERCISES

During strengthening exercises for the erector spinae and abdominal muscles, the loads on the spine can be high. Although such exercises must be effective for strengthening the trunk muscles concerned, they should be performed in such a way that the loads on the spine are adjusted to suit the condition of the individual.

The erector spinae muscles are intensely activated by arching the back in the prone position (Fig. 10-20A) (Pauly, 1966). Loading the spine in extreme positions such as this one produces high stresses on spine structures, in particular the spinous process (Adams et al., 1988). Although intradiscal pressure in a prone position with upper body support on the elbows is half that in standing (Wilke et al., 1999), it

is recommended for exercise that an initial position that keeps the vertebrae in a more parallel alignment is preferable when strengthening exercises for the erector spinae muscles are performed (Fig. 10-20B).

The importance of the abdominal muscles in spinal stability and interplay in the production of IAP reinforces the need for strong abdominal flexors. Sit-ups are a useful exercise for abdominal muscle strengthening, with many variations practiced and encouraged by health professionals, but certain variations are viewed as harmful to the low back. Although the most common belief has been that sit-ups with the knees flexed and feet unanchored will emphasize the abdominal contribution while minimizing psoas activity (Juker et al., 1998), this is not true. Both bent knee and straight leg sit-ups will produce comparable levels of psoas and abdominal activity, creating compressive spinal loading. Curl-ups, in which the head and shoulders are raised only to the point where the shoulder blades clear the table and lumbar spine motion is minimized (Fig. 10-21) and often emphasized in rehabilitation programs, are recommended for minimizing compressive lumbar loading (Axler & McGill, 1997; Juker et al., 1998). This modification of the exercise has been shown to be effective in terms of motor unit recruitment in the muscles (Ekholm et al., 1979; Flint, 1965; Partridge & Walters, 1959); all portions of the external oblique and rectus abdominis muscles are activated. Sit-ups with feet unanchored, legs elevated, or torso twisting do not significantly increase abdominal muscle activity (Axler & McGill, 1997). To limit the psoas activity, a reverse curl, wherein the knees are brought toward the chest and the buttocks are raised from the table, activates the internal and external oblique muscles and the rectus abdominis muscle (Partridge & Walters, 1959). If the reverse curl is performed isometrically, the disc pressure is lower than that produced during a sit-up, but the exercise is just as effective for strengthening the abdominal muscles (Fig. 10-22). It can be concluded that no single abdominal exercise can optimally train all trunk flexors while minimizing intervertebral joint loading. Instead, a varied program must be prescribed, tailored to the training objectives of the individual (Axler & McGill, 1997).

When designing a back strengthening exercise program, the most important consideration is the conclusion drawn by the Paris Task Force (Abenhaim et al., 2000). The guidelines set forth include recommendations that exercise is beneficial for subacute and chronic low back pain. No particular group or type of exercises has been shown to be most effective.

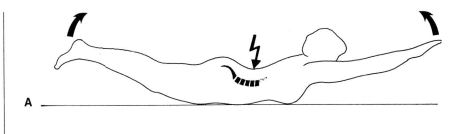

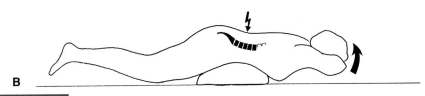

FIG. 10-20

A, Arching the back in the prone position greatly activates the erector spinae muscles but also produces high stresses on the lumbar discs, which are loaded in an extreme position. **B,** Decreasing the arch of the back by placing a pillow under the abdomen allows the discs to better resist stresses because the vertebrae are aligned with each other. Isometric exercise in this position is preferable.

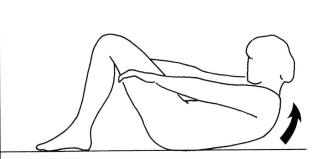

FIG. 10-21

Performing a curl to the point where only the shoulder blades clear the table minimizes the lumbar motion and hence the load on the lumbar spine is less than when a full sit-up is performed. A greater moment is produced if the arms are raised above the head or the hands are clasped behind the neck, as the center of gravity of the upper body then shifts farther away from the center of motion in the spine.

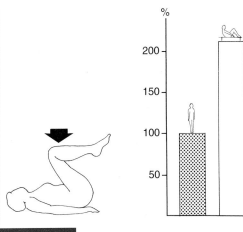

FIG. 10-22

A reverse curl, isometrically performed, provides efficient training of the abdominal muscles and produces moderate stresses on the lumbar discs. The relative loads on the third lumbar disc during a full sit-up and an isometric curl are compared with the load during upright standing, depicted as 100%. *Adapted with permission from Nachemson, A. (1975). Towards a better understanding of back pain: A review of the mechanics of the lumbar disc.* Rheumatol Rehabil, 14, 129.

MECHANICAL STABILITY OF THE LUMBAR SPINE

Mechanical stability for the lumbar spine can be achieved through several means: IAP, co-contraction of the trunk muscles, external support, and surgery. Surgical procedures for lumbar spine stability will not be covered in this section.

Intra-Abdominal Pressure

IAP is one mechanism that may contribute to both unloading and stabilization of the lumbar spine. IAP is the pressure created within the abdominal cavity by a coordinated contraction of the diaphragm and the abdominal and pelvic floor mus-

cles. Its unloading mechanism was first proposed by Bartelink in 1957 and Morris et al. in 1961. They suggested that IAP serves as a "pressurized balloon" attempting to separate the diaphragm and pelvic floor (Fig. 10-23, *A & B*). This creates an extensor moment that decreases the compression forces on the lumbar discs. The extensor moment produced by IAP has been calculated in several biomechanical models, with widely varying resulting reductions in extensor moment from 10 to 40% of the extensor load (Anderson et al., 1985; Chaffin, 1969; Eie, 1966; Lander et al., 1986; Morris et al., 1961).

Recent studies using fine-wire EMG of the deeper abdominal muscles found that the transversus abdominis is the primary abdominal muscle responsible for IAP generation (Cresswell, 1993;

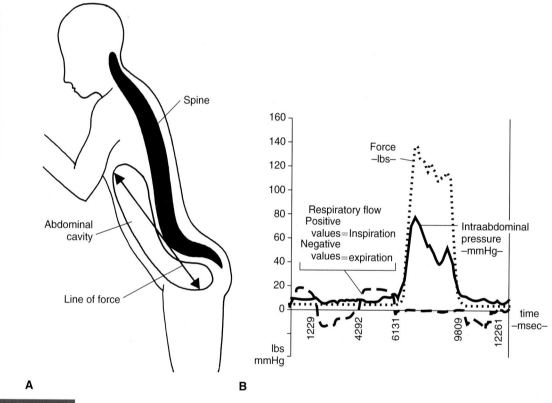

A

B

FIG. 10-23

A, Schematic illustration of the effect of intra-abdominal pressure. An increased pressure will create an extension moment on the lumbar spine. **B,** Intra-abdominal pressure (IAP) (measured by a nasogastric microtip transducer) and respiratory flow (measured through a Pneumotach) during stoop lift of 120 lbs. (approximately 60 kg). *Solid line,* IAP; *dotted line,* force exerted in lbs; *dashed line,* respiratory flow (negative values delineate expiration and positive values delineate inspiration). Note that the subject inspires before the lift and holds the breath throughout the lift. IAP increases and peaks together with the lifting force, helping to stabilize and unload the lumbar spine. *Courtesy of Markus Pietrek, MD and Marshall Hagins PT, MA. Program of Ergonomics and Biomechanics, New York University and Hospital for Joint Diseases, New York, NY, USA.*

Cresswell et al., 1994a; Cresswell et al., 1992; Hodges et al., 1999). As the transversus abdominis is horizontally oriented, it creates compression and an increase in IAP without an accompanying flexor moment. A recent experimental study gave the first direct evidence for a trunk extensor moment produced by elevated IAP (Hodges et al., 2000).

It has been demonstrated that the IAP contributes to the mechanical stability of the spine through a co-activation between the antagonistic trunk flexor and extensor muscles (Cholewicki et al., 1997, 1999a,b; Gardner-Morse & Stokes, 1998). As the abdominal musculature contracts, IAP increases and converts the abdomen into a rigid cylinder that greatly increases stability as compared with the multisegmented spinal column (McGill & Norman, 1987; Morris et al., 1961).

IAP increases during both static and dynamic conditions such as lifting and lowering, running and jumping, and unexpected trunk perturbations (Cresswell et al., 1992; Cresswell et al., 1994b; Cresswell & Thorstensson, 1994; Harman et al., 1988). Current research suggests that the transversus abdominis muscle, together with the diaphragm, plays an important role in stabilizing the spine in preparation for limb movement, regardless of the direction in which movement is anticipated. Transversus abdominis and diaphragmatic activity appear to occur independently, prior to activity of the primary limb mover or the other abdominal muscles (Hodges et al., 1997, 1999).

Trunk Muscle Co-Contraction

To understand the phenomenon of co-contraction during trunk loading, Krajcarski et al. (1999) studied the in vivo muscular response to perturbations at two rates causing a rapid flexion moment. The results of maximum trunk flexion angles and resulting extensor moments were compared. The results showed that with higher levels, co-contraction, spine compression, and trunk muscle stiffness increase. During unexpected loading, a 70% increase in muscle activity has been noted as compared with anticipated loading, which may lead to injury (Marras et al., 1987). Further investigation into the loading response has revealed that an inverse relationship (i.e., the shorter the warning time, the greater the peak trunk muscle response) exists between peak muscle response and warning time prior to loading (Lavender et al., 1989).

Loss of spine stability can be achieved through repetitive loading. This can be achieved through repetitive continuous motions that fatigue the trunk muscles. Muscle endurance is mechanically defined as the point at which fatigue of the muscles is observable, usually through a change in movement pattern. Parnianpour et al. (1988) used an isoinertial triaxial device to study force output and movement patterns when subjects performed a flexion and extension movement of the trunk until exhaustion. The results showed that with fatigue, coupled motion increased in the coronal and transverse planes during the flexion and extension movement. In addition, torque, angular excursion, and angular velocity of the motion decreased. The reduction in the functional capacity of the flexion-extension muscles was compensated for by secondary muscle groups and led to an increased couple motion pattern that is more injury prone. Figure 10-24, *A & B* shows the increase in axial rotation (torque and position) during flexion and extension of the trunk until exhaustion.

In an animal study, Solomonow et al. (1999) induced laxity of the spine in the ligaments, discs, and joint capsule by cyclic repetitive loading of feline in vivo lumbar spines. The cyclic loading resulted in desensitization of the mechanoreceptors with a significant decrease or complete elimination of reflexive stabilizing contractions of the multifidus muscle. This may lead to increased instability of the spine and a lack of protective muscular activity even before muscular fatigue is observed. A 10-minute rest period restored the muscular activity to approximately 25%.

External Stabilization

Restriction of motion at any level of the spine may increase motion at another level. The use of back belts as a means of preventing low back injury remains controversial. Originally it was believed to assist in increasing IAP as a way of unloading the spine during lifting; however, inconclusive evidence exists as to the biomechanical effectiveness of these devices (Perkins & Bloswick, 1995). The National Institute for Occupational Safety and Health has advised against the use of back belts to prevent low back injuries (NIOSH, 1994). As well, an orthotic worn to restrict thoracic and lumbar motion may result in compensatory motion at the lumbosacral level (Lumsden & Morris, 1968; Norton & Brown, 1957; Tuong et al., 1998).

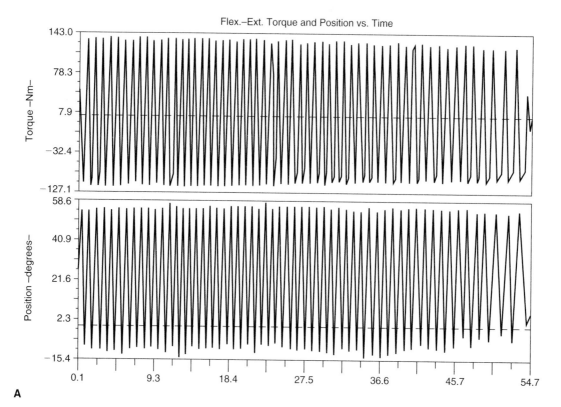

A

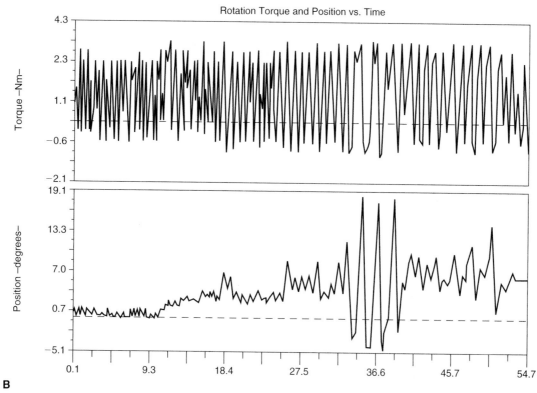

B

FIG. 10-24

Dynamic (isoinertial) flexion-extension trunk testing until exhaustion for one subject. Torque and position data is depicted for two planes, flexion-extension (**A**) and axial rotation (**B**). Note that flexion-extension torque production is diminishing as is the amount of performed extension of the trunk (**A**). Rotational torque and movement amplitude, increased accessory motion, and torque is shown in **B**.

Data for lateral flexion was similar to axial rotation and not shown here. *Adapted with permission from Parnianpour, M., Nordin, M., Kahanovitz, N., et al. (1988). The triaxial coupling of torque generation of trunk muscles during isometric exertions and the effect of fatiguing isoinertial movements on the motor output and movement patterns.* Spine, 13(9), 982-992.

Investigation into the effect of back belts on muscle activity has revealed no significant EMG activity differences in the back extensors during lifting with or without a back belt (Ciriello & Snook, 1995; Lee & Chen, 1999), while McGill et al. (1990) showed slightly increased EMG activity in the abdominal (except for the internal oblique muscles) and erector spinae muscles. Thomas et al. (1999) have verified a slight increase in EMG activity (2%) in the erector spinae during symmetric lifting with a back belt. Back belts have not been shown to significantly increase lifting capacity (Reyna et al., 1995).

Summary

1 The lumbar spine is a highly intricate and complex structure.

2 A vertebra-disc-vertebra unit constitutes a motion segment, the functional unit of the spine.

3 The intervertebral disc serves a hydrostatic function in the motion segment, storing energy and distributing loads. This function is reduced with disc degeneration.

4 The primary function of the facet joint is to guide the motion of the motion segment. The orientation of the facets determines the type of motion possible at any level of the spine. The facets may also sustain compressive loads, particularly during hyperextension.

5 Motion between two vertebrae is small and does not occur independently in vivo. Thus, the functional motion of the spine is always a combined action of several motion segments.

6 The instantaneous center of motion for the motion segments of the lumbar spine usually lies within the lumbar disc.

7 The trunk muscles play an important role in providing extrinsic stability to the spine; the ligaments and discs provide intrinsic stability.

8 Body position affects the loads on the lumbar spine. Any deviation from upright relaxed standing increases the load. Forward flexion and simultaneous twisting of the trunk produce high stresses on the lumbar spine.

9 Externally applied loads that are produced, for example, by lifting or carrying objects may subject the lumbar spine to very high loads. For the loads on the spine to be minimized during lifting, the distance between the trunk and the object lifted should be as short as possible.

10 IAP and co-contraction of trunk musculature increases the stability of the spinal column.

11 Trunk muscle fatigue may expose the spine to increased vulnerability as a result of loss of motor control and thereby increased stress on the surrounding ligaments, disc, and joint capsules.

12 Walking is an excellent exercise that poses a low load on the lumbar spine.

REFERENCES

Abenhaim, L., Rossignol, M., Valat, J.P., et al. (2000). The role of activity in the therapeutic management of back pain. Report of the International Paris Task Force on Back Pain. *Spine, 25,* 1S.

Adams, M.A., Dolan, P., & Hutton W.C. (1988). The lumbar spine in backward bending. *Spine, 13,* 1019

Adams, M.A. & Hutton, W.C. (1983). The mechanical functions of the lumbar apophyseal joints. *Spine, 8,* 327.

Allen, C.E.L. (1948). Muscle action potentials used in the study of dynamic anatomy. *Br J Phys Med, 11,* 66.

Anderson, C.K., Chaffin, D.B., Herrin, G.D., et al. (1985). A biomechanical model of the lumbosacral joint during lifting activities. *J Biomechanics, 18,* 57.

Andersson, E.A., Oddsson, L.I.E., Grundstrom, H., et al. (1996). EMG activities of the quadratus lumborum and erector spinae muscles during flexion-relaxation and other motor tasks. *Clinical Biomechanics, 11,* 392.

Andersson, G.B.J. & Lavender, S.A. (1997). Evaluation of Muscle Function. In J.W. Frymoyer (Ed.), *The Adult Spine. Principles and Practice* (2nd ed., pp. 341–380). New York: Lippincott-Raven.

Andersson, G.B.J., Ortengren, R., & Nachemson, A. (1976). Quantitative studies of back loads in lifting. *Spine, 1,* 178.

Andersson, G.B.J., Ortengren, R., & Nachemson, A. (1977). Intradiscal pressure, intra-abdominal pressure and myoelectric back muscle activity related to posture and loading. *Clin Orthop, 129,* 156.

Andersson, G.B.J., Ortengren, R., Nachemson, A., et al. (1974). Lumbar disc pressure and myoelectric back muscle activity during sitting. 1. Studies on an experimental chair. *Scand J Rehabil Med, 6,* 104.

Asmussen, E. & Klausen, K. (1962). Form and function of the erect human spine. *Clin Orthop, 25,* 55.

Axler, C.T. & McGill, S.M. (1997). Low back loads over a variety of abdominal exercises: Searching for the safest abdominal challenge. *Medicine & Science in Sports & Exercise, 29,* 804

Bartelink, D.L. (1957). The role of abdominal pressure in relieving the pressure on the lumbar intervertebral discs. *J Bone Joint Surg, 39B,* 718.

Basmajian, J.V. (1958). Electromyography of iliopsoas. *Anat Rec, 132,* 127.

Basmajian, J.V. & DeLuca, C.J. (1985). *Muscles Alive.* Baltimore: Williams & Wilkins.

Biering-Sorensen, F. (1984). Physical measurements as risk indicators for low-back trouble over a one-year period. *Spine, 9,* 106.

Callaghan, J.P., Patla, A.E., & McGill, S.M. (1999). Low back three-dimensional joint forces, kinematics, and kinetics during walking. *Clinical Biomechanics, 14,* 203.

Cappozzo, A. (1984). Compressive loads in the lumbar vertebral column during normal level walking. *J Orthop Res, 1,* 292.

Carlsöö, S. (1961). The static muscle load in different work positions: An electromyographic study. *Ergonomics, 4,* 193.

Chaffin, D.B. (1969). A computerized biomechanical model—Development of and use in studying gross body actions. *J Biomechanics, 2,* 429.

Chaffin, D.B. & Andersson, G.B.J. (1991). *Occupational Biomechanics* (2nd ed., pp. 171–263). New York: John Wiley & Sons, Inc.

Cheng, C.K., Chen, H.H., Chen, C.S., et al. (1998). Influences of walking speed change on the lumbosacral joint force distribution. *Biomed Mater Eng, 8,* 155.

Cholewicki, J., Juluru, K., & McGill, S.M. (1999a). Intra-abdominal pressure mechanism for stabilizing the lumbar spine. *J Biomech, 32,* 1–13.

Cholewicki, J., Juluru, K., Radebold, A., et al. (1999b). Lumbar spine stability can be augmented with an abdominal belt and/or increased intra-abdominal pressure. *European Spine Journal, 8,* 388.

Cholewicki, J., Panjabi, M.M., & Khachatryan, A. (1997). Stabilizing function of trunk flexor-extensor muscles around a neutral spine posture. *Spine, 22*(19), 2207.

Ciriello, V.M. & Snook, S.H. (1995). The effect of back belts on lumbar muscle fatigue. *Spine, 20,* 1271.

Cossette, J.W., Farfan, H.F., Robertson, G.H., et al. (1971). The instantaneous center of rotation of the third lumbar intervertebral joint. *J Biomech, 4*(149), 1971.

Creswell, A.G. (1993). Responses of intra-abdominal pressure and abdominal muscle activity during dynamic trunk loading in man. *Eur J Appl Physiol, 66,* 315.

Cresswell, A.G., Blake, P.L., & Thorstensson, A. (1994a). The effect of an abdominal muscle training program on intra-abdominal pressure. *Scand J Rehabil Med, 26,* 79.

Cresswell, A.G., Grundström, H., & Thorstensson, A. (1992). Observations on intra-abdominal pressure and patterns of abdominal intra-muscular activity in man. *Acta Physiol Scand, 144,* 409.

Cresswell, A.G., Oddsson, L., & Thorstensson, A. (1994b). The influence of sudden perturbations on trunk muscle activity and intra-abdominal pressure while standing. *Exper Brain Res, 98,* 336.

Cresswell, A.G., & Thorstensson, A. (1994). Changes in intra-abdominal pressure, trunk muscle activation and force during isokinetic lifting and lowering. *Eur J Appl Physiol, 68,* 315.

Dalstra, M. & Huiskes, R. (1995). Load transfer across the pelvic bone. *J Biomech, 28,* 715.

Davis, K.G., Marras, W.S., & Waters, T.R. (1998). Evaluation of spinal loading during lowering and lifting. *Clin Biomechanics, 13,* 141.

de Looze, M.P., Toussaint, H.M., van Dieen, J.H., et al. (1993). Joint moments and muscle activity in the lower extremities and lower back in lifting and lowering tasks. *J Biomech, 26,* 1067.

Eie, N. (1966). Load capacity of the low back. *J Oslo City Hosp, 16,* 73.

Ekholm, J., Arborelius, U., Fahlcrantz, A., et al. (1979). Activation of abdominal muscles during some physiotherapeutic exercises. *Scand J Rehabil Med, 11,* 75.

El-Bohy, A.A. & King, A.I. (1986). Intervertebral disc and facet contact pressure in axial torsion. In S.A. Lantz & A.I. King (Eds.), *1986 Advances in Bioengineering* (pp. 26–27). New York: American Society of Mechanical Engineers.

Farfan, H.F. (1975). Muscular mechanism of the lumbar spine and the position of power and efficiency. *Orthop Clin North Am, 6,* 135.

Flint, M.M. (1965). Abdominal muscle involvement during the performance of various forms of sit-up exercise. An electromyographic study. *Am J Phys Med, 44,* 224.

Floyd, W.F. & Silver, P.H.S. (1955). The function of the erectors spinae muscles in certain movements and postures in man. *J Physiol, 129,* 184.

Friedebold, G. (1958). Die AktiviUt normaler Rilckenstreckmuskulatur im Elektromyogramm unter verschiedenen Haltungsbedingungen; eine Studie zur Skelettmuskelmechanik. *Z Orthop, 90,* 1.

Fukuyama, S., Nakamura, T., Ikeda, T., et al. (1995). The effect of mechanical stress on hypertrophy of the lumbar ligamentum flavum. *J Spinal Disord, 8,* 126.

Galante, J.O. (1967). Tensile properties of the human lumbar annulus fibrosus. *Acta Orthop Scand Suppl, 100,* 1–91.

Gardner-Morse, M.G. & Stokes, I.A. (1998). The effects of abdominal muscle co-activation on lumbar spine stability. *Spine, 1*(23), 89.

Gertzbein, S.D., Seligmon, J., Holtby, R., et al. (1985). Centrode patterns and segmental instability in degenerative disc disease. *Spine, 10,* 257.

Granata, K.P. & Sanford, A.H. (1999). Lumbar-pelvic coordination is influenced by lifting task parameters. *Spine, 25*(11), 1413.

Gregersen, G.G. & Lucas, D.B. (1967). An in vivo study of the lumbar axial rotation of the human thoracolumbar spine. *J Bone Joint Surg, 49A,* 247–252.

Haher, T.R., O'Brien, M., Dryer, J.W., et al. (1994). The role of the lumbar facet joints in spinal stability. Identification of alternative paths of loading. *Spine, 19,* 26–67.

Harman, E.A., Frykman, P.N., Clagett, E.R., et al. (1988). Intra-abdominal and intra-thoracic pressures during lifting and jumping. *Med Sci Sports Exerc, 20,* 195.

Hasegawa, K., Takahashi, H.E., Koga, Y., et al. (1993). Mechanical properties of osteopenic vertebral bodies monitored by acoustic emission. *Bone, 14,* 737.

Haughton, V.M., Schmidt, T.A., Keele, K., et al. (2000). Flexibility of lumbar spinal motion segments correlated to type of tears in the annulus fibrosus. *J Neurosurg, 92,* 81.

Hodges, P.W., Cresswell, A., & Thortensson, A. (1999). Preparatory trunk motion accompanies rapid upper limb movement. *Exp Brain Res, 124,* 69.

Hodges, P.W. & Gandevia, S.C. (2000). Activation of the human diaphragm during a repetitive postural task. *J Physiol (Lond), 522,* 165.

Hodges P.W. & Richardson C.A. (1997). Feedforward contraction of transversus abdominis is not influenced by the direction of arm movement. *Exp Brain Res, 114,* 362.

Hutton, W.C. & Adams, M.A. (1982). Can the lumbar spine be crushed in heavy lifting? *Spine, 7,* 586.

Joseph, J. (1960). *Man's Posture: Electromyographic Studies.* Springfield: Charles C Thomas.

Juker, D., McGill, S., Kropf, P., et al. (1998). Quantitative intramuscular myoelectric activity of lumbar portions of psoas and the abdominal wall during a wide variety of tasks. *Med Sci Sports Exerc, 30,* 301.

King, A.I., Prasad, P., & Ewing, C.L. (1975). Mechanism of spinal injury due to caudocephalad acceleration. *Orthop Clin North Am, 6,* 19.

Klein, J.A., Hickey, D.S., & Huskins, D.W. (1983). Radial bulging of the annulus fibrosus and the function and failure of the intervertebral disc. *J Biomech, 16,* 211–217.

Krag, M.H., Seroussi, R.E., Wilder, D.G., et al. (1987). Internal displacement distribution from in vitro loading of human thoracic and lumbar spinal motion segments: Experimental results and theoretical predictions. *Spine, 12,* 1001–1007.

Krajcarski, S.R., Potvin, J.R., & Chiang, J. (1999). The in vivo response to the perturbations causing rapid flexion: Effects of pre-load and step input magnitude. *Clin Biomechanics, 14,* 54.

Kulak, R.F., Schultz, A.B., Belytschko, T., et al. (1975). Biomechanical characteristics of vertebral motion segments and intervertebral discs. *Orthop Clin North Am, 6,* 121.

Lander, J.E., Bates, B.T., & Devita, P.(1986). Biomechanics of the squat exercise using a modified center of mass bar. *Med Sci Sports Exerc, 18,* 469.

Lavender, S.A., Mirka, G.A., Schoenmarklin, R.W., et al. (1989). The effects of preview and task symmetry on trunk muscle response to sudden loading. *Human Factors, 31,* 101.

Lavender, S.A., Tsuang, Y.H., Andersson, G.B., et al. (1992). Trunk muscle co-contraction while resisting applied moments in a twisted posture. *Ergonomics, 36,* 1145.

Lee, Y.H. & Chen, C.Y. (1999). Lumbar vertebral angles and back muscle loading with belts. *Ind Health, 37,* 390.

Lucas, D.B. & Bresier, B. (1961). *Stability of the Ligamentous Spine.* Biomechanics Laboratory, University of California, San Francisco and Berkeley. Technical Report 40. San Francisco: The Laboratory.

Lumsden, R.M. & Morris, J.M. (1968). An in vivo study of axial rotation and immobilization at the lumbosacral joint. *J Bone Joint Surg, 50A,* 1591.

Marras, W.S. & Granata, K.P. (1995). A biomechanical assessment and model of axial twisting in the thoracolumbar spine. *Spine, 20,* 1440.

Marras, W.S. & Mirka, G.A. (1992). A comprehensive evaluation of trunk response to asymmetric trunk motion. *Spine, 17,* 318.

Marras, W.S., Rangarajulu, S.L., & Lavender, S.A. (1987). Trunk loading and expectation. *Ergonomics, 30,* 551.

McGill, S.M. & Norman, R.W. (1987). Reassessment of the role of intra-abdominal pressure in spinal compression. *Ergonomics, 30,* 1565.

McGill, S.M., Norman, R.W., & Sharratt, M.T. (1990). The effect of an abdominal belt on trunk muscle activity and intra-abdominal pressure during squat lifts. *Ergonomics, 33,* 147.

McGill, S.M., Yingling, V.R., & Peach, J.P. (1999). Three-dimensional kinematics and trunk muscle myoelectric activity in the elderly spine—a database compared to young people. *Clin Biomechanics, 14,* 389.

Miles, M. & Sullivan, W.E. (1961). Lateral bending at the lumbar and lumbosacral joints. *Anat Rec, 139,* 387.

Miller, J.A.A., Haderspeck, K.A., & Schultz, A.B. (1983). Posterior element loads in lumbar motion segments. *Spine, 8,* 331.

Moll, J.M.H. & Wright, V. (1971). Normal range of spinal mobility. An objective clinical study. *Ann Rheum Dis, 30,* 381.

Morris, J.M., Benner, G., & Lucas, D.B. (1962). An electromyographic study of the intrinsic muscles of the back in man. *J Anat Lond, 96,* 509–520.

Morris, J.M., Lucas, D.B., & Bresier, B. (1961). Role of the trunk in stability of the spine. *J Bone Joint Surg, 43A,* 327.

Mosekilde, L. (1993). Vertebral structure and strength in vivo and in vitro. *Calcif Tissue Int, 53,* S121.

Nachemson, A. (1960). Lumbar intradiscal pressure. *Acta Orthop Scand Suppl, 43,* 1–140.

Nachemson, A. (1963). The influence of spinal movements on the lumbar intradiscal pressure and on the tensile stresses in the annulus fibrosus. *Acta Orthop Scand, 33,* 183.

Nachemson, A. (1966). Electromyographic studies on the vertebral portion of the psoas muscle. With special reference to its stabilizing function of the lumbar spine. *Acta Orthop Scand, 37,* 177.

Nachemson, A. (1975). Towards a better understanding of back pain: A review of the mechanics of the lumbar disc. *Rheumatol Rehabil, 14,* 129.

Nachemson, A. & Elfström, G. (1970*). Intravital Dynamic Pressure Measurements in Lumbar Discs: A Study of Common Movements, Maneuvers and Exercises.* Stockholm: Almquist & Wiksell.

Nachemson, A.L. & Evans, J.H. (1968). Some mechanical properties of the third human lumbar interlaminar ligament (ligamentum flavum). *J Biomechanics, 1,* 211.

Nachemson, A. & Morris, J.M. (1964). In vivo measurements of intradiscal pressure. Discometry, a method for the determination of pressure in the lower lumbar discs. *J Bone Joint Surg, 46A,* 10/7.

National Institute for Occupational Safety and Health (1994). *Workplace Use of Back Belts.* DHHS (NIOSH), Number 94–122.

Nelson, J.M., Walmsley, R.P., & Stevenson, J.M. (1995). Relative lumbar and pelvic motion during loaded spinal flexion/extension. *Spine, 20,* 199.

Németh, G. (1984). On hip and lumbar biomechanics. A study of joint load and muscular activity. *Scand J Rehabil Med Suppl,* 10.

Norton, P.L. & Brown, T. (1957). The immobilizing efficiency of back braces. Their effect on the posture and motion of the lumbosacral spine. *J Bone Joint Surg, 39A,* 111.

Örtengren, R, Andersson, G.B.J., & Nachemson, A.L. (1981). Studies of relationships between lumbar disc pressure, myoelectric back muscle activity, and intra-abdominal (intragastric) pressure. *Spine, 6,* 98.

Osvalder, A.L., Neumann, P., Lovsund, P., et al. (1990). Ultimate strength of the lumbar spine in flexion—an in vitro study. *J Biomechanics, 23,* 453.

Panjabi, M.M., Goel, V.K., & Takata, K. (1982). Physiologic strains in the lumbar spinal ligaments. An in vitro biomechanical study. *Spine, 7,* 192.

Parnianpour, M., Nordin, M., Kahanovitz, N., et al. (1988). The triaxial coupling of torque generation of trunk muscles during isometric exertions and the effect of fatiguing isoinertial movements on the motor output and movement patterns. *Spine, 13*(9), 982–992.

Partridge, M.J. & Walters, C.E. (1959). Participation of the abdominal muscles in various movements of the trunk in man. An electromyographic study. *Phys Ther Rev, 39,* 791.

Pauly, J.E. (1966). An electromyographic analysis of certain movements and exercises. I. Some deep muscles of the back. *Anat Rec, 155*, 223.

Perkins, M.S. & Bloswick, D.S. (1995). The use of back belts to increase intraabdominal pressure as a means of preventing low back injuries: A survey of the literature. *Int J Occup Environ Health, 1*, 326.

Pope, M.H., Andersson, G.B.J., Broman, H., et al. (1986). Electromyographic studies of the lumbar trunk musculature during the development of axial torques. *J Orthop Res, 4*, 288–297.

Ranu, H.S. (1990). Measurement of pressures in the nucleus and within the annulus of the human spinal disc due to extreme loading. *Proc Inst Mech Eng (H), 204*, 141.

Reichmann, S. (1971). Motion of the lumbar articular processes in flexion-extension and lateral flexion of the spine. *Acta Morphol Neerl Scand 8*, 261.

Reichmann, S., Berglund, E., & Lundgren, K. (1972). Das Bewegungszentrum in der LendenwirbelsAule bei Flexion und Extension. *Z Anat Entwicklungsgesch, 138*, 283.

Reid, J.G. & Costigan, P.A. (1987). Trunk muscle balance and muscular force. *Spine, 12*, 783.

Reyna, J.R. Jr., Leggett, S.H., Kenney, K., et al. (1995). The effect of lumbar belts on isolated lumbar muscle. Strength and dynamic capacity. *Spine, 20*, 68.

Rolander, S.D. (1966). Motion of the lumbar spine with special reference to the stabilizing effect of posterior fusion. An experimental study on autopsy specimens. *Acta Orthop Scand, Suppl. 90*, 1–144.

Sato, K., Kikuchi, S., & Yonezawa, T. (1999). In vivo intradiscal pressure measurement in healthy individuals and in patients with ongoing back problems. *Spine, 24*, 2468.

Schultz, A., et al. (1982). Loads on the lumbar spine. Validation of a biomechanical analysis by measurements of intradiscal pressures and myoelectric signals. *J Bone Joint Surg, 64A*, 713.

Shirazi-Adl, A. (1994). Biomechanics of the lumbar spine in sagittal/lateral moments. *Spine, 19*, 2407.

Solomonow, M., Zhou, B.-H., Baratta, R.V., et al. (1999). Biomechanics of increased exposure to lumbar injury caused by cyclic loading: Part 1. Loss of reflexive muscular stabilization. *Spine, 24(23)*, 2426–2434.

Steffen, T., Baramki, H.G., Rubin, R., et al. (1998). Lumbar intradiscal pressure measured in the anterior and posterolateral annular regions during asymmetrical loading. *Clin Biomechanics, 13*, 495.

Sturesson, B., Selvik, G., & Uden, A. (1989). Movements of the sacroiliac joints. A roentgen stereophotogrammetric analysis. *Spine, 14*, 162.

Thomas, J.S., Lavender, S.A., Corcos, D.M., et al. (1999). Effect of lifting belts on trunk muscle activation during a suddenly applied load. *Human Factors, 41*, 670.

Tuong, N.H., Dansereau, J., Maurais, G., et al. (1998). Three-dimensional evaluation of lumbar orthosis effects on spinal behavior. *J Rehabil Res Dev, 35*, 34.

Urban, J.P.G. & McMullin, J.F. (1985). Swelling pressure of the intervertebral disc: Influence of proteoglycan and collagen contents. *Biorheology, 22*, 145.

van Dieën, J.H., Hoozemans, M.J.M., & Toussaint, H.M. (1999). Stoop or squat: A review of biomechanical studies on lifting technique. *Clin Biomechanics, 14*, 685.

Wang, M. & Dumas, G.A. (1998). Mechanical behavior of the female sacroiliac joint and influence of the anterior and posterior sacroiliac ligaments under sagittal loads. *Clin Biomechanics, 13*, 293.

White, A.A. (1969). Analysis of the mechanics of thoracic spine in man. An experimental study of autopsy specimens. *Acta Orthop Scand, Suppl 127*, 1–105.

White, A.A. & Panjabi, M.N. (1978). *Clinical Biomechanics of the Spine*. Philadelphia: J.B. Lippincott.

Wilke, H.J., Neef, P., Caimi, M., et al. (1999). New in vivo measurements of pressures in the intervertebral disc in daily life. *Spine, 24*, 755.

Wilder, D.G., Pope, M.H., & Frymoyer, J.W. (1980). The functional topography of the sacroiliac joint. *Spine, 5*, 575.

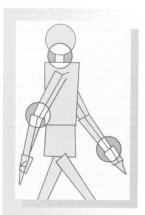

CHAPTER 11

Biomechanics of the Cervical Spine

Ronald Moskovich

Introduction

Knowledge of spinal biomechanics advanced exponentially during the second half of the twentieth century. A two-column model of the spine was described by Sir Frank Holdsworth (1963) and, later, a three-column model by Denis (1983), further refining the principle of spinal stability. The computer age has produced powerful methods for modern biomechanical modeling, the promise being the ability to assess the stability of a construct prior to implantation. Today, the application of cervical biomechanical knowledge spans many industries and supports improved medical diagnoses and treatment that is more effective. Future technological and electronic advances will continue to build on basic biomechanical principles, many of which will be outlined in this chapter.

Component Anatomy and Biomechanics

ANATOMY

The exquisite design of the cervical spine uniquely contributes to the structure of the human body and profoundly enhances its function. The cervical spine supports the skull and acts as a shock absorber for the brain. It also facilitates the transfer of weights and bending moments of the head. It protects the brainstem, spinal cord, and various neurovascular structures as they transit the neck and when they enter and exit the skull. The vertebral column also provides a multitude of muscle and ligamentous attachments for complex movement and stability. The neuromuscular control afforded by the muscle attachments combined with the numerous articulations of the cervical spine allows for a wide range of physiological motion that maximizes the range of motion of the head and neck and serves to integrate the head with the rest of the body and the environment.

The spine consists of 33 vertebrae divided into five regions: cervical (7) (Fig. 11-1), thoracic (12), lumbar (5), sacral (5 fused segments), and coccygeal (approximately 4). The two most cranial vertebrae, C1 (atlas) and C2 (axis), are atypical, with a unique structural role in the articulation between the head and the cervical spine. The atlanto-occipital joint, between C1 and the occipital bone of the skull, is also a functional part of the cervical spine. There

are five typical cervical vertebrae, C3–C7, which are similar in structure and function.

The spine has four curves when viewed in the sagittal plane. The cervical and lumbar regions are convex anteriorly (lordotic), while the thoracic and sacral regions are convex posteriorly (kyphotic). The lordotic curves develop after birth as the infant's spine straightens out, which facilitates development of a bipedal posture. Although there is a

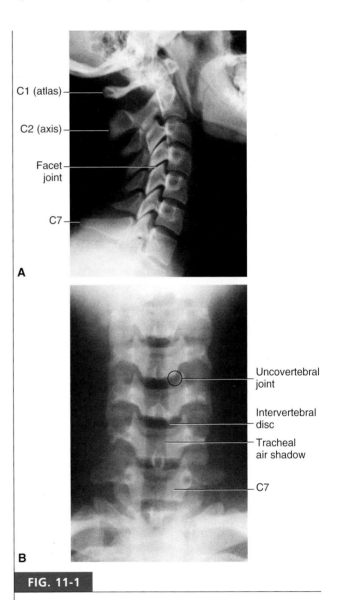

FIG. 11-1

A, Lateral roentgenogram of the cervical spine. Note the lordosis. The facet joints are aligned obliquely only to the frontal or coronal plane; hence, their excellent visualization in the lateral view. **B,** Anteroposterior view of the cervical spine.

harmonious progression of these curves from one to another, which may help distribute stresses and strains, injuries occur more commonly at the junctional areas because of differences in the relative stiffness of each anatomical segment of the spine. The physical structure of the anatomical elements modulates from the cervical to the sacral region in relation to the segmental function.

The lordosis in the cervical spine, like that in the lumbar spine, is maintained predominantly by slightly wedge-shaped intervertebral discs that are larger anteriorly than posteriorly. In contradistinction, thoracic kyphosis is maintained largely by the vertebral bodies themselves; because the posterior portion of the thoracic vertebral body is larger than the anterior portion, there is a relative kyphosis of the thoracic spine.

The conceptual biomechanical building block of the spinal column is the functional spinal unit or motion segment. It consists of two adjacent vertebrae and the intervening intervertebral discs and ligaments between the vertebrae. These ligaments are the anterior and posterior longitudinal ligaments; the intertransverse, interspinous, and supraspinous ligaments; and the facet capsular ligaments. As a result of the different functional demands of the various parts of the spinal column, segmental variation is expressed by changes in the size and shape of the vertebrae, the anatomy of the discoligamentous structures, and the alignment and structure of the facet joints.

Biological structures behave differently than do common engineering materials. Collagenous tissues exhibit both viscoelastic and anisotropic behavior. Viscoelastic properties are rate-dependent (time-dependent) behaviors under loading that are seen in both bone and soft tissues; mechanical strength increases with increased rates of loading. Anisotropy is the alteration in mechanical properties that is seen when bone is loaded along different axes. Anisotropic behavior occurs as a result of the dissimilar longitudinal and transverse microstructure.

Osseous Structures

The occiput–C1–C2 complex comprises the upper cervical spine and is responsible for approximately 40% of cervical flexion and 60% of cervical rotation. The occipital condyles articulate with the slightly concave lateral masses of the atlas. The primary motion permitted by this articulation is flexion and extension, accounting for a large portion of the

sagittal range of motion of the cervical spine. The C1–C2 articulation is the joint primarily responsible for rotation in the cervical spine.

The atlas, or C1, is a bony ring consisting of an anterior and posterior arch that is attached to the two lateral masses of the atlas (Fig. 11-2). The superior surfaces of the lateral masses, which face cranially and inward, form an articulation with the caudally and outward-facing occipital condyles of the skull (Fig. 11-3). Extension of the occipitocervical joint is limited by the bony anatomy; flexion is limited primarily by ligamentous structures, the tectorial membrane, and the longitudinal fibers of the cruciform ligament as well as by the posterior ligaments (Figs. 11-4 and 11-5). The anterior tubercle on the arch of C1 serves as an attachment for the longus colli muscle, a flexor of the neck. The posterior arch of the atlas is a modified lamina that is grooved on its superior surface for the passage of the vertebral arteries as they enter into the foramen magnum after piercing the posterior atlanto-occipital membrane.

Similar to the occipitocervical junction, there is no intervertebral disc between C1 and C2. Stability at this level is thus predicated on intact osseoligamentous structures. The articulation between C1 and C2 is primarily specialized for rotation. The body of C2 projects superiorly to form the odontoid process, or dens (Fig. 11-6). The projection of the body of C2 and the dens has a characteristic oblong appearance on lateral cervical radiographs and is

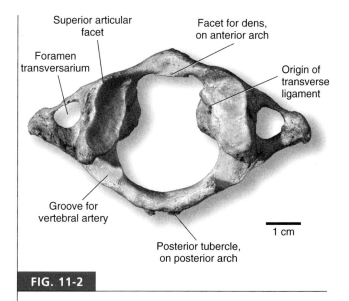

Superior articular facet

Facet for dens, on anterior arch

Foramen transversarium

Origin of transverse ligament

Groove for vertebral artery

Posterior tubercle, on posterior arch

1 cm

FIG. 11-2

Bony architecture of the atlas. Bar = 1 cm.

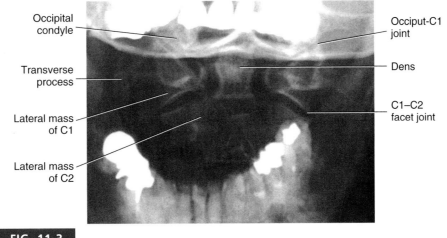

Occipital condyle

Transverse process

Lateral mass of C1

Lateral mass of C2

Occiput-C1 joint

Dens

C1–C2 facet joint

FIG. 11-3

The open-mouth radiograph demonstrates the occiput-C1 and the atlantoaxial articulations. Note the symmetric spacing between the lateral masses of C1 and the dens. Asymmetry or widening of these spaces may occur after rotatory disturbances or fractures of the C1 ring.

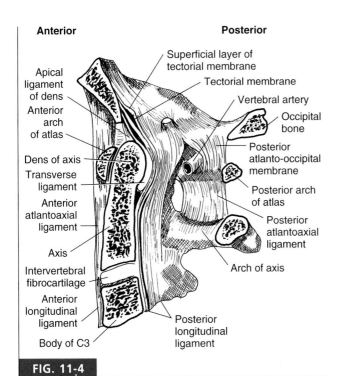

Anterior

Posterior

Superficial layer of tectorial membrane

Tectorial membrane

Vertebral artery

Occipital bone

Posterior atlanto-occipital membrane

Posterior arch of atlas

Posterior atlantoaxial ligament

Arch of axis

Apical ligament of dens

Anterior arch of atlas

Dens of axis

Transverse ligament

Anterior atlantoaxial ligament

Axis

Intervertebral fibrocartilage

Anterior longitudinal ligament

Body of C3

Posterior longitudinal ligament

FIG. 11-4

Median sagittal section through the occipital bone and the first three cervical vertebrae showing the articulations and surrounding ligaments.

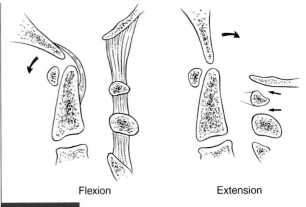

Flexion

Extension

FIG. 11-5

Tracings of lateral flexion and extension radiographs showing the occiput, C1, C2, and C3. The substantial relative motion between the occiput, C1, and C2 can be seen. *Large arrows* indicate the direction of motion. *Small arrows* indicate that approximation of the posterior elements limit occipitocervical extension. In contradistinction, maximum flexion is controlled by tautness of the ligaments. *Reprinted with permission from Moskovich, R. & Jones, D.A. (1999). Upper cervical spine instrumentation. Spine: State of the Art Reviews, 13(2), 233–253.*

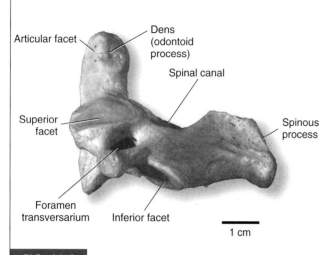

Articular facet

Dens (odontoid process)

Spinal canal

Superior facet

Spinous process

Foramen transversarium

Inferior facet

1 cm

FIG. 11-6

The axis vertebra, or C2. The superior facet articulation permits multiplanar motion while the inferior facet is aligned to articulate with a more typical cervical facet, which is more constrained. There is a smooth surface on the front of the dens for articulation with the anterior ring of C1. Bar = 1 cm.

often a helpful anatomical landmark. The dens articulates with and is restrained within a socket formed by the transverse ligament of C1 and the anterior arch of C1. The transverse ligaments run from the anterior arch of C1, behind the dens, and prevent anterior translation of C1 on C2. The other ligaments at the C1–C2 articulation are the alar, apical, and accessory alar ligaments. The alar ligaments, which are symmetrically placed on both sides of the dens, attach the dens to the occiput to prevent excessive rotation. The left alar ligament prevents right rotation and vice versa. To some extent, the alar ligaments also act to limit motion during side bending (Dvorak & Panjabi, 1987). The apical ligament also connects the dens to the occiput.

Unlike the two most cranial vertebrae, the anatomy of the third through the sixth cervical vertebrae is similar (Fig. 11-7). These four cervical vertebrae consist of a body, two pedicles, two lateral masses, two laminae, and a spinous process. The seventh cervical vertebra is slightly different in that it has a transitional form. It is called the vertebra prominens and has a larger spinous process that is not bifid like those of C3–C6.

The anterior components of a subaxial cervical motion segment are the vertebral bodies and the

disc. The cervical vertebral body is oval-shaped and is wider mediolaterally than anteroposteriorly. The transverse processes of the cervical spine are unique in that they all contain a transverse foramen for the passage of the vertebral artery. The transverse processes of the subaxial cervical vertebrae have two projections, the anterior and posterior tubercles, which serve as attachment points for anterior and posterior muscles, respectively. The large anterior tubercle of C6, referred to as the carotid tubercle, can be an important surgical landmark. The superior surface of the transverse process provides a groove for the exiting nerve root.

Each pedicle connects the vertebral body to a lateral mass, that portion of bone containing the superior and inferior facets. The facet joints regulate the movements of the spine and play a critical role in spinal stability. Those of the cervical spine are oriented at approximately 45° to the coronal plane and are located in the sagittal plane (Figs. 11-8 and 11-9). This orientation allows greater amounts of flexion than does lateral bending or rotation in the cervical spine. The facet joints resist most of the shear forces and approximately 16% of the compressive forces acting on the spine (Adams & Hutton, 1980). The laminae also arise from the lateral masses. The lateral masses have important surgical implications in the subaxial cervical spine because they contain a relatively large amount of bone and are easily accessible for the place-

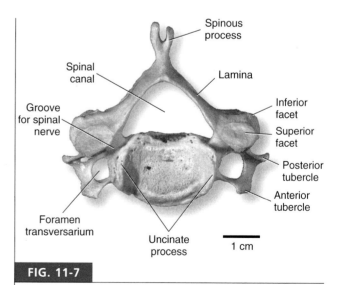

Spinous process

Spinal canal

Lamina

Groove for spinal nerve

Inferior facet

Superior facet

Posterior tubercle

Anterior tubercle

Foramen transversarium

Uncinate process

1 cm

FIG. 11-7

Superior view of a typical cervical vertebra, representative of C3–C6 (C7, the vertebra prominens, differs slightly in that it has a prominent nonbifid spinous process).

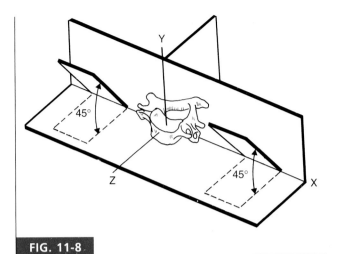

FIG. 11-8

Orientation of the facets of a typical cervical vertebra in three planes. The facets are oriented at a 45° angle to the transverse plane and the frontal plane, and are at right angles to the sagittal plane. Y indicates the craniocaudal axis, z the anteroposterior axis, and x the mediolateral axis. *Adapted with permission from White, A.A. III & Panjabi, M.M. (1990). Clinical Biomechanics of the Spine. Philadelphia: J.B. Lippincott.*

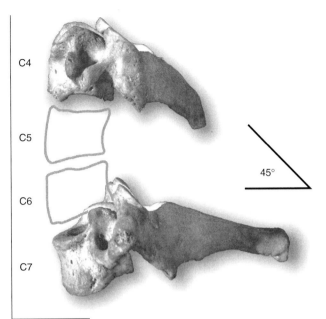

FIG. 11-9

Lateral photograph of a fourth and seventh cervical vertebra. The facet joint alignment is fairly close to 45° from the transverse plane. Note also the difference in size of the spinous processes, which are a reflection of the size and importance of the muscle attachments.

ment of screws, as opposed to the pedicles, which are difficult to cannulate safely in the neck.

The superior surfaces of the cervical vertebrae are saddle-shaped because of the uncinate processes, bony protuberances that arise from the lateral margins of the superior end plates (Fig. 11-10). The uncovertebral joints (joints of Luschka) develop during spinal maturation and play an important biomechanical role with respect to kinetics and stability.

Intervertebral Discs

The intervertebral discs are highly specialized structures that contribute up to one-third of the height of the vertebral column and form specialized joints between the cartilaginous end plates of the adjacent vertebral bodies. Activities such as running and jumping apply short-duration, high-amplitude loads to the intervertebral discs, whereas normal physical activity and upright stance result in the application of long-duration, low-magnitude loads to the disc. Discs are able to withstand greater than normal loads when compressive forces are rapidly applied based on the biomechanical principles of viscoelasticity. This property protects the disc from catastrophic failure until extremely high loads are applied.

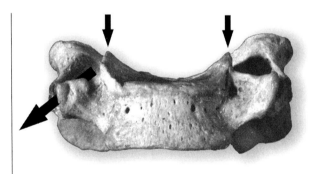

1 cm

FIG. 11-10

Anterior view of a sixth cervical vertebra. The *short arrows* indicate the uncinate processes and the *long arrow* indicates the pathway of the sixth cervical nerve root. The facet joints are located posteriorly. Bar = 1 cm.

The nucleus pulposus is centrally located within the disc and consists of almost 90% water in young individuals. The water content is highest at birth and decreases to approximately 70% as the disc degenerates with age. The rest of the nucleus pulposus consists of proteoglycan and collagen, which is exclusively type II collagen. Type II collagen fibrils are thought to be able to absorb compressive forces better than type I collagen fibrils.

Proteoglycans consist of a protein core attached to polysaccharide (glycosaminoglycan) chains. The polysaccharides are either keratin sulfate or chondroitin sulfate. The core protein, with its attached polysaccharides, is aggregated to hyaluronic acid through a link protein. The proteoglycans in the intervertebral discs are similar to those in articular cartilage, except that the proteoglycans present in the intervertebral discs have shorter polysaccharide chains as well as shorter core proteins. The nucleus pulposus contains more proteoglycan than does the annulus fibrosus. With increasing age and disc degeneration, the total proteoglycan content decreases.

The annulus fibrosus is the outer portion of the disc. Its water content is slightly less than that of the nucleus, being only approximately 78% water in younger individuals. With age, the water content falls to approximately 70%, like that of the nucleus pulposus in older persons. The annulus consists of collagen that is arranged in approximately 90 concentric lamellar bands. The collagen fibers in these sheets run at approximately 30° to the disc or 120° to each other in the adjacent bands. This unique orientation confers strength to the annulus while permitting some flexibility (Fig. 11-11). The composition of the collagen in the annulus is approximately 60% type II collagen and approximately 40% type I collagen. As the disc ages, the collagen undergoes irreducible cross-linking and the relative amount of type I collagen increases, replacing type II collagen in the disc.

MECHANICAL PROPERTIES

Vertebrae

The mechanical properties of the bone and soft tissues differ. Strength and stiffness and the relation of stress to strain are the key mechanical properties. Stress-strain curves are used to determine the relative loading behavior of bone. Stress is the load per unit area of a perpendicularly applied load. Strain is the change in length per unit of original length, usually expressed as a percentage.

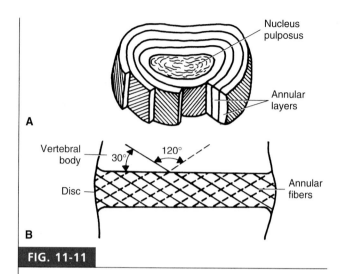

FIG. 11-11

Schematic drawings of an intervertebral disc showing the criss-cross arrangement of its fibers. **A,** Concentric layers of the annulus fibrosus are depicted as cut away to show the alternating orientation of the collagen fibers. **B,** The layers of the annular fibers are oriented at a 30° angle to the vertebral body and at 120° angles to each other. *Adapted with permission from White, A.A. III & Panjabi, M.M. (1990).* Clinical Biomechanics of the Spine. *Philadelphia: J.B. Lippincott.*

Cortical bone is stiffer than cancellous bone but can withstand greater stresses before failure. When the strain in vivo exceeds 2% of the original length, cortical bone fractures, but cancellous bone can withstand somewhat greater strains before fracturing. The greater ability to withstand strain is because of the structure of cancellous bone: its porosity varies from 30 to 90% compared with cortical bone with values of 5 to 30% (Carter & Hayes, 1977). Vertebral compression strength increases from the upper cervical to the lower lumbar levels.

Bone strength decreases with age as a result of the development of osteoporosis. The mineral content of vertebrae decreases with increasing age at a relatively constant rate (Hansson & Roos, 1986; Hansson et al., 1980). A 25% decrease in osseous tissue results in a more than a 50% decrease in the strength of the vertebrae (Bell, 1967). Because the cortical shell of a vertebra is responsible for only approximately 10% of its strength during compression, good quality cancellous bone is critically important (McBroom et al., 1985).

When bone is loaded in vivo, contraction of the muscles attached to the bone can alter the stress distribution in the bone. Bending moments are applied to the vertebral bodies during motions. During flexion, tensile stresses are applied to the posterior cortex and compression to the anterior cortex of the vertebral body. To perform lifting tasks, the back muscles are required to develop considerable forces (Schultz et al., 1982). Stresses in a typical cervical vertebra change from tensile to compressive in a region approximately 0.5 to 1 cm anterior to the posterior longitudinal ligament (Pintar et al., 1995). As bone is weaker and fails earlier in tension than in compression, posterior paraspinal muscle contraction can decrease the tensile stress on bone by producing a compressive stress that reduces or neutralizes the posterior cortical tensile stresses, allowing the vertebrae to sustain higher loads than would otherwise be possible. However, bone will often fail prior to damage occurring to the intervertebral disc under compressive loading. Finite element modeling of the cervical spine indicates that the increase in end plate stresses may be the initiating factor for failure of this component under compressive loads (Yoganandan et al., 1996a).

Intervertebral Discs

Intervertebral discs exhibit viscoelastic properties (creep and relaxation) and hysteresis (Kazarian, 1975). Creep occurs more slowly in healthy discs than in degenerated or herniated discs, suggesting that degenerated discs are less viscoelastic in nature (Kazarian, 1972).

Ligaments

Clinical stability of the spine depends primarily on the soft tissue components, especially in the cervical spine. The spinal ligaments are functional mainly in distraction along the line of their fibers. Ligament strength and limited extensibility help maintain stability, especially around the craniocervical junction. The alar ligaments have an in vitro strength of 200 N, and the transverse ligaments have an in vitro strength of 350 N (Dvorak et al., 1988a). The strength of the ligaments is related to both the anatomical demands and the flexibility required, which is a classic example of form following function.

The ligaments all have high collagen content except for the ligamentum flavum, which is exceptional in having a large percentage of elastin. The ligamentum flavum is under tension even when the spine is in a neutral position or somewhat extended, and thus pre-stresses the disc to some degree and provides some intrinsic support to the spine (Nachemson & Evans, 1968; Rolander, 1966). The elastic properties also assist in limiting the inward buckling of these ligaments during extension, which could potentially compress the neural elements.

Muscle

Muscular strength and control is imperative to maintain head and neck balance. In the cervical spine, muscle strength also has a role in reducing stresses on bones. Bending moments are applied to the vertebral bodies during various motions. During flexion, tensile stresses are applied to the posterior cortex and compression to the anterior cortex of the vertebral body. Substantial loads on the cervical spine have been calculated during neck flexion, particularly in the lower cervical motion segments.

Harms-Ringdahl (1986) calculated the bending moments generated around the axes of motion of the atlanto-occipital joint and the C7–T1 motion segment in seven subjects with the neck in five positions: full flexion, slight flexion, neutral, head upright with the chin tucked in, and full extension. The load on the junction between the occipital bone and C1 was lowest during extreme extension (ranging from an extension moment of 0.4 Nm to a flexion moment of 0.3 Nm). It was highest during extreme flexion (0.9 to 1.8 Nm), but this was only a slight increase over that produced when the neck was in the neutral position. The load on the C7–T1 motion segment was low with the neck in the neutral position but became even lower when the head was held upright with the chin tucked in (ranging from an extension moment of 0.8 Nm to a flexion moment of 0.9 Nm). The load increased somewhat during extreme extension (ranging from 1.1 to 2.4 Nm) and substantially during slight flexion (reaching 3.0 to 6.2 Nm). The greatest loads were produced during extreme extension, with moments ranging from 3.7 to 6.5 Nm.

In the same study, surface electrode electromyography was used to record activity over the erector spinae muscles of the cervical spine with the neck in the same five positions described above. Interestingly, the values obtained showed very low levels of muscle activity for all positions, even during extreme flexion in which the flexion moment on the C7–T1 motion segment increased more than threefold over the neutral position. The fact that the electromyographic levels over the neck extensors were low in this and other studies (Fountain et al., 1966; Takebe et al., 1974) suggests that the flexing moment is balanced by passive connective tissue structures, such as the joint capsules and ligaments. This phenomenon is seen in many other joints in which passive support is provided by the ligaments.

The values for the moments computed by Harms-Ringdahl (1986), however, are approximately 10% of the maximal values measured by Moroney and Schultz (1985) in 14 male subjects who resisted maximal and submaximal loads against the head while in an upright sitting position. The mean maximal voluntary moments were 10 Nm during axial rotation of the cervical spine, 12 to 14 Nm during flexion and lateral bending, and 30 Nm during extension. Calculation of the maximum (compressive) reaction forces on the C4–C5 motion segment ranged from 500 to 700 N during flexion, rotation, and lateral bending, and rose to 1,100 N during extension. Anteroposterior and lateral shear forces reached 260 N and 110 N, respectively. Calculated moments and forces generally correlated well with mean-measured myoelectric activities at eight sites around the perimeter of the neck at the C4 level.

Muscles play a critical role in basic postural homeostasis, as can be observed in both historical and present-day clinical settings. In unique observational studies in the 1950s of severely affected poliomyelitis patients, improvements in respiratory assistance for those with respiratory paralysis led to higher survival rates and a large number of patients who sustained complete paralysis of the cervical musculature. Patients with completely flail cervical spines were unable to support their heads unless adequate support was provided and actually remained in bed despite the good function of their extremities (Perry & Nickel, 1959). Similarly, severe cervical kyphosis occasionally is seen in elderly patients who do not have an obvious structural etiology when investigated radiologically. Some of these patients were found to have marked cervical extensor muscle weakness that has been attributed to senile cervical myopathy (Simmons & Bradley, 1988) (Fig. 11-12).

Neural Elements

Biomechanics of the neural elements have not been as well studied as the biomechanics of the osteoligamentous vertebral column, but our knowl-

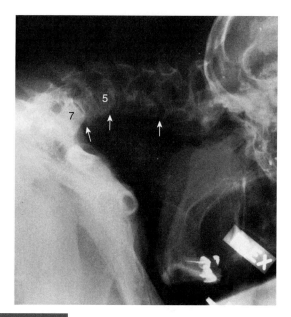

FIG. 11-12

Lateral cervical radiograph of a 68-year-old woman who presented with severe torticollis. She denied any history of injury and did not have evidence of a structural vertebral abnormality, infection, tumor, or inflammatory disease. Pseudosubluxations (arrows) are evident subaxially as a consequence of the marked kyphosis. Her neck was twisted only because she had a severe cervical flexion deformity, and she was unable to see forward except by turning her head to one side. She was neurologically intact. It was possible to extend her neck to a relatively neutral position using gentle traction. Following posterior fusion from C2 to C7, she returned to a normal independent life. Muscle biopsy was consistent with senile myopathy. *Reprinted with permission from Moskovich, R. (1997). Cervical instability (rheumatoid, dwarfism, degenerative, others). In K.H. Bridwell & R.L. DeWald (Eds.),* The Textbook of Spinal Surgery *(pp. 969–1009). Philadelphia: Lippincott-Raven Publishers.*

edge base is growing. To date, certain basic parameters have been established. The cervical spine undergoes significant changes in length during flexion and extension (Breig et al., 1966; Reill, 1960). Thus, while there is some longitudinal elasticity to the spinal cord, it tolerates axial translation poorly. It is the translatory forces that typically result in neurological injury. A compressive tolerance between 2.75 and 3.44 kN is estimated for the adult cervical spine before significant neurological injury occurs (Myers & Winkelstein, 1995).

Spinal cord injuries can also result from extreme or sudden flexion-extension movements, especially in the face of a shallow spinal canal. Head flexion alone has been shown to result in significant increases in the intramedullary spinal cord pressure in dogs (Kitahara et al., 1995). Neurological injuries may result from anteroposterior compression of the spinal cord and are more common if the spinal canal is stenotic. Flexion motions can result in injuries when the spinal cord makes contact with cervical osteophytes, and extension motions may result in a pincer-like compression of the cord between (anterior) osteophytes and (posterior) invaginated ligamentum flavum. Anterior or central spinal cord injuries may ensue.

Although a diagnosis of spinal stenosis may be made based on the absolute size of the spinal canal, imaging of the neuraxis itself may be of greater value. Contrast-enhanced computerized tomography, myelography, and magnetic resonance imaging can demonstrate actual impingement or distortion of the spinal cord. Studies performed in flexion and extension may enhance the value of the information by demonstrating the contribution of any dynamic soft tissue component to the impingement. The exact size of the bony cervical spinal canal and the vertebral body was measured in 368 cadaveric adult male vertebrae (Moskovich et al., 1996). This study used well-validated parametric statistical methods to determine that the mean sagittal diameter of the spinal canal for C3–C7 was close to 14 mm (14.07 ± 1.63 mm; N = 272) (Figs. 11-13 and 11-14). The mean ratio of the sagittal canal diameter to the vertebral body diameter (canal to body [c-b] ratio) was 86.68 ± 13.70. Thirty-one percent of subaxial vertebrae would be diagnosed as having spinal stenosis if a c-b ratio of less than 80% was considered abnormal. Another study also found a high false-positive error rate for the c-b ratio, with 49% of 80 asymptomatic football players having a c-b ratio of less than 80% at one or more cervical levels (Herzog et al., 1991). Yet another group evaluated the reliability of the c-b ratio using plain lateral radiographs and CT scans (Blackley et al., 1999). Results confirmed that a poor correlation exists between the true diameter of the canal and the ratio of its sagittal diameter to that of the vertebral body. The variability in anatomical morphology means that the use of ratios from anatomical measurements within the cervical spine is not reliable in determining the true diameter of the cervical canal.

Spinal cord injury without radiographic abnormalities (SCIWORA) have also been described,

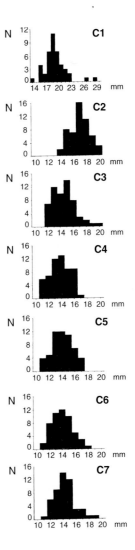

FIG. 11-13

Histograms of the C1–C7 sagittal canal diameters. Apart from the C1 plot, the same scale is used on all of the horizontal axes so that the distributions of the diameters can be compared. *Reprinted with permission from Moskovich, R., et al. (1996). Does the cervical canal to body ratio predict spinal stenosis? Bull Hosp Joint Dis, 55, 61–71.*

especially in children (Dickman et al., 1991; Osenbach & Menezes, 1989; Pang & Pollack, 1989). The etiology of such injuries is unknown, but one mechanism may be longitudinal traction. The unusually elastic biomechanics of the pediatric bony spine allows deformation of the musculoskeletal structures beyond physiological extremes, permitting direct cord trauma followed by spontaneous reduction of the bony spine (Kriss & Kriss, 1996). The isolated spinal cord resists tension poorly; axial tensile

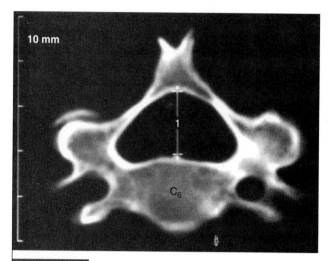

FIG. 11-14

Axial computerized tomographic scan of a sixth cervical vertebra, which was not part of the study detailed in the text. The anteroposterior diameter of the spinal canal measured 13.96 mm in this specimen.

forces to failure for three adult spinal cord specimens are reported to be 278 N ± 90 (Yoganandan et al., 1996b). Lower forces may result in direct neural injury or vascular disruption.

Kinematics

Kinematics is the study of motion of rigid bodies without taking into consideration other relevant forces. Kinematics of the spine describes the physiological and pathological motions that occur in the various spinal units. The traditional unit of study in kinematics is the motion segment, or the functional spinal unit. As described earlier, each motion segment consists of two adjacent vertebrae and their intervening soft tissues (Fig. 11-15).

Basic biomechanical testing involves the application of forces to a vertebral body and the subsequent measurement of the movements that occur (Fig. 11-16). Movements can be either rotational or translational. A degree of freedom is defined as a motion in which a rigid body can either translate back and forth along a straight line or rotate around a particular axis. Thus, each vertebral body may either translate or rotate in each of three orthogonal planes, for a total of six degrees of freedom (Panjabi et al., 1981) (Fig. 11-17). When either

rotation or translation of a body along one axis is consistently associated with a simultaneous rotation or translation along another axis, the motions are coupled. Coupled motions are normally expressed as displacements in the X, Y, or Z directions and rotations about the three orthogonal axes. Further analysis involving whole spines is more complex, and while it has yielded interesting results, motion segment analysis remains important for basic understanding.

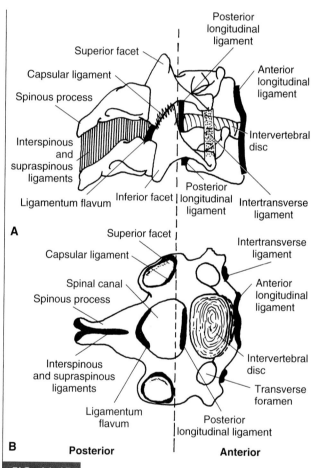

FIG. 11-15

Schematic representations of a cervical motion segment composed of two typical cervical vertebrae (C4 and C5), the intervertebral disc, and surrounding ligaments. The *broken line* divides the motion segment into anterior and posterior components. **A,** Lateral view. **B,** Superior view. *Adapted with permission from White, A.A. III, Johnson, R.M., Panjabi, M.M., et al. (1975). Biomechanical analysis of clinical stability in the cervical spine. Clin Orthop, 109, 85–96.*

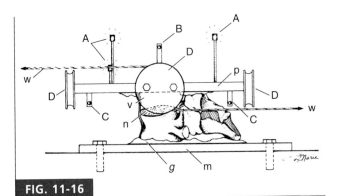

FIG. 11-16

Diagram of a test rig to evaluate a functional spinal unit using videophotogrammetry. This technique facilitates accurate measurements of motion without the measurements themselves having an effect on the displacements of the mobile vertebra. **A,** Light-emitting diodes (LEDs); **B** and **C,** Guide bars for application of tensile and compressive forces. **D,** Pulley for application of torques. Weights are attached to guide wires (w), which go around pulleys to produce torque on the upper vertebral body (v). n, intervertebral disc; g, acrylic cement that attaches lower aluminum plate (m) to test rig, which is rigidly bolted to the support frame. The upper plate (p) and upper vertebral body (v) are the moveable elements to which the loads and torques are applied. LEDs are rigidly attached to the upper plate and their movement is recorded by two video cameras. *Reprinted with permission from Raynor, R., Moskovich, R., Zidel, P., et al. (1987). Alteration in primary and coupled neck motions after facetectomy. Neurosurgery, 21(5), 681–687.*

RANGE OF MOTION

Measurements of cervical range of motion are based on radiographic studies or postmortem investigations. Inclinometers and various optoelectronic and electromagnetic devices used clinically for noninvasive evaluation of cervical spine motion are not as accurate; in particular, coupled motion is poorly quantified (Roozmon et al., 1993). The established range of active axial rotation to one side at C1–C2 is 27 to 49° (mean = 39°); passive rotation is 29 to 46° (mean = 41°) (Dvorak et al., 1987; Dvorak et al., 1988b; Penning & Wilmink, 1987). These measurements account for approximately 50% of the total cervical rotation.

Another stereoradiographic study of neck motion in adult men found a mean of 105° axial rotation between the occiput and the C7 vertebra. Seventy percent of the total axial rotation occurred between the occiput and the C2 vertebra. Each motion segment between the C2 and C7 vertebrae averaged from 4 to 8° rotation (Mimura et al., 1989). Less well appreci-

ated is the fact that a considerable amount of flexion and extension occurs at the C1–C2 articulation; 5 to 20° of flexion and extension occur with means of 12° (active) to 15° (passive) (Dvorak et al., 1988b).

Approximately 90° of axial rotation takes place in the subaxial cervical spine (C3–C7), about 45° to each side of neutral. Even greater lateral flexion is possible: approximately 49° to each side of neutral, giving a total of about 98°. The range of flexion and extension is approximately 64°: about 24° of extension and 40° of flexion. The motion in each plane is fairly evenly distributed throughout the motion segments (Lysell, 1969). The mean total range of anteroposterior translation in subaxial spinal motion segments is 3.5 ± 0.3 mm divided unequally: 1.9 mm for anterior shear and 1.6 mm for posterior shear. Lateral shear loading results in a mean total range of lateral motion of 3.0 mm ± 0.3 mm, divided equally between right and left; tension results in 1.1 mm of distraction and compression, 0.7 mm of loss of vertical height (Panjabi et al., 1986).

The great flexibility of the cervical spine allows the head to be positioned in a wide variety of ways,

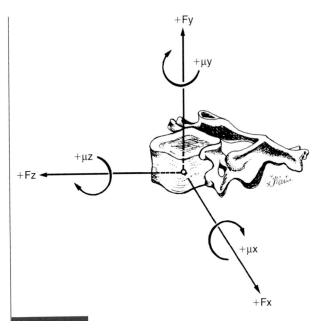

FIG. 11-17

A vertebral body showing the three primary Cartesian axes, x, y, and z. Along each axis a positive force, +F, is denoted by the direction of the *arrow.* The *curved arrows* indicate the direction of a positive torque, +μ. *Reprinted with permission from Raynor, R., Moskovich, R., Zidel, P., et al. (1987). Alteration in primary and coupled neck motions after facetectomy. Neurosurgery, 21(5), 681–687.*

permitting one, with equal ease, to gaze at an airplane overhead, glance over one's shoulder, or look for an object under a table. An analysis of the combined motion of the cervical spine using an electrogoniometer produced a remarkably large range of motion (Feipel et al., 1999): 122° ± 18° of flexion and extension, 144° ± 20° of axial rotation, and 88° ± 16° of lateral flexion. All primary motions were reduced with age. Sex had no influence on cervical motion range.

The active range of cervical spine motion required to perform daily functional tasks was studied in healthy adults (Bennett et al., 2000). A cervical spine range of motion device was fastened to the subject's head with a Velcro strap and a magnet was placed on the patient's shoulders to calibrate the instrument for measurement of cervical rotation and motion. Of the 13 daily functional tasks performed, tying shoes (flexion-extension 66.7°), backing up a car (rotation 67.6°), washing hair in the shower (flexion-extension 42.9°), and crossing the street (rotation head left 31.7° and rotation head right 54.3°) required the greatest active range of motion of the cervical spine. Of interest, several tasks were not found to produce the degrees of motion expected, and these included reading a newspaper (19.9° flexion-extension), writing at a table (26.2° flexion-extension), and reaching for objects overhead (4.3° flexion-extension). Side-bending was not found to be a significant movement in completion of the tasks but was coupled with rotation in one of the tasks (looking left and right to cross a street).

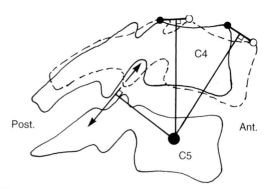

FIG. 11-18

Analysis of surface motion of the facet joints of the C4–C5 motion segment during flexion-extension. The schematic drawing represents superimposed roentgenograms of the motion segment in the neutral position and in slight flexion. The upper vertebra (C4) is considered to be the moving body and the subjacent vertebra (C5) is the base vertebra. Two points have been identified and marked on the moving body in the neutral position (*solid outline* of C4), and the same two points have been marked on the second roentgenogram with the motion segment slightly flexed (*dashed outline* of C4). Lines connecting the two sets of points have been drawn and their perpendicular bisectors have been added. The intersection of the perpendicular bisectors identifies the instant center of motion (*large solid dot*) for the degree of flexion under study. The perpendicular bisector (*arrowed line*) of a line drawn from the center of motion to the contact point of the facet joint surfaces indicates tangential motion, or gliding.

SURFACE JOINT MOTION

The motion between the joint surfaces of two adjacent vertebrae may be analyzed by means of the instant center technique of Reuleaux, described in Chapter 6. The method may be used to analyze surface motion of the cervical spine during flexion-extension and lateral flexion.

In a normal cervical spine, the instant center of flexion-extension is located in the anterior part of the lower vertebra in each motion segment. Instant center analysis indicates that tangential motion (gliding) takes place between the facet joints as the cervical spine is flexed and extended (Fig. 11-18). A consequence of these motions is that the size of the intervertebral foramina increases with flexion and decreases with extension (Fielding, 1957). These alterations have been quantified in a cadaver study that found there were statistically significant reductions of 10 and 13% in foraminal diameter, at 20 and

30° of extension, respectively. Conversely, in flexion there were statistically significant increases of 8 and 10% at 20 and 30° of flexion, respectively (Yoo et al., 1992). One practical application of this data relates to cervical collars used for the relief of neck pain. Conventional foam collars tend to place patients in slight extension, which may aggravate the symptoms. Turning a foam collar around, with the Velcro and narrow part anterior, puts the neck in slight flexion, which may increase the size of the intervertebral foramina and thereby relieve some of the pressure on an inflamed nerve root.

The instant center of motion of the cervical spine may be displaced as a result of pathological processes such as disc degeneration or ligament impairment. In such cases, instant center analysis may reveal distraction and jamming (compression) of the facet joint surfaces during flexion-extension instead of gliding (Fig. 11-19).

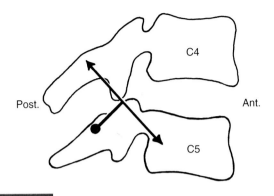

FIG. 11-19

Schematic drawing representative of a roentgenogram of the C4–C5 motion segment of a patient injured in a rear-end auto collision. The instant center of flexion-extension at this level (represented by the *large solid dot*) has been displaced from the anterior to the posterior part of C5 as a result of the injury process, which impaired the ligaments (compare with Fig. 11-18). The analysis of surface motion shows compression and distraction of the facet joints with flexion and extension.

COUPLED MOTION OF THE CERVICAL SPINE

Atlantoaxial Segment

The coupling characteristics of the atlantoaxial spinal motion segments are particularly important, as this area of the neck is extremely mobile. The dens is constrained within the osteoligamentous ring of the atlas, causing the C1–C2 lateral masses to articulate similarly to the condyles of the knee, with some sliding and rolling during flexion and extension. The instant centers of both rotation and flexion-extension lie in the center of the dens itself. Rotation at C1–C2 is coupled with both vertical translation along the Y axis (Fig. 11-20) and a degree of anteroposterior displacement (Werne, 1957). This implies that the C1–C2 joint is most stable in the neutral position, and, if rotated, attempts should be made to return it to the reduced position when performing an arthrodesis.

Subaxial Spine

The coupling patterns in the lower cervical spine are such that in lateral bending to the left, the spinous processes move to the right, and in lateral bending to the right, they move to the left (Lysell, 1969; Moroney et al., 1988) (Figs. 11-21 and 11-22). At C2,

there are 2° of coupled axial rotation for every 3° of lateral bending, which gives a ratio of 2:3 or 0.67. At C7, there is 1° of coupled axial rotation for every 7.5° of lateral bending, which gives a ratio of 2:15 or 0.13 (White & Panjabi, 1990). Results of finite element modeling indicate that the facet joints and uncovertebral joints are the major contributors to coupled motion in the lower cervical spine and that the uncinate processes effectively reduce motion coupling and primary cervical motion (in the same direction as load application), especially in response to axial rotation and lateral bending loads. Uncovertebral joints appear to increase primary cervical motion, showing an effect on cervical motion opposite to that of the uncinate processes (Clausen et al., 1997). Coupling of flexion-extension with transverse translation may be visualized roentgenographically (Fig. 11-23). During flexion, the vertebral body normally shifts forward; the facets glide up and over one another with pseudosubluxation. Changes in normal coupling patterns occur following pathological changes or surgical intervention.

Tensile load application to the cervical spine occurs in therapeutic traction, but more commonly so during trauma. Deployment of passive

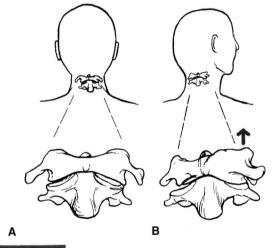

FIG. 11-20

Coupling of rotation and axial translation is depicted schematically. **A,** C1 and C2 are in the neutral position. **B,** C1 rises fractionally on C2 (*arrow*) as the head is rotated away from the midline. *Adapted with permission from Fielding, J.W. (1957). Cineroentgenography of the normal cervical spine.* J Bone Joint Surg, 39A, 1280–1288.

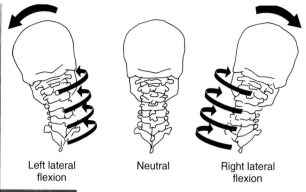

Left lateral flexion   Neutral   Right lateral flexion

FIG. 11-21

Coupled motion during lateral bending is depicted schematically. When the head and neck are flexed to the left, the spinous processes shift to the right, indicating rotation. The converse is also illustrated. *Adapted with permission from White, A.A. III & Panjabi, M.M. (1990).* Clinical Biomechanics of the Spine. *Philadelphia: J.B. Lippincott.*

vehicular restraint systems, such as airbags, may induce tensile forces in the neck. Isolated intervertebral discs fail at 569 N ± 54, and intact human cadaver cervical spines fail at 3373 N ± 464 (Yoganandan et al., 1996b). Active muscular contraction, however, is likely to raise these figures considerably.

Abnormal Kinematics

Abnormal kinematics generally refers to excessive motion within functional spinal units; however, abnormal kinematics may also refer to atypical patterns of motion such as abnormal coupling or paradoxical motion. Paradoxical motion is seen when the overall pattern of motion of one aspect of the spine is in one direction while the local pattern is the opposite. For instance, paradoxical flexion is seen when flexion occurs at a single functional spinal unit, although the spine as a whole is extended.

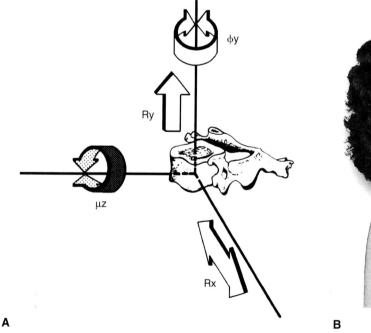

A

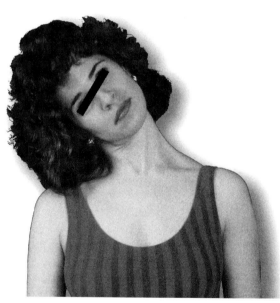

B

FIG. 11-22

A, This diagram illustrates some of the other coupled motions, which occur in response to a torque (μz) about the Z-axis (lateral bending). Lateral translation (Rx) and vertical motion (Ry) occur, as well as horizontal rotation (ϕy), which results in motion of the spinous processes to the right or the left. **B,** The subject is bending to her right, demonstrating the large range of normal cervical motion possible (approximately 50°).

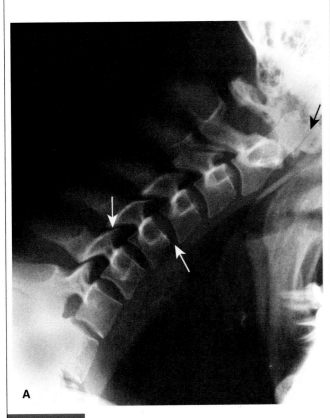

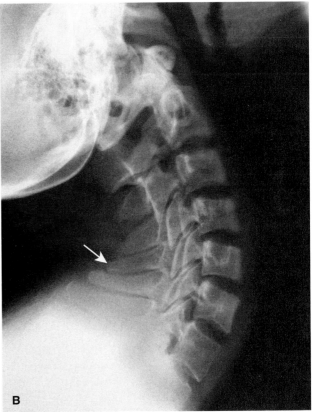

A

B

FIG. 11-23

Coupling of flexion-extension with transverse translation of the cervical spine is visible roentgenographically. **A,** During flexion the vertebral body shifts forward (small white arrow); the facets glide up and over one another with moderate subluxation at full flexion (large white arrow). Up to 2.5 mm of transverse translation may normally occur at the

C1–C2 articulation during flexion-extension; no translation is evident in this example (black arrow). **B,** During extension the reverse occurs, and the spinous processes limit motion as they touch at full extension (arrow). The size of the intervertebral foramina increases with flexion and decreases with extension.

These types of abnormal motions describe a pattern of movement known as instability.

Spinal Stability

The concept of spinal stability is an intriguing and sometimes confusing notion. Medical practitioners are frequently asked to look at a series of radiographs and make a determination whether the spine is stable. Exactly what is stability, how is it determined, and what happens if it is not present? The term spinal stability has acquired different meanings, depending on the setting in which it has been used. White and Panjabi describe the term clinically as the loss of the ability of the spine under physio-

logical loads to maintain its pattern of displacement so that there is no initial or additional neurological deficit, no major deformity, and no incapacitating pain (1990). Using this definition, physiological loads are those incurred during normal activity, and pain is not felt to be incapacitating if it can be controlled by non-narcotic drugs.

Stability is determined by many factors. There are different anatomical considerations in different regions of the spine. Certainly, ligamentous anatomy plays a large part in the stability of the spine, but the muscular and bony elements of the spine also play important roles.

Instability can be analyzed by considering kinematic instability and structural or component instability.

Kinematic instability focuses on either the quantity of motion (too much or too little) or the quality of motion present (alterations in the normal pattern), or both. Component instability addresses the clinical biomechanical role of the various anatomical components of the functional spinal unit. In this type of instability, loss or alteration of various anatomical portions determines the presence of instability (Box 11-1).

Sir Frank Holdsworth's account of a simple two-column concept of spinal stability provided a constructive basis for describing and analyzing the basic biomechanics of the spine:

> The synarthroses between the vertebral bodies rely for their stability upon the immensely strong annulus fibrosus. The diarthrodial apophyseal joints are stabilised by the capsule, by the interspinous and supraspinous ligaments and the ligamenta flava. This group of ligaments I call the 'posterior ligament complex.' It is upon this complex that the stability of the spine largely depends (Holdsworth, 1963).

Subsequently, Denis (1983) described a classification system for thoracolumbar fractures that can also be applied to a biomechanical analysis of spinal stability. In this description, the spinal elements are divided into three regions that form three spinal columns:

1. The anterior column consists of the anterior longitudinal ligament, the anterior annulus fibrosus, and the anterior half of the vertebral body.
2. The middle column consists of the posterior longitudinal ligament, the posterior half of the vertebral body, and the posterior annulus fibrosus.
3. The posterior column consists of the pedicles, facet joints, lamina, spinous processes, as well as the interspinous and supraspinous ligaments.
4. The anterior and middle columns form the primary weight-bearing column of the spine, with the posterior column providing the guiding and stabilizing elements.

Occipitoatlantoaxial Complex

The transverse ligament of the atlas completes the socket into which the dens is inserted. The ligament allows the dens to rotate, but limits its anterior translation. The ligament is inelastic and will not permit more than 2 to 3 mm of anterior subluxation of the first on the second vertebra (Field-

| BOX 11-1 | Conceptual Types of Instability |

Kinematic Instability
  Motion increased
  Instantaneous axes of rotation altered
  Coupling characteristics changed
  Paradoxical motion present
Component Instability
  Trauma
  Tumor
  Surgery
  Degenerative changes
  Developmental changes
Combined Instability
  Kinematic
  Component

ing et al., 1974). Anterior displacement of C1 on C2 of 3 to 5 mm is usually indicative of a rupture of the transverse ligament, while displacements of 5 to 10 mm suggest accessory ligament damage; displacement greater than 10 mm occurs with rupture of all the ligaments (Fielding et al., 1976). Anterior translations or displacements of C1 on C2 are assessed radiographically by measuring the distance from the anterior ring of the atlas to the back of the dens (atlantodental interval or ADI) (Fig. 11-24) (Case Study 11-1). Posterior subluxation of the atlas can only occur if the dens is fractured or if there is an os-odontoideum or hypoplastic dens.

Some diseases can weaken or destroy the transverse ligament. Most notably, synovitis in rheumatoid arthritis can create a pannus, which helps to destroy the atlantoaxial articulation as well as the transverse ligament (Figs. 11-25 and 11-26). Patients with Down syndrome are also susceptible to weakened transverse ligaments and must be carefully assessed clinically and radiographically before being allowed to participate in sporting events such as the Special Olympics.

Steel's "Rule of Thirds" is a guide to the amount of atlantoaxial displacement that can occur before spinal cord compression ensues (Steel, 1968). The internal anteroposterior diameter of the atlas is approximately 3 cm; of that, the dens occupies approximately 1 cm and the spinal cord approximately 1 cm, leaving 1 cm of space for soft tissue and for normal movement to occur (Fig. 11-27).

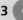

Subaxial Cervical Spine

Bailey (1963) stated that the musculature of the spine and the intervertebral discs were the most significant anatomical structures is providing cervical stability. Holdsworth (1963) emphasized the importance of the supraspinous and interspinous ligaments as well as the nuchal ligament. The nuchal ligament is thought to play a major role in

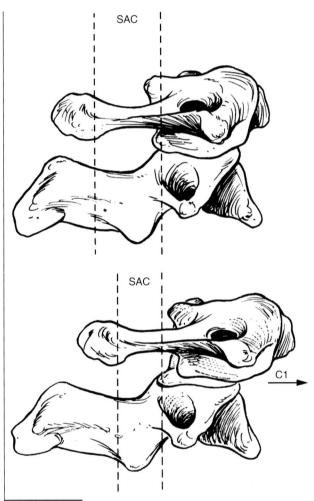

FIG. 11-24

The atlantodental interval (ADI) is inversely related to the space available for the spinal cord (SAC), which is denoted by the *dotted lines.* Anterior atlantoaxial subluxation causes a reduction in the SAC. Normal measurements for the ADI are less than 3 mm in adults or 4 mm in children. *Reprinted with permission from Moskovich, R. (1994). Atlantoaxial instability. Spine: State of the Art Reviews, 8(3), 531–549.*

CASE STUDY 11-1

Atlantoaxial Instability Without Fracture

A 30-year-old woman had a traumatic injury as a result of a forced flexion movement in a car accident. Continuous and severe neck pain occurred after the accident. She visited the emergency room and after a careful examination and x-ray evaluation, an anterior displacement of C1 on C2 was discovered (Fig. cs11-1-1).

A severe anterior dislocation of the atlas on the axis was confirmed after measuring the atlantodental interval (6 mm). For this case, no fracture of the atlas or the axis was detected and thus a deficiency of the transverse ligament may be assumed.

Clinical instability of the spine depends mainly on the soft tissue components. The cervical spine is a very mobile area, especially at the atlantoaxial level. Cervical subluxations and dislocations resulting from injuries of the osteoligamentous complex affect spinal stability and mobility at the cervical area. In addition, it may narrow the spinal canal and cause neurological impairment. Pure ligamentous injuries (as in this case) are less likely to heal and become stable, and therefore surgical procedures are likely to be considered.

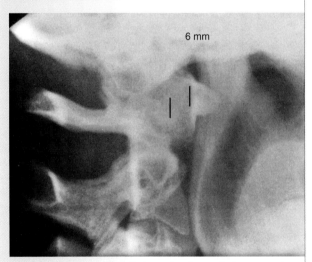

Case Study Figure 11-1-1. Lateral radiograph demonstrating an increased atlantodental interval of 6 mm after trauma.

proprioception and correct functioning of the erector spinae muscles. Experimental section of the ligaments in sequence from either anterior to posterior or posterior to anterior suggests that if a functional spinal unit has all of its anterior elements plus one additional structure or all of its posterior elements plus one anterior structure in-

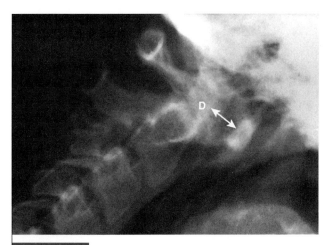

FIG. 11-25

Flexion lateral radiograph of a patient with rheumatoid arthritis. The dens (D) has been eroded and the transverse ligament is incompetent, resulting in atlantoaxial subluxation. The markedly widened atlanto-dens interval is indicated by the arrowed line.

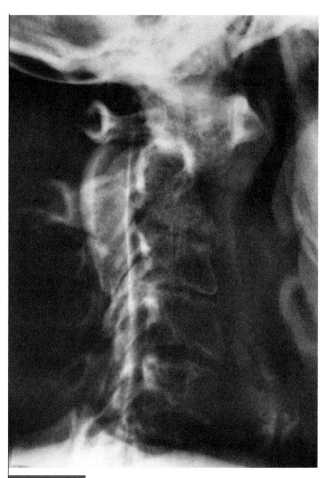

FIG. 11-26

Postmyelogram cervical radiograph in a patient with long-standing rheumatoid arthritis and fixed atlantoaxial subluxation. The space available for the cord has been reduced to 6.5 mm and compression of the proximal spinal cord is evident by examining the subdural space, which is outlined in white by the injected contrast medium. The patient developed cervical myelopathy, which necessitated decompression by transoral resection of the dens and posterior stabilization.

tact, it will probably remain stable under normal physiological loads. To provide for some clinical margin of safety, any motion segment should be considered unstable in which all of the anterior elements or all the posterior elements are destroyed or are unable to function (Panjabi et al., 1975; White et al., 1975). The clinical stability of various injuries must be assessed individually. The importance of clinical evaluation cannot be underestimated because significant spinal cord damage may occur after trauma even in the absence of fractures or ligamentous injuries (Gosch et al., 1972; Schneider et al., 1954). Valuable guidelines for the determination of clinical instability in the lower cervical spine have been provided in the form of a scoring system checklist (Box 11-2).

Using this scale, the measurement of translation takes into account variations in magnifications and is based on a tube-to-film distance of 183 cm. The 11° rotation is defined as 11° greater than the amount of rotation that exists at the motion segment above or below the functional spinal unit in question. The 3.5-mm value represents the radio-graphic measurement of the maximum permissible translation when the radiographic magnification is taken into account (Panjabi et al., 1986).

In case of questionable injury, when flexion and extension maneuvers should not be performed, a stretch test can be done to assess cervical integrity. A lateral cervical spine radiograph is taken at a standardized tube distance of 180 cm, and incremental 5-kg weights are applied as traction to the skull using cranial tongs (Fig. 11-28). Radiographs are taken after each additional weight has been applied. An abnor-

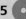

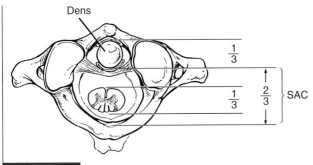

FIG. 11-27

Space available for the cord (*SAC*) is approximately two-thirds of the anteroposterior diameter of the spinal canal. One-third is taken up by the dens, one-third by the cord itself, and one-third is free space. *Reprinted with permission from Moskovich, R. (1994). Atlanto-axial instability. Spine: State of the Art Reviews, 8(3), 531–549.*

mal stretch test is defined as differences of greater than 1.7 mm interspace separation or greater than 7.5° change in angle between pre-stretch condition and the application of one-third body weight.

BOX 11-2	Checklist for the Diagnosis of Clinical Instability in the Middle and Lower Cervical Spine

Element	Point Value*
Anterior elements destroyed or unable to function	2
Posterior elements destroye or unable to function	2
Positive stretch test	2
Radiographic criteria	4
Flexion and extension x-rays	
Sagittal plane translation > 3.5 mm or 20% (2 pts)	
Sagittal plane rotation > 20° (2 pts)	
OR	
Resting x-rays	
Sagittal plane displacement > 3.5 mm or 20% (2 pts)	
Relative sagittal plane angulation > 11° (2 pts)	
Developmentally narrow spinal canal	1
Abnormal disc narrowing	1
Spinal cord damage	2
Nerve root damage	1
Dangerous loading anticipated	1

* Total of 5 or more = clinically unstable.

Modified from White, A.A. III & Panjabi, M.M. (1990). Clinical Biomechanics of the Spine (2nd ed., p. 314). Philadelphia: J.B. Lippincott.

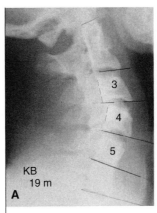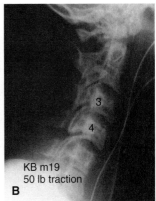

FIG. 11-28

Stretch test. **A,** Lateral radiograph of the cervical spine of a 19-year-old boy who was admitted with multiple injuries and neurological deficit compatible with an anterior cord syndrome. The radiograph shows increased angulation at C3–C4 and a block vertebra at C5–C6. Flexion-extension radiographs were contraindicated for fear of exacerbating his neurological injury. **B,** The stretch test was performed to ascertain whether significant instability existed. No abnormal distraction occurred at the interspace in question. His other injuries and fractures were treated routinely and he was given a soft collar to wear for 6 weeks. He made a slow but steady recovery with almost complete resolution of his upper extremity deficit, with no evidence of instability 1 year after the accident. *Reprinted with permission from Moskovich, R. (1997). Cervical instability (rheumatoid, dwarfism, degenerative, others). In K.H. Bridwell & R.L. DeWald (Eds.), The Textbook of Spinal Surgery (pp. 969–1009). Philadelphia: Lippincott-Raven Publishers.*

Applied Biomechanics

A thorough understanding of biomechanical principles is an important aspect of the treating physician's knowledge base because the normal structure and function of the spinal column is frequently altered during surgery. Whether treatment is a decompressive cervical laminectomy, a posterior foraminotomy with partial facetectomy, or an anterior cervical fusion, all of these interventions have certain ramifications with which one must be familiar. This knowledge not only benefits patient care but also is valuable in planning and executing treatment.

DECOMPRESSION

Cervical laminectomy often is performed to decompress the spinal cord. The compression may be caused by a stenotic process and can result in neurological symptoms such as radiculopathy or myelopathy. Other posterior decompressive procedures such as partial or full facetectomies for visualization or decompression of nerve root pathology also are commonly performed. Development of postlaminectomy kyphosis is well known in children and may develop in 17 (Miyazaki et al., 1989) to 25% of adults (Herkowitz, 1988). Postlaminectomy spinal deformity may occur in up to 50% of children who undergo laminectomies for spinal cord tumors (Lonstein, 1977). Simulated finite element analysis on cervical spines indicates that the primary cause of postlaminectomy deformity is resection of one or more spinous processes as well as the posterior ligamentous structures, such as the ligamentum flavum or interspinous or supraspinous ligaments. The removal of these structures causes the tensile forces normally present in the cervical spine to become unbalanced and place extra stress on the facet joints. Results indicate that either a kyphotic or a hyperlordotic cervical deformity may ensue, depending on the center of balance of the head (Saito et al., 1991).

Although reports exist of patients undergoing multiple-level cervical laminectomy with no evidence of clinical instability or deformity on long-term follow-up (Jenkins, 1973), most biomechanical studies indicate some degree of instability when the posterior elements are resected. Multilevel cervical laminectomy induces significant increases in total column flexibility associated with increased segmental flexural sagittal rotations. In a cadaveric laminectomy model, the mean stiffness of the intact cervical column was significantly greater than the mean stiffness for the laminectomized specimen, and there were consistently greater rotations as compared with the intact specimen (3.6 versus 8.0°) at every cervical spine level (Cusick et al., 1995).

The loss of facet joints alone causes a significant decrease in coupled motions that result from lateral bending. A moment about the anteroposterior axis results in a significant reduction in lateral displacement, a decrease in vertical displacement, and a decrease in rotation about the vertical axis. Partial facetectomy (<50%) did not, however, significantly alter flexion and extension movements (Raynor et al., 1987). Another anatomical study demonstrated that progressive laminectomy with resection of more than 25% of the facet joints resulted in significantly increased cervical flexion-extension, axial torsion, and lateral bending motion when compared with the intact spine (Nowinski et al., 1993).

A number of studies using three-dimensional finite element models showed that facetectomy has a greater effect on annulus stress than on intervertebral joint stiffness. Based on these models, it was concluded that a significant increase in annulus stresses and segmental mobility may occur when bilateral facet resection exceeds 50% (Kumaresan et al., 1997; Voo et al., 1997). Decompression by cervical laminoplasty, in which the facet joints are not sacrificed and the laminae are reconstructed, results in maintenance of flexion-extension and lateral bending stability, with a marginal increase in axial torsion. Iatrogenic injury is less likely to result if the capsules of the remaining facet joints and anterior elements remain intact.

Cervical subluxations and dislocations resulting from injury may narrow the spinal canal and cause neurological impairment. In some cases, adequate reduction and realignment of the vertebrae, followed by stabilization, may decompress the neural elements without resecting bone (Fig. 11-29).

ARTHRODESIS

Spinal arthrodesis is indicated in many disease processes such as spinal instability, neoplasm, posttraumatic and degenerative conditions of the spine. The goal of arthrodesis is to achieve a solid bony fusion in which two or more vertebrae solidly unite. In many cases, internal fixation is used to achieve initial stabilization as well as to correct deformity, if necessary.

An important principle regarding vertebral arthrodesis is that the stability established by internal fixation is a prelude to the biological process of fusion. Although fusion can occur without internal fixation, its appropriate use helps to increase the fusion rate and maintain structural alignment. Hardware by no means supplants the need for the surgeon to perform a thorough and careful preparation of the vertebrae and add bone graft to achieve fusion. With few exceptions, hardware that is not ultimately supported and protected by a solid fusion will fatigue and fail after a finite number of cycles. There is a race by the body to achieve a solid fusion mass before a fatigue failure of the implanted fixation device occurs.

The choice of a surgical approach to the cervical spine, as well as whether an anterior, posterior, or a combined arthrodesis should be performed, is dependent on the particular pathology present. When performing a fusion, it is important for the surgeon to understand the biomechanical properties of dif-

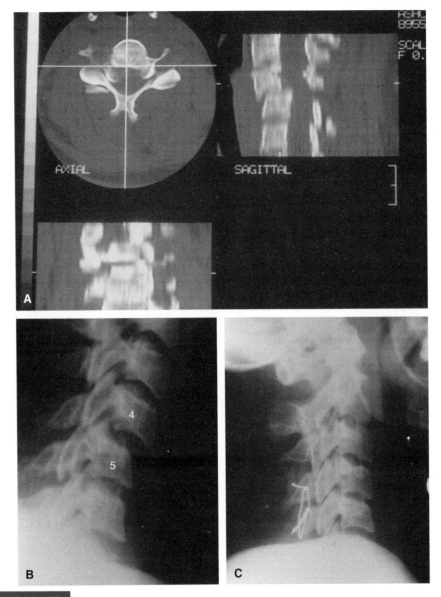

FIG. 11-29

Unilateral facet dislocation in a 24-year-old woman who was involved in a motor vehicle accident. The degree of vertebral subluxation is less than half the AP diameter of the vertebral body. Her spinal cord was compressed and she presented with an incomplete spinal cord injury. **A,** Computerized tomographic scans and reformatted images demonstrate the canal compromise at C5–C6. An attempt to realign the spine was made using longitudinal traction of up to approximately one-third of her body weight. **B,** The lateral radiograph with traction applied shows persistent malalignment. An open reduction was performed using a posterior exposure of the vertebra. Once the spine was realigned, the posterior tension band was recreated using interspinous wiring, and autogenous bone graft was inserted. **C,** The radiograph taken after the operation demonstrates restoration of normal vertebral relationships. The fixation provided good stability and enabled the patient to mobilize early. She had a good clinical outcome. *Reprinted with permission from Moskovich, R. (1997). Cervical instability (rheumatoid, dwarfism, degenerative, others). In K.H. Bridwell & R.L. DeWald (Eds.), The Textbook of Spinal Surgery (pp. 969–1009). Philadelphia: Lippincott-Raven Publishers.*

ferent types of fusion constructs. Cervical arthrodesis also has an affect on adjacent motion segments. Theoretically, there is an increase in motion at nearby unfused levels. Subsequent degeneration of other motion segments requiring additional levels of arthrodesis has been demonstrated in multiple studies (Cherubino et al., 1990; Hunter et al., 1980).

A recent study by Fuller et al. (1998) evaluated the distribution of motion across unfused cervical motion segments after a simulated segmental arthrodesis in cadaver cervical spines. The authors simulated one-, two-, and three-level fusions in human cervical spines. They then moved the cervical spines through a nondestructive 30° sagittal range of motion and compared this range of motion with that of unfused cervical spines. The findings of this study were interesting in that sagittal plane rotation was not increased disproportionately at the cervical motion segments immediately adjacent to a segmental arthrodesis. Although the authors acknowledged certain limitations of the study, they proposed that a cervical fusion causes a fairly uniform increase in motion across all remaining open cervical motion segments; therefore, an increased potential for degenerative change may exist at all cervical levels.

Another study was performed describing the incidence, prevalence, and radiographic progression of symptomatic adjacent level disease after cervical arthrodesis (Hilibrand et al., 1999). Adjacent level disease was defined as the development of a new radiculopathy or myelopathy that was referable to a motion segment adjacent to the site of a prior anterior cervical arthrodesis. The findings revealed that symptomatic adjacent level disease occurred at a relatively constant incidence of 2.9% per year. A survivorship analysis revealed that approximately 26% of patients who had an anterior cervical arthrodesis would have new disease at an adjacent level within 10 years of the operation. The study also demonstrated that more than two-thirds of the patients who developed adjacent level cervical disease experienced failure of nonoperative treatment and needed an additional procedure performed.

Cervical Spine Fixation

Arthrodesis of the cervical spine may be indicated for a number of reasons, most commonly for trauma and degenerative diseases. Much research has been performed to analyze the biomechanical advantages of anterior approaches, posterior approaches, or a combined procedure. With the advent of newer technologies, internal fixation systems have become available that can satisfactorily stabilize the cervical spine from either approach.

When an anterior approach is used, a discectomy or a vertebrectomy at one or more levels is commonly performed, usually followed by an anterior cervical arthrodesis. The excised disc or bone must be replaced with a structural graft or prosthesis to restore anterior column support to the spine. Osseous replacement may be in the form of autogenous or allogenic bone, commonly from the iliac crest if autogenous or from the fibula or iliac crest if allogenic (Fig. 11-30). The more cortical nature of fibula grafts may result in delayed incorporation compared with iliac crest grafts, which, therefore, are preferred clinically. The immediate postoperative strength of any of these bone grafts under axial compression on a material testing machine reveals that they will adequately support the loads required in the cervical spine. The physical properties of human bank bone seem to be preferable to autologous bone grafts, especially in

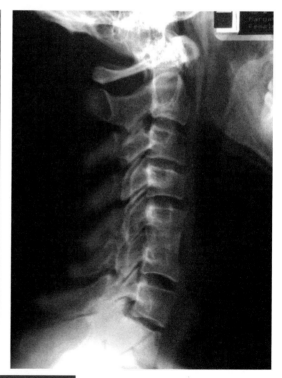

FIG. 11-30

Lateral radiograph of the cervical spine of a 35-year-old female who had an anterior cervical discectomy at C5–C6 and interbody arthrodesis using autogenous iliac crest tricortical bone graft. Note the maintenance of lordosis at the fused segment and the integration and remodeling of the graft.

TABLE 11-1

Compressive Strength of Various Interbody Graft Materials

Graft Type	Mean ± Standard Deviation	
Fibular strut	5,070 ± 3,250 N	Fibular strut significantly stronger than crest or rib grafts: $P < 0.05$
Anterior iliac crest	1,150 ± 487 N	
Posterior iliac crest	667 ± 311 N	
Rib	452 ± 192 N	
Hydroxylapatite 200 μm pore size	1,420 ± 480 N	Pore size of 200 μm significantly stronger than 500 μm pore size: $P < 0.05$
Hydroxylapatite 500 μm pore size	338 ± 78 N	

Adapted with permission from Wittenberg, R.H., Moeller, J., & White, A.A. III. (1990). Compressive strength of autogenous and allogenous bone grafts for thoracolumbar and cervical spine fusion. *Spine, 15*(10), 1073–1077.

older patients (Wittenberg et al., 1990). The biological incorporation of allograft appears to be satisfactory and its use obviates the need to harvest autologous bone from the iliac crest, sparing patients additional surgical trauma and potential complications.

Calcium phosphate (bone) ceramics form a strong bond with host bone because of a zone of apatite microcrystals deposited perpendicular to the hydroxylapatite ceramic surface (Jarcho, 1981). Synthetic hydroxylapatite blocks used for interbody cervical arthrodesis in goats produced similar fusion rates and biomechanical stiffness when compared with autogenous bone (Pintar et al., 1994). It is interesting to note that the goat holds its head erect, and thus loads the cervical spine similarly to human bipeds. Goat models for cervical spine biological/biomechanical testing are, therefore, popular.

A canine thoracic anterior arthrodesis model yielded contrary results when tested biomechanically: autogenous iliac crest grafts were stiffer in all motions than were ceramic graft substitutes (Emery et al., 1996). Naturally grown coral is also a useful bone graft substitute once it has been processed. It is available commercially in two different porosities (200 μm and 500 μm pore size). The grafts of lower porosity had a compressive strength comparable with bicortical iliac crest grafts, although they were much more brittle. They can therefore be considered appropriate for clinical use with respect to their compressive strength (Table 11-1). An increasing variety of prosthetic interbody cages are becoming available (Shono et al., 1993); long-term clinical results are eagerly awaited. Additional anterior (Fig. 11-31) or posterior internal fixation using plates and screws for added support may be used.

Posterior arthrodeses of the cervical spine are commonly performed after trauma but may also be used to treat degenerative, inflammatory, or neoplastic conditions. Unlike anterior fixation devices, which are solely used in the subaxial cervical spine, posterior fixation devices can extend up to the occiput (Fig. 11-32). Posterior fixation has commonly consisted of various wiring methods, which are used as a tension band posteriorly (Sutterlin et al., 1988). Within the past decade, however, techniques utilizing screws in both the atlantoaxial and subaxial spine have become more popular.

Techniques for atlantoaxial fixation have evolved from onlay bone grafting alone to ever-more sophisticated methods of internal fixation. Interlaminar clamp fixation is clinically reliable and safe (Moskovich & Crockard, 1992). Screw fixation techniques may confer increased translational and axial rotational stability, but with greater surgical risks. A biomechanical evaluation of four commonly used techniques for posterior atlantoaxial fixation was performed (Grob et al., 1992). Cadaver C1–C2 functional spinal units were tested in flexion-extension, lateral bending, and rotation, while intact as well as after a complete ligamentous injury. The fixation techniques used were:

1. Sublaminar wire with one median graft (Gallie type)
2. Wire fixation with two bilateral grafts (Brooks type)
3. Transarticular screw fixation (Magerl)
4. Two bilateral posterior Halifax clamps (Fig. 11-33)

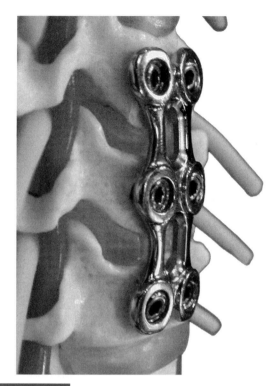

FIG. 11-31

An example of an anterior cervical plate applied over two motion segments on a model of the cervical spine (Peak cervical plate, DePuy Acromed, Inc., Raynham, MA). The screws do not penetrate the posterior cortex and are locked to the plate to prevent backing out.

strated similar or improved fusion rates compared with stand-alone bone grafts.

Another group assessed the biomechanical stability of seven different cervical reconstruction methods using 24 calf cervical spine segments (Kotani et al., 1994). They studied three posterior-only techniques, anterior-only cervical plates, anterior bone graft alone, and a combined anterior plate with posterior triple wiring. The results demonstrated that for one-level instability, the stiffness values of reconstruction with an anterior procedure alone were significantly smaller than those of all the other constructs tested. Interestingly, stiffness was restored to pre-injury levels in specimens with two-level injury patterns reconstructed using any of the three anterior methods. The findings do not support the use of exclusive anterior methods in either posterior or

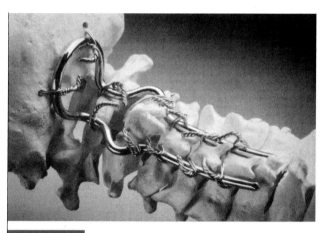

FIG. 11-32

Posterior occipitocervical fixation using a highly modified stainless steel loop (Ransford loop, Surgicraft; Redditch, Worcs., U.K.) wired into place on a skeleton model. The cranial loop is attached to the occiput using wires that pass through paired full-thickness burr holes. The wires are not passed around the foramen magnum. The loop is pre-bent to conform to the posterior craniocervical angle and may be adjusted intraoperatively. The limbs of the loop are attached via sublaminar wires at each level. Note how the axis laminar wires are tightened **below** the flare of the loop, which serves to maintain distraction between the occiput and the axis vertebra. Sublaminar wire use is one of many techniques available to achieve segmental posterior fixation. *Reprinted with permission from Moskovich R., et al. (2000). Occipitocervical stabilization for myelopathy in patients with rheumatoid arthritis. Implications of not bone grafting.* J Bone Joint Surg, 82A, 349–365.

The Gallie technique allowed significantly more rotation in flexion, extension, axial rotation, and lateral bending than did the other three fixation techniques. No significant differences were noted in the amount of rotation between the other three fixation techniques, although the Magerl transarticular screw fixation tended to permit the least amount of rotation, as might be expected.

A variety of anterior cervical plating systems are currently available, and many have been subject to biomechanical analyses. Investigators demonstrated that in a single-level procedure, an anterior cervical plate serves as a load-sharing device rather than as a load-shielding device, enabling graft consolidation as observed in other clinical studies (Rapoff et al., 1999). Bone union may be expected to occur at a lower rate if the bones are shielded from compressive forces; however, clinical experience with anterior cervical plates has generally demon-

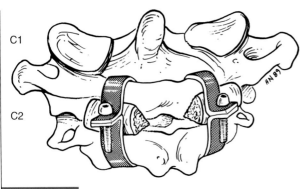

FIG. 11-33

Diagram of a skeletonized atlantoaxial motion segment viewed from its posterior aspect. The method of application of the interlaminar clamps can be seen. The bone grafts lie under the Halifax clamps and allow the posterior construct to be locked tightly, providing immediate stability. *Reprinted with permission from Moskovich, R., & Crockard, H.A. (1992). Atlantoaxial arthrodesis using interlaminar clamps. An improved technique.* Spine, 17, 261–267.

three-column instability. In three-column or multi-level instability, combined front and back procedures utilizing an anterior plate and posterior triple wiring demonstrated clear biomechanical advantages. Clinical use of anterior plate fixation without posterior fixation for three-column cervical injuries, however, resulted in satisfactory clinical outcomes (Ripa et al., 1991). These results underscore the need for good clinical evaluation and studies that take into account the fourth-dimension—time. Fusion is a biological process that occurs over time and supercedes the importance of in vitro or computer-simulated biomechanical studies.

BIOMECHANICS OF CERVICAL TRAUMA

Airbag Injuries

Motor vehicle accidents continue to be the leading cause of injury-related deaths in the United States. In 1984, the National Highway Traffic Safety Administration (NHTSA) required that automatic occupant protection devices (airbags or automatic seat belts) be placed in all automobiles in the 1987–1990 model years. In 1993, the passenger-side airbag was introduced. Studies generally concluded that front seat occupants are adequately protected against frontal impact if belts are worn in an airbag-

equipped vehicle (King & Yang, 1995). However, not long after airbag devices became available, airbag injuries involving front seat passengers began to be described and by late 1997, 49 child deaths and 19 serious injuries had been attributed to passenger-side airbags (Marshall et al., 1998).

A retrospective review was performed by three pediatric radiologists to determine if a pattern of injury was common to this new mechanism of pediatric trauma (Marshall et al., 1998). Their findings, as well as the findings of other studies, demonstrated that passenger-side airbags pose a lethal threat to children riding in the front seat of an automobile (Giguere et al., 1998; McCaffrey et al., 1999; Mohamed & Banerjee, 1998). Many of the children killed in these accidents were front seat passengers involved in low-speed collisions in which the driver sustained no or only minor injuries; the pattern of injury seen is different in the rear-facing infant car seat versus the forward-facing child car seat. In the former, the injury to the infant was often massive skull injury and cerebral hematoma as a result of the proximity of their heads to the airbag, while in the latter, children sustained many more cervical injuries. Two of the older children had autopsy findings of atlanto-occipital dislocation and one sustained a "near decapitation" injury, demonstrating the vulnerability of the pediatric cervical spine to the explosive forces of an expanding airbag that hyperextends the child's fragile neck. Recent guidelines from the NHTSA (Box 11-3) were prompted by reports of airbag injuries to children and emphasize that children of any age should be properly secured in the back seat (National Highway Traffic Safety Administration, 1996).

A mathematical simulation was performed to study the potential of head and neck injury to an un-belted driver restrained by an airbag (Yang et al.,

| BOX 11-3 | National Highway Traffic Safety Administration Guidelines Regarding Airbags & Children |

The back seat is the safest place for children of any age to ride.

Never put an infant (less than 1 year old) in the front of a car with a passenger-side airbag.

Infants must always ride in the back seat, facing the rear of the car.

Make sure everyone is buckled up. Unbuckled occupants can be hurt or killed by an airbag.

1992). It was found that when the standard 20° angle steering wheel was used, neck joint torques were decreased by 22%. The resultant head acceleration increased 41% from the baseline study when a vertical steering wheel was used. If the vertical dimension of the airbag was reduced by 10%, neck joint torques were increased by 14%, while head acceleration showed a slight decrease of 9%. Although ideal dimensions and inflation rates for airbags remain elusive, their use has resulted in a significant reduction in head and neck injuries.

Whiplash Syndrome

Whiplash syndrome is a complex set of symptoms that may present after an acceleration hyperextension injury. These injuries typically occur when a car is struck from behind, but may also be caused by lateral or frontal collisions (Barnsley et al., 1994) (Case Study 11-2). The acceleration of the car seat pushes the torso of the occupant forward with the result that the unsupported head falls backward, resulting in an extension strain to the neck. A secondary flexion injury may occur if the vehicle just struck then strikes another vehicle in front and just as suddenly decelerates again, throwing the occupant forward once more. Crowe coined the term 'whiplash' in 1928 in a lecture on neck injuries caused by rear-end automobile collisions in the United States but later reported that he regretted using the term (Breck & Van Norman, 1971) because it describes only the manner in which a head was moved suddenly to produce a sprain in the neck and not a specific injury pattern. Therefore, we refer to this clinical entity as whiplash *syndrome*, not as whiplash *injury*.

Although whiplash injuries are a common traumatic event, the pathology is poorly understood. Often the severity of the whiplash trauma does not correlate with the seriousness of the clinical problem, which can include neck and shoulder pain, dizziness, headache, and blurring of vision (Brault et al., 1998; Ettlin et al., 1992; Panjabi et al., 1998a; Sturzenegger et al., 1994). Apart from a frequently observed loss of physiological lordosis, a radiographic examination of the cervical spine is often normal. Even newer technology such as MRI is not always able to reveal a soft tissue injury. MRI examination of the cerebrum and cervical spinal column performed 2 days after a whiplash neck sprain injury in 40 patients did not detect any pathology connected to the injury, nor was the MRI able to predict symptom development or outcome (Borchgrevink et al., 1997). Injuries that have been documented include interspinous ligament tears, spinous process fractures, disc rupture, ligamentum flavum rupture, facet joint disruption, and stretching of the anterior muscles. The diagnosis and management of whiplash injuries are often confounded by concomitant psychosocial and medicolegal issues as well (Wallis et al., 1998).

One of the early (unpublished) biomechanical studies of whiplash injury was done by the late Dr. Irving Tuell, an orthopaedic surgeon in Seattle, Washington. He used a ciné camera to photograph himself driving as he was rammed from behind by his surgical resident driving another car. Frames drawn from that movie clearly demonstrate the hyperextension of his neck over the seatback of his car (Fig. 11-34). One can also see the effect of inertial forces on the mandible as his jaw snaps open while the acceleration forces his head backwards. This mechanism may explain the temporomandibular injuries that are a common accompaniment of cervical whiplash injuries.

A recent study of rear-end collisions quantitatively elucidated the actual neck movements that take place (Castro et al., 1997). After being rammed from behind, the mean acceleration of the target vehicles was from 2.1 to 3.6 g. Maximal extension was reached when the head contacted the headrest; the angle between the head and upper body varied from 10 to 47° (mean = 20°). In the absence of a headrest, the maximal recorded extension was 80°. Follow-up clinical and MRI examinations were performed. The study concluded that the "limit of harmlessness" for stresses arising from rear-end impacts with regard to the velocity changes lies between 10 and 15 km/h. In studies, a reproducible whiplash trauma model using whole cervical spine specimens mounted on a bench top sled was used to simulate rear-end collision with increasing horizontal accelerations applied to the sled (Panjabi et al., 1998a,b). Both sled and head kinematics can be measured using potentiometers and accelerometers. Using this whiplash model, an S-shaped curve was described in whiplash injuries in which the lower cervical spine hyperextended and the upper cervical spine flexed (Grauer et al., 1997). The investigators felt that the injury was incurred during the hyperextension phase in the lower cervical spine.

Correct positioning of adjustable headrests behind the skull, not behind the neck, is important. Tests using a Hyge sled and a Hybrid III dummy were performed by other investigators to determine

CASE STUDY 11-2

Whiplash Syndrome

A 32-year-old man was injured in a car accident. The traumatic event happened after being struck from behind. In this case, the inertia of the head and the flexible spine resulted in marked hyperextension movement of the head. The acceleration of the car seat pushed the torso of the occupant forward with the result that the unsupported head fell backward, resulting in an extension strain to the neck.

The patient presented with severe neck and shoulder pain accompanied by sleep disturbance. The right sternocleidomastoid muscle was approximately twice as large as the left sternocleidomastoid muscle. After muscle testing against resistance, the pain increased (Fig. cs11-2-1).

To decelerate the posterior rotating head, a moment and a force must be developed by active and passive stabilizers, joint surfaces, and the intervertebral disc. The moment and force give rise to tension, compression, and shear stresses and strains in various parts of the neck causing, damage. During the collision, the muscle tension increases with the velocity of lengthening. A tension inappropriate for the length-tension curve occurs and partial rupture of the sterno-cleidomastoid muscle is produced. *Reprinted with permission from Frankel, V.H. (1972). Whiplash injuries to the neck. In C. Hirsh & Y. Zotterman (Eds.),* Cervical Pain *(pp. 97–111). New York: Pergamon Press.*

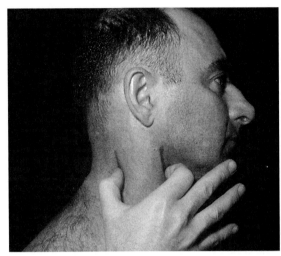

Case Study Figure 11-2-1.

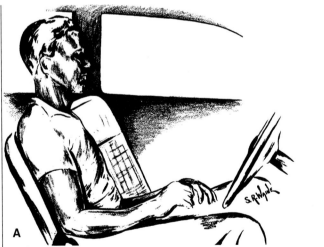

A

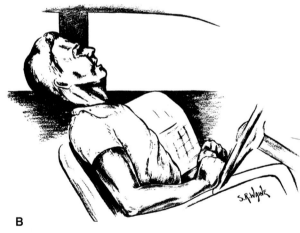

B

FIG. 11-34

Hand-drawn cells traced from two frames of a ciné movie of Dr. Irving Tuell driving his car.
(A) Before and **(B)** after being rammed from behind by another car driven by his resident.

biomechanical responses for the various conditions observed in normal driving (Viano & Gargan, 1996). Risk of injury was assumed to be proportional to neck extension. A low headrest position carries a relative injury risk of 3.4 in rear-end crashes, compared with 1.0 for the favorable condition. If all adjustable headrests were placed in the up position, the relative risk would be lowered to 2.4, a 28.3% reduction in whiplash injury risk.

Significantly more complex acceleration injuries ascribed to high G-force activities are now occurring. There is a report in the literature of cervical injury in pilots of F-16 fighter planes, citing a 1-year prevalence of neck injury of 56.6% and a career prevalence of neck injury of 85.4% (Albano & Stanford, 1998).

Maintenance of neurological homeostasis and protection of the spinal cord, nerves, and vessels and support and protection of the skull are the ultimate tasks of the cervical spine. An appreciation of the principles presented should afford a greater understanding to physicians and allied health professionals involved in the treatment of cervical spine pathology. With increasing technological advances in our society, we remain vulnerable not only to common types of cervical trauma but also to idiosyncratic methods of injury related to these new technologies. Acceleration injuries have been occurring for decades but cervical spine injuries caused by airbags have only recently been described, and our involvement in increasingly greater speeds and higher risk activities places us in increasing jeopardy. As our body of knowledge expands, we continue to discover new methods of injury. It is critical to pursue rational treatments for these disorders based on sound biomechanical principles.

Summary

1 A functional spinal unit or motion segment consists of two adjacent vertebrae and the intervening intervertebral discs and ligaments between the vertebrae.

2 When either rotation or translation of a body along one axis is consistently associated with a simultaneous rotation or translation along another axis, the motions are coupled.

3 Intervertebral disks exhibit viscoelastic properties (creep and relaxation) and hysteresis.

4 Discs are able to withstand greater than normal loads when compressive forces are rapidly applied, which protects the disc from catastrophic failure until extremely high loads are applied.

5 Vertebral body compression strength increases from upper cervical to lower lumbar levels.

6 The mean sagittal diameter of the male adult spinal canal for C3–C7 is close to 14 mm; the spinal cord diameter is about 10 mm.

7 Ligamentum flavum is under tension even when the spine is in a neutral position or somewhat extended, prestressing the disc and providing some intrinsic support to the spine.

8 Muscles play a critical role in basic postural homeostasis. Patients with paralyzed cervical muscles are unable to support their heads.

9 The spinal cord has some longitudinal elasticity but it tolerates axial translation poorly. It is the translatory forces that typically result in neurological injury.

10 Instant center analysis indicates that tangential motion (gliding) takes place between the facet joints as the cervical spine is flexed and extended. The size of the intervertebral foramina increases with flexion and decreases with extension.

11 Kinematic instability refers to the quantity of motion (too much or too little) or the quality of motion present (alterations in the normal pattern), or both. Component instability addresses the clinical biomechanical role of the various anatomic structures of the functional spinal unit.

12 Any motion segment in which all of the anterior elements or all the posterior elements are destroyed or are unable to function should be considered unstable.

13 A significant increase in annulus stresses and segmental mobility may occur when bilateral facet resection exceeds 50%.

14 Appropriate use of internal fixation helps to increase the fusion rate and maintain structural alignment.

15 Front seat occupants are adequately protected against frontal impact if seatbelts are worn in an airbag equipped vehicle. Passenger-side air bags pose a lethal threat to children riding in the front seat of an automobile.

16 Whiplash syndrome is a complex set of symptoms that may present after an acceleration hyperextension injury.

REFERENCES

Adams, M.A. & Hutton, W.C. (1980). The effect of posture on the role of the apophysial joints in resisting intervertebral compressive forces. *J Bone Joint Surg, 62B*, 358–62.

Albano, J.J. & Stanford, J.B. (1998). Prevention of minor neck injuries in F-16 pilots. *Aviat Space Environ Med, 69*, 1193–1199.

Bailey, R.W. (1963). Observations of cervical intervertebral disc lesions in fractures and dislocations. *J Bone Joint Surg, 45A*, 461.

Barnsley, L., Lord, S., & Bogduk, N. (1994). Whiplash injury. *Pain, 58*, 283–307.

Bell, G.H. (1967). Variation in the strength of vertebra with age and their relation to osteoporosis. *Calcif Tissue Res, 1*, 75.

Bennett, S.E., Schenk, R.J., & Simmons, E.D. (2000). Active range of motion utilized in the cervical spine to perform daily functional tasks (Abstract). *Association of Bone and Joint Surgeons 52nd Annual Meeting.* San Antonio, TX, May 2000.

Blackley, H.R., Plank, L.D., & Robertson, P.A. (1999). Determining the sagittal dimensions of the canal of the cervical spine. The reliability of ratios of anatomical measurements. *J Bone Joint Surg, 81B*, 110–112.

Borchgrevink, G., Smevik, O., Haave, I., et al. (1997). MRI of cerebrum and cervical columna within two days after whiplash neck sprain injury. *Injury, 28*, 331–335.

Brault, J.R., Wheeler, J.B., Siegmund, G.P., et al. (1998). Clinical response of human subjects to rear-end automobile collisions [published erratum appears in Arch Phys Med Rehabil 1998 Jun;79(6):723]. *Arch Phys Med Rehabil, 79*, 72–80.

Breck, L.W. & Van Norman, R.W. (1971). Medicolegal aspects of cervical spine sprains. *Clin Orthop, 74*, 124–8.

Breig, A., Turnbell, I., & Hassler, O. (1966). Effect of mechanical stress on the spinal cord in cervical spondylosis. *J Neurosurg, 25*, 45–56.

Carter, D.R. & Hayes, W.C. (1977). The compressive behavior of bone as a two-phase porous structure. *J Bone Joint Surg, 59A*, 954–962.

Castro, W.H., Schilgen, M., Meyer, S., et al. (1997). Do "whiplash injuries" occur in low-speed rear impacts? *Eur Spine J, 6*, 366–375.

Cherubino, P., Benazzo, F., Borromeo, U., et al. (1990). Degenerative arthritis of the adjacent spinal joints following anterior cervical spinal fusion: Clinicoradiologic and statistical correlations. *Ital J Orthop Traumatol, 16*, 533–543.

Clausen, J.D., Goel, V.K., Traynelis, V.C., et al. (1997). Uncinate processes and Luschka joints influence the biomechanics of the cervical spine: Quantification using a finite element model of the C5–C6 segment. *J Orthop Res, 15*, 342–347.

Cusick, J.F., Pintar, F.A., & Yoganandan, N. (1995). Biomechanical alterations induced by multilevel cervical laminectomy. *Spine, 20*, 2392–2398.

Denis, F. (1983). The three column spine and its significance in the classification of acute thoracolumbar spinal injuries. *Spine, 8*, 817–831.

Dickman, C.A., Zabramski, J.M., Hadley, M.N., et al. (1991). Pediatric spinal cord injury without radiographic abnormalities: Report of 26 cases and review of the literature. *J Spinal Disord, 4*, 296–305.

Dvorak, J., Froehlich, D., Penning, L., et al. (1988b). Functional radiographic diagnosis of the cervical spine: Flexion/extension. *Spine, 13*(7), 748–755.

Dvorak, J., Hayek, J., & Zehnder, R. (1987). CT-functional diagnostics of the rotatory instability of the upper cervical spine. Part II. An evaluation of healthy adults and patients with suspected instability. *Spine, 12*(8), 726–731.

Dvorak, J. & Panjabi, M.M., (1987). Functional anatomy of the alar ligaments. *Spine, 12*, 183–189.

Dvorak, J., Schneider, E., Saldinger, P., et al. (1988a). Biomechanics of the craniocervical region: The alar and transverse ligaments. *J Orthop Res, 6*, 452–461.

Emery, S.E., Fuller, D.A., & Stevenson, S. (1996). Ceramic anterior spinal fusion. Biologic and biomechanical comparison in a canine model. *Spine, 21*, 2713–2719.

Ettlin, T.M., Kischka, U., Reichmann, S., et al. (1992). Cerebral symptoms after whiplash injury of the neck: A prospective clinical and neuropsychological study of whiplash injury. *J Neurol Neurosurg Psychiatry, 55*, 943–948.

Feipel, V., Rondelet, B., Le Pallec, J., et al. (1999). Normal global motion of the cervical spine: An electrogoniometric study. *Clin Biomech, 14*, 462–470.

Fielding, J.W. (1957). Cineroentgenography of the normal cervical spine. *J Bone Joint Surg, 39A*, 1280–1288.

Fielding, J.W., Cochran, G.v.B., Lawsing, J.F. III, et al. (1974). Tears of the transverse ligament of the atlas: A clinical and biomechanical study. *J Bone Joint Surg, 56A*, 1683–1691.

Fielding, J.W., Hawkins, R.J., & Ratzan, S.A. (1976). Spine fusion for atlanto-axial instability. *J Bone Joint Surg, 58A*, 400–407.

Fountain, F.P., Minear, W.L., & Allison, R.D. (1966). Function of longus colli and longissimus cervicis muscles in man. *Arch Phys Med, 47*, 665–669.

Frankel, V.H. (1972). Whiplash injuries to the neck. In C. Hirsh & Y. Zotterman (Eds.), *Cervical Pain* (pp. 97–111). New York: Pergamon Press.

Fuller, D.A., Kirkpatrick, J.S., Emery, S.E., et al. (1998). A kinematic study of the cervical spine before and after segmental arthrodesis. *Spine, 23*, 1649–1656.

Giguere, J.F., St-Vil, D., Turmel, A., et al. (1998). Airbags and children: A spectrum of C-spine injuries. *J Pediatr Surg, 33*, 811–816.

Gosch, H.H., Gooding, E., & Schneider, R.C. (1972). An experimental study of cervical spine and cord injuries. *J Trauma, 12*, 570–575.

Grauer, J.N., Panjabi, M.M., Cholewicki, J., et al. (1997). Whiplash produces an S-shaped curvature of the neck with hyperextension at lower levels. *Spine, 22*, 2489–2494.

Grob, D., Crisco, J.J. III, Panjabi, M.M., et al. (1992). Biomechanical evaluation of four different posterior atlantoaxial fixation techniques. *Spine, 17*(5), 480–490.

Hansson, T. & Roos, B. (1986). Age changes in the bone mineral of the lumbar spine in normal women. *Calcif Tissue Int, 38*, 249–251.

Hansson, T., Roos, B., & Nachemson, A. (1980). The bone mineral content and ultimate compressive strength of lumbar vertebrae. *Spine, 5*, 46–55.

Harms-Ringdahl, K. (1986). On assessment of shoulder exercise and load-elicited pain in the cervical spine. *Biomechanical Analysis of Load—EMG—Methodological Studies of Pain Provoked by Extreme Position.* Karolinska Institute, University of Stockholm.

Herkowitz, H.N. (1988). A comparison of anterior cervical fusion, cervical laminectomy, and cervical laminoplasty for the surgical management of multiple level spondylotic radiculopathy. *Spine, 13,* 774–780.

Herzog, R.J., Wiens, J.J., Dillingham, M.F., et al. (1991). Normal cervical spine morphometry and cervical spinal stenosis in asymptomatic professional football players. Plain film radiography, multiplanar computed tomography, and magnetic resonance imaging. *Spine, 16,* S178–S186.

Hilibrand, A.S., Carlson, G.D., Palumbo, M.A., et al. (1999). Radiculopathy and myelopathy at segments adjacent to the site of a previous anterior cervical arthrodesis. *J Bone Joint Surg, 81A,* 519–28.

Holdsworth, F.W. (1963). Fractures, dislocations, and fracture-dislocations of the spine. *J Bone Joint Surg, 45B,* 6–20.

Hunter, L., Braunstein, E., & Bailey, R. (1980). Radiographic changes following anterior fusion. *Spine, 5,* 399–401.

Jarcho, M. (1981). Calcium phosphate ceramics as hard tissue prosthetics. *Clin Orthop, 157,* 259–278.

Jenkins, D.H. (1973). Extensive cervical laminectomy. Long-term results. *Br J Surg, 60,* 852–854.

Kazarian, L.E. (1975). Creep characteristics of the human spinal column. *Orthop Clin North Am, 6,* 3.

Kazarian, L. (1972). Dynamic response characteristics of the human intervertebral column: An experimental study of autopsy specimens. *Acta Orthop Scand, 146,* 146.

King, A.I. & Yang, K.H. (1995). Research in biomechanics of occupant protection. *J Trauma, 38,* 570–576.

Kitahara, Y., Iida, H., & Tachibana, S. (1995). Effect of spinal cord stretching due to head flexion on intramedullary pressure. *Neurol Med Chir, 35,* 285–288.

Kotani, Y., Cunningham, B.W., Abumi, K., et al. (1994). Biomechanical analysis of cervical stabilization systems. An assessment of transpedicular screw fixation in the cervical spine. *Spine, 19,* 2529–2539.

Kriss, V.M. & Kriss, T.C. (1996). SCIWORA (spinal cord injury without radiographic abnormality) in infants and children. *Clin Pediatr, 35,* 119–124.

Kumaresan, S., Yoganandan, N., Pintar, F.A., et al. (1997). Finite element modeling of cervical laminectomy with graded facetectomy. *J Spinal Disord, 10,* 40–46.

Lonstein, J.E. (1977). Post-laminectomy kyphosis. *Clin Orthop, 128,* 93–100.

Lysell, E. (1969). Motion in the cervical spine. An experimental study on autopsy specimens. *Acta Orthop Scand, Suppl 123,* 1–61.

Marshall, K.W., Koch, B.L., & Egelhoff, J.C. (1998). Air bag-related deaths and serious injuries in children: Injury patterns and imaging findings. *Am J Neuroradiol, 19,* 1599–607.

McBroom, R.J., Hayes, W.C., Edwards, W.T., et al. (1985). Prediction of vertebral body compressive fracture using quantitative computed tomography. *J Bone Joint Surg, 67A,* 1206–1214.

McCaffrey, M., German, A., Lalonde, F., et al. (1999). Air bags and children: A potentially lethal combination. *J Pediatr Orthop, 19,* 60–64.

Mimura, M., Moriya, H., Watanabe, T., et al. (1989). Three-dimensional motion analysis of the cervical spine with special reference to the axial rotation. *Spine, 14,* 1135–1139.

Miyazaki, K., Tada, K., Matsuda, Y., et al. (1989). Posterior extensive simultaneous multisegmental fusion for cervical myelopathy with cervical instability and kyphotic and/or S-shaped deformities. *Spine, 14*(11), 1160–1170.

Mohamed, A.A. & Banerjee, A. (1998). Patterns of injury associated with automobile airbag use. *Postgrad Med J, 74,* 455–458.

Moroney, S.P. & Schultz, A.B. (1985). Analysis and measurement of loads on the neck. *Trans Orth Res Soc, 10,* 329.

Moroney, S.P., Schultz, A.B., Miller, J., et al. (1988). Load displacement properties of lower cervical spine motion segments. *J Biomech, 21,* 769–779.

Moskovich, R. (1994). Atlanto-axial instability. *Spine: State of the Art Reviews, 8*(3), 531–549.

Moskovich, R. (1997). Cervical instability (rheumatoid, dwarfism, degenerative, others). In K.H. Bridwell & R.L. DeWald (Eds.), *The Textbook of Spinal Surgery* (pp. 969–1009). Philadelphia: Lippincott-Raven Publishers.

Moskovich R., et al. (2000). Occipitocervical stabilization for myelopathy in patients with rheumatoid arthritis. Implications of not bone grafting. *J Bone Joint Surg, 82A,* 349–365.

Moskovich, R. & Crockard, H.A. (1992). Atlantoaxial arthrodesis using interlaminar clamps. An improved technique. *Spine, 17,* 261–267.

Moskovich, R. & Jones, D.A. (1999). Upper cervical spine instrumentation. *Spine: State of the Art Reviews, 13,* 233–253.

Moskovich, R., Shott, S., & Zhang, Z.H. (1996). Does the cervical canal to body ratio predict spinal stenosis? *Bull Hosp Joint Dis, 55,* 61–71.

Myers, B.S. & Winkelstein, B.A. (1995). Epidemiology, classification, mechanism, and tolerance of human cervical spine injuries. *Crit Rev Biomed Eng, 23,* 307–409.

Nachemson, A. & Evans, J.H. (1968). Some mechanical properties of the third human lumbar interlaminar ligament (ligamentum flavum). *J Biomech, 1,* 201.

National Highway Traffic Safety Administration. (1996). Air bag alert. *Ann Emerg Med, 28,* 242.

Nowinski, G.P., Visarius, H., Nolte, L.P., et al. (1993). A biomechanical comparison of cervical laminoplasty and cervical laminectomy with progressive facetectomy. *Spine, 18,* 1995–2004.

Osenbach, R.K. & Menezes, A.H. (1989). Spinal cord injury without radiographic abnormality in children. *Pediatr Neurosci, 15,* 168–174.

Pang, D. & Pollack, I.F. (1989). Spinal cord injury without radiographic abnormality in children—The SCIWORA syndrome. *J Trauma, 29,* 654–664.

Panjabi, M.M., Cholewicki, J., Nibu, K., et al. (1998b). Simulation of whiplash trauma using whole cervical spine specimens. *Spine, 23,* 17–24.

Panjabi, M.M., Cholewicki, J., Nibu, K., et al. (1998a). Capsular ligament stretches during in vitro whiplash simulations. *J Spinal Disord, 11,* 227–232.

Panjabi, M.M., Kraig, M.H., & Goel, V.K. (1981). A technique for measurement and description of three-dimensional six degree-of-freedom motion of a body joint with an application to the human spine. *J Biomechanics, 14,* 447–460.

Panjabi, M.M., Summers, D.J., Pelker, R.R., et al. (1986). Three-dimensional load-displacement curves due to forces on the cervical spine. *J Orthop Res, 4,* 152–161.

Panjabi, M.M., White, A.A. III, & Johnson, R.M. (1975). Cervical spine mechanics as a function of transection of components. *J Biomechanics, 8,* 327–336.

Penning, L. & Wilmink, J.T. (1987). Rotation of the cervical spine. A study in normal people. *Spine 12,* 732–738.

Perry, J. & Nickel, V.L. (1959). Total cervical-spine fusion for neck paralysis. *J Bone Joint Surg, 41A,* 37–60.

Pintar, F.A., Maiman, D.J., Hollowell, J.P., et al. (1994). Fusion rate and biomechanical stiffness of hydroxylapatite versus autogenous bone grafts for anterior discectomy. An in vivo animal study. *Spine, 19,* 2524–2528.

Pintar, F.A., Yoganandan, N., Pesigan, M., et al. (1995). Cervical vertebral strain measurements under axial and eccentric loading. *J Biomech Eng, 117,* 474–478.

Rapoff, A.J., O'Brien, T.J., Ghanayem, A.J., et al. (1999). Anterior cervical graft and plate load sharing. *J Spinal Dis, 12,* 45–49.

Raynor, R.B., Moskovich, R., Zidel, P., et al. (1987). Alteration in primary and coupled neck motions after facetectomy. *Neurosurgery, 21,* 681–687.

Reill, J. (1960). Effects of flexion-extension movement of the head and spine on the spinal cord and nerve roots. *J Neurol Neurosurg Psychiatr, 23,* 214–221.

Ripa, D.R., Kowall, M.G., Meyer, P.R. Jr., et al. (1991). Series of ninety-two traumatic cervical spine injuries stabilized with anterior ASIF plate fusion technique. *Spine, 16*(3), 46–55.

Rolander, S.D. (1966). Motion of the lumbar spine with special reference to the stabilizing effect of posterior fusion. An experimental study on autopsy specimens. *Acta Orthop Scand, 90,* 1–144.

Roozmon, P., Gracovetsky, S.A., Gouw, G.J., et al. (1993). Examining motion in the cervical spine. I: Imaging systems and measurement techniques. *J Biomed Eng, 15,* 5–12.

Saito, T., Yamamuro, T., Shikata, J., et al. (1991). Analysis and prevention of spinal column deformity following cervical laminectomy. I. Pathogenetic analysis of post-laminectomy deformities. *Spine, 16,* 494–502.

Schneider, R.C., Cherry, G., & Pantek, H. (1954). The syndrome of acute central cervical spinal cord injury with special reference to the mechanism involved in hyperextension injuries of the cervical spine. *J Neurosurg, 11,* 546–577.

Schultz, A., Anderson, G., Örtengren, R., et al. (1982). Loads on the lumbar spine: Validation of a biomechanical analysis by measurements of intradiscal pressure and myoelectric signals. *J Bone Joint Surg, 64A,* 713–720.

Shono, Y., McAfee, P.C., Cunningham, B.W., et al. (1993). A biomechanical analysis of decompression and reconstruction methods in the cervical spine. Emphasis on a carbon-fiber-composite cage. *J Bone Joint Surg, 75A,* 1674–1684.

Simmons, E.H. & Bradley, D.D. (1988). Neuro-myopathic flexion deformities of the cervical spine. *Spine, 13,* 756–762.

Steel, H.H. (1968). Anatomical and mechanical considerations of atlanto-axial articulation. In Proceedings of the American Orthopaedic Association. *J Bone Joint Surg, 50A,* 1481–1482.

Sturzenegger, M., DiStefano, G., Radanov, B.P., et al. (1994). Presenting symptoms and signs after whiplash injury: The influence of accident mechanisms. *Neurology, 44,* 688–693.

Sutterlin, C.E., McAfee, P.C., Warden, K.E., et al. (1988). A biomechanical evaluation of cervical spinal stabilization methods in a bovine model. Static and cyclical loading. *Spine, 13,* 795–802.

Takebe, K., Vitti, M., & Basmajian, J.V. (1974). The functions of semispinalis capitis and splenius capitis muscles: An electromyographic study. *Anat Rec, 179,* 477–480.

Viano, D.C. & Gargan, M.F. (1996). Headrest position during normal driving: Implication to neck injury risk in rear crashes. *Accident Anal Prev, 28,* 665–674.

Voo, L.M., Kumaresan, S., Yoganandan, N., et al. (1997). Finite element analysis of cervical facetectomy. *Spine, 22,* 964–969.

Wallis, B.J., Lord, S.M., Barnsley, L., et al. (1998). The psychological profiles of patients with whiplash-associated headache. *Cephalalgia, 18,* 101–105.

Werne, S. (1957). Studies in spontaneous atlas dislocation. *Acta Orthop Scand, 23* Suppl.

White, A.A. III, Johnson, R.M., Panjabi, M.M., et al. (1975). Biomechanical analysis of clinical stability in the cervical spine. *Clin Orthop, 109,* 85–96.

White, A.A. III & Panjabi, M.M. (1990). *Clinical Biomechanics of the Spine.* Philadelphia: J.B. Lippincott.

Wittenberg, R.H., Moeller, J., & White, A.A. III (1990). Compressive strength of autogenous and allogenous bone grafts for thoracolumbar and cervical spine fusion. *Spine, 15*(10), 1073–1077.

Yang, K.H., Latouf, B.K., & King, A.I. (1992). Computer simulation of occupant neck response to airbag deployment in frontal impacts. *J Biomech Eng, 114,* 327–331.

Yoganandan, N., Kumaresan, S.C., Voo, L., et al. (1996a). Finite element modeling of the C4–C6 cervical spine unit. *Med Eng Phys, 18,* 569–574.

Yoganandan, N., Pintar, F.A., Maiman, D.J., et al. (1996b). Human head-neck biomechanics under axial tension. *Med Eng Phys, 18,* 289–294.

Yoo, J.U., Zou, D., Edwards, W.T., et al. (1992). Effect of cervical spine motion on the neuroforaminal dimensions of human cervical spine. *Spine, 17,* 1131–1136.

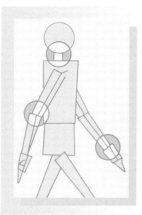

CHAPTER 12

Biomechanics of the Shoulder

Craig J. Della Valle, Andrew S. Rokito, Maureen Gallagher Birdzell,
Joseph D. Zuckerman

Introduction

The shoulder links the upper extremity to the trunk and acts in conjunction with the elbow to position the hand in space for efficient function. It consists of the glenohumeral, acromioclavicular, sternoclavicular, and scapulothoracic articulations and the musculature structures that act on them to produce the most dynamic and mobile joint in the body (Fig. 12-1). An absence of bony constraints allows a wide range of motion at the expense of stability, which is provided for instead by the various ligamentous and muscular structures.

The biomechanics of the shoulder are complex, and a complete discussion necessitates an analysis of the four aforementioned articulations that make up the shoulder complex. This chapter describes the anatomy of the various aspects of the shoulder complex and shows how their structure allows for efficient biomechanical function.

Kinematics and Anatomy

To produce the intricate motions necessary for normal functioning of the shoulder complex, the four articulations with their associated components act together in a way that produces mobility greater than that afforded by any one individual articulation. The ability of the shoulder complex to position the humerus and the remainder of the upper extremity in space is further augmented by movement of the spine. A discussion follows of the types and ranges of motion for the shoulder complex as a whole, with subsequent sections discussing the manner in which motion is achieved at each of the articulations.

RANGE OF MOTION OF THE SHOULDER COMPLEX

Shoulder range of motion is traditionally measured in terms of flexion and extension (elevation or movement of the humerus away from the side of the thorax in the sagittal plane), abduction (elevation in the coronal plane), and internal-external rotation (axial rotation of the humerus with the arm held in an adducted position) (Fig. 12-2). Although during functional activities these pure motions are rarely seen, we can better understand the complex motions of the shoulder by analyzing the separate components needed to achieve any one position.

Although forward elevation of 180° is theoretically possible, the average value in men is 167° and in women it is 171°. Extension or posterior elevation averages 60° (Boone & Azen, 1979). These values are limited by capsular torsion. Abduction in the coronal plane is limited by bony impingement of the greater tuberosity on the acromion. Forward elevation in the plane of the scapula, therefore, is considered to be more functional because in this plane the inferior portion of the capsule is not twisted and the musculature of the shoulder is optimally aligned for elevation of the arm (Fig. 12-3). Although shoulder range of motion normally decreases as part of the aging process, physical activity can counteract this process (Murray et al., 1985).

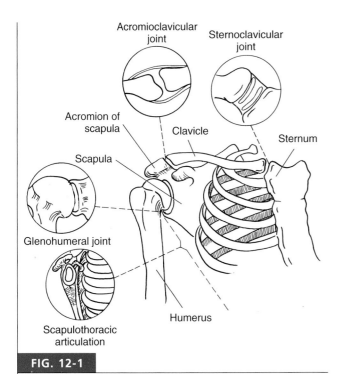

FIG. 12-1

Schematic depiction of the bony structures of the shoulder and their four articulations. The circular insets show front views of the three synovial joints—sternoclavicular, acromioclavicular, and glenohumeral—and a lateral view of the scapulothoracic joint, a bone-muscle-bone articulation. *Adapted with permission from De Palma, A.F. (1983). Biomechanics of the shoulder. In* Surgery of the Shoulder *(3rd ed., pp.65–85). Philadelphia: J.B. Lippincott.*

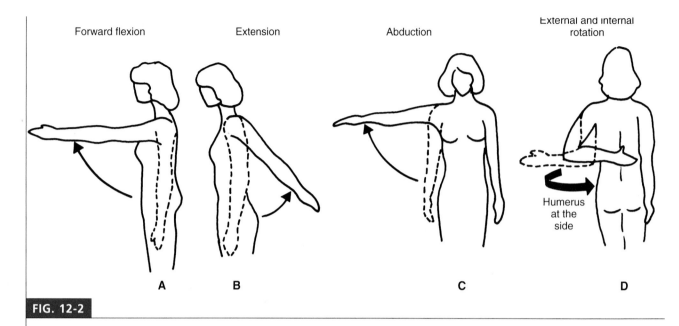

FIG. 12-2

A, Forward flexion. The humerus is in the sagittal plane. **B,** Extension. The humerus is in the sagittal plane. **C,** Abduction. The humerus is in the frontal plane. **D,** Rotation around the long axis of the humerus. External and internal rotation with the humerus at the side. Internal rotation is shown with the arm behind the back, which is a functionally important form of this motion.

STERNOCLAVICULAR JOINT

The sternoclavicular joint consists of the enlarged medial end of the clavicle and the most superolateral aspect of the manubrium, linking the upper extremity directly to the thorax. In addition, a small facet is present inferiorly that articulates with the

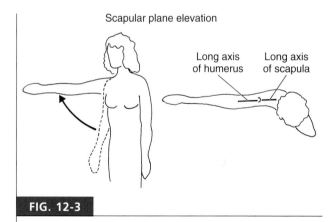

FIG. 12-3

Elevation in the scapular plane, which is midway between forward flexion and abduction. The humerus is in the plane of the scapula.

first rib. This is a true synovial joint that has a saddle-like shape and contains a fibrocartilaginous articular disc or meniscus that divides it into two compartments.

Although the joint itself has little intrinsic stability, the articular disc in conjunction with anterior, posterior, costoclavicular, and interclavicular ligaments maintains joint apposition (Fig. 12-4). The anterior and posterior sternoclavicular ligaments resist anterior and posterior translations (as well as superior displacement), while the costoclavicular ligament, which runs between the undersurface of the medial end of the clavicle and the first rib, resists upward as well as posterior displacement of the clavicle (via its anterior portion) and is thought to be the major constraint in limiting sternoclavicular motion. The interclavicular ligament connects the superomedial aspect of the clavicles and assists in restraining the joint superiorly. The posterior portion of the interclavicular ligament also assists with anterior restraint of the sternoclavicular joint. Specifically, the interclavicular ligament tightens with arm depression and is lax when the arm is elevated (Morrey & An, 1990). The disc prevents medial displacement of the clavicle, which may occur when carrying objects at the side, as well as inferior

Sternoclavicular Joint

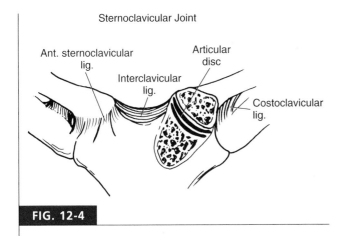

FIG. 12-4

Demonstration of the anatomy of the sternoclavicular joint. *Reprinted with permission from DeLee J. & Drez, D. (1994). Orthopaedic Sports Medicine. Principles and Practice (p. 464). Philadelphia: W.B. Saunders Co.*

displacement via articular contact. Although these structures act as important stabilizers, they still allow for significant motion including up to 50° of axial rotation and 35° of both superior-inferior elevation and anterior-posterior translation (Fig. 12-5).

ACROMIOCLAVICULAR JOINT

The acromioclavicular joint (Fig. 12-6) lies between the lateral end of the clavicle and the acromion of the scapula (the lateral and anterior extension of the scapular spine) and is subject to the high loads transmitted from the chest musculature to the upper extremity. It too is a synovial joint, but has a planar configuration. A wedge-shaped articular disc, whose function is poorly understood, is found within the joint originating from the superior aspect. Both sides of the articular surface are covered with fibrocartilage and the joint itself slopes inferomedially, causing the lateral end of the clavicle to slightly override the acromion.

A weak fibrous capsule encloses the joint and is reinforced superiorly by the acromioclavicular ligament. The acromioclavicular ligament acts primarily to restrain both axial rotation and posterior translation of the clavicle. The majority of the joint's vertical stability is provided by the coracoclavicular ligaments that suspend the scapula from the clavicle (Fukuda et al., 1986). The coracoclavicular ligaments consist of the posteromedi-

ally directed coroid and the anterolaterally directed trapezoid ligaments, which are distinct structures that serve different biomechanical functions. The smaller coroid ligament acts to limit superior-inferior displacement of the clavicle. The quadrilaterally shaped trapezoid is the larger and stronger of the two ligaments and is found lateral to the coroid; it resists axial compression or motion about a horizontal axis. The

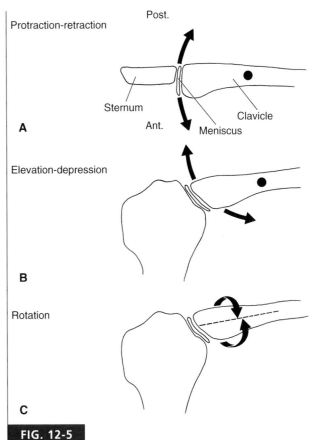

FIG. 12-5

Motion at the sternoclavicular joint. **A,** Top view showing the clavicular protraction and retraction (anteroposterior gliding) in the transverse plane around a longitudinal axis (*solid dot*) through the costoclavicular ligament, not shown. Motion takes place between the sternum and the meniscus. **B,** Anterior view showing clavicular elevation and depression (superoinferior gliding) in the frontal plane around a sagittal axis (*solid dot*) through the costoclavicular ligament, not shown. Motion occurs between the clavicle and the meniscus. **C,** Anterior view depicting the clavicular rotation around the longitudinal axis of the clavicle.

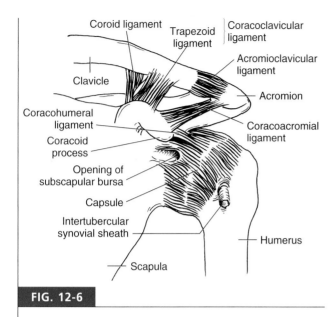

FIG. 12-6

The coracoclavicular ligament complex consists of the larger and heavier trapezoid ligament, which is oriented laterally, and the smaller coroid ligament, situated more medially. *Reproduced with permission from Hollinshead, W.H. (1969). Anatomy for Surgeons (Vol. 3). New York: Harper & Row.*

coracoacromial ligament lies on the lateral side of the acromioclavicular joint and runs from the most lateral aspect of the coracoid to the medial aspect of the acromion.

Although clavicular rotation does occur with arm elevation, Rockwood (1975) found little relative motion between the clavicle and acromion. This has been attributed to synchronous clavicular and scapular rotation with little resultant relative motion at the acromioclavicular joint; the majority of scapulothoracic motion occurs via the sternoclavicular joint. Thus, rigid fixation or fusion of the acromioclavicular joint produces little loss of overall shoulder function while sternoclavicular fixation leads to restricted motion or, more commonly, implant failure.

CLAVICLE

The clavicle lies between the two aforementioned articulations, acting as a strut connecting the thorax to the upper extremity. It is an S-shaped, double-curved bone: the medial two thirds of the body convex anteriorly while the lateral end is concave. It protects the underlying brachial plexus and

vascular structures and serves as an attachment site for many of the muscles that act on the shoulder. The clavicle also provides for the normal appearance and contour of the upper chest. Elevation of the upper extremity is accompanied by rotation as well as elevation of the clavicle, with approximately 4° of clavicular elevation for every 10° of arm elevation, with the majority of this motion occurring at the sternoclavicular joint (Inman, Saunders, & Abbott, 1944).

GLENOHUMERAL JOINT AND RELATED STRUCTURES

Although motion at the acromioclavicular, sternoclavicular, and scapulothoracic articulations is vital to the overall function of the shoulder complex, the central player is the glenohumeral joint. The articular surface of the proximal humerus forms a 120° arc and is covered with hyaline cartilage as is the glenoid fossa. The humeral head is retroverted or posteriorly directed 30° with respect to the intercondylar plane of the distal humerus and has an upward or medial inclination of 45°; this configuration gives the humerus an overall more anterior and lateral orientation (Fig. 12-7). The greater and lesser tuberosities lie lateral to the articular surface of the proximal humerus that serves as the attachment site for the rotator cuff musculature. The long head of the biceps tendon traverses the bicipital groove

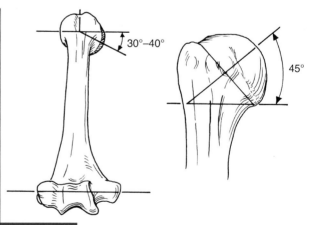

FIG. 12-7

The two-dimensional orientation of the articular surface of the humerus with respect to the bicondylar axis. *Reprinted with permission from Rockwood, C. & Matsen, F. (1990). The Shoulder (p. 219). Philadelphia: W.B. Saunders Co.*

(which lies between the tuberosities) beneath the transverse humeral ligament (Fig. 12-8).

The proximal humerus articulates with the glenoid fossa, which itself is retroverted 7° and superiorly inclined 5° relative to the plane of the scapula (Fig. 12-9, *A & B*). This slight superior inclination provides a significant degree of geometric stability, helping to resist inferior subluxation or dislocation (Itoi et al., 1992). The glenoid fossa is shallow and is able to contain only approximately one third of the diameter of humeral head. The bony architecture is augmented by the cartilaginous surface, which is thicker peripherally than it is centrally, acting to slightly but significantly increase the depth of the

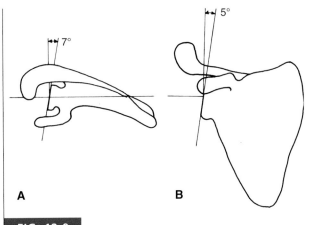

A   **B**

FIG. 12-9

A, The glenoid is retroverted 7° with respect to the plane perpendicular to the scapular plane. **B,** The glenoid faces superiorly approximately 5°. *Reprinted with permission from Simon, S.R. (Ed). (1994). Orthopaedic Basic Science (p. 526–527). Rosemont, IL: AAOS.*

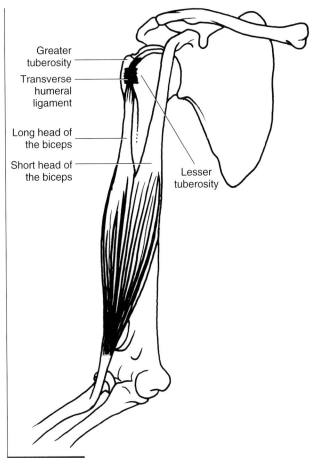

Greater tuberosity

Transverse humeral ligament

Long head of the biceps

Short head of the biceps

Lesser tuberosity

FIG. 12-8

The long head of the biceps goes in the bicipital groove between the greater and lesser tuberosities. The transverse humeral ligament helps stabilize the biceps tendon in the groove. *Reprinted with permission from Neer, C. (1990). Shoulder Reconstruction (p. 29). Philadelphia: W.B. Saunders Co.*

glenoid as a whole. Although the congruity between the articular surfaces of the proximal humerus and glenoid was previously thought to be somewhat imprecise, stereophotogrammetric studies (whereby a fine grid is projected onto an object that is then photographed from two different directions in the context of known reference targets, allowing for a three-dimensional reconstruction) have shown this articulation to be precise, with the deviation from sphericity of the convex humeral articular surface and concave glenoid articular surface being less than 1% (Soslowsky et al., 1992). Less than 1.5 mm of translation of the humeral head on the glenoid surface has been demonstrated in normal subjects during a 30° arc of motion (Poppen & Walker, 1976); thus, motion at the glenohumeral joint is almost purely rotational. Given the paucity of bony constraint, stability is instead provided by the capsular, ligamentous, and muscular structures that surround the glenohumeral joint.

Glenoid Labrum

The glenoid labrum (Fig. 12-10) is a fibrocartilaginous rim that acts to deepen the glenoid, providing 50% of the overall depth of the glenohumeral joint (Warner, 1993). It has a triangular configuration when viewed in cross-section and has firm attach-

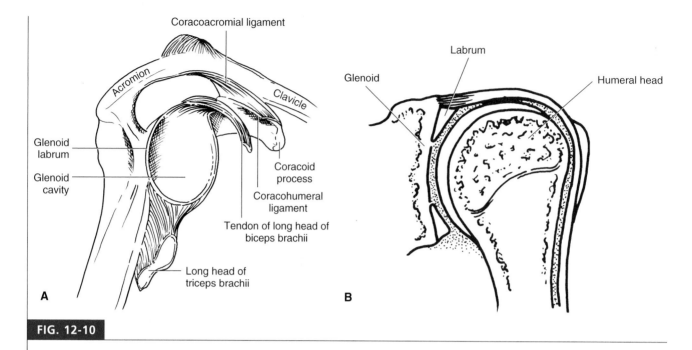

FIG. 12-10

A, The glenoid labrum is attached to the underlying bony glenoid and is confluent at its area with the long head of the biceps tendon. **B,** The labrum has a triangular configuration when viewed in cross-section and serves to effectively deepen the glenoid, increasing the stability of the gleno-humeral joint.

ments inferiorly to the underlying bone, having more variable and looser attachments in its superior and anterosuperior portions. The superior portion of the glenoid labrum is confluent with the tendon of the long head of the biceps and, along with the adjacent supraglenoid tubercle, serves as its site of insertion (Moore, 1999).

Measurements of the force needed to dislocate the humeral head under constant compressive pressure have shown that with an intact labrum, the humeral head resists tangential forces of approximately 60% of the compressive load; resection of the labrum reduces the effectiveness of compression-stabilization by 20% (Lippitt et al., 1993). Detachment of the superior labrum with anterior-posterior extension (i.e., "SLAP lesion") can occur from traction (repetitive overhead activities or a sudden pull on the arm) or compression (a fall onto an outstretched arm). This lesion can be a cause of severe pain and shoulder instability (Itoi, Hsu, & An, 1996) as a result of significant increases in glenohumeral translation when compared with the intact shoulder (Pagnani et al., 1995). (Fig. 12-11).

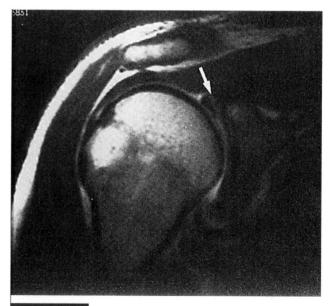

FIG. 12-11

Oblique coronal image showing a tear involving the insertion of the long head of the biceps tendon and the superior labrum (*arrow*).

Joint Capsule

The glenohumeral joint capsule has a significant degree of inherent laxity with a surface area that is twice that of the humeral head (Warner, 1993). This redundancy allows for a wide range of motion. Medially, the capsule attaches both directly onto (anteroinferiorly) and beyond the glenoid labrum and laterally it reaches to the anatomical neck of the humerus. Superiorly, it is attached at the base of the coracoid, enveloping the long head of the biceps tendon and making it an intra-articular structure (Fig. 12-11).

The capsule also has a stabilizing role, tightening with various arm positions. In adduction, the capsule is taut superiorly and lax inferiorly; with abduction of the upper extremity, this relationship is reversed and the inferior capsule tightens. As the arm is externally rotated, the anterior capsule tightens while internal rotation induces tightening posteriorly. The posterior capsule in particular has been shown to be crucial in maintaining glenohumeral stability, acting as a secondary restraint to anterior dislocation (particularly in positions of abduction) as well as acting as a primary posterior stabilizing structure (Itoi, Hsu, & An, 1996).

Glenohumeral and Coracohumeral Ligaments

The three glenohumeral ligaments (superior, middle, and inferior) are discrete extensions of the anterior glenohumeral joint capsule and are critical to shoulder stability and function (Fig. 12-12). The superior glenohumeral ligament originates from the anterosuperior labrum, just anterior to the long head of the biceps, and inserts onto the lesser tuberosity. It is present in the majority of shoulders but only well developed in 50%. The superior glenohumeral ligament acts as the main restraint to inferior translation with the arm in the resting or adducted position (Warner et al., 1992).

The coracohumeral ligament originates from the lateral side of the base of the coracoid to insert on the anatomical neck of the humerus (Fig. 12-6) (Cooper et al., 1993). This structure lies anterior to the superior glenohumeral ligament and reinforces the superior aspect of the joint capsule. These ligaments span the rotator interval between the subscapularis and supraspinatus. Some research indicates that these structures have a secondary role in preventing inferior translation of the shoulder while in the adducted, neutrally rotated position. The functional significance of the coracohumeral ligament, however, seems to be related to the overall development of the glenohumeral ligaments in a given individual, having a larger role in those with a less-developed superior glenohumeral ligament (Warner et al., 1992).

The middle glenohumeral ligament originates inferior to the superior glenohumeral ligament (at the 1 o'clock to 3 o'clock position, right shoulder) and inserts further laterally on the lesser tuberosity. Great variability in the anatomy of this structure has been demonstrated, being absent in as many as 30% of shoulders (Curl & Warren, 1996). It may originate from the anterosuperior portion of the labrum, the supraglenoid tubercle, or the scapular neck. Morphological variants have been described, including a cord-like variant (clearly distinct from the anterior band of the inferior glenohumeral ligament) and a sheet-like variant (blending with the anterior band of the inferior glenohumeral ligament). Functionally, the middle glenohumeral ligament acts as a secondary restraint to inferior translations of the glenohumeral joint with the arm in the abducted and externally rotated position (Warner et al., 1992). It also serves as a restraint to anterior translation, having its maximal effect with the arm abducted 45°.

The inferior glenohumeral ligament originates from the inferior aspect of the labrum and inserts on the anatomical neck of the humerus. It has been shown to have three distinct components (O'Brien et al., 1990): an anterior band originating from 2 to 4 o'clock (right shoulder), a posterior component originating from 7 to 9 o'clock (right shoulder), and an axillary pouch (Fig. 12-12). The inferior glenohumeral ligament has the greatest functional significance, acting as the primary anterior stabilizer of the shoulder with the arm in 90° of abduction. As the arm is abducted and externally rotated, the anterior band of the inferior glenohumeral ligament tightens, resisting anterior translation. With internal rotation of the abducted arm, the posterior band becomes taut and posterior translation is resisted. The inferior gleno-humeral ligament complex also serves to resist inferior translation of the glenohumeral joint with the arm in the abducted position. Variability as to the size and attachment sites of the glenohumeral ligaments has been demonstrated (Warner et al., 1992); however, the clinical significance of this has yet to be fully elucidated although it has been suggested that absence of the middle glenohumeral ligament may predispose to instability (Steinbeck et al., 1998).

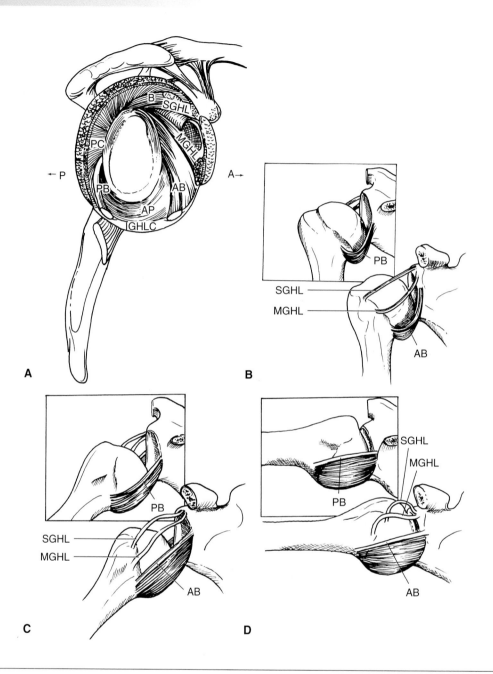

FIG: 12-12

A, Schematic drawing of the shoulder capsule illustrating the location and extent of the inferior glenohumeral ligament complex (IGHLC). *A,* anterior; *P,* posterior; *B,* biceps tendon; *SGHL,* superior glenohumeral ligament; *MGHL,* middle gleno-humeral ligament; *AB,* anterior band; *AP,* axillary pouch; *PB,* posterior band; *PC,* posterior capsule. *Reprinted with permission from O'Brien, S.J., Neves, M.C., Amoczky, S.P., et al. (1990). The anatomy and histology of the inferior glenohumeral ligament complex of the shoulder.* Am J Sports Med, 18, 579–584. **B,** The superior glenohumeral ligament is the primary restraint to inferior translation in the adducted shoulder at neutral rotation. In this position, the middle glenohumeral ligament and the anterior and posterior bands of the inferior gleno-

humeral ligament complex remain lax. **C,** The anterior band is the primary restraint resisting inferior translation of the shoulder at 45° abduction and neutral rotation. In this position, the superior glenohumeral ligament, the middle gleno-humeral ligament, and posterior band are lax. **D,** At 90° ab-duction, the anterior and posterior bands of the inferior glenohumeral ligament cradle the humeral head to prevent inferior translation. The posterior band is more significant in external rotation, whereas the anterior band plays a greater role in internal rotation. *Reprinted with permission from Warner, J.P., Deng, X.H., Warren, R.F., et al. (1992). Static capsuloligamen-tous restraints to superior-inferior translations of the glenohumeral joint.* Am J Sports Med, 20, 675–678.

Experimental Techniques: Ligament Cutting Studies

Ligament cutting studies have been instrumental in furthering our knowledge regarding the contribution of a given anatomical structure to overall glenohumeral stability (Curl & Warren, 1996). In this technique, cadaveric specimens are biomechanically tested before and after selectively cutting sequential structures. A force is then applied in a given arm position, and the translation that occurs is measured. From this information, the relative contribution that a given structure provides to overall stability can be determined. When a particular pattern of shoulder instability is then identified, the physician can infer which anatomical structures may be deficient or disrupted so that a rational plan of physical therapy or surgical repair can be implemented.

Additional Constraints to Glenohumeral Stability

Synovial fluid acts via cohesion and adhesion to further stabilize the glenohumeral joint. Synovial fluid adheres to the articular cartilage overlying the glenoid and proximal humerus, causing the two surfaces to slide along one another. The synovial fluid provides a cohesive force between these two, making it difficult to pull them apart (Simon, 1994). Under normal conditions, the intra-articular pressure within the glenohumeral joint is negative, acting to pull the overlying capsule and glenohumeral ligaments inward. If the integrity of the glenohumeral joint capsule is compromised (e.g., venting the capsule) or if a significant effusion exists (normally the glenohumeral joint contains less than 1 cc of fluid), significant increases in translation are observed (Kumar & Balasubramaniam, 1985). Specifically, venting the capsule reduces the force needed for anterior humeral head translation by 55%, for posterior translation by 43%, and for inferior translation by 57% (Gibb et al., 1991) (Case Study 12-1).

SCAPULOTHORACIC ARTICULATION

The scapula is a flat, triangular bone that lies on the posterolateral aspect of the thorax between the second and seventh ribs. It is angled 30° anterior to the coronal plane of the thorax and is rotated slightly toward the midline at its superior end and tilted anteriorly with respect to the sagittal plane

CASE STUDY 12-1

Shoulder Instability

A 21-year-old man fell while skiing onto his right upper extremity, causing forceful abduction and external rotation. He noted acute pain in the arm and was unable to move it. Physical examination revealed loss of the normal contour of the shoulder and painful range of motion. Radiographs showed an anterior dislocation with posterior superior humeral head impaction fracture. The patient underwent closed reduction. Postreduction radiographs confirmed reduction of the humeral head with a small bony avulsion fracture of the anterior-inferior glenoid rim, which represents a detachment of the anterior labrum in the area of the superior band of the glenohumeral ligament insertion (Case Study Figure 12-1-1).

Structural alteration of bony geometry, ligaments, and labrum resulted in shoulder instability. The detachment of the anterior labrum and the superior band of the ligament insertion affected primarily the resistance to anterior translation of the humeral head, resulting in anterior dislocation. In addition, a concomitant capsule lesion affected the intra-articular negative pressure necessary to pull the humeral head inward. After conservative management, the patient did well for 6 months until he sustained a recurrent dislocation. The patient subsequently opted for operative treatment that included repair of the fracture and capsule and a complete period of rehabilitation with emphasis on joint stability and proprioception.

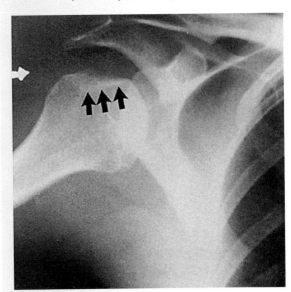

Case Study Figure 12-1-1.

(Fig. 12-13) (Laumann, 1987). The spine of the scapula gives rise laterally to the acromion process that articulates with the distal clavicle at the acromioclavicular joint. The coracoclavicular ligaments and muscular attachments help to support the scapula and stabilize it against the thorax (Fig. 12-6). There is, however, no osseous connection with the axial skeleton. This allows for a wide range of scapular motion, including protraction, retraction, elevation, depression, and rotation.

The scapulothoracic articulation involves gliding of the scapula on the posterior aspect of the thorax. Interposed between the scapula and the thoracic wall lie the subscapularis (arising from the costal surface of the body of the scapula) and the serratus anterior, which help to stabilize the scapula against the chest wall and thus prevent "scapular winging" (Fig. 12-14). These two muscles glide along one another to provide greatly enhanced mobility of the shoulder complex as a whole.

Elevation of the arm involves motion at both the glenohumeral joint and the scapulothoracic articulation. Although the contribution from each varies according to arm position and the specific task being performed, the average ratio of glenohumeral to scapulothoracic motion is 2:1 (Tibone et al., 1994). Elevation of the arm also induces complex rotatory motion of the scapula, with anterior rotation during the first 90° followed by posterior rotation with a total arc of approximately 15° (Morrey & An, 1990).

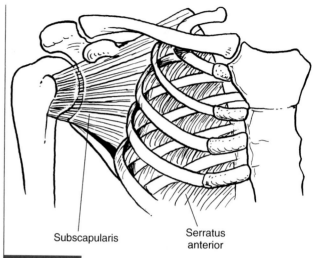

Subscapularis   Serratus anterior

FIG. 12-14

Anterior view of the scapulothoracic articulation, a bone-muscle-bone articulation between the scapula and thorax. During scapular motion, the subscapularis muscle, which attaches broadly to the costal surface of the scapula, glides on the serratus anterior muscle, which originates on the first eight ribs and inserts into the costal surface of the scapula along the length of its vertebral border.

SPINAL CONTRIBUTION TO SHOULDER MOTION

Although often overlooked, motion of the thoracic and lumbar spine contributes to the ability to position the upper extremity in space, thereby enhancing the overall motion and function of the shoulder complex. Flexion of the spine away from an extremity attempting to reach an object overhead enhances the range of motion attainable (Fig. 12-15). The importance of spinal motion in overhead activities such as throwing and racquet sports has also been demonstrated.

Kinetics

Numerous muscles act on the various components of the shoulder complex to provide both mobility and dynamic stability. Dynamic stabilization occurs via several possible mechanisms (Moffey & An, 1990), including passive muscle tension, or via a barrier effect of the contracted muscle, compressive forces brought about by muscular contraction, joint motion that induces tightening of

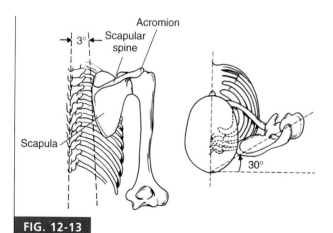

Acromion
Scapular spine
3°
Scapula
30°

FIG. 12-13

Scapular orientation on the chest wall. *Left,* 30° anterior. *Right,* 3° upward. Reprinted with permission from Warner JJP: The gross anatomy of the joint surfaces, ligaments, labrum, and capsule. In: Matsen, F.A., Fu, F.H., Hawkins, R.J. (Eds.) The Shoulder: A Balance of Mobility and Stability. Rosemont, IL: American Academy of Orthopaedic Surgeons, 1993.

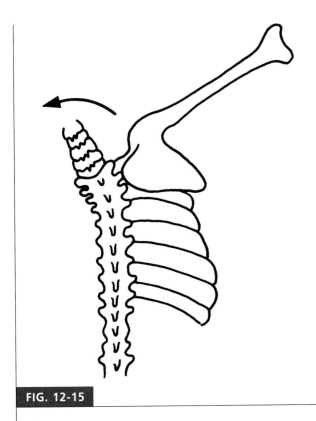

Lateral bending of the spine enhances the ability to position the upper extremity. *Reprinted with permission from Rockwood, C. & Matsen, F. (1990). The Shoulder (p. 219). Philadelphia: W.B. Saunders Co.*

activated differently for specific activities. The deltoid originates from the lateral third of the clavicle, acromion, and scapular spine and inserts on the anterolateral aspect of the humerus. The anterior head acts as a strong flexor and internal rotator of the humerus, the middle head as an abductor, and the posterior head as an extensor and external rotator. The pectoralis major lies over the anterior chest wall and has two heads, a clavicular head originating from the side of the clavicle and a sternocostal head originating from the sternum, manubrium, and the upper costal cartilages. The two heads converge at the sternoclavicular joint. The pectoralis major inserts at the intertubercular groove of the humerus between the tuberosities and acts to adduct and internally rotate the humerus. Secondarily, the clavicular head acts as a flexor or forward elevator of the humerus while the sternocostal head extends the humerus. The pectoralis minor lies deep to the pectoralis major, functioning as an important scapular stabilizer. The pennate subclavius muscle lies inferior to the clavicle and may assist in clavicular motions. It has a tendinous origin from the anteromedial aspect of the first rib and inserts on

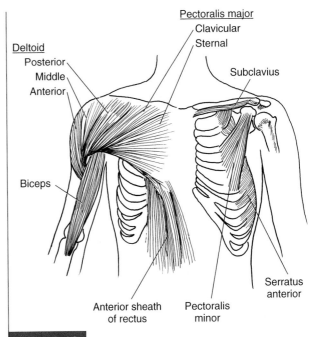

Anterior view showing the superficial muscles (left shoulder) and the deep muscles beneath the deltoid and pectoralis muscles (right shoulder).

the passive or ligamentous constraints, or via a redirection of the joint force toward the center of the glenoid.

To understand muscle function and force transmission, one must consider a given muscle's orientation, size, and activity. Given the multiple articulations present in the shoulder complex, any given muscle may span several different joints, and depending on the position of the upper extremity, its relationship with regard to any one articulation may change, altering its effect on that joint and the resultant forces or motions produced.

MUSCULAR ANATOMY

The shoulder musculature can be thought of in layers. The outermost layer consists of the deltoid and pectoralis major muscles (Fig. 12-16). The deltoid forms the normal, rounded contour of the shoulder and is triangular in shape, with anterior, middle, and posterior heads. Each portion of the deltoid is the undersurface of the medial clavicle (Morrey & An, 1990).

Beneath this outer layer lies the rotator cuff musculature: the supraspinatus, infraspinatus, subscapularis, and teres minor (Fig.12-17). These four muscles act to abduct and rotate the humerus and act as important glenohumeral stabilizers via both passive muscle tension and dynamic contraction. The supraspinatus originates from the supraspinatus fossa of the scapula and inserts on the greater tuberosity of the proximal humerus. It forms a force couple with the deltoid during abduction of the humerus. The infraspinatus and teres minor originate from the inferior aspect of the scapula and insert on the greater tuberosity. These muscles act as external rotators of the humerus. The subscapularis lies on the costal surface of the scapula and inserts on the lesser tuberosity of the proximal humerus. It functions as an important internal rotator of the humerus. The subscapularis, along with the middle and inferior glenohumeral ligaments, has also been shown to act as an important anterior stabilizer of the glenohumeral joint, particularly with the arm held at 45° of abduction. The teres major muscle (Fig. 12-18), while not part of the rotator cuff, also originates from the scapula, but at its inferior angle coursing inferior to the teres minor and then passing anteriorly to insert on the humerus at the intertubercular groove. It functions to assist with arm adduction and internal rotation.

The biceps muscle is also involved with motion of the shoulder complex. It is composed of two heads: a short head that originates from the tip of the coracoid process of the scapula and a long head that originates from the superior glenoid labrum and supraglenoid tubercle (Fig. 12-8). The tendon of the long head of the biceps lies within the glenohumeral joint and descends between the greater and lesser tuberosities, joining the short head to insert on the bicipital tuberosity of the radius. The biceps functions to flex and supinate the forearm and elevates the humerus. The long head of the biceps also acts as a humeral head depressor and, as such, plays a role in maintaining glenohumeral stability (Itoi et al., 1994).

Several muscles lie on the back and act directly on the scapula (Fig. 12-18). The outermost layer consists of the trapezium that covers the posterior neck and uppermost portion of the trunk, inserting on the superior aspect of the lateral one third of the clavicle, acromion, and scapular spine. The trapez-

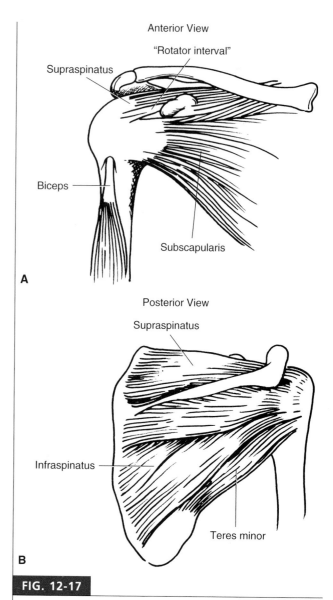

A, Anterior view. The "rotator interval" is a term introduced in 1970 to indicate the space between the supraspinatus and subscapularis tendons. The coracohumeral ligament lies superficially along its anterior edge, where it is readily available for release as indicated. The long head of the biceps lies deep along its posterior edge and serves as a guide to this interval during surgery. *Reprinted with permission from Neer, C. (1990). Shoulder Reconstruction (p. 29). Philadelphia: W.B. Saunders Co.* **B,** Posterior view. The two external rotators of the humerus, the infraspinatus and teres minor muscles, which are also the posterior wall of the rotator cuff. Note the median raphe of the infraspinatus, which is often mistaken at surgery for the border between the infraspinatus and the teres minor. *Reprinted with permission from Rockwood, C. & Matsen, F. (1990). The Shoulder (p. 219). Philadelphia: W.B. Saunders Co.*

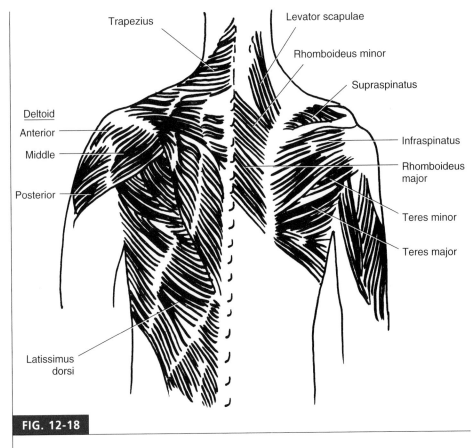

FIG. 12-18

Posterior view showing the superficial muscles (left shoulder) and underlying muscles (right shoulder).

ium serves to elevate, retract, and rotate the scapula. The latissimus dorsi covers the inferior portion of the back, inserting on the intertubercular groove of the humerus. It acts to extend, adduct, and internally rotate the humerus.

Below these muscles lie the levator scapulae superiorly, which elevate and inferiorly rotate the scapula, and the rhomboid muscles below, which retract and rotate the scapula. Both of these muscle groups act to assist the serratus anterior (which lies laterally on the chest and intercostal muscles inserting onto the medial border of the anterior surface of the scapula) in keeping the scapula fixed to the trunk.

INTEGRATED MUSCULAR ACTIVITY OF THE SHOULDER COMPLEX

Electromyography allows for the quantification of muscular activity during dynamic conditions. This permits insight into the level of muscular ac-

tivity but does not directly indicate forces generated. A complete understanding of the latter requires knowledge of the moment arm (measured as the distance between the instantaneous center of rotation of the joint and the distance of muscular pull) and the physiological cross-section of the involved muscle (measured as the muscular volume divided by its length). In the shoulder complex, each motion is associated with movement at multiple articulations and the constantly changing relationships of the muscular origins and insertions.

Given the paucity of osseous stability at the glenohumeral joint, force generated by one muscle (the primary agonist) requires the activation of an antagonistic muscle so that a dislocating force does not result (Simon, 1994). The antagonist usually accomplishes this via an eccentric contraction whereby the muscle is lengthened while actively contracting or via the production of a neutralizing force of equal magnitude but in the opposite direction. The relationship between two such muscles is also referred to as a force couple (Fig. 12-19). Around the glenohumeral joint, there is a force couple in the coronal plane (between the deltoid and the inferior portion of the rotator cuff) and in the transverse plane between the subscapularis muscle anteriorly and the posterior rotator cuff musculature (the infraspinatus and teres minor).

Relative motion is produced by an imbalance between the agonist and antagonist that produces torque. The degree of torque and the resultant angular velocity produced is determined by the relative activation of two such muscles or muscle groups. Resultant muscular forces are determined via an understanding of the cross-sectional area of the activated muscles involved and their orientation at the time of activation.

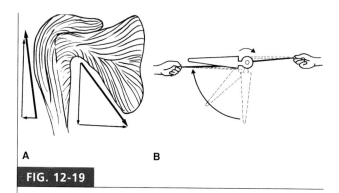

A   **B**

FIG. 12-19

The deltoid and the oblique rotator cuff muscles (infraspinatus, subscapularis, and teres minor) combine to produce elevation of the upper extremity by means of a force couple (two forces equal in magnitude but opposite in direction). With the arm at the side (**A**), the directional force of the deltoid is upward and outward with respect to the humerus while the force of the oblique rotator cuff muscles is downward and inward. These two rotational forces can be resolved into their respective vertical and horizontal components. The horizontal force of the deltoid acting below the center of rotation of the glenohumeral joint is opposite in direction to the horizontal force of the oblique rotators, which is applied above the center of rotation. These forces acting in opposite directions on either side of the center of rotation produce a powerful force couple, as illustrated by the arm signal (**B**). The vertical forces offset each other, thereby stabilizing the humeral head on the glenoid and allowing elevation to take place. *Adapted with permission from Lucas, D.B. (1973). Biomechanics of the shoulder joint. Arch Surg, 107, 425.*

Forward Elevation

The most basic motion of the shoulder complex involves elevation of the arm in the scapular plane. This motion has been studied in depth via both electromyography and stereophotogrammetry. The muscles of the shoulder girdle have subsequently been grouped according to relative importance with regard to this motion. The first grouping includes the deltoid (specifically the anterior and middle heads), trapezium (inferior portion), supraspinatus, and serratus anterior (Simon, 1994). The second grouping consists of the middle portion of the trapezium, the infraspinatus, and the long head of the biceps. A third group consists of the posterior head of the deltoid, the clavicular head of the pectoralis major, and the superior portion of the trapezium. The fourth and final group includes the sternal head of the pectoralis major, the latissimus dorsi, and the long head of the triceps.

The inter-relationship between the muscular forces involved in shoulder elevation was first studied by Inman, who found that the deltoid and supraspinatus work synergistically while the remainder of the rotator cuff musculature provides a humeral depressing force to counter subluxation of the humeral head (Inman, Saunders, & Abbott, 1944). Thus, the vertically oriented pull of the deltoid is offset by a net inferior force created by the infraspinatus, subscapularis, and teres minor.

Electromyographic studies have shown that both the supraspinatus and deltoid are active throughout the range of arm elevation. The supraspinatus, however, is felt to have a larger role in initiating abduction. As the arm is progressively elevated from the side, the moment arm of the deltoid improves, resulting in a larger force in relation to the supraspinatus (Fig. 12-20). The percentage of shearing or vertical force created by the deltoid likewise decreases with increasing amounts of abduction. The angle of pull of the supraspinatus is more constant at approximately 75°, acting not only to elevate or abduct the arm but also to compress the humeral head within the glenoid. The remaining rotator cuff muscles pull at approximately 45°, which is directed inferiorly (slightly higher in the teres minor at 55°), resulting in forces that equally compress and depress the humeral head to maintain glenohumeral stability (Fig. 12-21).

Selective anesthetic block of the axillary nerve (and resulting deltoid paralysis) demonstrates that forward elevation is possible albeit significantly weakened. Likewise, a suprascapular nerve block

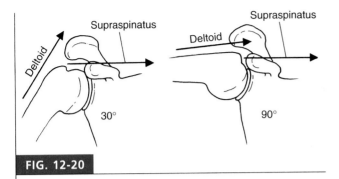

FIG. 12-20

As the arm is abducted to 90°, the direction of pull of the deltoid approximates that of the supraspinatus. Therefore, patients with a large tear of the rotator cuff often can actively maintain the arm abducted to 90° but may not be capable of actively abducting to 90°. *Reprinted with permission from Simon, S.R. (Ed). (1994). Orthopaedic Basic Science (p. 527). Rosemont, IL: AAOS.*

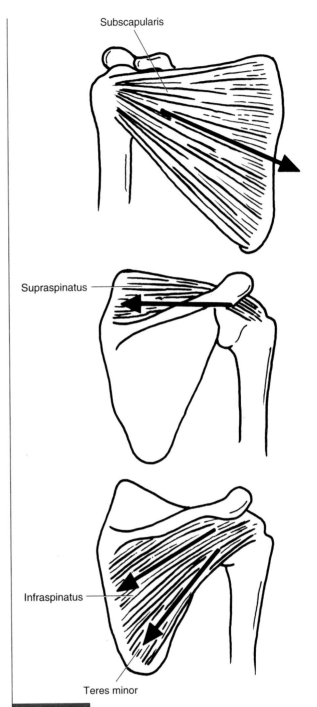

FIG. 12-21

The angle of pull of the subscapularis (*top*) is approximately 45°. The angle of pull of the infraspinatus (*bottom*) is also approximately 45°, and the teres minor (*bottom*) is approximately 55°. These vectors result in nearly equal glenohumeral joint compression and humeral head depression. The supraspinatus (*center*) is essentially horizontal in its orientation, resulting in compression of the glenohumeral joint.

and the resultant supraspinatus paralysis induced has a similar effect. However, a block of both nerves results in a loss of arm elevation (Colachis, & Strohm, 1971; Howell et al., 1986) (Case Study 12-2).

When pure abduction is compared with pure forward elevation, the same basic relationships are seen with the rotator cuff acting to stabilize the glenohumeral joint while the deltoid provides the necessary torque. Forward flexion results in activation of the anterior and middle deltoid (73 and 62% activity, respectively) with stability provided mainly by the supraspinatus, infraspinatus, and latissimus dorsi, the latter being particularly active (25% activation) with forward flexion beyond 90°. Pure abduction requires similar muscular activity; however, the subscapularis shows increased activation as it acts as the prime stabilizer via eccentric contraction.

External Rotation

The primary external rotator of the humerus is the infraspinatus, with significant contributions made by the posterior head of the deltoid and the teres minor. With any given amount of shoulder abduction, electromyography reveals the prime external rotator to be the infraspinatus. The subscapularis is similarly active but serves an antagonistic role as the main stabilizer preventing anterior displacement of

Subacromial Impingement Syndrome and Rotator Cuff Tear

A 63-year-old right-hand-dominant woman who presents right shoulder pain of 6 months' duration. The patient noted increasing pain at night and with overhead activities of daily living such as putting on a shirt and brushing her hair. The pain is unresponsive to pain killers. Physical examination revealed diffuse tenderness over the shoulder and deltoid with painful forward elevation above 60° and internal rotation limited to her ipsilateral greater trochanter. She had a positive Neer sign (painful forward elevation between 60 and 120°) and a positive Hawkins sign (pain with passive abduction and internal rotation). A subacromial impingement test was positive with near complete relief of pain and restoration of forward elevation to 150° but persistent weakness on resisted shoulder abduction. A diagnosis of subacromial impingement syndrome is made. The patient was initially managed with conservative treatment. At 6 weeks follow-up, the patient had persistent pain and an MRI of her shoulder revealed a full thickness tear of the supraspinatus tendon. The patient opted for operative management (Case Study Fig.12-1-1).

Biomechanically, rotator cuff tears have been likened to a suspension bridge, whereby the free margin of the tear corresponds to the cable and the residual attachments correspond to the supports at each end of the cable's span. This configuration allows the muscle that has been torn at its insertion to still exert its effects by way of the "spans" of the bridge. Thus, patients may have a "functional" rotator cuff tear in which they are still able to perform overhead activities. If the tearing force present at the two supports is great enough, however, worsening of the tear will occur.

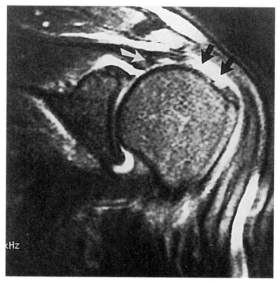

Case Study Figure 12-2-1.

the humeral head with external rotation. As the amount of shoulder abduction is increased, the posterior deltoid increases in efficiency as an accessory external rotator of the humerus secondary to improvement of its moment arm.

Internal Rotation

Internal rotation of the shoulder is accomplished by the subscapularis, sternal head of the pectoralis major, latissimus dorsi, and teres major. The subscapularis is active during all phases of internal rotation, with decreased relative activity seen with extremes of abduction. In the same way, activity of the sternal head of the pectoralis major and the latissimus dorsi decreases with abduction. However, the posterior and middle heads of the deltoid compensate with increased eccentric activity during internal rotation while the arm is abducted.

Extension

Extension of the upper extremity is accomplished by the posterior and middle heads of the deltoid. The supraspinatus and subscapularis are also continually active throughout arm extension, resisting forces via eccentric activity that would tend to cause anterior dislocation.

Scapulothoracic Motion

Motion at the scapulothoracic articulation allows maintenance of deltoid tension, allowing it to maintain optimal power regardless of arm position. With forward elevation at the arm, the scapula rotates, increasing stability at the glenohumeral joint and decreasing the tendency for impingement of the rotator cuff beneath the acromion (Fig. 12-22). A rotational force couple (two equal, noncollinear, parallel but oppositely direct forces) between the upper trapezium, levator scapulae, and upper serratus anterior with concomitant contraction of the lower trapezium and serratus anterior leads to scapular rotation that is necessary for full forward elevation (Fig. 12-23) (Simon, 1994).

LOADS AT THE GLENOHUMERAL JOINT

The glenohumeral joint is considered to be a major load-bearing joint. Although calculations of the exact forces acting on it are challenging given the large number of involved muscular structures and possible positions attainable, several simplifying assumptions allow an estimation of the magnitude of these forces. A free-body diagram of a person holding the upper extremity held at 90° of abduction can be utilized as an example; it is assumed that only the deltoid muscle is active and that it acts at a distance of 3 cm from the center of rotation of the humeral head. Three forces are then considered: the deltoid muscle force (D), the weight of the arm (equivalent to 0.05 body weight [BW] acting at the center of gravity of the limb, 3 cm), and the joint-reactive force at the glenohumeral joint (J). The joint reactive force and the force of the deltoid, being nearly parallel, are considered to be a force couple and are of equal but opposite magnitude. The force on the glenohumeral joint when holding the arm at 90° of abduction can be estimated to be one-half of body weight (Calculation Box 12-1, Case A). If a weight (W) of 2 kg is added (equivalent to 0.025 body weight of an 80-kg male) to the hand of the outstretched extremity held at 90° of abduction, a similar calculation can be made (Calculation Box 12-1, Case B).

Experimentally, loads at the glenohumeral joint and the forces necessary for arm elevation have been determined. These forces have been found to be greatest at 90° of elevation, with the deltoid force equivalent to 8.2 times the weight of the arm and

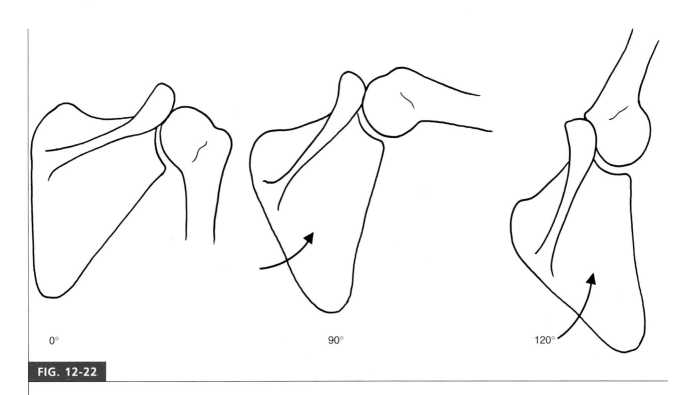

0°   90°   120°

FIG. 12-22

Forward elevation or abduction 0–120° of the arm requires synchronous rotation of the scapula. *Reprinted with permission from Simon, S.R. (Ed). (1994).* Orthopaedic Basic Science *(p. 527–535). Rosemont, IL: AAOS.*

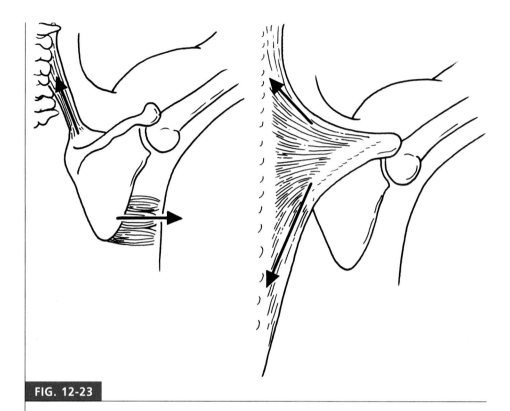

FIG. 12-23

Rotation of the scapula is produced by the synergistic contractions of the lower portion of the serratus anterior and the lower trapezius, with the upper trapezius, levator scapulae, and upper serratus anterior. *Reprinted with permission from Simon, S.R. (Ed). (1994). Orthopaedic Basic Science (p. 527–535). Rosemont, IL: AAOS.*

the joint reactive force equivalent to 10.2 times the weight of the arm (Inman, Saunders, & Abbott, 1944). More recent investigations of these same forces utilizing the assumption that the muscular force is proportional to its area multiplied by its activity as determined by electromyography have yielded similar values, with a maximal joint reactive force of 89% of body weight seen at 90° of elevation in the scapular plane (Poppen, & Walker, 1978).

THE BIOMECHANICS OF PITCHING

Pitching has been divided into five stages: wind up, early cocking, late cocking, acceleration, and follow-through (Tibone et al., 1994). The deltoid has been found to be responsible for elevation and abduction of the humerus in the early phases, followed by increased activation of the rotator cuff musculature in the late cocking phase acting both to rotate the humerus and prevent anterior subluxation of the glenohumeral joint (Bames & Tullos, 1978). Specifically, the supraspinatus acts in the late cocking phase to draw the humeral head toward the glenoid, the infraspinatus and teres minor pull the humeral head posteriorly, and the subscapularis both prevents excessive external rotation of the humerus and contracts eccentrically to relieve stress on the anterior shoulder (Tibone et al., 1994). The importance of scapular (and thus glenoid) stabilization has also been recognized, and the serratus anterior has been shown to fire actively in the late cocking phase; this provides a stable platform for humeral motion. Thus, coordinated, sequential activation of the shoulder musculature is needed to prevent anterior subluxation of the glenohumeral joint and the overuse tendinitis that can ensue.

CALCULATION BOX 12-1

Calculation of Reaction Forces

Estimates of the reaction force on the glenohumeral joint are obtained with the use of simplifying assumptions (Poppen & Walker, 1978).

Case A. In this example, the arm is in 90° of abduction, and it is assumed that only the deltoid muscle is active. The force produced through the tendon of the deltoid muscle (D) acts at a distance of 3 cm from the center of rotation of the joint (indicated by the *hollow circle*). The force produced by the weight of the arm is estimated to be 0.05 times body weight (BW) and acts at a distance of 30 cm from the center of rotation. The reaction force on the glenohumeral joint (J) may be calculated with the use of the equilibrium equation that states that for a body to be in moment equilibrium, the sum of the moments must equal zero. In this example, the moments acting clockwise are considered to be positive and counterclockwise moments are considered to be negative.

$$\Sigma M = 0$$
$$(30 \text{ cm} \times .05\text{BW}) - (D \times 3 \text{ cm}) = 0$$
$$D = \frac{30 \text{ cm} \times .05 \text{ BW}}{3 \text{ cm}}$$
$$D = 0.5 \text{ BW}$$

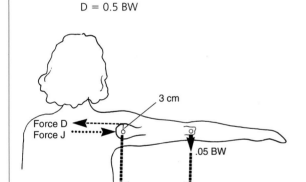

Calculation Box Figure 12-1-1.

D is approximately one-half body weight. Because D and J are almost parallel but opposite, they form a force couple and are of equal magnitude; thus, the joint reaction force is also approximately one-half body weight.

Case B. Similar calculations can be made to determine the value for D when a weight equal to 0.025 times body weight is held in the hand with the arm in 90° of abduction.

$$\Sigma M = 0$$
$$(30 \text{ cm} \times .05 \text{ BW}) + (60 \text{ cm} \times .025 \text{ BW}) - (D \times 3 \text{ cm}) = 0$$
$$D = \frac{(30 \text{ cm} \times .05 \text{ BW}) + (60 \text{ cm} \times .025 \text{ BW})}{3 \text{ cm}}$$
$$D = 1 \text{ BW}$$

Once again, D and J are essentially equal and opposite, forming a force couple. Thus, the joint reaction force is approximately equal to body weight.

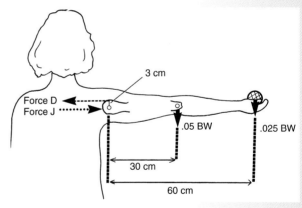

Calculation Box Figure 12-1-2.

Summary

1 The shoulder consists of the glenohumeral, acromioclavicular, sternoclavicular, and scapulothoracic articulations and the muscular structures that act on them to produce the most mobile joint in the body.

2 The sternoclavicular joint, which connects the medial end of the clavicle to the manubrium, links the upper extremity to the thorax. The articular disc within the joint and the ligaments that surround it provide stability while allowing for significant rotation of the clavicle. Little relative motion is seen between the clavicle and acromion at the acromioclavicular joint.

3 The glenohumeral joint, while known to be a precise articulation, is inherently unstable because the glenoid fossa is shallow and is able to contain only approximately one third of the diameter of the humeral head. Stability is instead provided by the capsular, muscular, and ligamentous structures that surround it.

4 The three glenohumeral ligaments (superior, middle, and inferior) are discrete extensions of the anterior glenohumeral joint capsule and are critical to shoulder stability and function.

5 The inferior glenohumeral ligament has the most functional significance (particularly the anterior band), acting as the primary anterior stabilizer of the shoulder when the arm is abducted 90°.

6 The integrity of the shoulder capsule and the negative intra-articular force it maintains also plays an integral part in maintaining shoulder stability.

7 Elevation of the arm involves motion at both the glenohumeral joint and the scapulothoracic articulation.

8 Movements of the spine assist the shoulder in positioning the upper extremity in space.

9 The muscles around the shoulder contribute to stability via a barrier effect by producing compressive forces on the glenohumeral joint and by eccentric contraction.

10 The glenohumeral joint is a major load-bearing joint with forces equivalent to one-half body weight produced when holding the arm in an outstretched position.

REFERENCES

Agur, A.M.R., Lee, M., & Grant, J.C. (1991). *Atlas of Anatomy* (9th ed.). Baltimore: Williams & Wilkins.

Bames, D.A. & Tullos, H.S. (1978). An analysis of 100 symptomatic baseball players. *Am J Sports Med, 6,* 62–67.

Boone, D.C. & Azen, S.P. (1979). Normal range of motion of joints in male subjects. *J Bone Joint Surg, 61,* 756–759.

Colachis, S.C. Jr. & Strohm, B.R. (1971). Effect of suprascapular and axillary nerve blocks on muscle force in upper extremity. *Arch Phys Med Rehabil, 52,* 22–29.

Cooper, D.E., O'Brien, S.J., Amoczky, S.P., et al. (1993). The structure and function of the coracohumeral ligament: An anatomic and microscopic study. *J Shoulder Elbow Surg, 2,* 70–77.

Curl, L.A. & Warren, R.F. (1996). Glenohumeral joint stability: Selective cutting studies on the static capsular restraints. *Clin Orthop, 330,* 54–65.

DeLee J. & Drez, D. (1994). *Orthopaedic Sports Medicine. Principles and Practice* (p. 464). Philadelphia: W.B. Saunders.

De Palma, A.F. (1983). Biomechanics of the shoulder. In *Surgery of the Shoulder* (3rd ed., pp.65–85). Philadelphia: J.B. Lippincott.

Fukuda, K., Craig, E.V., An, K., et al. (1986). Biomechanical study of the ligamentous system of the acromioclavicular joint. *J Bone Joint Surg, 68,* 434–440.

Gibb, T.D., Sidles, J.A., Harryman, D.T., et al. (1991). The effect of capsular venting on glenohumeral laxity. *Clin Orthop, 268,* 120–127.

Hollinshead, W.H. (1969). *Anatomy for Surgeons* (Vol. 3). New York: Harper & Row.

Howell, S.M., Imobersteg, A.M., Seger, D.H., et al. (1986). Clarification of the role of the supraspinatus muscle in shoulder function. *J Bone Joint Surg, 68A,* 398–404.

Inman, V.T., Saunders, J.B., & Abbott, L.C. (1944). Observations on the function of the shoulder joint. *J Bone Joint Surg, 26A,* 1–30.

Itoi, E., Hsu, H.C., & An, K.N. (1996). Biomechanical investigation of the glenohumeral joint. *J Shoulder Elbow Surg, 5,* 407–424.

Itoi, E., Motzkin, N.E., Morrey, B.F., et al. (1994). Stabilizing function of the long head of the biceps in the hanging arm position. *J Shoulder Elbow Surg, 3,* 135–142.

Itoi, E., Motzkin, N.E., Morrey, B.F., et al. (1992). Scapular inclination and inferior stability of the shoulder. *J Shoulder Elbow Surg, 1,* 131–139.

Kumar, V.P. & Balasubramaniam, P. (1985). The role of atmospheric pressure in stabilizing the shoulder: An experimental study. *J Bone Joint Surg, 67B,* 719–721.

Laumann, U. (1987). Kinesiology of the shoulder joint. In R. Kolbel, et al. (Eds.), *Shoulder Replacement.* Berlin: Springer-Verlag, 1987.

Lippitt, S.B., Vanderhooft, J.E., Harris, S.L., et al. (1993). Glenohumeral stability from concavity-compression: A quantitative analysis. *J Shoulder Elbow Surg, 2,* 27–35.

Lucas, D.B. (1973). Biomechanics of the shoulder joint. *Arch Surg, 107,* 425.

Matsen, F., Fu, F., & Hawkins, R. (Eds.) (1992). *The Shoulder: A Balance of Mobility and Stability.* Rosemont, IL: AAOS. [Vail, Colorado: Workshop Supported by the American Academy of Orthopaedic Surgeons, the National Institute of Arthritis and Musculoskeletal Skin Diseases, the American Shoulder and Elbow Surgeons, the Orthopaedic Research and Education Foundation.]

Moffey, B.F. & An, K.N. (1990). Biomechanics of the shoulder. In C.A. Rockwood & F.A. Matsen III (Eds.), *The Shoulder* (pp. 208–245). Philadelphia: W.B. Saunders.

Moore, K.L. (1999). *Clinically Oriented Anatomy* (4th ed.). Philadelphia: Lippincott Williams & Wilkins.

Morrey, B.F. & An, K.N. (1990). Biomechanics of the shoulder. In C.A. Rockwood & F.A. Matsen III (Eds.), *The Shoulder.* Philadelphia: W.B. Saunders.

Murray, M.P., Gore, D.R., Gardner, G.M., et al. (1985). Shoulder motion and muscle strength of normal men and women in two age groups. *Clin Orthop, 192,* 195.

Neer, C. (1990). *Shoulder Reconstruction* (p. 29). Philadelphia: W.B. Saunders Co.

O'Brien, S.J., Neves, M.C., Amoczky, S.P., et al. (1990). The anatomy and histology of the inferior glenohumeral ligament complex of the shoulder. *Am J Sports Med, 18,* 579–584.

Pagnani, M.J., Deng, X.H., Warren, R.F., et al. (1995). Effect of lesions of the superior portion of the glenoid labrum on glenohumeral translations. *J Bone Joint Surg, 77A,* 103–110.

Poppen, N.K. & Walker, P.S. (1978). Forces at the glenohumeral joint in abduction. *Clin Orthop, 135,* 165–170.

Poppen, N.K. & Walker, P.S. (1976). Normal and abnormal motion of the shoulder. *J Bone Joint Surg, 58A,* 195–201.

Rockwood, C.A. Jr. (1975). Dislocations about the shoulder. In C.A. Rockwood Jr. & D.P. Green (Eds.), *Fractures* (1st ed., Vol 1, pp. 624–815). Philadelphia: J.B. Lippincott.

Rockwood, C. & Matsen, F. (1990). *The Shoulder* (p. 219). Philadelphia: W.B. Saunders Co.

Simon, S.R. (Ed). (1994). *Orthopaedic Basic Science* (p. 527). Rosemont, IL: AAOS.

Soslowsky, L.J., Flatow, E.L., Bigliani, L.U., et al. (1992). Articular geometry of the glenohumeral joint. *Clin Orthop, 285,* 181–190.

Steinbeck, J., Liljenqvist, U., & Jerosh, J. (1994). The anatomy of the glenohumeral ligamentous complex and its contribution to anterior shoulder stability. *J Shoulder Elbow Surg, 7*(2),122–6.

Tibone, J., Patek, R., Jobe, F.W., et al. (1994). The Shoulder: Functional anatomy, biomechanics and kinesiology. In J.C. DeLee & D. Drez (Eds.), *Orthopaedic Sports Medicine.* Philadelphia: W.B. Saunders Co.

Warner, J.P. (1993). The gross anatomy of the joint surfaces, ligaments, labrum and capsule. In F.A. Matsen, F.H. Fu, & R.J. Hawkins (Eds.), *The Shoulder: A Balance of Mobility and Function* (pp. 7–27). Rosemont, IL: AAOS.

Warner, J.P., Deng, X.H., Warren, R.F. et al. (1992). Static capsuloligamentous restraints to superior-inferior translations of the glenohumeral joint. *Am J Sports Med, 20,* 675–678.

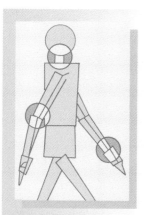

CHAPTER 13

Biomechanics of the Elbow

Laith M. Jazrawi, Andrew S. Rokito, Maureen Gallagher Birdzell,
Joseph D. Zuckerman

Introduction

The elbow is a complex joint that functions as a fulcrum for the forearm lever system that is responsible for positioning the hand in space. A detailed understanding of the biomechanics of elbow function is essential for the clinician to effectively treat pathological conditions affecting the elbow joint.

Anatomy

The elbow joint complex allows two types of motion: flexion-extension and pronation-supination. The humeroulnar and humeroradial articulations allow elbow flexion and extension and are classified as ginglymoid or hinged joints. The proximal radioulnar articulation allows forearm pronation and supination and is classified as a trochoid joint. The elbow joint complex, when considered in its entirety, is therefore a trochleoginglymoid joint. The trochlea and capitellum of the distal humerus are internally rotated 3 to 8° (Fig. 13-1*C*) and in 94 to 98° of valgus with respect to the longitudinal axis of the humerus (Fig. 13-1*A*). The distal humerus is anteriorly angulated 30° along the long axis of the humerus (Fig. 13-1*B*). The articular surface of the ulna is oriented in approximately 4 to 7° of valgus angulation with respect to the longitudinal axis of its shaft (Fig. 13-2*A*).

The distal humerus is divided into medial and lateral columns that terminate distally with the trochlea connecting the two columns (Fig. 13-3). The medial column diverges from the humeral shaft at a 45° angle and ends approximately 1 cm proximal to the distal end of the trochlea. The distal one third of the medial column is composed of cancellous bone, is ovoid in shape, and represents the medial epicondyle. The lateral column of the distal humerus diverges at a 20° angle from the humerus at the same level as the medial column and ends with the capitellum. The trochlea is in the shape of a spool and is comprised of medial and lateral lips with an intervening sulcus. This sulcus articulates with the semilunar notch of the proximal ulna. The articular surface of the trochlea is covered by hyaline cartilage in an arc of 330°. The capitellum, comprising almost a perfect hemisphere, is covered by hyaline cartilage forming an arc of approximately 180°.

The articular surface of the ulna is rotated 30° posteriorly with respect to its long axis. This matches the 30° anterior angulation of the distal humerus, which helps provide stability to the elbow joint in full extension

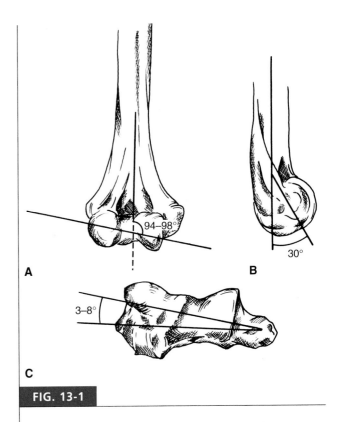

FIG. 13-1

Angular orientation of the distal humerus in the anteroposterior (**A**), lateral (**B**), and axial (**C**) projections.

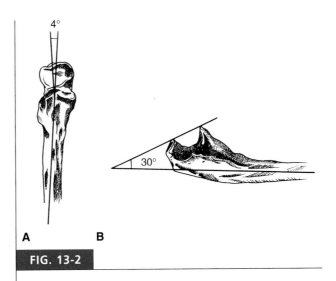

FIG. 13-2

Angular orientation of the proximal ulna in the anteroposterior (**A**) and lateral (**B**) planes.

341

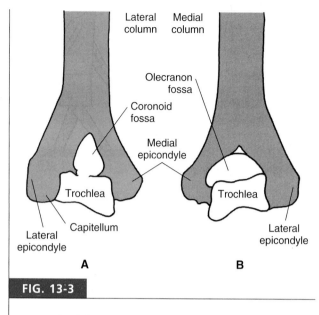

Lateral column   Medial column

Olecranon fossa

Coronoid fossa

Medial epicondyle

Trochlea

Capitellum

Lateral epicondyle

Lateral epicondyle

Trochlea

A   **B**

FIG. 13-3

Anterior (**A**) and posterior (**B**) projections of the distal humerus highlighting the medial and lateral columns.

(Fig13-2). The arc of articular cartilage of the greater sigmoid notch is 180°, but this is often not continuous in its midportion. In more than 90% of individuals, this area is comprised of fatty, fibrous tissue (Walker, 1977). As Morrey noted, this anatomical feature explains the propensity for fractures to occur in this area, as this portion of the greater sigmoid notch is not supported by stronger subchondral bone (Morrey, 1986).

The radial neck is angulated 15° from the long axis in the anterior-posterior plane away from the bicipital tuberosity (Fig. 13-4). Four fifths of the radial head is covered by hyaline cartilage. The anterolateral one fifth lacks articular cartilage and strong subchondral bone, explaining the increased propensity for fractures to occur in this region.

Kinematics

Elbow flexion and extension take place at the humeroulnar and humeroradial articulation. The normal range of flexion-extension is from 0 to 146° with a functional range of 30 to 130°. The normal range of forearm pronation-supination averages from 71° of pronation to 81° of supination (Morrey et al., 1981). Most activities are accomplished within the functional range of 50° pronation to 50° supination. Clinically, patients can tolerate flexion

contractures of up to 30°, which is consistent with the functional range values described above. Flexion contractures greater than 30° are associated with complaints of significant loss of motion. There is a considerable and rapid loss of the ability to reach in space with flexion contractures greater than 30° (Fig. 13-5) (An & Morrey, 1991).

The axis of rotation for flexion-extension has been shown by several investigators to be at the center of the trochlea, supporting the concept that elbow flexion can be represented as a uniaxial hinge. Ewald and Ishizaki, conversely, discovered a changing axis of rotation with elbow flexion (Ewald, 1975; Ishizuki, 1979). London demonstrated that the axis of rotation passes through the center of concentric arcs outlined by the bottom of the trochlear sulcus and the periphery of the capitellum (London, 1981). He also noted that the surface joint motion during flexion-extension was primarily of the gliding type and that with the extremes of flexion-extension (the final 5 to 10° of both flexion and extension), the axis of rotation changed and the gliding/sliding joint motion changed to a rolling type motion. The rolling occurs at the extremes of flexion and extension as the coronoid process comes into contact with the floor of the humeral olecranon fossa and the olecranon contacts the floor of the olecranon fossa. In addition,

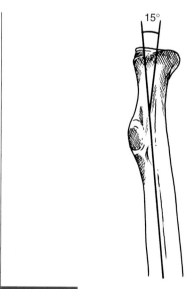

15°

FIG. 13-4

Angulation of the radial head/neck in relation to the radial shaft.

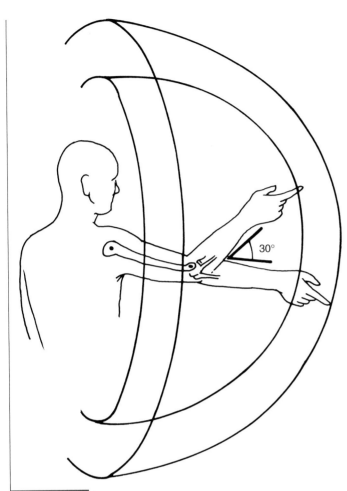

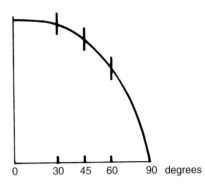

Motion loss	Function (volume) loss
30°	28%
45°	39%
60°	60%

Function = Volume
$$V = 4/3\ \pi r^3$$

FIG. 13-5

Diagram depicts the dramatic loss of effective reach area with flexion contractures of the elbow greater than 30°

internal axial rotation of the ulna has been shown to occur during early flexion and external axial rotation during terminal flexion, demonstrating that the elbow cannot be truly represented as a simple hinge joint. In conclusion, evidence suggests that the elbow has a changing center of rotation during flexion-extension and functions in a more complex manner than would a simple uniaxial hinge.

Despite variation in findings among investigators, Morrey, Tanaka, and An (1991) have stated that the deviation of the center of joint rotation is minimal and the reported variation is probably the result of limitations in experimental design. Therefore, the ulnohumeral joint could be assumed to move as a uniaxial articulation except at the extremes of flexion-extension. The axis of rotation of flexion-extension occurs about a tight locus of points measuring 2 to 3 mm in its broadest dimension and is in the center of the trochlea and capitellum on the lateral view. It is approximated by a line passing through the center of the lateral epicondyle and trochlea and then through the anteroinferior aspect of the medial epicondyle (Fig. 13-6) (Morrey & Chao, 1976). These factors should be taken into account during joint replacement procedures of the elbow as well as when placing hinged external fixators across the elbow joint (Figgie, Inglis, & Mow, 1986).

Pronation and supination take place primarily at the humeroradial and proximal radioulnar joints with the forearm rotating about a longitudinal axis passing through the center of the capitellum and

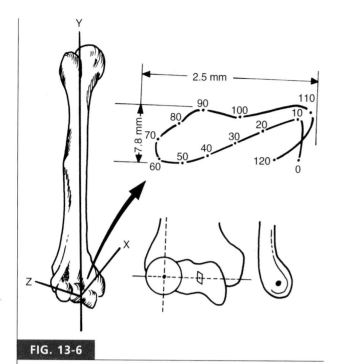

FIG. 13-6

Dimensions of the locus of the instant center of rotation. As depicted, the axis of rotation runs through the center of the trochlea and capitellum.

radial head and the distal ulnar articular surface. This axis is oblique in relation to the anatomical axis of the radius and ulna. During pronation-supination, the radial head rotates within the annular ligament and the distal radius rotates around the distal ulna in an arc outlining the shape of a cone. Carret et al. (1976) studied the instant centers of rotation at the proximal and distal radioulnar joints with the forearm in varying degrees of pronation and supination. They found that the proximal instant center of rotation varied with differences in the curvature of the radial head among individuals. Chao and Morrey (1978) investigated the effect of pronation and supination on the position of the ulna and found no significant axial rotation or valgus deviation of this bone during forearm rotation when the elbow was fully extended. O'Driscoll et al. (1991) has demonstrated that internal axial rotation of the ulna occurs with pronation while external axial rotation occurs with supination. Kapandji (1982) has suggested that both the distal radius and ulna rotate about the axis of pronation-supination, with the ulnar arc of rotation being significantly smaller than the radial arc of

rotation. Ray et al. (1951) demonstrated some varus-valgus movement of the distal ulna with rotation on an axis extending from the radial head through the index finger (Fig. 13-7).

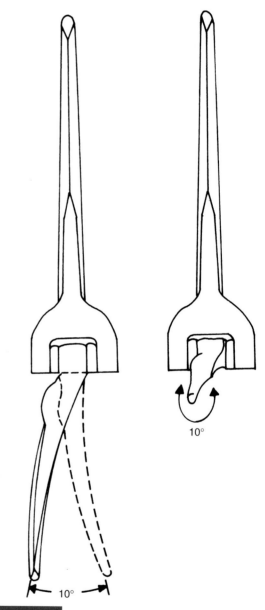

FIG. 13-7

Diagram of semiconstrained total elbow replacement allowing a variable amount of toggle in the varus/valgus and axial planes. The design takes into consideration the fact that the motion of the elbow cannot be purely represented as a simple hinge.

Palmer et al. (1982) have demonstrated proximal radial migration with forearm pronation. This finding has been supported by observations at elbow arthroscopy. In addition, as a result of the ovoid shape of the radial head, its axis is displaced laterally in pronation by 2 mm to allow space for the medial rotation of the radial tuberosity (Kapandji, 1982).

Carrying Angle

The valgus position of the elbow in full extension is commonly referred to as the carrying angle. The carrying angle is defined as the angle between the anatomical axis of the ulna and the humerus measured in the anteroposterior plane in extension or simply the orientation of the ulna with respect to the humerus, or vice versa, in full extension (Fig. 13-8). The angle is less in children than

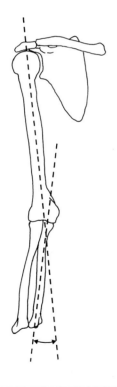

FIG. 13-8

The carrying angle of the elbow, formed by the interception of the long axes of the humerus and the ulna with the elbow fully extended and the forearm supinated. Valgus angulation normally ranges from 10 to 15°.

in adults and greater in females than in males, averaging 10 and 13° of valgus, respectively, with a wide distribution in both (Atkinson & Elftman, 1945; Mall, 1905). Steindler (1955) reported a gradual increase in the carrying angle with age but found no statistical difference between men and women in this rate of increase or the carrying angle. Controversy exists regarding the change in the carrying angle as the elbow is flexed. An et al. (1984) have noted that this controversy arises from the various references systems employed to determine the carrying angle. They noted that when the carrying angle is defined as either the angle formed between the long axis of the humerus and ulna on a plane containing the humerus or vice versa, the carrying angle changes minimally with flexion. If the carrying angle is defined as the abduction-adduction angle of the ulna relative to the humerus using Eulerian angles to describe arm motion, the carrying angle decreases with joint flexion changing to varus in extreme flexion (Fig. 13-9).

Elbow Stability

Valgus forces at the elbow are resisted primarily by the anterior band of the medial collateral ligament (MCL) complex. The MCL complex consists of an anterior bundle, a posterior bundle, and the transverse ligament (Fig. 13-10). The anterior bundle tightens in extension while the posterior bundle tightens in flexion. This occurs because the MCL complex does not originate at the center of the axis of elbow rotation (Fig. 13-11). The anterior band of the MCL complex originates from the inferior surface of the medial epicondyle of the distal humerus and inserts along the medial edge of the olecranon. With an intact anterior band, the radial head does not offer significant additional resistance to valgus stress. However, with a transacted or disrupted anterior band, the radial head becomes the primary restraint to valgus stress, emphasizing its function as a secondary stabilizer in elbows with an intact MCL (Palmer, Glisson, & Werner, 1982). Despite studies by Morrey (Morrey, An, & Stormont, 1988; Morrey, Tanaka, & An, 1991) demonstrating the secondary valgus stabilizing effect of the radial head, several investigators have noted increased valgus laxity after radial head excision (Coleman, Blair, & Shurr, 1987; Gerard, Schernburg, & Nerot, 1984; Johnston,

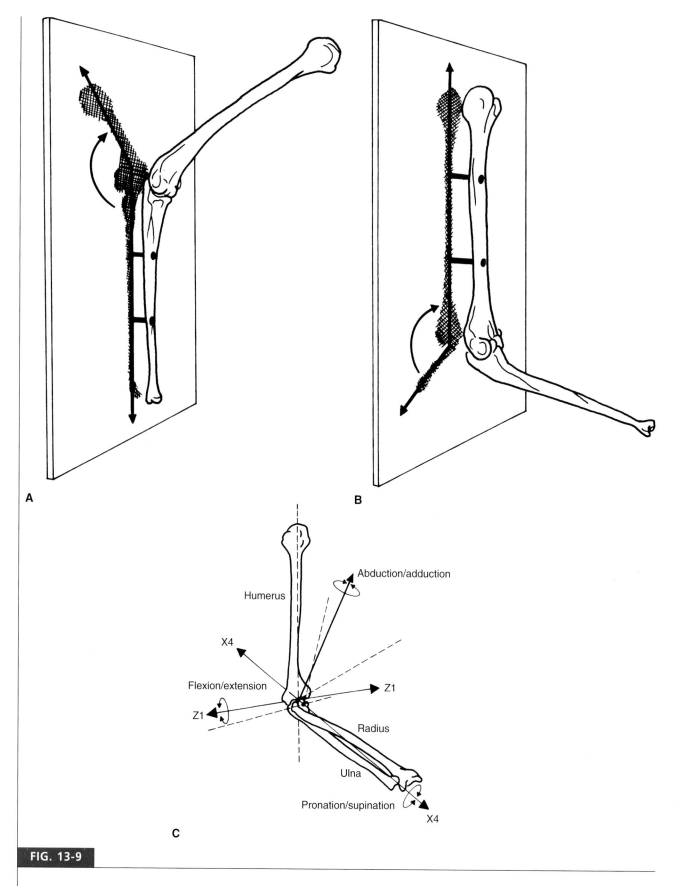

FIG. 13-9

A, Carrying angle measured as the angle between the long axis of the ulna and the long axis of projection of the humerus on the plane containing the ulna. **B,** Carrying angle measured as the angle formed between the long axis of the humerus and the long axis of the projection of the ulna on the plane containing the humerus. **C,** Eulerian angle measurement of ulnar motion in reference to the humerus. Abduction-adduction rotates about the axis orthogonal to both the Z and X4 axes; flexion-extension rotates about the Z1 axis; forearm axial rotation takes place about the X4 axis.

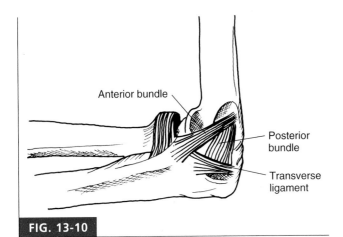

FIG. 13-10

Medial collateral ligament complex containing anterior and posterior bundles as well as a transverse component.

1962; Morrey, Chao, & Hui, 1979). However, this does not seem to be clinically disabling (Hotchkiss, 1997).

Selective ligament transection studies have shown that in extension, resistance to valgus stress is shared equally by the MCL complex, capsule, and joint articulation. In flexion, the primary resistor to valgus stress is the MCL complex (Morrey & An, 1983). In extension, the elbow articulation provides most of the resistance to varus stress, followed by the anterior capsule. In flexion, the elbow articulation remains the primary restraint to varus stress followed by the anterior capsule and the lateral collateral ligament (LCL) complex, respectively, with the LCL complex contributing only 9% (Table 13-1). Elbow extension is limited primarily by the anterior capsule and anterior bundle of the MCL complex. Excision of the olecranon fossa fat pad has been shown to provide 5° of additional extension (Walker, 1977). Furthermore, Morrey et al. (1991) have demonstrated an almost linear decrease in ulno-humeral joint stability with serial removal of 25 to 100% of the olecranon.

The LCL complex consists of the radial collateral ligament that originates from the lateral epicondyle and inserts on the annular ligament, the lateral ulnar collateral ligament that originates from the lateral epicondyle and passes superficial to the annular ligament inserting onto the supinator crest of the ulna, and the accessory LCL complex (Fig. 13-12). The origin of the LCL complex lies at the center of the axis of elbow rotation, explaining its consistent length throughout the flexion-extension arc (Fig. 13-13). Although Morrey and An (1983) have demonstrated only a minimal contribution of the LCL complex to varus stability, others have shown the LCL complex to be an important stabilizer of

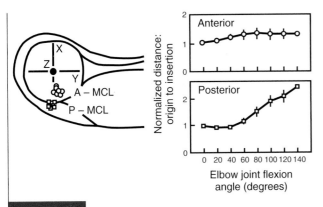

FIG. 13-11

Origin of the anterior and posterior bundles of the medial collateral ligament (MCL) complex. As the MCL does not originate on the axis of elbow rotation, there are changes in its length as a function of elbow flexion. The anterior bundle, which is closer to the axis of rotation, is the most isometric.

TABLE 13-1

Percent Contribution of Restraining Force During Displacement (Rotational or Distractional)

Position	Stabilizing Element	Distraction	Varus	Valgus
Extension	MCL	12	–	31
	LCL	10	14	–
	Capsule	70	32	38
	Articulation	–	55	31
Flexion	MCL	78	–	54
	LCL	10	9	–
	Capsule	8	13	10
	Articulation	–	75	33

MCL, medial collateral ligament complex; LCL, lateral collateral ligament complex

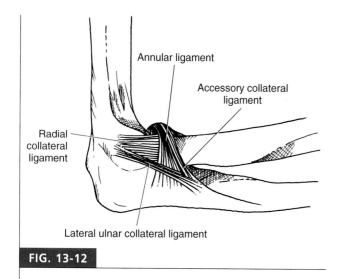

FIG. 13-12

The lateral collateral ligament complex.

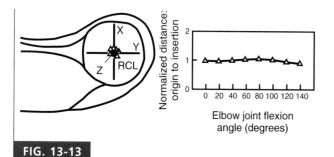

FIG. 13-13

Origin of the lateral collateral ligament complex at the elbow axis of rotation. The ligament remains isometric throughout the flexion-extension range of the elbow. *RCL,* radial collateral ligament.

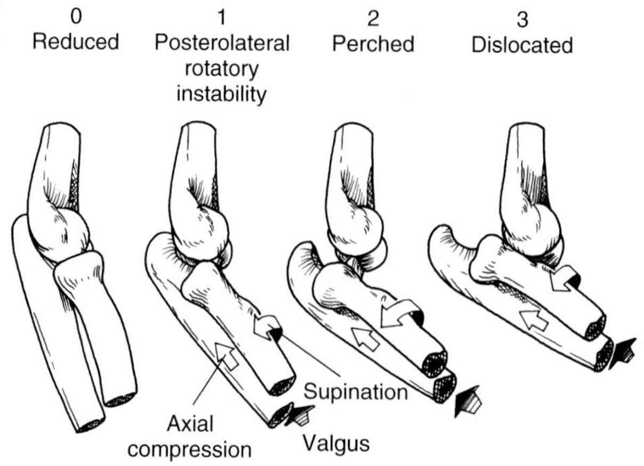

FIG. 13-14

Clinical stages of posterolateral rotatory instability of the elbow.

the humeroulnar joint with forced varus and external rotation (Daria et al., 1990; Durig et al., 1979; Josefsson, Johnell, & Wenderberg, 1987; O'Driscoll, Morrey, & An, 1990a; Osborne & Cotterhill, 1966) .

O'Driscoll and colleagues (1990a) described the entity of posterolateral rotatory instability of the elbow in which the ulna supinates on the humerus and the radial head dislocates in a posterolateral direction (Fig. 13-14). It has been shown that the elbow can dislocate posterolaterally or posteriorly with an intact MCL complex. This can occur with combined valgus and external rotation loads across the elbow joint (Sojbjerg, Helmig, & Jaersgaard-Andersen, 1989). The lateral ulnar collateral is the primary restraint to posterolateral rotatory instability of the elbow, followed by the radial collateral ligament and capsule. O'Driscoll et al. (1990b) also noted a small but significant effect of the inherent negative intra-articular pressure of the elbow joint to varus and rotation stresses (Case Study 13-1).

Structures limiting passive flexion include the capsule, triceps, coronoid process, and radial head. Structures limiting elbow extension include the olecranon process and the anterior band of the MCL complex. Passive resistance to pronation-supination is provided in large part by the antagonist muscle group on stretch, not by the ligamentous structures (Braune & Flugel, 1842). Others have shown that the quadrate ligament provides restraint to forearm rotation (Spinner & Kaplan, 1970).

Longitudinal stability of the forearm is provided by both the interosseous membrane and the triangular fibrocartilage. Lee et al. (1992) demonstrated marked proximal migration of the radius only after 85% of the interosseous membrane was sectioned. Hotchkiss et al. (1989) demonstrated increased stiffness of the interosseous membrane with forearm supination and noted that the triangular fibrocartilage complex (TFCC) was responsible for 8% of longitudinal forearm stiffness, while the central band of the interosseous membrane provided 71%. Reardon et al. (1991) demonstrated in cadavers that with removal of the radial head alone, proximal radial migration was 0.4 mm. When combined with interosseous membrane transaction alone, proximal

CASE STUDY 13-1

Elbow Fracture Dislocation

A 16-year old male gymnast falls onto an outstretched arm, producing abnormal loads in the elbow complex. The axial loading during the fall onto the outstretched position caused a fracture on the radial head, altering the articular congruity of the radiocapitellum joint and the stability of the elbow (Fig. cs13-1-1).

Instability of the joint occurs in posterolateral dislocation. The ulna supinates onto the humerus, the radial head dislocates in the posterolateral direction, and the lateral ulnar collateral ligament is injured, as is the radial collateral ligament and capsule. All these abnormalities lead to an increase in stress within the joint and a loss of stability and congruency necessary for normal joint kinematics.

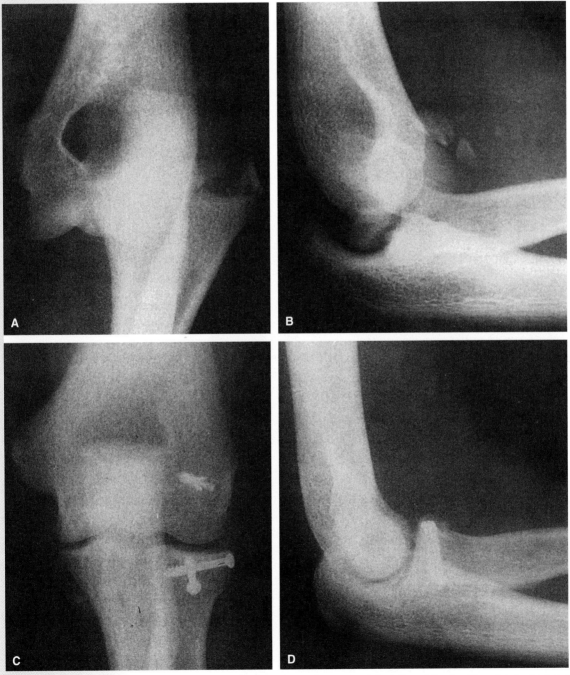

Case Study Figure 13-1-1.   Figure A: Antero-posterior X-rays that confirms postero-lateral elbow dislocation. Figure B: Lateral radiography that shows fracture on the radial head and capitellum. Figures C, D: Posterior and lateral view. Post-operative x-rays. Congruence of the joint has been achieved.

radial migration increased to 4.4 mm. Radial head resection when combined with TFCC transaction caused 2.2 mm of proximal radial migration. The combination of radial head resection, interosseous membrane transaction, and TFCC transaction led to the greatest increase in proximal radius migration of 16.8 mm.

Kinetics

The primary flexor of the elbow is the brachialis, which arises from the anterior aspect of the humerus and inserts on the anterior aspect of the proximal ulna (Fig. 13-15). The biceps arises via a long head tendon from the supraglenoid tubercle and a short head tendon from the coracoid process of the scapula and inserts on the bicipital tuberosity of the radius. It is active in flexion when the forearm is supinated or in the neutral position. The brachioradialis, which originates from the lateral two thirds of the distal humerus and inserts on the distal aspect of the radius near the radial styloid, is active during rapid flexion movements of the elbow and when weight is lifted during a slow flexion movement (Basmajian & Latif, 1957). The brachialis, biceps, brachioradialis, and extensor carpi radialis are the major flexors of the elbow, the brachialis possessing the greatest work capacity (An et al., 1981).

The primary extensor of the elbow, the triceps, is composed of three separate heads. The long head originates from the infraglenoid tubercle and the medial and lateral heads originate from the posterior aspect of the humerus (Fig. 13-15). The three heads coalesce to form one tendon that inserts onto the olecranon process of the ulna. The medial head is the primary extensor and the lateral and long heads act in reserve (Basmajian, 1969). The anconeus muscle, which arises from the posterolateral aspect of the distal humerus and inserts onto the posterolateral aspect of the proximal ulna, is also active in extension. This muscle is active in initiating and maintaining extension. While the triceps, anconeus, and flexor carpi ulnaris are active in extension, the triceps has the largest work capacity of all the elbow extensors (An et al., 1981).

Muscles involved in supination of the forearm include the supinator, biceps, and lateral epicondylar extensors of the wrist and fingers. The primary muscle involved in supination is the biceps brachii. The supinator arises from the lateral epicondyle of the humerus and the proximal lateral aspect of the ulna and inserts into the anterior aspect of the supinated proximal radius.

Muscles involved in pronation include the pronator quadratus and pronator teres. The pronator quadratus originates from the volar aspect of the distal ulna and inserts onto the distal and lateral aspect of the supinated radius. The pronator teres is more proximally located, arising from the medial epicondyle of the humerus and inserting onto the lateral aspect of the midshaft of the supinated radius. The pronator quadratus is the primary pronator of the forearm regardless of its position. The pronator teres is a secondary pronator when rapid pronation is required or during resisted pronation (Basmajian, 1969).

In a study examining elbow strength in normal individuals, supination strength was shown to be 20 to 30% greater than pronation strength (Askew et al., 1986). Consistent with muscle cross-sectional area and moment arms, flexion strength was 30% greater than extension strength. Lastly, males were consistently 40% stronger than females in elbow strength testing.

Electromyography

Electromyography has been helpful in defining the contributions of elbow musculature during activities of daily living and specifically defined tasks. The biceps brachii is only minimally active during elbow flexion when the forearm is pronated (Basmajian & Latif, 1957; Funk et al., 1987; Maton & Bouisset, 1977; Stevens et al., 1973). Brachialis activity, however, is not affected by forearm rotation during flexion (Funk et al., 1987; Stevens et al., 1973). The brachioradialis also is active during flexion. This activity is enhanced when the forearm is in a neutral or pronated position (Basmajian & Travill, 1961; DeSousa, DeMoraes, & DeMoraes, 1961; Funk et al., 1987; Stevens et al., 1973). Electromyographic data demonstrates that the medial head of the triceps and anconeus is active during elbow extension, with the lateral and long heads of the triceps serving as secondary extensors. Morrey (1993) concluded the following from the electromyographic data: (1) the biceps is generally less active in full pronation of the forearm, secondary to its role as a supinator; (2) the brachialis is active throughout flexion and is believed to be the workhorse of flexion; (3) electrical activity of the triceps

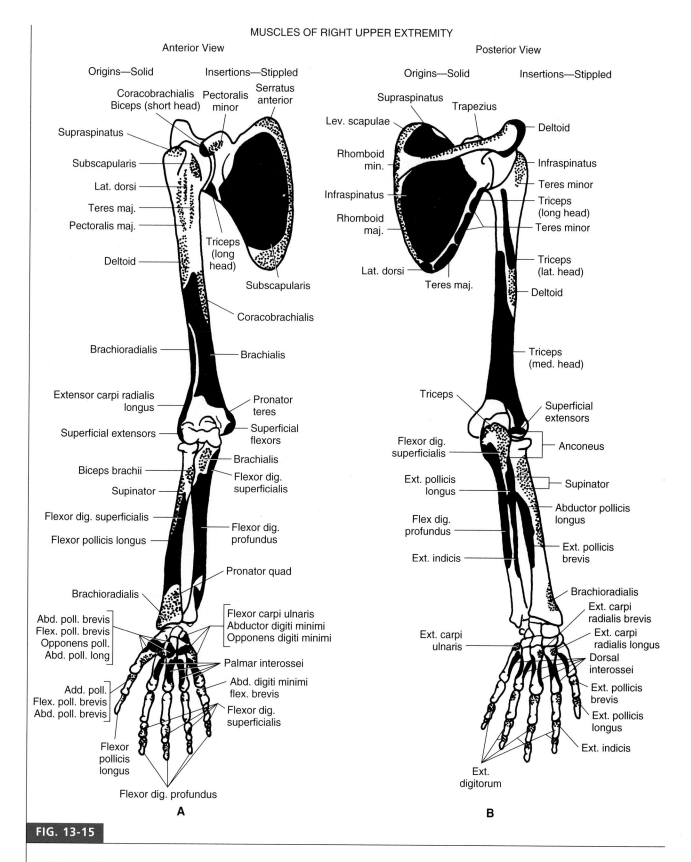

MUSCLES OF RIGHT UPPER EXTREMITY

Anterior View

Origins—Solid   Insertions—Stippled

Coracobrachialis Pectoralis Serratus
Biceps (short head) minor anterior

Supraspinatus

Subscapularis

Lat. dorsi

Teres maj.

Pectoralis maj.

Deltoid

Triceps
(long
head)

Subscapularis

Coracobrachialis

Brachioradialis   Brachialis

Extensor carpi radialis   Pronator
longus   teres

Superficial extensors   Superficial
flexors

Biceps brachii   Brachialis

Supinator   Flexor dig.
superficialis

Flexor dig. superficialis

Flexor pollicis longus   Flexor dig.
profundus

Brachioradialis   Pronator quad

Abd. poll. brevis   Flexor carpi ulnaris
Flex. poll. brevis   Abductor digiti minimi
Opponens poll.   Opponens digiti minimi
Abd. poll. long

Palmar interossei

Add. poll.   Abd. digiti minimi
Flex. poll. brevis   flex. brevis
Abd. poll. brevis   Flexor dig.
superficialis

Flexor
pollicis
longus

Flexor dig. profundus

A

Posterior View

Origins—Solid   Insertions—Stippled

Supraspinatus   Trapezius

Lev. scapulae   Deltoid

Rhomboid   Infraspinatus
min.
          Teres minor
Infraspinatus   Triceps
          (long head)
Rhomboid   Teres minor
maj.
          Triceps
Lat. dorsi   (lat. head)
          Deltoid
Teres maj.

          Triceps
          (med. head)

Triceps   Superficial
          extensors

Flexor dig.   Anconeus
superficialis

Ext. pollicis   Supinator
longus
          Abductor pollicis
Flex dig.   longus
profundus
          Ext. pollicis
Ext. indicis   brevis

          Brachioradialis
          Ext. carpi
          radialis brevis
          Ext. carpi
          radialis longus
Ext. carpi   Dorsal
ulnaris   interossei
          Ext. pollicis
          brevis
          Ext. pollicis
          longus
          Ext. indicis

Ext.
digitorum

B

Origin and insertions of muscles of the upper extremity. **A,** Anterior view. **B,** Posterior view.

increases with increased elbow flexion as a result of the stretch reflex; and (4) the anconeus is active in all positions and is considered to be a dynamic joint stabilizer.

Elbow Joint Forces

Halls and Travill (1964) demonstrated that in intact cadaver forearms, 43% of longitudinal forces are transmitted through the ulnotrochlear joint and 57% are transmitted through the radiocapitellar joint. Ewald et al. (1977) determined that the elbow joint compressive force was eight times the weight held by an outstretched hand. An and Morrey (1991) determined that during strenuous weight-lifting, the resultant force at the ulnohumeral joint ranges from one to three times body weight. Force transmission through the radial head is greatest between 0 and 30° of flexion and is greater in pronation than in supination (Morrey, An, & Stormont, 1988). This is secondary to the "screw home" mechanism of the radius with respect to the ulna with proximal migration occurring during pronation and distal translation occurring during supination. As mentioned previously, the radial head bears the load at the radiocapitellar joint. Disruption of the TFCC and the interosseous membrane in the presence of an intact radial head does not result in proximal radioulnar migration. Absence of the radial head as a result of fracture or resection and a concomitant disruption of the TFCC and interosseous membrane will result in proximal migration of the radius (Sowa, Hotchkiss, & Weiland, 1995).

The force generated at the elbow joint is greatest when flexion is initiated. Increased flexion strength and decreased elbow forces are seen with the elbow at 90° of flexion. This is because of the improved mechanical advantage of the elbow flexors secondary to lengthening of the flexion moment arm. Interestingly, the resultant force vector direction at the elbow changes by more than 180° through the entire flexion-extension (Pearson, McGinley, & Butzel, 1963). Clinically, this change in the resultant vector should be taken into consideration when considering internal fixation of the distal humerus fractures (Morrey, 1994; Pearson et al., 1963) as well as when considering total joint replacement (Goel, Lee, & Blair, 1989).

During elbow flexion, the ulna is posteriorly translated as contact occurs at the coronoid. Dur-

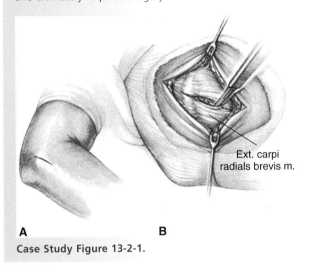
ing the forced extension that occurs during the follow-through phase of the throwing motion, impaction of the olecranon against the olecranon fossa has been demonstrated in the overhead athlete. This impaction may result in the formation of osteophytes at the olecranon tip (Tullos et al., 1972).

The force generated in the elbow has been shown to be up to three times body weight with certain activities (An et al., 1981). Nicol et al. (1977), using three-dimensional biomechanical analysis, found that during dressing and eating activities the joint reaction forces were 300 N. Rising from a chair resulted in a joint reaction force of 1700 N and pulling a table, 1900 N, which is almost three times body weight (Case Study 13-2).

Articular Surface Forces

Contact areas of the elbow occur at four locations; two are located at the olecranon and two on the coronoid (Fig. 13-16) (Stormont et al., 1985). The humeroulnar contact area increases from elbow extension to flexion. The radial head also increases its contact area with the capitellum from extension to flexion. During valgus-varus loads to the elbow, Morrey et al. (1988) demonstrated the varus-valgus pivot point to be located at the midpoint of the lateral aspect of the trochlea.

Calculation of Joint Reaction Forces at the Elbow

As several muscles participate in producing flexion and extension of the elbow, a few simplifying assumptions must be made in order for joint reaction forces to be estimated in certain static and dynamic

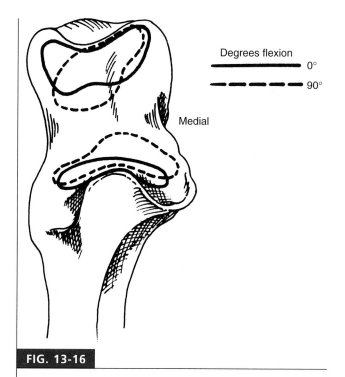

Degrees flexion

———————— 0°

– – – – – – – – 90°

Medial

FIG. 13-16

Contact areas in the sigmoid fossa during elbow flexion demonstrating that the contact areas move toward the center of the sigmoid fossa during elbow flexion.

situations. In the following static example, the simplified free-body technique for coplanar forces is used to calculate the joint reaction force at the elbow during flexion with and without an object in the hand (Calculation Box 13-1). The elbow is flexed 90°; it is assumed that the predominant elbow flexors are the brachialis and the biceps and that the force produced through the tendons of these muscles (B) acts perpendicular to the longitudinal axis of the forearm. The distance between the center of rotation of the elbow joint and point of insertion of the tendons of these muscles (the lever arm of B) is approximately 5 cm. The mass of the forearm (2 kg) produces a gravitational force (W) equal to 20 N. The lever arm of W, the distance from the center of rotation of the elbow to the midpoint of the forearm, is 13 cm. The force produced by any weight held in the hand (P) acts at a distance of 30 cm from the center of rotation of the elbow joint.

The muscle force required to keep the elbow in the flexed position (B) is calculated with the equilibrium equation for moments. The equilibrium equation for forces is then used to calculate the joint reaction force on the trochlear fossa (J). When no object is held in the hand, the muscle force is calculated to be 52 N and the joint reaction force, 32 N. By contrast, when a 1-kg weight is held in the hand, producing a gravitational force (P) of 10 N at a distance of 30 cm from the center of elbow rotation, the required muscle forces (B) rise to 112 N and the joint reaction force more than doubles, reaching 82 N. Thus, small loads applied to the hand dramatically increase the elbow joint reaction force.

An estimation of the joint reaction force also can be made for the elbow during extension. In the case study, the elbow is held in 90° of flexion with the forearm positioned over the head and parallel to the ground (Calculation Box 13-2). In this position, action of the elbow extensors is required to offset the gravitational force on the forearm. It is assumed that the triceps is the predominant extensor and that the force through the tendon of this muscle acts perpendicular to the longitudinal axis of the forearm. Therefore, the three main coplanar forces acting on the elbow include the force produced by the weight of the arm (W), the tensile force exerted through the tendon of the triceps muscle (T), and the joint reaction force on the trochlear fossa of the ulna (J). The distance between the center of rotation of the elbow and the point of insertion of the tendon of the triceps muscle (the lever arm of T) is approximately 3 cm.

CALCULATION BOX 13-1

Joint Reaction Force: Elbow Flexion

The reaction force on the elbow joint during elbow flexion with and without an object in the hand can be calculated by means of the simplified free-body technique for coplanar forces and the equilibrium equations that state that the sum of the moments and the sum of the forces acting on the elbow joint must be zero. The primary elbow flexors are assumed to be the biceps and the brachialis muscles. The force produced through the tendons of these muscles (B) acts at a distance of 5 cm from the center of rotation of the joint (indicated by the hollow circle). The force produced by the weight of the forearm (W), taken to be 20 N, acts at a distance of 13 cm from the center of rotation. The force produced by any weight held in the hand (P) acts at a distance of 30 cm from the center of rotation.

Case A. No object is held in the hand. B is calculated with the equilibrium equation for moments. Clockwise moments are considered to be positive, whereas counterclockwise moments are considered to be negative.

$$\Sigma M = 0.$$
$$(13 \text{ cm} \times P) + (30 \text{ cm} \times P) - (5 \text{ cm} \times B) = 0$$
If W = 20 N and P = 0.
$$B = \frac{13 \text{ cm} \times 20 \text{ N}}{5 \text{ cm}}$$

B is calculated to be 52 N.

J, the reaction force on the trochlear fossa of the ulna, can now be calculated by means of the equilibrium equation for forces. Gravitational forces are negative; forces in the opposite direction are positive.

$$\Sigma F = 0$$
$$B - J - W - P = 0$$
$$J = 52 \text{ N} - 20 \text{ N} - 0 \text{N}.$$

J is found to be 32 N.

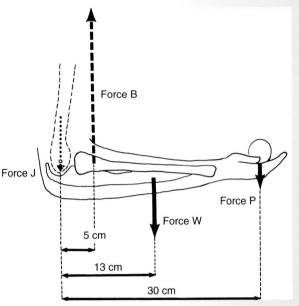

Force B

Force J

Force P

Force W

5 cm

13 cm

30 cm

Calculation Box Figure 13-1-1.

Case B. An object of 1 kg is held in the hand, producing a force of 10 N (P).

$$\Sigma M = 0$$
If W = 20 N and P = 10 N.
$$(13 \text{ cm} \times 20 \text{N}) + (30 \text{ cm} \times 10 \text{N}) - (5 \text{ cm} \times B) = 0$$
$$B = \frac{260 \text{ Ncm} + 300 \text{ Ncm}}{5 \text{ cm}}$$

B is found to be 112 N.

The joint reaction force can now be calculated.

$$\Sigma F = 0$$
$$B - W - P - J = 0$$
$$J = B - W - P$$
$$J = 112 \text{ N} - 20 \text{ N} - 10 \text{ N}.$$

J is found to be 82 N. Thus, in this example, a 1-kg object held in the hand with the elbow flexed 90° increases the joint reaction force by 50 N.

T and J are calculated with the equilibrium equations. The joint reaction force for the elbow in extension is 107 N, compared with 32 N in flexion. This more than threefold increase can be explained by the fact that the lever arm for the elbow extensor force is shorter than that for the flexor force—3 cm as opposed to 5 cm. Thus, a greater muscle force (87 N as opposed to 52 N) is required for the forearm to be maintained in the extended position, and as a result the joint reaction force is greater.

CALCULATION BOX 13-2

Joint Reaction Force: Elbow Extension

The joint reaction force during elbow extension can be calculated by means of the same method:

$$\Sigma M = 0$$
$$(13 \text{ cm} \times W) - (3 \text{ cm} \times T) = 0$$
$$\text{If } W = 20 \text{ N}$$
$$T = \frac{13 \text{ cm} \times 20 \text{ N}}{3 \text{ cm}}$$
T is found to be 87 N.

$$\Sigma F = 0$$
$$J - T - W = 0$$
$$J = T + W$$
$$J = 87 \text{ N} + 20 \text{ N}.$$

J is found to be 107 N. Thus, in this example, the joint reaction force during elbow extension is 75 N greater than during elbow flexion.

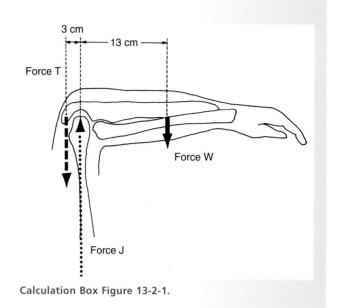

Calculation Box Figure 13-2-1.

Summary

A clear understanding of elbow mechanics and function is critical to gain a broader understanding of problems affecting the elbow joint. This knowledge will provide the basis for management of elbow disorders.

1 The elbow joint complex consists of three articulations: the humeroulnar, humeroradial, and proximal radioulnar. It allows two types of motion, flexion-extension and pronation-supination.

2 The functional range of elbow motion is 30 to 130° of flexion-extension and 50 to 50° of pronation-supination, with most activities of daily living accomplished within this range. There is a significant and rapid loss of the ability to reach in space with flexion contractures of the elbow greater than 30°.

3 The axis of rotation for flexion-extension occurs about a tight locus of points measuring 2 to 3 mm in its broadest dimension and is located in the center of the trochlea and capitellum in the lateral view.

4 The elbow has a changing center of rotation during flexion-extension and cannot be truly represented as a simple hinge joint.

5 The carrying angle of the elbow is defined as the angle between the anatomical axis of the ulna and humerus in the anteroposterior plane and in full elbow extension. It averages between 10 and 15° of valgus.

6 The primary stabilizer to valgus stress at the elbow is the anterior band of the MCL complex, with the radial head acting as a secondary stabilizer. The primary restraint to varus stress is the elbow articulation. The lateral ulnar collateral ligament is the main stabilizer to posterolateral rotatory instability of the elbow.

7 The primary flexor of the elbow is the brachialis while the primary extender is the triceps. The anconeus is active in initiating and maintaining flexion and is considered to act as a dynamic joint stabilizer. The main source of supination is the biceps brachii. The pronator quadratus is the primary pronator of the forearm regardless of position of the forearm or degree of elbow flexion.

8 Force generated in the elbow has been shown to be up to three times body weight when performing activities of daily living.

REFERENCES

An, K.N., Hui, F.C., Morrey, B.F., et al. (1981). Muscles across the elbow joint: A biomechanical analysis. *J Biomech, 14,* 659-69.

An, K.N. & Morrey, B.F. (1991). Biomechanics. In B.F. Morrey (Ed.), *Joint Replacement Arthroplasty* (pp 257-73). New York: Churchill Livingstone.

An, K.N., Morrey, B.F., & Chao, E.Y.S. (1984). Carrying angle of the human elbow. *Joint J Orthop Res, 1,* 369-378.

Askew, L.J., An, K.N., Morrey, B.F., et al. (1986). Isometric strength in normal individuals. *Clin Orthop, 222,* 261-266.

Atkinson, W.B. & Elftman, H. (1945). The carrying angle of the human arm as a secondary sex character. *Anat Record, 91,* 49-52.

Basmajian, J.V. (1969). Recent advances in the functional anatomy of the upper limb. *Am J Phys Med, 48,* 165.

Basmajian, J.V. & Latif, S. (1957). Integrated actions and functions of the chief flexors of the elbow. *J Bone Joint Surg, 39A,* 1106.

Basmajian, J.V. & Travill, A.A. (1961). Electromyography of the pronator muscles in the forearm. *Anat Rec, 139,* 45.

Braune, W. & Flugel, A. (1842). Uber pronation and supination des menschlichen voderarms und der hand. *Arch Anat Physiol Anat Rbt.*

Carret, J.P., Fischer, L.P., Gonon, G.P., et al. (1976). Etude cinematique de la prosupination au niveau des articulations radiocubitales (radio ulnaris). *Bull Assoc Anat,* 279-295.

Chao, E.Y. & Morrey, B.F. (1978). Three dimensional rotation of the elbow. *J Biomech, 11,* 57-73.

Coleman, D.A., Blair, W.F., & Shurr, D. (1987). Resection of the radial head for fracture of the radial head: A long-term follow-up of seventeen cases. *J Bone Joint Surg, 69A,* 385-392.

Daria, A., Gil, E., Delgado, E., et al. (1990). Recurrent dislocation of the elbow. *Int Orthop, 14,* 41-45.

DeSousa, O.M., DeMoraes, J.L., & DeMoraes, V.F.L. (1961). Electromyographic study of the brachioradialis muscle. *Anat Rec, 139,* 125.

Durig, M., Muller, W., Ruedi, T.P., et al. (1979). The operative treatment of elbow dislocation in the adult. *J Bone Joint Surg, 61A,* 239-244.

Ewald, F.C. (1975). Total elbow replacement. *Orthop Clin North Am, 6,* 685-696.

Ewald, F.C., Thomas, W.H., Sledge, C.B., et al. (1977). Non-constrained metal to plastic total elbow arthroplasty in rheumatoid arthritis. In *Joint Replacement in the Upper Limb* (pp. 77-81). London: I Mech Eng Publications.

Figgie, H.E. III, Inglis, A.E., & Mow, V.C. (1986). A critical analysis of alignment factors affecting functional outcome in total elbow arthroplasty. *J Arthroplasty, 1,* 169.

Funk, D.A., An, K.N., Morrey, B.F., et al. (1987). Electromyographic analysis of muscles across the elbow joint. *J Orthop Res, 5(4),* 529.

Gerard, Y., Schernburg, F., & Nerot, C. (1984). Anatomical, pathological and therapeutic investigation of fractures of the radial head in adults [abstract]. *J Bone Joint Surg, 64B,* 141.

Goel, V.K., Lee, I.K., & Blair, W.F. (1989). Stress distribution in the ulna following a hinged elbow arthroplasty. *J Arthroplasty, 4,* 163.

Halls, A.A. & Travill, A. (1964). Transmission of pressures across the elbow joint. *Anat Rec, 150,* 243-248.

Hotchkiss, R.N. (1997). Displaced fractures of the radial head: Internal fixation or excision? *J Am Acad Orthop Surg, 5,* 1-10.

Hotchkiss, R.N., An, K.N., Sowa, D.T., et al. (1989). An anatomic and mechanical study of the interosseous membrane of the forearm: Pathomechanics of proximal migration of the radius. *J Hand Surg, 14A,* 256-261.

Ishizuki, M. (1979). Functional anatomy of the elbow joint and three dimensional quantitative motion analysis of the elbow joint. *J Jpn Orthop Assn, 53,* 989-996.

Johnston, G.W. (1962). A follow-up of one hundred cases of fracture of the head of the radius with a review of the literature. *Ulster Med J, 31,* 51-56.

Josefsson, P.O., Johnell, O., & Wenderberg, B. (1987). Ligamentous injuries in dislocations of the elbow joint. *Clin Orthop, 221,* 221-225.

Kapandji, I.A. (1982). *The Physiology of Joints* (Vol. 1). Edinburgh: Churchill Livingstone.

Lee, D.H., Greene, K.S., Bidez, M.W., et al. (1992). Role of the forearm interosseous membrane. *47th Annual Meeting of the American Society for Surgery of the Hand.* Phoenix, Arizona, p. 42.

London, J.T. (1981). Kinematics of the elbow. *J Bone Joint Surg, 63A,* 529-535.

Mall, F.P. (1905). On the angle of the elbow. *Am J Anat, 4,* 391-404.

Maton, B. & Bouisset, S. (1977). The distribution of activity among the muscles of a single group during isometric contraction. *Eur J Appl Physiol, 37,* 101.

Morrey, B.F. (1986). Applied anatomy and biomechanics of the elbow joint. In *AAOS Instructional Course Lecture* (Ch. 8, Vol. 35, pp. 59-68). St. Louis: C.V. Mosby.

Morrey, B.F. (1994). Biomechanics of the elbow and forearm. In J.C. Delee & D. Drez (Eds.), *Orthopaedic Sports Medicine* (Ch. 17). Philadelphia: W.B. Saunders.

Morrey, B.F. (1993). *The Elbow and Its Disorders* (2nd ed.). Philadelphia: W.B. Saunders.

Morrey, B.F. & An, K.N. (1983). Articular and ligamentous contributions to stability of the elbow joint. *Am J Sports Med, 11,* 315-319.

Morrey, B.F., An, K.N., & Stormont, T.J. (1988). Force transmission through the radial head. *J Bone Joint Surg, 70A,* 250-256.

Morrey, B.F., Askew, L.J., An, K.N., & Chao, E.Y. (1981). A Biomechanical study of functional elbow motion. *J Bone Joint Surg, 63A,* 872.

Morrey, B.F. & Chao, E.Y. (1976). Passive motion of the elbow joint. *J Bone Joint Surg, 58A,* 501.

Morrey, B.F., Chao, E.Y., & Hui, F.C. (1979). Biomechanical study of the elbow following excision of the radial head. *J Bone Joint Surg, 61A,* 63-68.

Morrey, B.F., Tanaka, S., & An, K.N. (1991). Valgus stability of the elbow. *Clin Orthop, 265,* 187.

Nicol, A.C., Berme, N., & Paul, J.P. (1977). A biomechanical analysis of elbow joint function. In *Joint Replacement in the Upper Limb* (pp. 45-51). London: Institution of Mechanical Engineers.

O'Driscoll, S.W., Bell, D.F., & Morrey, B.F. (1991). Posterolateral rotatory instability of the elbow. *J Bone Joint Surg, 73A(3),* 440.

O'Driscoll, S.W., Morrey, B.F., & An, K.N. (1990b). Intra-articular pressure and capacity of the elbow. *Arthroscopy, 6(2),* 100.

O'Driscoll, S.W., Morrey, B.F., & An, K.N. (1990a). The pathoanatomy and kinematics of posterolateral instability (pivot-shift) of the elbow. *Orthop Trans, 14*, 306.

Osborne, G. & Cotterill, P. (1966). Recurrent dislocation of the elbow. *J Bone Joint Surg Br, 48B*, 340-346.

Palmer, A.K., Glisson, R.R., & Werner, F.W. (1982). Ulnar variance determination. *J Hand Surg, 7*, 376.

Pearson, J.R., McGinley, D.R., & Butzel, L.M. (1963). A dynamic analysis of the upper extremity: Planar motions. *Human Factors, 5*, 59.

Ray, R.D., Johnson, R.J., & Jameson, R.M. (1951). Rotation of the forearm. An experimental study of pronation and supination. *J Bone Joint Surg, 33A*, 993-996.

Reardon, J.P., Lafferty, M., Kamaric, E., et al. (1991). Structures influencing axial stability to the forearm: The role of the radial head, interosseous membrane, and distal radioulnar joint. *Orthop Trans, 15*, 436-437.

Sojbjerg, J.O., Helmig, P., & Jaersgaard-Andersen, P. (1989). Dislocation of the elbow: An experimental study of the ligamentous injuries. *Orthopedics, 12*, 461-463.

Sowa, D.T., Hotchkiss, R.N., & Weiland, A.J. (1995). Symptomatic proximal translation of the radius following radial head resection. *Clin Orthop, 317*, 106-113.

Spinner, M. & Kaplan, E.B. (1970). The quadrate ligament of the elbow: Its relationship to the stability of the proximal radioulnar joint. *Acta Orthop Scand, 41*, 632.

Steindler, A. (1955). In *Kinesiology of the Human Body Under Normal and Pathological Conditions*. Springfield: Charles C. Thomas.

Stevens, A., Stijns, H., Peybrouck, T., et al. (1973). A polyelectromyographical study of the arm muscles at gradual isometric loading. *Electromyogr Clin Neurophysiol, 13*, 46S.

Stormont, T.J., An, K.N., Morrey, B.F., et al. (1985). Elbow joint contact study: A comparison of techniques. *J Biomech, 18(5)*, 329.

Tullos, H.S., Erwin, W., Woods, G.W., et al. (1972). Unusual lesions of the throwing arm. *Clin Orthop, 88*, 169.

Walker, P.S. (1977). In *Human Joints and Their Artificial Replacement*. Springfield, IL: Charles C. Thomas, Publisher.

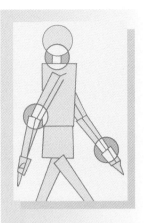

CHAPTER 14

Biomechanics of the Wrist and Hand

Ann E. Barr, Jane Bear-Lehman
adapted from Steven Stuchin, Fadi J. Bejjani

Introduction

The wrist, or carpus, is the collection of bones and soft tissue structures that connects the hand to the forearm. This joint complex is capable of a substantial arc of motion that augments hand and finger function, yet it possesses a considerable degree of stability. The wrist functions kinematically by allowing for changes in the location and orientation of the hand relative to the forearm and kinetically by transmitting loads from the hand to the forearm and vice versa.

Although the function of all joints of the upper extremity is to position the hand in space so that it can perform the activities of daily living, the wrist appears to be the key to hand function. Stability of the wrist is essential for proper functioning of the digital flexor and extensor muscles, and wrist position affects the ability of the fingers to flex and extend maximally and to grasp effectively during prehension.

The hand is a highly complex and multifaceted mobile organ. It is valued and judged for its performance and appearance in delicate prehensile tasks to powerful grasp patterns. It is remarkably mobile and adaptable as it conforms to the shape of objects to be grasped or studied, emphasizes or gestures an idea to be expressed, or shows an act of love or affection (Tubiana, 1984).

The hand is the final link in the mechanical chain of levers that begins at the shoulder. The mobility and stability of the shoulder, the elbow, and the wrist, all operating in different planes, allows the hand to move within a large volume of space and to reach all parts of the body with relative ease. The unique arrangement and mobility of the 19 bones and 14 joints of the hand provide the structural foundation for the hand's extraordinary functional adaptability.

Anatomy of the Wrist and Hand

WRIST ARTICULATIONS

The wrist joint complex consists of the multiple articulations of the eight carpal bones with the distal radius, the structures within the ulnocarpal space, the metacarpals, and each other (Fig. 14-1). The soft tissue structures surrounding the carpal bones include the tendons that cross the carpus or attach to it and the ligamentous structures that connect the carpal bones to each other and to the bony elements of the hand and forearm.

The eight carpal bones are divided into the proximal and distal rows. The bones of the distal row from radial to ulnar are the trapezium, trapezoid, capitate, and hamate. The distal carpal row forms a relatively immobile transverse unit that articulates with the metacarpals to form the carpometacarpal joints. All four bones in the distal row fit tightly against each other and are held together by stout interosseous ligaments. The more mobile proximal row consists of the scaphoid, lunate, and triquetrum. This row articulates with the distal radius to form the radiocarpal joint (scaphoid fossa of radius, 46%; lunate fossa of radius, 43%; ulnar soft tissue structures, 11%) (Simon et al., 1994). The scaphoid spans both rows anatomically and functionally and articulates exclusively with the radius. The lunate articulates in part with the ulnar soft tissue structures. The eighth carpal bone, the pisiform, is a sesamoid bone that mechanically enhances the wrist's most powerful motor, the flexor carpi ulnaris, and forms its own small joint with the triquetrum. Between the proximal and distal rows of carpal bones is the midcarpal joint, and between adjacent bones of these rows are the intercarpal joints (Fig. 14-1). The palmar surface of the carpus as a whole is concave, constituting the floor and walls of the carpal tunnel (Fig. 14-2).

The distal radius, lunate, and triquetrum articulate with the distal ulna through a ligamentous and cartilaginous structure, the ulnocarpal or triangular fibrocartilage complex (TFCC). The components of this complex are illustrated in Figure 14-3, and its functional role will be discussed in detail along with ligamentous function.

HAND ARTICULATIONS

The finger and thumb are the elementary components of the hand (Fig. 14-4). Because each digital unit extends into the middle of the hand, the term digit ray is used to indicate the entire chain, composed of one metacarpal and three phalanges (two in the thumb). The digital rays are numbered from the radial to the ulnar side: I (thumb), II (index finger), III (middle finger), IV (ring finger), and V (little finger). Each finger ray articulates proximally with a particular carpal bone in a carpometacarpal (CMC) joint. The next joint in each ray—the metacarpophalangeal (MCP) joint—links the metacarpal

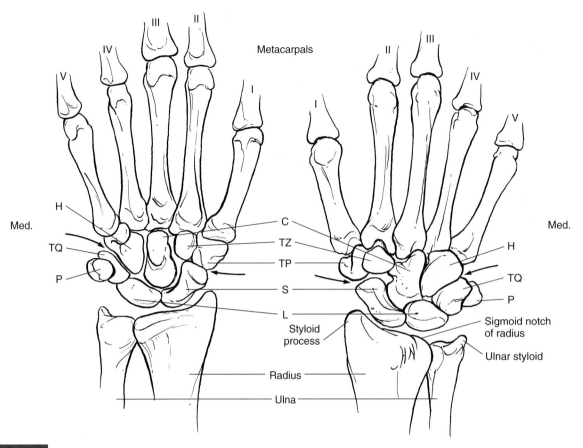

FIG. 14-1

Schematic drawings of the wrist joint complex showing the eight carpal bones and their articulations with the distal radius, the metacarpal bones of the hand, and each other. Palmar view (*left*) and dorsal view (*right*) of the right hand. *H,* hamate; *C,* capitate; *TZ,* trapezoid; *TP,* trapezium; *TQ,* triquetrum; *P,* pisiform; *L,* lunate; *S,* scaphoid. The *arrows* indicate the line of the midcarpal joint. *Adapted with permission from Taleisnik, J. (1985).* The Wrist. *New York: Churchill Livingstone.*

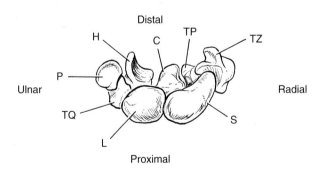

FIG. 14-2

Longitudinal view of the right hand from proximal to distal showing the palmar surface of the bones. This concave surface constitutes the floor and walls of the carpal tunnel, through which the median nerve and flexor tendons pass. The carpal tunnel is bordered laterally by the prominent tubercle of the trapezium and medially by the hook of the hamate. The motor branch of the ulnar nerve (not shown) winds around the base of the hook before entering the deep palmar compartment. *S,* scaphoid; *L,* lunate; *TQ,* triquetrum; *P,* pisiform; *H,* hamate; *C,* capitate; *TP,* trapezium; *TZ,* trapezoid. *Adapted with permission from Taleisnik, J. (1985).* The Wrist. *New York: Churchill Livingstone.*

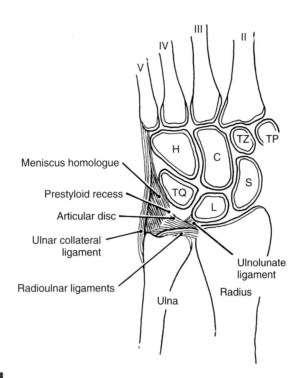

FIG. 14-3

Longitudinal section (frontal plane) of the right wrist and hand viewed from the palmar side. The components of the triangular fibrocartilage complex are visible between the distal ulna and the lunate and triquetrum. *S,* scaphoid; *L,* lunate; *TQ,* triquetrum (the pisiform is not shown); *H,* hamate; *C,* capitate; *TZ,* trapezoid, *TP,* trapezium. *Adapted with permission from Palmer, A.K. & Werner, F.W. (1981). The triangular fibrocartilage complex of the wrist—anatomy and function.* J Hand Surg, 6, 153.

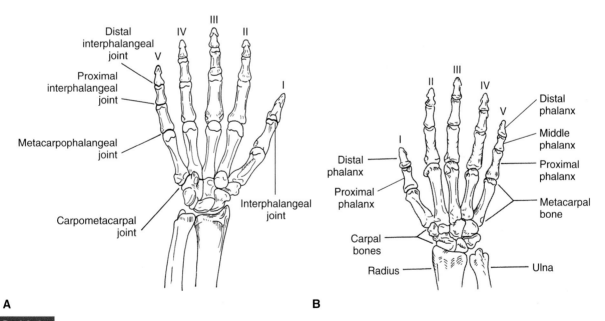

A **B**

FIG. 14-4

Schematic drawing of the skeleton of the hand. The finger rays are numbered from the radial (medial) to the ulnar (lateral) side. **A,** Palmar (anterior) view of the right hand. The joints are labeled. **B,** Dorsal (posterior) view of the right hand. The bones are labeled.

bone to the proximal phalanx. Between the phalanges of the fingers, a proximal (PIP) and a distal (DIP) interphalangeal joint are found; the thumb has only one interphalangeal (IP) joint. The thenar eminence at the palmar side of the first metacarpal is formed by the intrinsic muscles of the thumb. Its ulnar counterpart, the hypothenar eminence, is created by muscles of the little finger and an overlying fat pad.

ARCHES OF THE HAND

The bones of the hand are arranged in three arches (Fig. 14-5), two transverse and one longitudinal (Flatt, 1974; Tubiana, 1984). The proximal transverse arch, with the capitate as its keystone, lies at the level of the distal carpus and is relatively fixed. The distal transverse arch, with the head of the third metacarpal as its keystone, passes through all of the metacarpal heads and is more mobile. The two transverse arches are connected by the rigid portion of the longitudinal arch, composed of the four digital rays and the proximal carpus. The second and third metacarpal bones form the central pillar of this arch (Flatt, 1974). The longitudinal arch is completed by the individual digital rays, and the mobility of the thumb and fourth finger and fifth finger

rays around the second and third fingers allows the palm to flatten or cup itself to accommodate objects of various sizes and shapes (Strickland, 1987).

Although the extrinsic flexor and extensor muscles are largely responsible for changing the shape of the working hand, the intrinsic muscles of the hand are primarily responsible for maintaining the configuration of the three arches (refer to Table 14-1 for a listing of the muscles of the wrist and the hand as well as the corresponding muscle actions). A collapse in the arch system resulting from bone injury, rheumatic disease, or paralysis of the intrinsic muscles can contribute to severe disability and deformity.

NERVE AND BLOOD SUPPLY OF THE WRIST AND HAND

The covering of the hand is important because of its physical qualities, sensory properties, and microcirculation (Tubiana, 1984). The skin on the dorsum or the back of the hand differs and is distinct from the skin that covers the palmar surface. Dorsal skin is mobile, often regarded as very fine, and highly flexible, allowing for a wide array of articular movements. In contrast, palmar skin is thick, glabrous, and inelastic. Palmar skin plays a significant role in hand perceptibility or the perception of touch, safety of the upper limb through sensory protection, and in providing support for the limb as in weight-bearing.

The wrist and the hand are innervated for motor and sensory function by three peripheral nerves descending from the brachial plexus: radial, median, and ulnar (Fig. 14-6). The radial nerve primarily supplies innervation to those muscles that facilitate extension of the wrist and the digits, namely the long wrist extensors. Impairment or injury to the radial nerve will cause wrist drop and instability at the wrist that impedes effective hand grasp. In terms of sensory function, the radial nerve supplies the skin along the radial sphere of the forearm and the hand, and sensory impairment in radial nerve denervation minimally impedes hand function. The median nerve primarily innervates the long flexors of the wrist and the hand. Impairment of the median nerve affects the radial flexor muscles of the hand more greatly than it does those on the ulnar side. The median nerve is most critical to fine motor hand function in terms of the motor supply that it provides, as well as its sensory supply. The median nerve is often regarded as the eyes of the hand because it is responsible for the innervation of the first

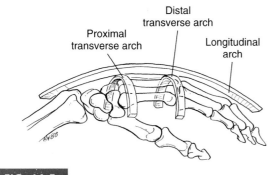

Proximal
transverse arch

Distal
transverse arch

Longitudinal
arch

FIG. 14-5

The three skeletal arches of the hand (mediolateral view). The relatively fixed proximal transverse arch passes through the distal carpus at the level of the distal carpal row. The more mobile distal transverse arch passes through the metacarpal heads. The longitudinal arch is composed of the four finger rays and the proximal carpus. *Adapted with permission from Strickland, J.W. (1987). Anatomy and kinesiology of the hand. In E.E. Fess & C.A. Philips (Eds.),* Hand Splinting: Principles and Methods *(2nd ed., pp. 3–41). St. Louis: C.V. Mosby.*

TABLE 14-1

Muscles of the Wrist and Hand

Muscles of the Wrist

Muscle	Action
Flexors	
Flexor carpi ulnaris	Flexion of wrist; ulnar deviation of hand
Flexor carpi radialis	Flexion of wrist; radial deviation of hand
Palmaris longus	Tension of the palmar fascia
Extensors	
Extensor carpi radialis longus and brevis	Extension of wrist; radial deviation of hand
Extensor carpi ulnaris and brevis	Extension of wrist; ulnar deviation of hand
Pronators-Supinators	
Pronator teres	Forearm pronation
Pronator quadratus	Forearm pronation
Supinator	Forearm supination
Brachioradialis	Pronation or supination, depending on position of forearm

Muscles of the Hand

Muscle	Action
Extrinsic Muscles	
Flexors	
Flexor digitorum superficialis	Flexion of PIP and MCP joints
Flexor digitorum profundus	Flexion of DIP, PIP, and MCP joints
Flexor pollicis longus	Flexion of IP and MCP joints of thumb
Extensors	
Extensor pollicis longus	Extension of IP and MCP joints of thumb; secondary adduction of the thumb
Extensor pollicis brevis	Extension of MCP joint of thumb
Abductor pollicis longus	Abduction of thumb
Extensor indicis proprius	Extension of index finger
Extensor digitorum communis	Extension of fingers
Extensor digiti quinti proprius	Extension of V finger
Intrinsic Muscles	
Interossei (all)	Extension of PIP and DIP joints and flexion of MCP joints
Dorsal interossei	Spread of index and ring fingers away from long finger
Palmar interossei	Adduction of index, ring, and little fingers toward long finger
Lumbricals	Extension of PIP and DID joints and flexion of MCP 2–5 finger
Thenar Muscles	
Abductor pollicis brevis	Abduction of thumb
Flexor pollicis brevis	Flexion and rotation of thumb
Opponens pollicis	Rotation of first metacarpal toward palm
Hypothenar muscles	
Abductor digiti quinti	Abduction of little finger (extension of PIP and DIP joints)
Flexor digiti quinti brevis	Flexion of proximal phalanx of little finger and forward rotation of fifth metacarpal
Adductor pollicis	Adduction of thumb

Modified from Strickland, J.W. (1987). Anatomy and kinesiology of the hand. In E.E. Fess & C.A. Philips (Eds.), *Hand Splinting: Principles and Methods* (2nd ed., pp. 3–41). St. Louis: C.V. Mosby.

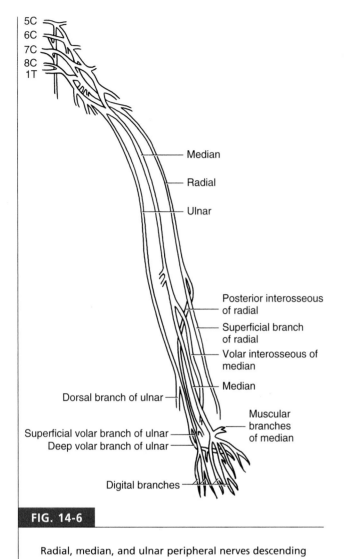

5C
6C
7C
8C
1T

Median

Radial

Ulnar

Posterior interosseous of radial

Superficial branch of radial

Volar interosseous of median

Median

Dorsal branch of ulnar

Muscular branches of median

Superficial volar branch of ulnar

Deep volar branch of ulnar

Digital branches

FIG. 14-6

Radial, median, and ulnar peripheral nerves descending from the brachial plexus.

three digits of the hand on the palmar surface. Without adequate sensation in these digits, fine motor skill is compromised or lost (Case Study 14-1).

The ulnar nerve is regarded as the power source for the grip. It innervates the muscles along the ulnar sphere and the ulnar hand flexors and the majority of the hand intrinsics, particularly those responsible for digital adduction and abduction. The ulnar nerve is known for its ability to protect the upper limb as it innervates the skin surface along the ulnar border. The majority of resting patterns for the upper limb or hand use is performed with the upper limb positioned so that the ulnar borders of the forearm, wrist, and hand are in direct contact

with the environment or giving support to the body by direct and sustained weight-bearing or contact onto a surface.

The hand as an organ of touch has a myriad of receptors of all kinds in its palmar skin. Microscopic study of the palmar skin shows that it possesses

CASE STUDY 14-1

Carpal Tunnel Syndrome in a Clerical Worker

A 26-year-old female who works as an administrative assistant presented with complaints of right hand and wrist discomfort of gradual onset and intermittent severity over the past 2 years. Her symptoms are worsened by prolonged hours of typing on her computer keyboard. A detailed examination shows numbness and tingling of the volar aspect of the distal right forearm and wrist, swelling of the wrist, grip weakness, and positive Phalen's and Tinel's tests. The evaluation suggests compression of the median nerve within the carpal tunnel producing associated motor and sensory changes. A nerve conduction velocity test later confirmed a diagnosis of carpal tunnel syndrome (CTS). The patient was placed on light duty with restrictions on typing tasks and was scheduled for CTS release surgery (Case Study Fig. 14-1-1).

This case illustrates the potential influence of work tasks involving highly repetitive hand and finger movements for prolonged periods of time on the delicate structures of the hand and wrist. The increased intracompartmental pressure within the carpal tunnel associated with ergonomic risk factors such as repetitive loading and awkward wrist positions are major factors contributing to median nerve compression in this case.

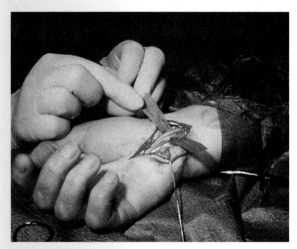

Case Study Figure 14-1-1.

highly specialized Pilary ridges with many types of sensory receptors and nerve fiber properties (Cauna, 1954). The sensory receptors change from free nerve ending to encapsulated receptors or mechanoreceptors. There are more receptors than nerve fibers, and each fiber is connected to several receptors (Mount Castle, 1968). Furthermore, sensory information is transmitted over quickly or slowly adapting nerve fiber properties. It is also known that sensation does not have the same value within the hand; certain zones or regions have more receptivity to a stimulus than do others. For example, the sensory acuity is considered to be of a more specialized quality in the specific anatomical regions required for very fine motor prehension: the ulnar half of the digital pulp of the thumb, the radial half of the digital pulp of both the index and middle fingers, and the ulnar border of the little finger. It is essential to be aware of these specialized regions and their critical role in terms of the restoration of hand function following injury (Tubiana, 1984).

Blood is dually supplied to the wrist and the hand by the ulnar and radial arteries, which join or communicate together after each has individually entered into the hand. The skin of the hand is supplied by both a deep and a superficial plexus. The general pattern of the blood supply to the wrist and the hand does not differ from that which is found in other parts of the body. What differs in terms of cutaneous circulation relates to the hand's distal location from the heart and to its constant exposure to thermal and postural variations (Tubiana, 1984). Similar to the highly complex and varied sensory receptors noted within the hand, particularly within the palmar skin, the hand hosts a complex and dense capillary system (Cauna, 1954). This dense system allows for more variation in capillary pressure than in other parts of the body. Capillary pressure depends on a number of factors such as arteriolar tone, venous return, the position of the wrist and the hand, and temperature (Cauna, 1954; Tubiana, 1984). Hand injury or disease that alters or threatens the cycle of vasodilatation-vasoconstriction can cause progressive wrist and hand edema that leads to stiffness or causalgia.

Control of the Wrist and Hand

Active control of the wrist and hand is achieved through coordinated action of both extrinsic musculature, originating from the forearm and humeral segments, and intrinsic musculature, originating from the carpal and hand segments. This muscular control fulfills needs for both mobility and stability during functional wrist and hand activities. The muscles of the wrist and hand are summarized in Table 14-1. No muscles are intrinsic to the carpus; therefore, passive mechanisms derived from bony morphology, ligamentous function, and tendinous expansions play major roles in controlling carpal and digital movements during hand activities. In this sense, the carpus acts as a bridge for muscle action and load transmission between the hand and forearm segments.

A number of anatomical features contribute to the stability and control of the various articulations of the hand. The coordinated actions of the extrinsic and intrinsic muscles of the hand permit control of the digit rays; a dorsal tendinous complex known as the extensor assembly contributes to the control and stability of the joints and a well-developed flexor tendon sheath pulley system facilitates smooth and stable flexion of these joints. The bony and ligamentous asymmetry of the MCP joints lends the hand its functional versatility. The IP joints gain their stability from the shape of their articular contours and from special ligamentous restraints.

PASSIVE CONTROL MECHANISMS
Bony Mechanisms

The PIP and midcarpal joints in the wrist create a double-hinged system. This bimuscular, biarticular construction is subject to collapse under compressive load (Landsmeer, 1976). Because virtually no muscles insert on the carpus to provide dynamic stability, the compressive forces of the long flexors and extensors tend to cause the carpus to buckle at the PIP and midcarpal joints. Intricate ligamentous constraints and the precise opposition of multifaceted articular surfaces counteract these tendencies and afford stability.

In the sagittal plane of the wrist, both the scaphoid and the lunate are wedge-shaped with the palmar aspect of both bones being wider than the dorsal aspect (Kauer, 1980). Because compression tends to squeeze a wedge to its narrowest portion, both the lunate and the scaphoid would tend to be displaced palmward and rotate into extension with contraction of the long flexors and extensors.

As both the scaphoid and lunate tend to be forced into extension, stabilization forces must be directed primarily toward flexion. It is here that the contribution of the scaphoid spanning both distal and proximal carpal rows can be appreciated. The natural tendency of the scaphoid to extend is stabilized at the midcarpal level; the trapezium and trapezoid articulate with the dorsal aspect of the scaphoid, pushing its distal pole down into flexion. Hence, the scaphoid counteracts the extension tendency of the lunate, lending some stability to the biarticular carpal complex (Fig. 14-7).

This arrangement has an advantage over a symmetrical biarticular system because instability is focused in only one direction and can be countered by a single force applied in the opposite direction or flexion (Kauer, 1980; Kauer & Landsmeer, 1981). This mechanism is consistent with the use of the finger and wrist flexors during hand function.

Ligamentous Mechanisms

WRIST LIGAMENTS

As in other joints, the function of the wrist ligaments is to restrict joint motion and appose joint surfaces. In addition, the ligaments of the wrist are capable of inducing bony displacements and of transmitting loads originating in proximal or distal segments (Taleisnik, 1985). The palmar ligaments (Fig. 14-8A) are thick and strong, whereas the dorsal ligaments (Fig. 14-8B) are much thinner and fewer in number (Taleisnik, 1976, 1985).

The highly developed, complex ligamentous system of the wrist can be divided into extrinsic and intrinsic components (Table 14-2). The extrinsic ligaments run from radius to carpus and from carpus to metacarpals. The intrinsic ligaments originate and insert on the carpus.

The palmar extrinsic ligaments include the radial collateral ligament, the palmar radiocarpal ligaments, and components of the Triangular fibrocartilage complex (TFCC). The radial collateral ligament is actually more palmar than lateral and is viewed as the most lateral of all palmar radiocarpal fascicles rather than as a collateral ligament per se, because the function of a true collateral ligament is not functionally advantageous in the wrist.

The palmar radiocarpal ligaments are arranged in superficial and deep layers. In the superficial layer, most fibers assume a V shape, providing restraint and support. The deep ligaments are three strong fascicles named according to their points of origin and insertion: the radioscaphocapitate (or radiocapitate) ligament, which supports the waist of the scaphoid; the radiolunate ligament, which supports the lunate; and the radioscapholunate ligament, which connects the scapholunate articulation with the palmar portion of the distal radius. This ligament checks scaphoid flexion and extension. Studies of the tensile strength of carpal ligaments suggest that the weakest link between the carpus and the forearm is through the radioscaphocapitate and radial collateral ligaments, both of which are on the radial side of the wrist (Mayfield et al., 1979).

The dorsal extrinsic ligaments include the three bands of the dorsal mediocarpal ligament. Originating from the rim of the radius, these three fascicles insert firmly into the lunate, triquetrum, and scaphoid, respectively.

The intrinsic ligaments can be grouped into three categories (short, long, and intermediate) according to their length and the relative intercarpal movement they allow. Overall, the palmar intrinsic ligaments are thicker and stronger than the dorsal ones.

The three short intrinsic ligaments—palmar, dorsal, and interosseous—are stout, unyielding fibers that bind the adjacent carpal bones tightly. These strong ligaments are responsible for maintaining the four bones of the distal carpal row as an immobile functional unit (Taleisnik, 1976; Weber, 1984). Three intermediate intrinsic ligaments are located between the lunate and triquetrum, the scaphoid and lunate, and the scaphoid and trapezium.

Of the two long intrinsic ligaments—dorsal intercarpal and palmar intercarpal—the palmar is the more important. Also called the deltoid, or V, ligament, it stabilizes the capitate because it attaches to its neck and fans out proximally to in-

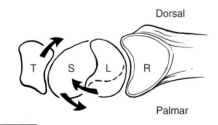

FIG. 14-7

Schematic drawing of the trapezoid (T), scaphoid (S), lunate (L), and radius (R) in a sagittal view. The tendency of the wedge-shaped lunate (palmar pole larger than dorsal pole) to rotate into extension is counteracted by the scaphoid, which provides a palmar-flexing force induced by the trapezium and trapezoid. *Adapted with permission from Taleisnik, J. (1985). The Wrist. New York: Churchill Livingstone.*

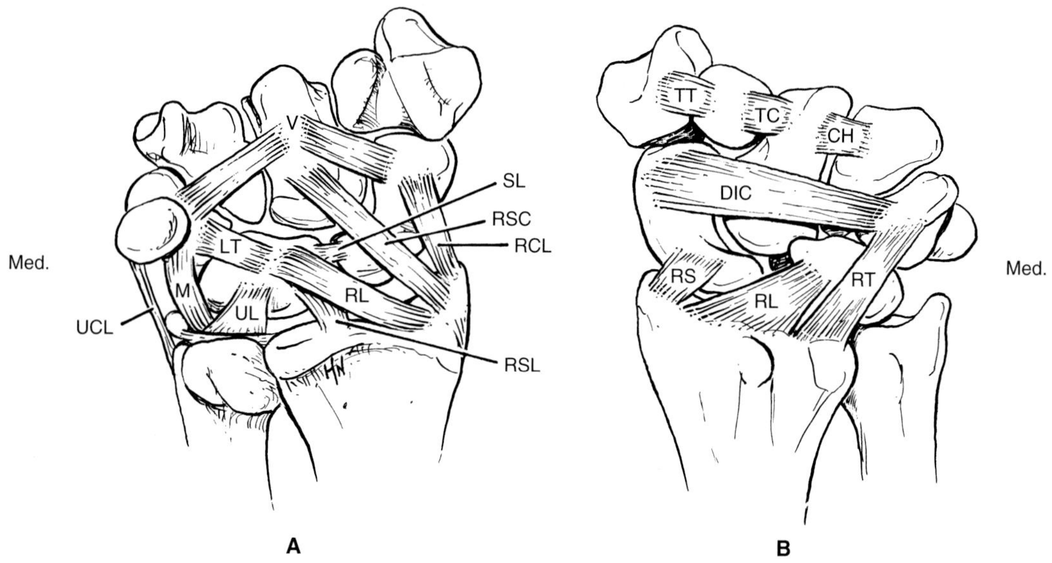

FIG. 14-8

The ligaments of the wrist. **A,** The palmar wrist ligaments (right hand). Extrinsic ligaments: *RSC,* radioscaphocapitate ligament; *RCL,* radial collateral ligament; *RL,* radiolunate ligament; *RSL,* radioscapholunate ligament; *UL,* ulnolunate ligament; *M,* meniscus homologue (radiotriquetral ligament); *UCL,* ulnar collateral ligament; the superficial palmar radiocarpal ligament and the triangular fibrocartilage are not shown. Intrinsic ligaments: *SL,* scapholunate ligament; *LT,* lunotriquetral ligament; *V,* palmar intercarpal (deltoid, or V)

ligament. The short palmar intrinsics are not shown. **B,** The dorsal wrist ligaments of the right hand. Extrinsic ligaments: *RT,* radiotriquetral; *RL,* radiolunate; and *RS,* radioscaphoid fascicles of the dorsal radiocarpal ligament. Intrinsic ligaments: *DIC,* dorsal intercarpal; *TT,* trapeziotrapezoid; *TC,* trapeziocapitate; and *CH,* capitohamate fascicles of the short intrinsic ligaments. The scaphotrapezium ligament is not shown. *Adapted with permission from Taleisnik, J. (1985). The Wrist. New York: Churchill Livingstone.*

TABLE 14-2

Ligaments of the Wrist

Extrinsic Ligaments	Intrinsic Ligaments
Proximal (radiocarpal)	Short
Radiocollateral	Palmar
Palmar radiocarpal	Dorsal
Superficial	Intermediate
Deep	Lunotriquetral
Radioscaphocapitate (radiocapitate)	Scapholunate
Radiolunate	Scaphotrapezium
Radioscapholunate	Long
Ulnocarpal complex	Palmar intercarpal (V, deltoid)
Meniscus homologue (radiotriquetral)	Dorsal intercarpal
Triangular fibrocartilage (articular disc)	
Ulnar collateral ligament	
Ulnolunate ligament	
Dorsal radiocarpal	
Distal (carpometacarpal)	

Modified from Taleisnik, J. (1985). *The Wrist.* New York: Churchill Livingstone.

sert into the scaphoid and triquetrum. The dorsal intercarpal ligament originates from the triquetrum and courses laterally and obliquely to insert on the scaphoid and trapezium (Testut & Latarjet, 1951).

TRIANGULAR FIBROCARTILAGE COMPLEX

The components of the TFCC are the radiotriquetral ligament (meniscus homologue), the triangular fibrocartilage (articular disc), the ulnolunate ligament, the ulnar collateral ligament, and the poorly distinguishable dorsal and palmar radioulnar ligaments (Fig. 14-3). The meniscus homologue and the triangular fibrocartilage have a strong common origin from the dorsoulnar corner (sigmoid notch) of the radius. From there the meniscus courses toward the palm and around the ulnar border of the wrist to insert firmly into the triquetrum, while the triangular fibrocartilage extends horizontally to insert into the base of the ulnar styloid process. Between the meniscus homologue and the triangular fibrocartilage there is often a triangular area, the prestyloid recess, which is filled with synovium. Dorsally, the TFCC has a weak attachment to the carpus except where some of its fibers join the tendon sheath of the flexor carpi ulnaris dorsolaterally. The ulnolunate ligament connects the palmar border of the triangular fibrocartilage with the lunate. The ulnar collateral ligament arises from the ulnar styloid process and extends distally to the base of the fifth metacarpal bone.

Volz et al. (1980) analyzed the pattern of contact between the proximal carpal row and the distal radial and ulnar surfaces while the radiocarpal joint complex was subjected to compressive loads in a position of neutral wrist flexion and extension. With small loads, the initial contact area was between the scaphoid, lunate, and distal radial plate, but with increasing loads the contact area extended to the TFCC. Removal of the TFCC diminished the contact area between the lunate and the distal radial-ulnar surface, thus increasing the stress per unit area between these structures.

Volz's group (1980) concluded that compressive loads are directed across the carpus along a vector force pattern that passes through the head of the capitate to the scapholunate junction and then to the distal radial-ulnar triangular fibrocartilage surfaces. They suggested that any alteration in the alignment of the structures of the proximal and distal carpal rows might provoke an increase in stress in localized areas, which would then accelerate articular cartilage wear.

HAND LIGAMENTS

The hand has an intricate retinacular system that encloses, compartmentalizes, and restrains the joint and tendons as well as the skin, nerves, and blood vessels (Smith et al., 1996). This interconnecting structural system encircles each digit to create balanced forces of the intrinsic and extrinsic musculature and stability and control of the hand.

All of the digital articulations have one essential feature in common: they are designed to function in flexion. Each joint has firm collateral ligaments bilaterally and a thick anterior capsule reinforced by a fibrocartilaginous structure known as the palmar (volar) plate. By comparison, the dorsal capsule is thin and lax. The palmar tendinous apparatus, composed of the two flexor tendons, is much stronger than the dorsal extensor assembly, and even the skin is thicker on the palmar side.

Digital Flexor Tendon Sheath Pulley System

Most tendons in the hand are restrained to some extent by sheaths and retinacula that keep them close to the skeletal plane so that they maintain a relatively constant moment arm, rather than bowstringing across the joints. The pulley system of the flexor tendon sheath in the finger is the most highly developed of these restraints.

As they extend from their muscles, the digital flexor tendons pass through the carpal tunnel, along with the tendon of the flexor pollicis longus and the median nerve, before fanning out toward their respective digits. The flexor superficialis tendon inserts on the middle phalanx and the flexor profundus inserts on the distal phalanx. In each digit, these two tendons, surrounded by their synovial sheaths, are held against the phalanges by a fibrous sheath. At strategic locations along the sheath are five dense annular pulleys (designated as Al, A2, A3, A4, and A5) and three thinner cruciform pulleys (Cl, C2, and C3) (Fig. 14-9). These pulleys allow for a smooth curve so that no sharp or angular bends exist in the course of the tendon. Local points of high pressure, stress raisers, between tendon and sheath are therefore minimized.

At the point where the A3 pulley traverses the PIP joint, the tension in the tendon generated by joint flexion either pulls the pulley away from its attachment to the bone or pulls the bone away from the joint. This is no problem in a normal, stable joint, but when the joint becomes unstable, as in a patient

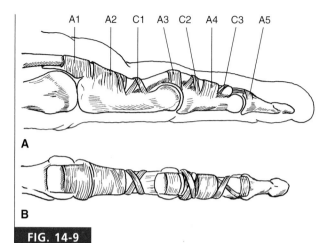

A1 A2 C1 A3 C2 A4 C3 A5

A

B

FIG. 14-9

Schematic drawings of the components of the digital flexor tendon sheath. The five strong annular pulleys (A1, A2, A3, A4, A5) are important in assuring efficient digital motion by apposing the tendons to the phalanges. The three thin, pliable cruciate pulleys (C1, C2, C3) allow flexibility of the sheath while maintaining its integrity. **A,** Mediolateral view. **B,** Palmar view of the sheath without its tendons. *Adapted with permission from Doyle, J.R. & Blythe, W. (1975). The finger flexor tendon sheath and pulleys: Anatomy and reconstruction.* In AAOS Symposium on Tendon Surgery in the Hand. *St. Louis: C.V. Mosby; and Strickland, J.W. (1987). Anatomy and kinesiology of the hand. In E.E. Fess & C.A. Philips (Eds.),* Hand Splinting. Principles and Methods *(2nd ed., pp. 3–41). St. Louis: C.V. Mosby.*

with rheumatoid arthritis, there could be a danger of severe PIP subluxation.

To appreciate the magnitude of these subluxating forces and how they increase with increased flexion, consider two separate flexed positions of a PIP joint: 60° and then 90°. At 60°, the two limbs of the flexor tendon form an angle of 120° (Calculation Box Fig. 14-1-1). At that point, the tension in the restraining pulley must equal the tension in the tendon for the system to be in equilibrium. At 90° of flexion, however, the pulley must sustain 40% more tension than the tendon (Calculation Box Fig. 14-1-2) (Brand, 1985; Brand & Hollister, 1992).

Digital Collateral Ligaments
The common essential feature of the articulations of the digits is that they function in the direction of flexion and have two firm collateral ligaments and a thick reinforced anterior capsule. The anterior fibrocartilage is known as the palmar or volar plate (Tubiana, 1984). There are significant differences between the interphalangeal and metacar-

pophalangeal articulations of the digits as well as significant differences between the same level for each digit (Hakstian & Tubiana, 1967; Kucynski, 1968; Landsmeer, 1955; Smith & Kaplan, 1967; Tubiana, 1984).

A unique feature of the MCP joint is its asymmetry, which is apparent both in the bony configuration of the metacarpal head (Fig. 14-10) and in the location of the radial and ulnar collateral ligament attachments to it (Landsmeer, 1955). The collateral ligaments of the MCP joint extend obliquely forward from the proximal attachment at the dorsolateral aspect of the metacarpal head to their insertion on the palmolateral aspect of the base of the proximal phalanx. The bilateral asymmetry in the site of the attachment of these ligaments manifests itself particularly in the asymmetric range of abduction-adduction in these joints. The asymmetric bilateral arrangement of the interossei also contributes to the overall asymmetry of the MCP joints (Fig. 14-11).

Quantification of the length changes in the collateral ligaments during MCP joint motion was accomplished by Minami and associates (1984), who used biplanar roentgenographic techniques to analyze the lengths of the dorsal, middle, and palmar thirds of the radial and ulnar collateral ligaments of

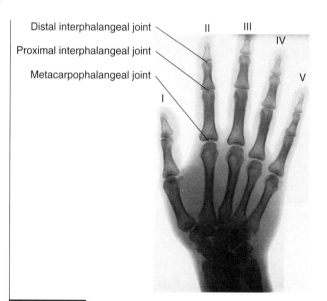

Distal interphalangeal joint
Proximal interphalangeal joint
Metacarpophalangeal joint

FIG. 14-10

Posteroanterior roentgenogram of the right hand and wrist revealing asymmetry in the configuration of the metacarpal heads. Also apparent is the disparity in the diameters of the proximal and distal surfaces of the PIP joints, the distal surfaces being considerably wider.

Flexor Tendon Sheath Pulley System at the PIP Joint

Magnitude of subluxating forces and increment with flexion position at the PIP joint.

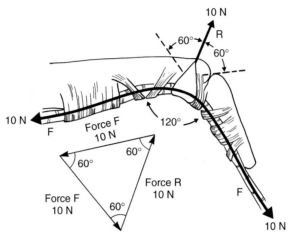

Calculation Box Figure 14-1-1. Lateral view. The PIP joint is flexed 60°. With the system in equilibrium, the resultant force (R) in the pulley system is equal to the vector sum of the two components of the tensile force (F) in the flexor tendon (i.e., 10 N). These three forces are presented graphically in an equilateral triangle of forces.

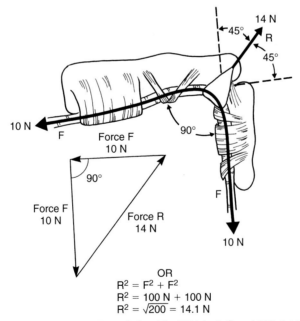

$$OR$$
$$R^2 = F^2 + F^2$$
$$R^2 = 100\ N + 100\ N$$
$$R^2 = \sqrt{200} = 14.1\ N$$

Calculation Box Figure 14-1-2. Lateral view. The PIP joint is flexed 90°. A triangle of forces shows that the resultant force R in the pulley system equals 14 N. Therefore, R equals 1.4 F. The value for R is also found by use of the Pythagorean theorem, which states that in a right triangle, the square of the hypotenuse equals the sum of the squares of the sides. Adapted with permission from Brand, P.W. (1985). *Clinical Mechanics of the Hand* (pp. 30–60). St. Louis: C.V. Mosby.

the index finger at various degrees of joint flexion. When the MCP joint was flexed from 0 to 80°, the dorsal portion of the ligaments lengthened 3 to 4 mm, the middle portion elongated slightly, and the palmar portion shortened 1 to 2 mm. When the MCP joint moved into hyperextension, the dorsal portion of the ligaments shortened 2 to 3 mm, the middle third shortened slightly, and the palmar third lengthened slightly. Thus, the dorsal portions of both collateral ligaments appear to provide the principal restraining force when the MCP joint is

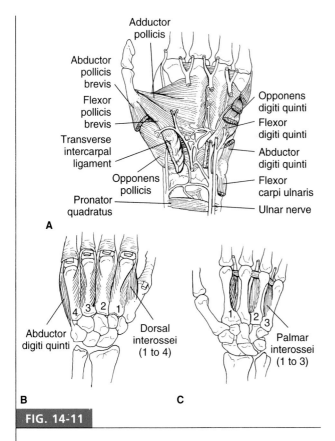

A

B   **C**

FIG. 14-11

The intrinsic muscles of the hand. **A,** Palmar view of the left hand. **B,** Dorsal view of the left hand showing the four dorsal interossei and the abductor digiti quinti. These muscles abduct the fingers (i.e., move them away from the midline of the hand). **C,** Palmar view of the left hand showing the three palmar interossei. These muscles adduct the second, fourth, and fifth fingers, flex the MCP joint, and extend the PIP joint. *Adapted with permission from Strickland, J.W. (1987). Anatomy and kinesiology of the hand. In E.E. Fess & C.A. Philips (Eds.), Hand Splinting. Principles and Methods (2nd ed., pp. 3–41). St. Louis: C.V. Mosby; and Caillet, R. (1982). Hand Pain and Impairment (3rd ed.). Philadelphia: F.A. Davis.*

flexed, while the palmar portions provide a restraining force during MCP extension. This study supports the rationale for positioning the MCP joint in 50 to 70° of flexion to prevent extension contracture when immobilization is required.

The collateral ligaments are found to be slack when the MCP joints are held positioned in extension and taut when the MCPs are positioned in flexion. By placing the MCPs into full flexion, the cam configuration of the metacarpal head tightens the collateral ligaments and the lateral mobility or "play" observed when the MCPs were held into extension is limited (Strickland, 1987). Therefore, the fingers cannot be spread or abducted unless the hand is open, or flattened (Agur, 1991).

The transverse intermetacarpal ligament, which connects the palmar plates, gives additional stability to the MCP region (Fig. 14-12). The extensor tendons are linked to this transverse structure by the transverse laminae, which hold them in position on the dorsal side of the MCP joint.

Volar Plate

In addition to the role of the collateral and accessory collateral ligament, attention is brought to the function of the palmar or volar plate (Fig. 14-13). The accessory collateral ligaments are just palmar to the radial and ulnar collateral ligaments, which originate from the metacarpal and insert into the thick palmar fibrocartilaginous plate. This plate on the volar surface of the MCP is firmly attached to the base of the proximal phalanx and it is loosely attached to the volar surface of the neck of the metacarpal. It serves to reinforce the joint capsule anteriorly and to prevent impingement of the flexor tendons during MCP flexion. This anatomical alignment allows for the volar plate to slide proximally like a moving visor during MCP flexion (Agur, 1991; Strickland, 1987). The volar plate also limits hyperextension of the MCP joint. The volar plates are connected by the transverse intermetacarpal ligaments that then connect each plate to its neighbor (Strickland, 1987).

Tendinous Mechanisms

DIGITAL EXTENSOR ASSEMBLY SYSTEM

The long extensor tendons are flat structures that emerge from their synovial sheaths at the dorsal side of the carpus and run over the MCP joint; they are held in this position by the sagittal bands. At the dorsum of the proximal phalanx, these extensor tendons and parts of the interossei interweave so as to

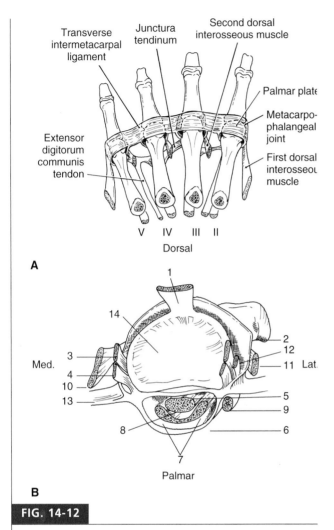

A, Fibrous structures of the proximal transverse (MCP) arch (palmar view of the right hand). Adapted with permission from Tubiana, R. (1984). Architecture and functions of the hand. In R. Tubiana, J.-M. Thomine, & E. Mackin (Eds.), *Examination of the Hand and Upper Limb* (pp. 1–97). Philadelphia: W.B. Saunders. **B,** Capsuloligamentous structures of the MCP joint (transverse view of the proximal phalangeal joint surface, middle finger, left hand). 1, extensor digitorum communis tendon; 2, sagittal band; 3, collateral ligament; 4, accessory collateral ligament; 5, volar plate; 6, flexor tendon sheath; 7, flexor digitorum superficialis tendon; 8, flexor digitorum profundus tendon; 9, lumbrical muscle; 10, dorsal interosseous muscle; 11, dorsal interosseous muscle; 12, insertion of dorsal interosseous muscle into base of phalanx; 13, transverse intermetacarpal ligament; 14, articular surface of proximal phalanx. *Adapted with permission from Zancolli, E. (1979). Structural and Dynamic Bases of Hand Surgery (2nd ed., pp. 3–63). Philadelphia: J.B. Lippincott.*

FIG. 14-12

form a tendinous complex, the extensor assembly (also known as the extensor mechanism), which extends over both IP joints (Fig. 14-14).

Trifurcation of the long extensor tendon and fanning of interosseous fibers result in the formation of one medial and two lateral bands. The medial band (or central slip) runs dorsally over the trochlea of the proximal phalanx and inserts into the base of the middle phalanx. The two lateral bands course alongside the shoulders of the PIP joint. These bands pursue their way distally and merge over the dorsum of the middle phalanx, forming the terminal tendon, which inserts into the dorsal tubercle of the distal phalanx. This terminal tendon is linked to the proximal phalanx by means of the oblique retinacular ligaments. These ligaments originate from the proximal phalanx and run laterally around the PIP joint, just palmar to the center of motion of this joint in the extended position, to join the terminal tendon.

Illustrating the action of the extensor assembly in coupling PIP and DIP joint motion, Landsmeer

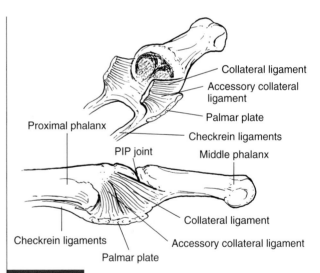

FIG. 14-13

Oblique (*top*) and mediolateral (*bottom*) views of the PIP joint. This joint gains stability from a string, three-sided ligamentous support system produced by the collateral ligament, the accessory collateral ligament, and the palmar fibrocartilaginous plate (volar plate), which is anchored to the proximal phalanx by proximal and lateral extensions know as the checkrein ligaments. *Adapted with permission from Strickland, J.W. (1987). Anatomy and kinesiology of the hand. In E.E. Fess & C.A. Philips (Eds.), Hand Splinting. Principles and Methods (2nd ed., pp. 3–41). St. Louis: C.V. Mosby.*

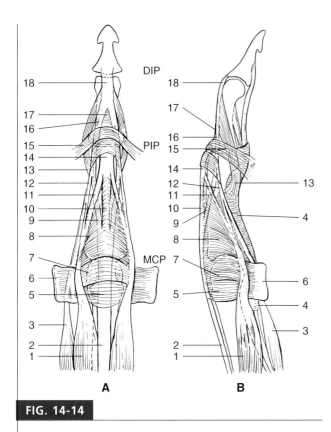

DIP

18

17
16
15
14
13
12
11
10
9
8

7

6
5

3

2
1

PIP

MCP

18

17

16
15

14

12
11
10
9
8

7

5

2
1

13

4

6

4

3

A   **B**

FIG. 14-14

Schematic drawing of the digital extensor assembly. *MCP,* metacarpophalangeal joint; *PIP,* proximal interphalangeal joint; *DIP,* distal interphalangeal joint. 1, interosseous muscle; 2, extensor digitorum communis tendon; 3, lumbrical muscle; 4, flexor tendon fibrous sheath; 5, sagittal band; 6, intermetacarpal ligament; 7, transverse fibers of interosseous hood; 8, oblique fibers of interosseous hood; 9, lateral band of long extensor tendon; 10, medial band of long extensor tendon; 11, central band of interosseous tendon; 12, lateral band of interosseous tendon; 13, oblique retinacular ligament; 14, medial band of long extensor tendon in central slip; 15, transverse retinacular ligament; 16, lateral band of long extensor tendon; 17, triangular ligament; 18, terminal tendon. **A,** Dorsal view. Just proximal to the PIP joint, the long extensor tendon (extensor digitorum communis tendon) within the central slip trifurcates into one medial and two lateral bands. The medial band inserts into the base of the middle phalanx. The lateral bands converge over the dorsum of the middle phalanx to form the terminal tendon, which inserts on the distal phalanx. **B,** Sagittal view. The oblique retinacular ligaments, which originate from the proximal phalanx, course laterally around the PIP joint just palmar to the center of rotation of flexion-extension, then join the terminal tendon. *Adapted with permission from Tubiana, R. (1984). Architecture and functions of the hand. In R. Tubiana, J.-M. Thomine, & E. Mackin (Eds.),* Examination of the Hand and Upper Limb *(pp. 1–97). Philadelphia: W.B. Saunders*

(1949) described the "release of the distal phalanx" (Fig. 14-15). If a finger is flexed at the PIP joint only, the whole trifurcated extensor assembly is pulled distally, following the central slip. This slip alone is taut because the distal pull occurs at the middle phalanx; the lateral bands remain slack but are allowed to shift distally over the same distance. Only part of the slack of the lateral bands is required for flexion of the PIP joint because these bands run closer to the center of motion of this joint than does the central slip. Therefore, some of the slack will remain, allowing passive or active flexion of the distal phalanx but no active extension. The "released" distal phalanx is the functional basis for the coupled flexion and extension of the DIP and PIP joints.

Conversely, if the DIP is actively flexed, the entire extensor assembly is displaced distally. This relaxes the central slip and simultaneously increases the tension in the oblique retinacular ligaments, a tension that creates a flexion force at the PIP joint. Because the central slip is already unloaded, flexion of this joint is then unavoidable. The release of the distal phalanx is fundamental for pulp-to-pulp pinch. It also allows, through intermittent contraction of the flexor profundus, a change from pulp-to-pulp to tip-

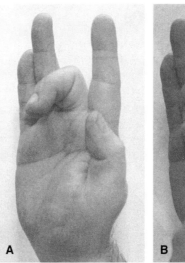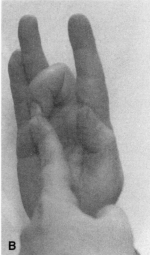

A   **B**

FIG. 14-15

Release of the distal phalanx. **A,** All fingers are extended, and the PIP joint of the middle finger is flexed. The DIP joint of this finger is totally out of control. **B,** The DIP joint is very loose and can be flexed or extended only passively.

to-tip pinch, a mechanism used in precision handling such as needlework and active tactile exploration.

Sarrafian and coworkers (1970) used strain gauges to measure the tension in different parts of the extensor mechanism during finger flexion and further elaborated on this phenomenon. They found an increase in the central slip tension beyond 60° of PIP flexion; at 90° of flexion there was total relaxation of the lateral bands.

ACTIVE CONTROL MECHANISMS

Muscular Mechanisms of the Wrist

The wrist joint complex is surrounded at its periphery by the 10 wrist tendons, whose muscles and their actions are listed in Table 14-1. The three flexors and three extensors are the motors of the wrist, controlling radial and ulnar deviation as well as wrist flexion and extension. Four additional muscles control pronation and supination of the forearm. Eight of the muscles originate from the forearm, and two, the brachialis and extensor carpi radialis longus, originate above the elbow. Except for the flexor carpi ulnaris tendon, which attaches to the pisiform, all of the wrist muscle tendons traverse the carpal bones to insert on the metacarpals.

Each wrist tendon has a substantial amplitude of excursion. The extensor carpi radialis brevis and longus each have a maximal excursion of approximately 37 mm. The flexor carpi radialis excursion is approximately 40 mm, and that of the flexor carpi ulnaris is approximately 33 mm. The pronator teres excursion is approximately 50 mm (Boyes, 1970). Impairment of the excursion of any of these tendons owing to adhesions after trauma or surgery can seriously limit wrist motion.

The arrangement of digital and wrist extensor and flexor systems around the wrist axis makes for antagonist groupings of motor forces that afford positional stability. The extensor digitorum communis and extensor indicis proprius pair against the flexor carpi radialis and flexor pollicis longus. The extensor carpi ulnaris works against the extensor pollicis brevis, and the abductor pollicis longus and extensor carpi radialis longus pair against the flexor carpi ulnaris and the flexor digitorum pollicis (Steindler, 1955).

The contributions of the extensor carpi ulnaris, extensor pollicis brevis, and abductor pollicis

longus were assessed electromyographically during wrist flexion (Kauer, 1979, 1980). In addition to demonstrating their expected muscle actions, these muscles were found to function as a dynamic "adjustable collateral system" that acts as a true collateral support, the extensor carpi ulnaris for the ulnar side of the wrist and the extensor pollicis brevis and abductor pollicis longus for the radial side. In this way, active control mechanisms serve to fulfill the void left by the lack of collateral ligamentous restrictions while still affording considerable positional variability for functional hand activities (Case Study 14-2).

CASE STUDY 14-2

de Quervain's Tenosynovitis

A 50-year-old female school teacher complains of pain on active radial abduction of the thumb after performing a prolonged, continuous paper cutting task. The pain extends proximally from the radial styloid along the dorsoradial aspect of the wrist and increases with passive stretch of the abductor pollicis longus (Finkelstein's test). After a careful examination, de Quervain's tenosynovitis is confirmed.

In this case, overuse by performance of a repetitive, forceful task involving abduction of the thumb while the wrist is ulnar deviated contributed to the development of the tenosynovitis. Another contributing factor is the anatomical structure of this first dorsal compartment of the wrist. The restrictive volume of this compartment along with the multiaxial movements of the thumb render the tendons of the abductor pollicis longus and the extensor pollicis brevis susceptible to inflammation following exposure to high frictional loads.

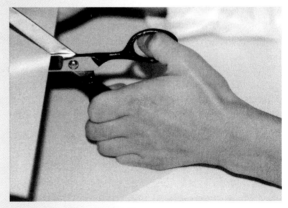

Case Study Figure 14-2-1.

Muscular Mechanisms of the Hand

The digital rays are controlled by the extrinsic and intrinsic muscles (Table 14-1). The extrinsic muscles originate in the arm and forearm. The intrinsic muscles are entirely confined to the hand (Fig. 14-11). Although the contribution of each system is distinctly different, the coordinated functioning of intrinsic and extrinsic muscle systems is essential for the satisfactory performance of the hand in a wide range of tasks.

The values most often cited for the strengths of the extrinsic muscles of the hand were reported by Von Lanz and Wachsmuth (1970). Their values (Table 14-3) show that the strength of the finger flexors is over twice that of the extensors.

Kinematics

The multiplicity of wrist articulations and the complexity of carpal motion make it difficult to calculate the instant center of motion for the primary axes of flexion-extension or radial-ulnar deviation. Various studies have placed the instant center of rotation in the head of the capitate, with the flexion-extension axis oriented from the radial to the ulnar styloid process and the radial-ulnar deviation axis oriented orthogonal to the flexion-extension axis. This kinematic model is undoubtedly an oversimplification of the complex carpal motions during wrist movement, but it appears to adequately describe functional wrist movement (Brumbaugh et al., 1982, Landsmeer, 1961; MacConaill, 1941; Volz et al., 1980; von Bonin, 1929; Wright, 1935/1936; Youm & Yoon, 1979).

The hand is an extremely mobile organ that can coordinate an infinite variety of movements in relation to each of its components. The blending of hand and wrist movements enables the hand to mold itself to the shape of an object being palpated or grasped. The great mobility of the hand is the result of the articular contours, the position of the bones in relation to one another, and the actions of an intricate system of muscles.

WRIST RANGE OF MOTION

The articulations of the wrist joint complex allow motion in two planes: flexion-extension (palmar flexion and dorsiflexion) in the sagittal plane and radial-ulnar deviation (abduction-adduction) in the frontal plane. Combinations of these motions are also possible, the greatest range of wrist motion taking place from radial deviation and extension to ulnar deviation and palmar flexion.

TABLE 14-3

Strength Values of the Extrinsic Muscles of the Hand

Muscle	Strength (Nm)
Flexor pollicis longus	12
Extensor pollicis longus	1
Abductor pollicis longus	
As a wrist flexor	1
As a wrist abductor	4
Extensor pollicis brevis	1
Flexor digitorum superficialis	48
Flexor digitorum profundus communis	45
Extensor digitorum communis	17
Extensor indicis proprius	5

Data from Von Lanz, T. & Wachsmuth, W. (1970). Functional anatomy. In J.H. Boyes (Ed.), *Bunnell's Surgery of the Hand* (5th Ed.). Philadelphia: J.B. Lippincott.

Although small amounts of axial rotation are possible and may exist in some individual wrists, from a practical standpoint such rotation does not occur through the carpal complex (Volz, 1976; Youm et al., 1978). Axial rotation of the hand, expressed as pronation and supination, results instead from motion arising at the proximal and distal radioulnar and the radiohumeral joints (Volz et al., 1980).

Flexion and Extension

The normal wrist range of motion is 65 to 80° of flexion and 55 to 75° of extension, but it can vary widely among individuals. Owing to a slight palmar tilt of the distal radial plates, flexion exceeds extension by an average of 10°.

Investigators have found various values for the contribution of the proximal and distal carpal rows to the total arc of flexion and extension. Sarrafian and coworkers (1977) noted that approximately 60% of flexion occurs at the midcarpal joint and 40% in the radiocarpal joint, while approximately 67% of extension takes place at the radiocarpal joint and 33% at the midcarpal joint (Fig. 14-16).

Radial and Ulnar Deviation

The total arc of radial-ulnar deviation is approximately 65°, 15 to 25° radialward and 30 to 45° ulnarward (Simon et al., 1994; Volz et al., 1980; Youm et al., 1978). The distal carpal row follows the finger rays during both radial and ulnar deviation, whereas the proximal carpal row glides in the direction opposite to hand movement with greater excursion during ulnar deviation.

During radial deviation, the scaphoid undergoes flexion (palmward rotation of its distal pole) as a result of its encroachment on the radial styloid process (Fig. 14-17A). This scaphoid motion is transmitted across the proximal row through the scapholunate ligament. Thus, in radial deviation the scaphoid flexes and so does the proximal carpal row. This conjunct movement of the scaphoid and proximal carpal row is reversed toward extension during ulnar deviation (Fig. 14-17C). During ulnar deviation, the triquetrum is displaced palmward by the proximal migration of the hamate. The motion of the triquetrum in turn causes the lunate to extend.

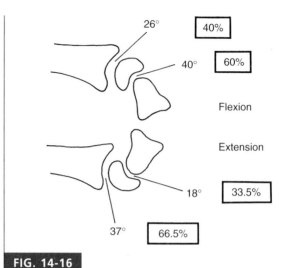

FIG. 14-16

Approximately 60% of wrist flexion (*top*) occurs at the midcarpal joint, whereas approximately two thirds of wrist extension (*bottom*) arises at the radiocarpal joint. *Adapted with permission from Sarrafian, S.K., Melamed, J.L., & Goshgarian, G.M. (1977). Study of wrist motion in flexion and extension.* Clin Orthop, 126, *153.*

A double-V system formed by the palmar intercarpal ligament and the radiolunate and ulnolunate ligaments renders support during radial-ulnar deviation (Fig. 14-18). The apex of the proximal V is at the lunate and that of the distal V at the capitate. In ulnar deviation, the medial arm of the proximal V, the ulnolunate ligament, becomes somewhat transverse and inhibits radial displacement of the lunate, while the lateral arm, the radiolunate ligament, orients longitudinally and limits lunate extension. The V configuration is now an L. The distal V also becomes an L, but in the opposite direction. The lateral intrinsic ligamentous fibers connecting the scaphoid and capitate become somewhat transverse to check the central ulnar translation of the capitate during this motion. The medial fibers from triquetrum to capitate shift longitudinally and control capitate flexion. In radial deviation, the opposite configurations apply (Taleisnik, 1985).

Forearm Pronation and Supination

The motions of forearm pronation and supination through the PIP and distal radioulnar and mediohumeral joints, although not part of wrist motion proper, play an intricate role in hand and wrist function. Average range of motion of pronation-supination is 150° (60–80° of pronation and 60–85° of supination). In a biomechanical study, Youm et al. (1979) found the axis of pronation-supination to lie oblique to both the radius and the ulnar, passing through the center of the humeral capitulum and the midpoint of the head of the ulna. Modest lateral movement of

the ulnar head of up to 9° in the direction opposite that of the distal radius has been demonstrated during this motion (Ray et al., 1951), and the ulnar head glides in the sigmoid notch of the radius from a dorsal distal position to a palmar proximal position as the forearm moves from full pronation into full supination (Bunnell, 1956; Palmer & Wemer, 1984; Rose-Innes, 1990; Vesely, 1967).

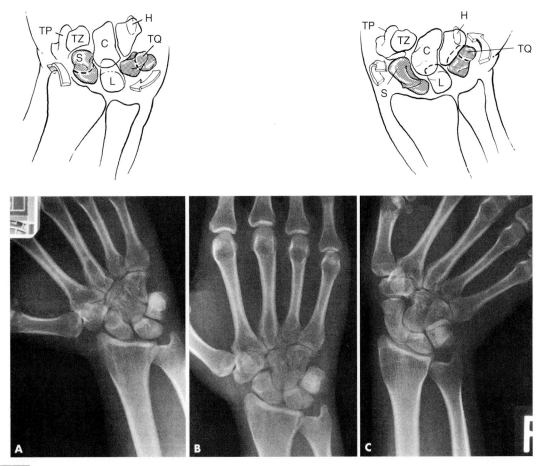

FIG. 14-17

Roentgenograms of the right wrist and hand (dorsal view) showing the position of the carpal bones in radial deviation (**A**), in the neutral position (**B**), and in ulnar deviation (**C**). *Arrows* in the schematic drawings above roentgenograms **A** and **C** indicate general movement of the bones of the proximal row with wrist motion. In radial deviation, the bones of the proximal row are flexed toward the palm. The scaphoid appears foreshortened, the lunate appears triangular, and the

triquetrum is proximal in relation to the hamate. In ulnar deviation, the bones of the proximal row are extended. The scaphoid appears elongated, the shape of the lunate appears trapezoidal, and the triquetrum is distal in relation to the hamate. *TP*, trapezium; *TZ*, trapezoid; *C*, capitate; *H*, hamate; *TQ*, triquetrum; *L*, lunate; *S*, scaphoid. Roentgenogram courtesy of Alex Norman, M.D.; *drawings adapted with permission from Taleisnik, J. (1985). The Wrist. New York: Churchill Livingstone.*

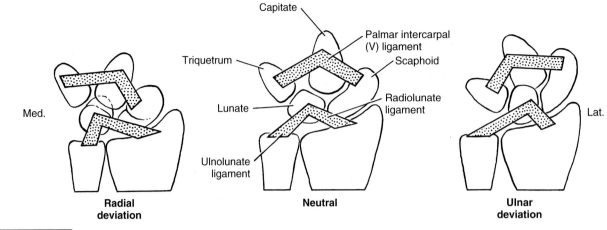

FIG. 14-18

Diagrammatic representation of the changes in alignment of the double-V system formed by the ulnolunate and radiolunate ligaments and the palmar intercarpal (V, or deltoid) ligament with the wrist in radial deviation, the neutral position, and ulnar deviation (palmar view of right hand). *Adapted with permission from Taleisnik, J. (1985). The Wrist. New York: Churchill Livingstone.*

DIGITAL RANGE OF MOTION

The varying shapes of the CMC, MCP, and IP joints of the fingers are responsible for the differences in degrees of freedom at these joints. The unique orientation of the thumb, the large web space, and the special configuration of the thumb CMC joint affords this digit great mobility and versatility.

Fingers

The second and third metacarpals are linked to the trapezoid and capitate and to each other by tight-fitting joints that are basically immobile (Fig. 14-19). As a result, these metacarpal and carpal bones constitute the "immobile unit" of the hand. The articulations of the fourth and fifth metacarpals with the hamate permit a modest amount of motion: 10 to 15° of flexion-extension at the fourth CMC joint and 20 to 30° at the fifth. Limited palmar displacement, or descent, of these metacarpals may take place. This motion allows cupping of the hand and is essential for gripping.

The MCP joints of the four fingers are unicondylar diarthrodial joints (Figs. 14-10 and 14-19), allowing motion in three planes: flexion-extension (sagittal plane), abduction-adduction (frontal plane), and slight pronation-supination (transverse plane), which is coupled with abduction-adduction (Hagert, 1981).

The range of MCP flexion from the zero position is approximately 90° (Fig. 14-20A), but this value differs among the fingers. The fifth finger demonstrates the most flexion (approximately 95°) and the second (index) finger, approximately 70° (Batmanabane & Malathi, 1985). Extension beyond the zero position varies considerably and depends on joint laxity.

The PIP and distal joints of the four digits are bicondylar hinge joints as a result of the tongue-and-groove fit of their articular surfaces (Figs. 14-10 and 14-19). These surfaces are closely congruent throughout the range of flexion-extension, which is the only motion possible in these joints. Flexion is measured from the zero position with the finger in the plane of the hand. The largest range of flexion, 110° or more, occurs in the PIP joint (Fig. 14-20B). Flexion of approximately 90° takes place in the DIP joint (Fig. 14-20C). Extension beyond the zero position, termed hyperextension, is a regular feature of the DIP and PIP joints, although it depends largely on ligamentous laxity, especially in the PIP joint.

The range of motion of the MCP, PIP, and DIP joints is often reported individually for each of the three joints. In addition to this, composite measurements scores are often reported. These summation scores for either active or passive movement—TAM (total active movement) or TPM (total passive movement)—represent the summation of the total available degrees of flexion at the MCP, PIP, and DIP joints for a given digit minus the extension deficit for each of the represented three joints.

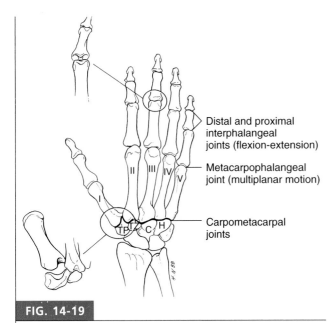

Distal and proximal interphalangeal joints (flexion-extension)

Metacarpophalangeal joint (multiplanar motion)

Carpometacarpal joints

FIG. 14-19

Schematic representations of the joints of the finger rays (dorsal view of the right hand). The CMC joint between the first metacarpal and trapezium (TP) is composed of two saddle-shaped surfaces, the convexity of one fitting tightly into the concavity of the other (*inset* shows enlargement). This arrangement allows for movement of the thumb in a wide arc of motion. The tight-fitting joints that link the second and third metacarpals with the trapezoid (TZ) and capitate (C), respectively, and with each other are relatively immobile, rendering these four bones the "immobile unit" of the hand. The joints between the fourth and fifth metacarpals and the hamate (H) permit a modest amount of flexion and extension. The unicondylar configuration of the MCP joints of the four fingers allows motion in three planes and combinations thereof. By contrast, the tongue-and-groove articular contours of the bicondylar hinge joints between the phalanges limit motion to one plane (flexion-extension) and contribute to the stability of these joints in resisting shear and rotary forces (*inset* shows enlargement of a typical IP joint in an oblique view). *Adapted with permission from Strickland, J.W. (1987). Anatomy and kinesiology of the hand. In E.E. Fess & C.A. Philips (Eds.),* Hand Splinting: Principles and Methods *(2nd ed., pp. 3–41). St. Louis: C.V. Mosby; and Van Zwieten, K.J. (1980). The extensor assembly of the finger in man and non-human primates: A morphological, functional, and comparative anatomical study. Unpublished Thesis, University of Leiden, The Netherlands.*

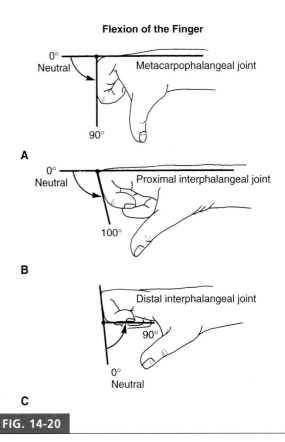

Flexion of the Finger

0° Neutral

Metacarpophalangeal joint

90°

A

0° Neutral

Proximal interphalangeal joint

100°

B

Distal interphalangeal joint

90°

0° Neutral

C

FIG. 14-20

Flexion of the three joints of the finger, beginning with the neutral position in which the extended fingers are in the plane of the dorsal hand and wrist. **A,** Flexion of the MCP joint, averaging 70 to 90°. **B,** Flexion at the PIP joint, averaging 100° or more. **C,** Flexion at the DIP joint, averaging 90°. *Adapted with permission from American Academy of Orthopaedic Surgeons (1965).* Joint Motion: Method of Measuring and Recording. *Chicago: AAOS. [Reprinted by the British Orthopaedic Association, 1966.]*

Thumb

At the CMC level, the base of the thumb metacarpal forms a saddle joint with the trapezium (Fig. 14-19). This configuration allows the thumb metacarpal a wide range of motion through a conical space extending from the plane of the hand palmarly to the radial direction. Motion of the first metacarpal is described in degrees of abduction, either radial or palmar, from the second metacarpal, thereby defining the plane in which this motion is carried out with respect to the plane of the hand. The terms flexion and extension with respect to the thumb are reserved for motions of the MCP and IP joints.

Functionally, the most important motion of the thumb is opposition, in which abduction coupled with rotation at the CMC joint moves the thumb toward the pad of the little finger; flexion at the MCP and IP joints then brings the thumb closer to the fingertips (Fig. 14-21). Full opposition is then noted when the pad of the thumb touches the pad of the fifth finger. A lateral orientation of the thumb to the fifth finger represents use of flexion and adduction, for it is the use of the opponens muscles that defines thumb opposition, which is only considered complete when pad to pad contact is made.

The MCP joint of the thumb resembles those of the fingers. The range of flexion from the zero position varies considerably among individuals, from as little as 30° to as much as 90°; extension from the zero position is approximately 15° (Batmanabane & Malathi, 1985). The IP joint of the thumb, the most distal joint, resembles and performs similarly to the analogous distal joints in the fingers.

FUNCTIONAL WRIST MOTION

Because the joints proximal to the wrist may provide compensatory motion, even a considerable loss of wrist motion may not interfere significantly with activities of daily living. An electrogoniometric study of the range of wrist flexion-extension required for accomplishing 14 activities showed that an arc of 45° (10° of flexion to 35° of extension) was sufficient for performing most of them (Brumfield & Champoux, 1984). Seven activities of personal care that require placing the hand at various locations on the body were accomplished within a range of 10° of flexion to 15° of extension, and most were performed with the wrist slightly flexed. Other necessary activities requiring an arc of wrist motion, such as eating, drinking, using a telephone, and reading,

OPPOSITION OF THE THUMB
Composite of Three Motions

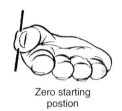

Zero starting
postion

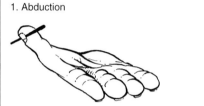

1. Abduction

2. Rotation

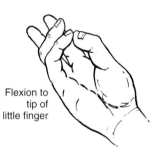

3. Flexion

Flexion to
tip of
little finger

FIG. 14-21

Opposition of the thumb, which begins with the extended thumb in line with the index finger, is the combined motions of abduction and rotation of the (CMC) joint. Flexion in the metacarpophalangeal (MCP) and interphalangeal (IP) joints then brings the tip of the thumb closer to the fifth finger. Palmar displacement, or descent, of the fourth and fifth metacarpals and flexion in the MCP and IP joints of the fifth finger result in tip-to-tip contact between the thumb and fifth finger. *Adapted with permission from the American Academy of Orthopaedic Surgeons (1965).* Joint Motion: Method of Measuring and Recording. *Chicago: AAOS. [Reprinted by the British Orthopaedic Association, 1966.]*

were accomplished by motion of 5° of flexion to 35° of extension. Nearly all of these continuous tasks required only extension. Rising from a chair employed the greatest arc of motion, nearly 63°. Volz and coworkers (1980) also found that loss of wrist mobility did not seriously impede performance of the activities of daily living. Volunteers with wrists immobilized in four different positions were asked to rate their performance on 10 activities, and performance averages were then computed for each position of immobilization. The results disclosed the least compromise of hand function with wrists immobilized in 15° of extension (88% of normal performance) and the greatest disability with the wrists placed in 20° of ulnar deviation (71% of normal function).

Interaction of Wrist and Hand Motion

Wrist motion is essential for augmenting the fine motor control of the fingers and hand. Positioning the wrist in the direction opposite that of the fingers alters the functional length of the digital tendons so that maximal finger movement can be attained. Wrist extension is synergistic to finger flexion and increases the length of the finger flexor muscles, allowing increased flexion with stretch (Fig. 14-22A) (Tubiana, 1984). Conversely, some flexion of the wrist puts tension on the long extensors, causing the fingers to open automatically and aiding full finger extension (Fig. 14-22B).

The synergistic movements of the wrist extensors and the more powerful digital flexors are facilitated by the architecture of the wrist. The digital flexor tendons cross the wrist within the depths of the carpal arch and are held close to the axis of wrist flexion-extension, affecting wrist position minimally. By contrast, the extrinsic wrist flexors and extensors are positioned widely about the periphery to provide maximal moment arms for positioning the wrist.

As the wrist changes its position and the functional lengths of the digital flexor tendons are altered, the resultant forces in the fingers vary, affecting the ability to grip. Volz and associates (1980) evaluated electromyographically the relationship of grip strength and wrist position. Grip strengths of 67, 134, 201, and 268 N were analyzed with the wrist in five positions: 40 and 20° of flexion, neu-

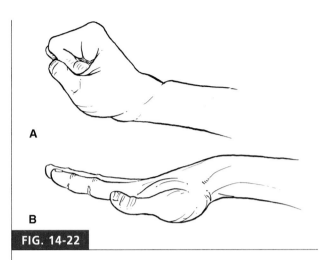

A

B

FIG. 14-22

Role of wrist position in finger function. **A,** Slight extension of the wrist allows the flexor muscles to attain maximal functional length, permitting full flexion. **B,** Slight flexion of the wrist places tension on the digital extensor tendons automatically opening the hand and aiding full finger extension.

tral, and 20 and 40° of extension. They found that grip strength was greatest at approximately 20° of wrist extension and least at 40° of wrist flexion. With the wrist in 40° of extension and in the neutral position, grip strength was slightly less than the maximal values.

Studies by Hazelton and coworkers (1975) of the influence of wrist position on the force produced at the middle and distal phalanges revealed that the greatest force was generated with the wrist in ulnar deviation, the next greatest in extension, and the least in palmar flexion. Taken together, the results of Volz and associates (1980) and Hazelton et al. (1975) suggest that for grip to be effective and have maximal force, the wrist must be stable and must be in slight extension and ulnar deviation. This conclusion is consistent with the findings concerning load transmission through the ulnar TFCC structures.

The position of the wrist also changes the position of the thumb and fingers, thus affecting the ability to grip. When the wrist is flexed with the hand relaxed, the pulp of the thumb reaches only the level of the DIP of the index finger; with the wrist extended, the pulps of the thumb and index finger are passively in contact, creating an optimal situation for gripping or patching (Fig. 14-23).

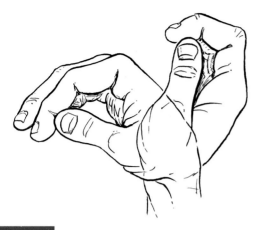

FIG. 14-23

When the wrist is flexed, the tip of the thumb is level with the distal interphalangeal joint of the index finger. With the wrist in extension, the pulps of the thumb and index finger come passively into contact. *Adapted with permission from Tubiana, R. (1984). Architecture and functions of the hand. In R. Tubiana, J.-M. Thomine, & E. Mackin (Eds.), Examination of the Hand and Upper Limb (pp. 1–97). Philadelphia: W. B. Saunders.*

Patterns of Prehensile Hand Function

Prehensile movements of the hand are those in which an object is seized and held partly or wholly within the compass of the hand. Such movements are used in a broad range of purposive activities involving handling of objects of all shapes and sizes. Efficient prehensile function depends on a multitude of factors, the most important of which are:

1. Mobility of the first CMC joint and, to a lesser extent, of the fourth and fifth MCP joints
2. Relative rigidity of the second and third CMC joints
3. Stability of the longitudinal finger and thumb arches
4. Balanced synergism and antagonism between the long extrinsic muscles and the hand intrinsic muscles
5. Adequate sensory input from all areas of the hand
6. The precise relationships among the length, mobility, and position of each digital ray.

Many attempts have been made to classify different patterns of prehensile hand function. Napier (1956) identified two distinct patterns of prehensile movement in the normal hand: power grip and precision grip. He emphasized that the fundamental requisite to prehension, stability, can be met by either posture.

Power grip, or power grasp, is a forceful act performed with the finger flexed at all three joints so that the object is held between the finger and the palm, with the thumb positioned on the palmar side of the object to force it securely into the palm (Fig. 14-24*A*). It is usually performed with the wrist deviated ulnarly and dorsiflexed slightly to augment the tension in the flexor tendons.

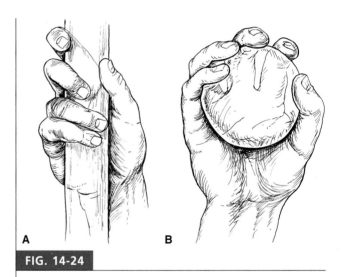

A **B**

FIG. 14-24

The two fundamental patterns of prehensile hand function. **A,** A typical power grip. The adducted thumb forms a clamp with the partly flexed fingers and the palm. The palmar descent of metacarpals IV and V and additional flexion in their respective MCP joints enable these fingers to hold the object firmly against the palm. Counter-pressure is applied by the thumb, which lies approximately in the plane of the palm. The wrist is deviated ulnarward and dorsiflexed slightly to increase the tension in the flexor tendons. Grip of an object along the oblique palmar axis (palmar groove), as shown here, involves a larger area of contact, and thus more control, than does grip along the transverse palmar axis. **B,** A typical precision maneuver. The object is pinched between the flexor aspects of the fingers and the thumb. The fingers are semiflexed and the thumb is abducted and opposed. The wrist is dorsiflexed. *Adapted with permission from Landsmeer, J.M.F. (1955). Anatomical and functional investigations on the articulation of the human fingers. Acta Anat Suppl, 24.*

Precision grip involves the manipulation of small objects between the thumb and the flexor aspects of the fingers in a finely controlled manner (Fig. 14-24B). The wrist position varies so as to increase the manipulative range. The fingers are generally in a semiflexed position, and the thumb is palmarly abducted and opposed. Certain prehensile activities involve both power and precision grips (Fig. 14-25).

As a refinement of Napier's classification, Landsmeer (1962) suggested that the precision grip be termed "precision handling" because it involves no forceful gripping of the object and is a dynamic process without a static phase. In both power grip and precision handling, full opposition of the thumb to the ring and little fingers is obtained via palmar displacement of the metacarpals of these digits.

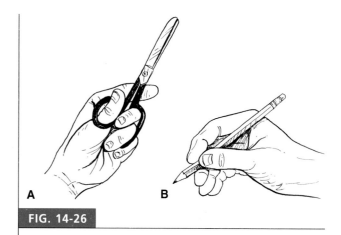

FIG. 14-26

The "dynamic tripod," a type of precision handling where the thumb, index finger, and middle finger work in close synergy for precision handling of the object while the ring finger and the little finger provide support and static control. This functional configuration is demonstrated in the use of scissors (**A**) and a pencil (**B**).

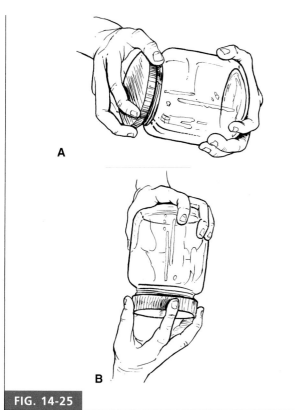

FIG. 14-25

The two fundamental patterns of hand function are used in unscrewing the lid of a tightly closed jar. **A,** As the motion is begun, the right hand assumes a power grip posture. **B,** As the lid loosens, the hand assumes a precision posture to perform the final stages of unscrewing. *Adapted with permission from Napier, J.R. (1956). The prehensile movements of the human hand.* J Bone Joint Surg, 38B, 902–913.

A variant of precision handling is the often used "dynamic tripod" (Capener, 1956), wherein the thumb, index finger, and middle finger have a dynamic action, working in close synergy for precision handling of the object, while the ring and little fingers are used largely for support and static control (Fig. 14-26). A further refinement is pinching a small object between the thumb and index finger. Such maneuvers are commonly classified as tip pinch, palmar pinch, lateral (or key) pinch, and pulp (or ulnar) pinch, depending on the parts of the phalanges brought to bear on the object being handled (Fig. 14-27).

Another important distinction between power grip and precision handling is the fundamentally different position of the thumb in each posture. In the power grip, the thumb is adducted; in precision handling, it is palmarly abducted (Fig. 14-24). The relationship of the hand to the forearm also differs strikingly. In the power grip (Fig. 14-24A), the hand is usually deviated ulnarly and the wrist is held approximately in a neutral position so that the long axis of the thumb coincides with that of the forearm. In this way, pronation and supination can be transmitted from the forearm to the object. In precision handling (Fig. 14-24B), the hand is generally held midway between wrist radial and ulnar deviation, and the wrist is markedly reflected in the posture of the thumb. When the demand for precision is minimal or absent, the thumb is wrapped over the dorsum of the middle phalanges of the digits and acts purely as a reinforcing mechanism. When an element of precision is required in what is predominately a power grip, such as the fencing grip (Fig. 14-28A), the thumb is adducted and aligned with the long axis of the cylinder so that, by means of small

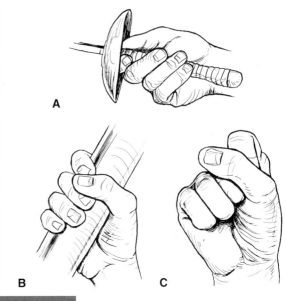

FIG. 14-28

The fencing grip (**A**) is a power grip in which the element of precision plays a large part. Instead of being wrapped over the dorsum of the digits, the thumb is aligned with the long axis of the cylinder so that it can control the direction in which the force is applied. In so doing, the thumb loses its effect as a powerful buttress on the radial side of the hand. Hence, some of the power grip is sacrificed in the interest of precision. The coal-hammer grip (**B**) and the bunched fist (**C**) are examples of a string power grip with no element of precision. The ulnar deviation characteristic of a power grip is apparent in both cases. *Adapted with permission from Napier, J.R. (1956). The prehensile movements of the human hand.* J Bone Joint Surg, 38B, 902–913.

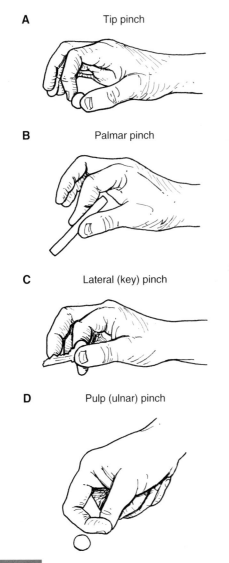

A Tip pinch

B Palmar pinch

C Lateral (key) pinch

D Pulp (ulnar) pinch

FIG. 14-27

Examples of precision handling in which small objects are pinched between the thumb and index finger. These grips are classified according to the parts of the phalanges brought to bear on the object handled. **A,** Tip-to-tip pinch. **B,** Palmar pinch. **C,** Lateral (key) pinch. **D,** Pulp (ulnar) pinch.

adjustments of posture, it can control the direction in which the force is being applied. At the other extreme of the power grip range is the coal-hammer grip (Fig. 14-28B), the crudest form of prehensile function, where the thumb is wholly occupied in reinforcing the clamping action of the digits. An example of this extreme in an empty hand is the bunched fist (Fig. 14-28C).

Rotating the thumb into an opposing position is a requirement of almost every hand function, whether it be a strong grip or a delicate precision pinch. In some instances, however, the thumb may not be involved at all, as in the hook grip in which the fingers are flexed so that their pads lie parallel and slightly away from the palm, together forming a hook. This posture requires relatively little muscle activity to maintain and is used when precision requirements are minimal and when power must be exerted continuously for long periods. Functionally, the hook grip pattern has limited potential and is not used very often. An example of its use is to carry an attaché case or a suitcase by its handle. In contrast, the individual whose hand intrinsic muscles are paralyzed or severely weakened relies on the hook grasp for all functional task completion. The hook grasp is the only grasp pattern available when the hand intrinsics are not working.

Summary

1 The wrist is a complicated joint complex consisting of the multiple articulations of the eight carpal bones with the distal radius, the structures of the TFCC, the metacarpals, and each other. The carpal bones are conventionally divided into a proximal and a distal row.

2 Motions at the wrist include flexion-extension and radial-ulnar deviation. Stability during radial-ulnar deviation is provided by a double-V system formed by the palmar intrinsic ligament and the radiolunate and ulnolunate ligaments.

3 The proximal and distal carpal rows form a bimuscular, biarticular chain that is subject to collapse under compression. Stability is provided by precise opposition of the articular surfaces and intricate intrinsic and extrinsic ligament constraints.

4 The extensor carpi ulnaris, extensor pollicis brevis, and abductor pollicis longus act as a dynamic collateral system to provide wrist stability during functional hand movements.

5 Wrist position affects the ability of the fingers to flex and extend maximally and to grasp effectively.

6 The TFCC plays a significant role in cushioning compressive loads across the wrist joint.

7 The flexor carpi ulnaris is the most powerful wrist motor and tends to place the wrist in a position of flexion and ulnar deviation.

8 The finger rays of the hand are arranged in three arches: one longitudinal and two transverse. Derangement or collapse of the arch system as a result of bone injury, rheumatic disease, or paralysis of the intrinsic muscles of the hand can contribute to severe disability and deformity.

9 The hand is the principal instrument of touch. The combination of sensibility and motor function gives the hand its great importance as an organ of information and accomplishment.

10 The trapezoid, capitate, and second and third metacarpals, with their tight-fitting articulations, form the immobile unit of the hand. In their articulation with the hamate, the fourth and fifth metacarpals are permitted a modest amount of palmar displacement, a motion essential for gripping.

11 The most important motion of the thumb is opposition, in which abduction coupled with rotation at the CMC joint moves the thumb toward the tip of the little finger.

12 The finger rays are controlled by the coordinated action of the extrinsic and intrinsic muscle systems. The operation of each ray is not completely independent of its neighbor's.

13 The components of the digital extensor assembly, especially the oblique retinacular ligaments, account for the release of the distal phalanx and the coupling of PIP and DIP joint motion.

14 A unique feature of the MCP joints is their asymmetry, reflected in the bony configuration of the metacarpal heads, in the attachments of the collateral ligaments, and in the arrangement of the interossei.

15 The MCP joints are stabilized primarily by the radial and ulnar collateral ligaments and also by the transverse intermetacarpal ligament, which links the palmar plates to each other.

16 The digital flexor tendon sheath pulley system is essential for maintaining a relatively constant moment arm for the finger flexors and for minimizing stress raisers between tendon and sheath. The second and fourth annular pulleys play a particularly important role in this respect.

17 The flexor superficialis tendon has a greater overall excursion than does the flexor profundus. The excursion of the flexors is larger than that of the extensors, and the excursion of the extrinsic muscle tendons is generally greater than that of the intrinsic tendons.

18 Extra excursion required at any one joint owing to disruption of the pulley system results in inadequate excursion and subsequent weakness in the more distal joints.

19 The strength of the finger flexors is over twice that of the extensors.

20 Efficient prehensile function depends on the mobility of the thumb CMC joint and the fourth and fifth MCP joints, relative rigidity of the second and third CMC joints, balanced synergism-antagonism between the extrinsic and intrinsic muscles, and adequate sensory input. The relative lengths of the metacarpals and phalanges and the finger rays as a whole are also important.

21 The position of the thumb and the relationship between hand and forearm are the most important differences between power grip and precision handling.

REFERENCES

Agur, A. (1991). *Grant's Atlas of Anatomy* (9th ed.). Baltimore: Williams & Wilkins.

American Academy of Orthopaedic Surgeons (1965). *Joint Motion. Method of Measuring and Recording.* Chicago: AAOS. [Reprinted by the British Orthopaedic Association, 1966.]

Batmanabane, M. & Malathi, S. (1985). Movements at the carpometacarpal and metacarpophalangeal joints of the hand and their effect on the dimensions of the articular ends of the metacarpal bones. *Anat Rec, 213,* 102.

Boyes, J.H. (Ed.) (1970). *Bunnell's Surgery of the Hand* (5th ed.). Philadelphia: J.B. Lippincott.

Brand, P.W. (1985). *Clinical Mechanics of the Hand* (pp. 30–60). St. Louis: C.V. Mosby.

Brand, P.W. & Hollister, A. (1992) *Clinical Mechanics of the Hand* (2nd ed.). St. Louis: C.V. Mosby.

Brumbaugh, R.B., Crowninshield, R.D., Blair, W.F., et al. (1982). An in vivo study of normal wrist kinematics. *J Biochem Eng, 104,* 176.

Brumfield, R.H. & Champoux, J.A. (1984). A biomechanical study of normal functional wrist motion. *Clin Orthop, 187,* 23.

Bunnell, S. (1956). *Surgery of the Hand* (3rd Ed.). Philadelphia: J.B. Lippincott.

Caillet, R. (1982). *Hand Pain and Impairment* (3rd Ed.). Philadelphia: F.A. Davis.

Capener, N. (1956). The hand in surgery. *J Bone Joint Surg, 38B,* 128.

Cauna, N. (1954). Nature and functions of the papillary ridges of the digital skin. *Anat Rec, 119,* 449.

Doyle, J.R. & Blythe, W. (1975). The finger flexor tendon sheath and pulleys: Anatomy and reconstruction. In *AAOS Symposium on Tendon Surgery in the Hand.* St. Louis: C.V. Mosby.

Flatt, A.E. (1974). *The Care of the Rheumatoid Hand* (pp. 12–32). St. Louis: C.V. Mosby.

Hakstian, R.W. & Tubiana, R. (1967). Ulnar deviation of the fingers. The role of joint structure and function. *J Bone Joint Surg., 49A,* 299–316.

Hagert, C.-G. (1981). Anatomical aspects on the design of metacarpophalangeal implants. *Reconstr Surg Traumatol, 18,* 92.

Hazelton, F.T., Smidt, G.L., Flatt, A.E., et al. (1975). The influence of wrist position on the force produced by the finger flexors. *J Biomech, 8,* 301.

Kauer, J.M.G. (1979). The collateral ligament function in the wrist joint. *Acta Morphol Neer Scand, 17,* 252.

Kauer, J.M.G. (1980). Functional anatomy of the wrist. *Clin Orthop, 149,* 9.

Kauer, J.M.G. & Landsmeer, J.M.F. (1981). Functional anatomy of the wrist. In R. Tubiana (Ed.), *The Hand* (Vol. 1). Philadelphia: W.B. Saunders.

Kucynski, K. (1968). The upper limb. In R. Passmore & J. S. Robson (Eds.), *A Companion to Medical Studies* (Vol. I). Oxford: Blackwell Scientific Publications.

Landsmeer, J.M.F. (1955). Anatomical and functional investigations on the articulation of the human fingers. *Acta Anat, Suppl 24,* 1–69.

Landsmeer, J.M.F. (1949). The anatomy of the dorsal aponeurosis of the human finger and its functional significance. *Anat Rec, 104,* 31.

Landsmeer, J.M.F. (1976). *Atlas of Anatomy of the Hand.* Edinburgh: Churchill Livingstone.

Landsmeer, J.M.F. (1962). Power grip and precision handling. *Ann Rheum Dis, 21,* 164.

Landsmeer, J.M.F. (1961). Studies in the anatomy of articulation. I. The equilibrium of the "intercalated" bone. *Acta Morphol Neerl-Scand, 3,* 287.

MacConaill, M.A. (1941). The mechanical anatomy of the carpus and its bearings on some surgical problems. *J Anat, 75,* 166.

Mayfield, J.K., et al. (1979). Biomechanical properties of human carpal ligaments. *Orthop Trans, 3,* 143.

Minami, A., et al. (1984). Ligamentous structures of the metacarpophalangeal joint: A quantitative anatomic study. *J Orthop Res, 1,* 361.

Mount Castle, V. (1968). *Medical Physiology* (Vol. II, 12th ed., pp. 1345–1371). St. Louis: C.V. Mosby.

Napier, J.R. (1956). The prehensile movements of the human hand. *J Bone Joint Surg, 38B,* 902–913.

Palmer, A.K. & Werner, F.W. (1981). The triangular fibrocartilage complex of the wrist—anatomy and function. *J Hand Surg, 6,* 153.

Palmer, A.K. & Werner, F.W. (1984). Biomechanics of the distal radioulnar joint. *Clin Orthop, 187,* 26.

Ray, R.D., Johnson, R.J., & Jameson, R.M. (1951). Rotation of the forearm. An experimental study of pronation and supination. *J Bone Joint Surg, 33A,* 993.

Rose-Innes, A.P. (1990). Anterior dislocation of the ulna at the inferior radio-ulnar joint. *J Bone Joint Surg, 42B,* 515.

Sarrafian, S.K., Melamed, J.L., & Goshgarian, G.M. (1977). Study of wrist motion in flexion and extension. *Clin Orthop, 126,* 153.

Sarrafian, S.K., et al. (1970). Strain variation in the components of the extensor apparatus of the finger during flexion and extension: A biomechanical study. *J Bone Joint Surg, 52A,* 80.

Simon, S.R., et al. (1994). *Kinesiology.* In S.R. Simon (Ed.), *Orthopaedic Basic Science* (pp. 536–558). Rosemont, IL: AAOS.

Smith, L.K., Weiss, E.L., & Lemkuhl, L.D. (1996). *Brunnstrom's Clinical Kinesiology* (5th ed.). Philadelphia: F.A. Davis.

Smith, R.J. & Kaplan, E.B. (1967). Rheumatoid deformities at the metacarpo-phalangeal joints of the fingers: A correlative study of anatomy and physiology. *J Bone Joint Surg, 49A,* 31.

Steindler, A. (1955). *Kinesiology of the Human Body* (p. 534). Springfield: Charles C Thomas.

Strickland, J.W. (1987). Anatomy and kinesiology of the hand. In E.E. Fess & C.A. Philips (Eds.), *Hand Splinting: Principles and Methods* (2nd ed., pp. 3–41). St. Louis: C.V. Mosby.

Taleisnik, J. (1976). The ligaments of the wrist. *J Hand Surg, 1,* 110.

Taleisnik, J. (1985). *The Wrist.* New York: Churchill Livingstone.

Testut, L. & Latarjet, A. (1951). *Tratado de Anatomia Humana* (Vol. 1., 9th ed.). Buenos Aires: Salvat Editores.

Tubiana, R. (1984). Architecture and functions of the hand. In R. Tubiana, J.-M. Thomine, & E. Mackin (Eds.), *Examination of the Hand and Upper Limb* (pp. 1–97). Philadelphia: W.B. Saunders.

Vesely, D.G. (1967). The distal radioulnar joint. *Clin Orthop, 51,* 75.

Volz, R.G. (1976). The development of a total wrist arthroplasty. *Clin Orthop, 116,* 209.

Volz, R.G., Lieb, M., & Benjamin, J. (1980). Biomechanics of the wrist. *Clin Orthop, 149,* 112.

von Bonin, G. (1929). A note on the kinematics of the wrist-joint. *J Anat, 63,* 259.

Von Lanz, T. & Wachsmuth, W. (1970). Functional anatomy. In J.H. Boyes (Ed.), *Bunnell's Surgery of the Hand* (5th Ed.). Philadelphia: J.B. Lippincott.

Weber, E.R. (1984). Concepts governing the rotational shift of the intercalated segment of the carpus. *Orthop Clin North Am, 15,* 193.

Wright, R.D. (1935/36). A detailed study of the movement of the wrist joint. *J Anat, 70,* 137.

Youm, Y., Dryer, R.F., Thambyrajah, K., et al. (1979). Biomechanical analyses of forearm pronation-supination and elbow flexion-extension. *J Biomech 12,* 245.

Youm, Y., McMurtry, R.Y., Flatt, A.E., et al. (1978). Kinematics of the wrist. *J Bone Joint Surg, 60A*(4), 423–31.

Youm, Y. & Yoon, Y.S. (1979). Analytical development in investigation of wrist kinematics. *J Biomech, 12,* 613.

Zancolli, E. (1979). *Structural and Dynamic Bases of Hand Surgery* (2nd ed., pp. 3–63). Philadelphia: J.B. Lippincott.

PART III

Applied Biomechanics

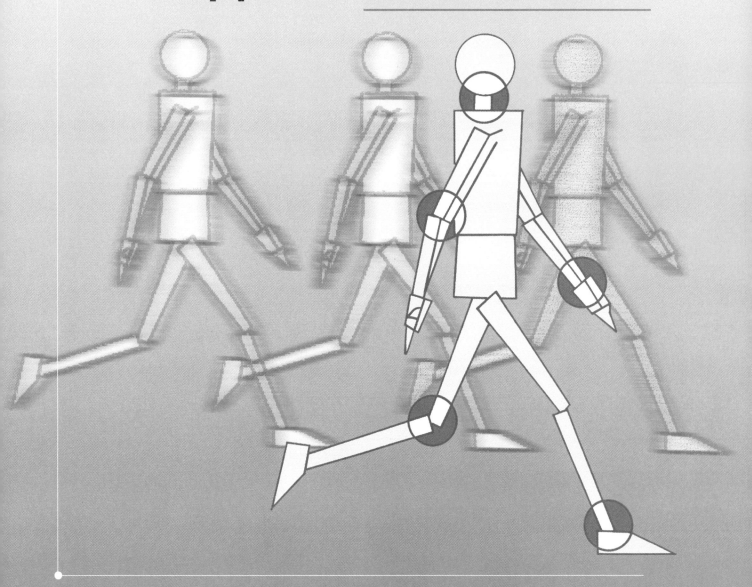

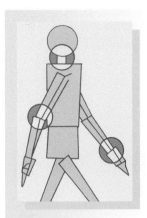

CHAPTER 15

Introduction to the Biomechanics of Fracture Fixation

Frederick J. Kummer

Introduction

The study of fracture fixation biomechanics can be divided into two main areas: (1) criteria for achieving fracture stability and promotion of bone healing and (2) the characterization of techniques and devices intended to mechanically stabilize a fracture. An understanding of the biomechanical principles involved in these areas will aid the engineer in implant design and enable the surgeon in selection of the most effective technique and device to obtain successful results in patients.

Fracture Stability and Healing

The clinical goal of effective fracture treatment is rapid healing, without significant deformity or limb shortening, to restore the patient to a pre-fracture level of function. In the elderly, rapid mobilization is essential to prevent deleterious consequences of bed stay. The first goal of treatment is fracture stabilization. This is determined by the location and type of fracture, the muscle and body forces acting on it, and the various passive soft tissue constraints such as ligaments and fascia. Some simple fractures are inherently stable with low loading and thus require minimal treatment, such as sling (clavicle), while others, such as midshaft comminuted femur fracture, require major surgical intervention and insertion of an internal fixation device for adequate fixation. Although an osteotomy (a surgically created fracture for correction of deformity) allows close approximation of fracture ends, typical fractures are often fragmented and usually lack inherent stability. The interdigitation of the bone ends can facilitate stability, such as when a tapered bone end is inserted into the medullary cavity (creating a displacement deformity, however).

Traditional methods for the treatment of fractures are externally applied and include traction, cast, and braces. External forces or constraints applied to the injured limb act to stabilize the fracture (by limiting muscle or soft tissue forces leading to deformity) and maintain alignment of the limb. However, in many cases, as a result of the nature of the fracture or the patient's condition, an internal or external fixation device attached directly to the bone is required to achieve adequate fracture stabilization. The designs and use of these fixation devices rely on an understanding of bone healing and the loads and forces to which the device is subjected.

FRACTURE HEALING

Currently, controversy exists about whether completely rigid fixation is the optimal condition for bone healing. Micromotion has been shown to aid healing. Healing results even in cases of gross motion such as that seen in rib fractures. Rigid fixation may lead to delayed healing, bone atrophy, and a lack of external stimuli necessary for the healing process.

Although gross motion between two or more bone fragments usually leads to nonunion and fibrocartilage tissue formation, there is a low level of displacement (micromotion) that appears advantageous to healing by providing a mechanical signal that stimulates the biological repair processes. The amount of local strain in the healing region (change in length divided by the original length) seems to determine the nature of the tissues formed (e.g., fibrocartilage or bone). The optimal frequency, wave form, and total number of cycles of this signal currently are being investigated. Several methods to promote healing by externally stimulating a fracture with ultrasound or electromagnetic fields are in clinical use (Case Study 15-1). Concern also exists regarding the process of stress shielding that occurs when the fixation device carries most or all of the mechanical load and thus, by Wolff's law, promotes localized osseous resorption as a result of the resultant unloading of the bone around the device. This is often referred to as load bearing versus load sharing. Much of the initial osteopenia seen beneath fracture plates, however, is thought to be caused by vascular disruption during their application.

Bone healing in the presence of a gap with minimal movement passes through several stages of repair with a concomitant increase in mechanical strength as mineralization increases: hematoma and inflammation, callus formation, replacement by woven bone, and finally remodeling into lamellar or trabecular bone. Callus can form both periosteally and endosteally and enlarges the diameter of the bone at the fracture site. Although callus is less strong and stiff than mature bone, this increased diameter can increase stiffness in bending and torsion at the fracture site as a result of the increased moments of inertia. Direct bone apposition by compression with rigid fixation, in which the initial repair stages are eliminated or minimized, heals by a remodeling process and can take longer because vascularity must be re-established.

The other important factor for healing is adequate blood supply that necessitates the surgeon

CASE STUDY 15-1

Ultrasound Treatment for Fracture Healing

A 40-year-old female involved in a motor vehicle collision in December sustained a left tibiofibular fracture treated with external fixation. Case Study Fig. 15-1-1, in January, low-intensity pulsed ultrasound (US) was initiated to promote fracture healing. Case Study Fig. 15-1-2, in March, 3 months postfracture and 2 months after initiation of pulsed US application, early healing is detected (arrow). Case Study Fig. 15-1-3, in May, 5 months after injury and 4 months following initiation of US, the bone healing is successful.

Pulsed low-intensity ultrasound has been successfully used for fracture repair (Frankel, 1998). Ultrasound is an acoustic radiation at frequencies above the limit of human hearing. Its acoustic radiation, in the form of pressure waves, provides micromechanical stress and force to the bone and surrounding tissue. This mechanical stimulation plays a major role in bone healing because bone reacts to the amount and direction of force and remodels to adapt to the applied stress and its direction. Reprinted with permission from Wolff, J. (1986). *Das Gesetz der Transformation der Knochen* [The law of bone remodeling]. P. Maquet & R. Fulong (Trans.). Berlin: Springer-Verlag. (Original work published in 1892).

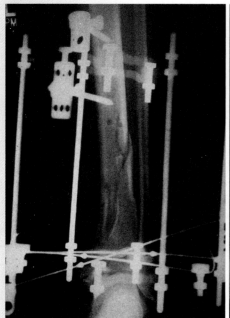

Case Study Figure 15-1-1.

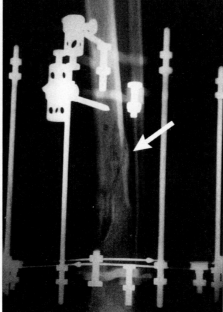

Case Study Figure 15-1-2.

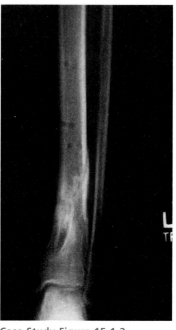

Case Study Figure 15-1-3.

preserving the vascular supply of the bone (e.g., periosteum) and providing conditions for early revascularization by careful operative technique (e.g., soft tissue preservation). Numerous studies have demonstrated a direct relationship between the quantity and quality of microvascular structures in the healing region and the rate of formation and resultant mechanical properties of the new bone.

SURGICAL FACTORS

Many factors determine the optimal fixation method for a specific fracture application. First are mechanical considerations, specifically the types (tension, bending, and/or torsion) and magnitude of forces to which the fixation will be subjected and whether these forces will be cyclic, requiring additional strength of fixation to account for possible device fatigue (Case Study 15-2). The second factor is the bone quality, which determines the strength available to support the fixation device. Other factors are related to surgical and anatomical considerations, for example, the exposure (possible scarring and vascular compromise), whether the device will fit adequately within the soft tissues, and if neurovascular structures are at risk. The nature of the original injury and the amount of soft tissue damage also determine treatment techniques.

Fixation Plate Failure

An internal contemporary fixation plate inserted into the arm of a 25-year-old male who sustained a fracture of the radius. The plate was fractured as a result of fatigue 20 years later. Repeated loading and unloading of a material will cause it to fail, even if the loads are below the ultimate stress (Simon, 1994). Each loading cycle produces a minute amount of microdamage that accumulates with repetitive loads until the material fails. Mechanical considerations as to the magnitude and repetition of the loads to which the fixation will be subjected should be considered, along with the fatigue life of the material. This is recorded on a curve of stress versus number of cycles. Thus, higher stresses produce failure in fewer cycles (loading to the ultimate stress produces failure in one cycle), while lower stresses are tolerated for an extended period.

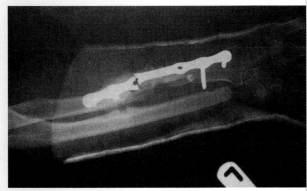

Case Study Figure 15-2-1.

Evaluation of fixation strength can be accomplished by laboratory testing of actual implants in cadaver bone. One difficulty of such testing is in adequately simulating in the test model the complex in vivo, cyclic forces on the device. Another difficulty is in simulating the biological repair processes that would act to stabilize the fixation over time. Cadaver studies also can determine the anatomical structures at risk. Computer modeling such as finite element analysis can be used as an initial method to evaluate fixation methods and device designs but requires quantified parameters of bone modulus and strength, which may be lacking, for an exact solution.

Clinical trials is the other major method used to evaluate the efficacy of a particular fixation method. However, care must be taken to adopt the appropriate techniques to quantify data and design the trial (number of patients, adequate follow-up) so that the many variables can be properly analyzed and proper statistical significance determined.

Fixation Devices and Methods

Wires, staples, pins, plates, and screws are the common implant devices used to achieve fracture fixation. These are usually made of stainless steel (316L), sometimes of titanium alloy (Ti-6A1-4V), or occasionally of cobalt-chromium alloy. Each metal has advantages and disadvantages such as strength, modulus (stiffness), corrosion resistance, and ease of imaging (MRI, CAT). Sometimes there is a "race" between healing of the bone and fracture, usually by fatigue, of the device. There is a recent interest in the clinical application of biodegradable polymers such as polylactic acid. Polymers are more flexible than metals and would lead to greater load bearing by the healing fracture; biodegradable materials do not have to be removed in a secondary operation and their mechanical properties gradually decrease with time, thus avoiding stress shielding. However, their mechanical strength is much less than that of metal and some of the degradation products have shown untoward biological responses. Research continues into the use of various glues, cements, and adhesives for fracture fixation, some of which are also biodegradable.

Wire fixation used as cerclage or a bone suture is a common application; in both cases multiple wires are required to provide stable, three-dimensional fixation. This requires achieving equal tension during tightening because loosening at one or more sites can provide a locus for motion and possible nonunion or cause malpositioning. Problems with wire fracture fixation include the necessity and surgical complexity of making a bone hole and passing the wire, breakage during tightening or later as a result of fatigue (cyclic loading), and cut-through of the bone. For cerclage applications, there is concern about compromise of the periosteal blood supply and the resulting increased healing time required for revascularization.

Some recent developments are wire tensioning/twisting instruments and the use of crimping systems to avoid the problems with twisting or knot tying. There are also new oriented polymers (Spectra) that do not stretch as traditional suture materials do that can be used with a suture anchor system to eliminate the difficulty of looping a suture through bone and suture abrasion against the bone.

Staples alone usually do not provide sufficient mechanical stability for permanent fixation and their use often requires pre-drilling holes for the staple legs; pneumatic-driven staples can be used to rapidly tack fragments prior to a more rigid fixation but need careful control of the insertion driving force to prevent untoward damage to the bone. Some staple designs have been developed that can effect compression during insertion, such as staple fabrication from nitinol (an alloy that changes shape when heated to body temperature).

Kirschner wires are normally used to hold fragments of bone prior to rigid fixation and for percutaneous pinning of small bone fractures but, in general, lack sufficient mechanical stability for their use as a primary fixation in weight-bearing bones. At least two wires should be used for each bone fragment, and they should not be inserted in a parallel manner to prevent "pistoning" of the bone fragment along the wires (Fig. 15-1). Threaded pins provide additional stability because they minimize sliding of the bone fragments, but their removal is more difficult. Occasionally, pinning is used in combination with sutures looped and tightened around the pin ends or through loops in the pins. This "tension band" technique provides significantly increased mechanical stability of the fixation.

The major intrinsic factors that influence screw-holding power are outer thread diameter, thread configuration, and thread length; extrinsic factors are bone quality, type, and screw insertion orientation and driving torque (Fig. 15-2). The two basic types of screws are cortical and cancellous and are distinguished by their thread design; cancellous screws have a greater distance between adjacent threads (pitch) and the ratio of outer thread diameter to body diameter (Fig. 15-3).

The inherent holding power of a screw is a function of the outer thread diameter times the length of its threads within the bone. When used to hold two bone fragments together, screws commonly are used in a lag modality in which the proximal portion of the screw remains free within one fragment (either by using a screw design having no proximal threads or by enlargement of the hole in the proximal fragment, which should require the use of a washer under the screw head for adequate support). Insertion torque determines the force with which bone fragments are held together, which, in turn, creates the friction that prevents their motion. Control of torque (torque-limiting screwdriver) is im-

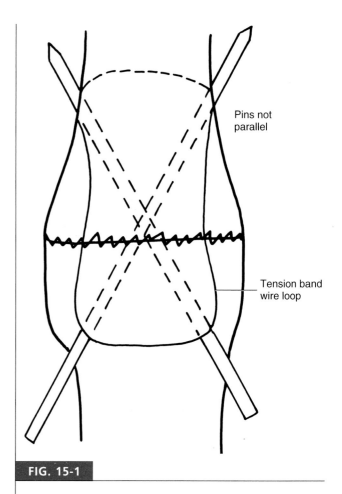

Pins not parallel

Tension band wire loop

FIG. 15-1

Tension band wiring of two K-wires; tightening the wire loop applies compression to the fixation. K-wires are inserted in a skewed configuration for stability.

portant to prevent stripping of the bone or screw head torsional failure.

Because of anatomical constraints or surgical exposure, screws cannot always be inserted perpendicular to the bone axis or the orientation of the ends of the bone fragments is not perpendicular to the screw axis. In this case, the holding power of the screw is decreased and a shear component of the holding force is created, which acts to destabilize alignment. Pre-tapping of the screws usually is not necessary and has been shown to have minimal effect on their holding ability; many screws are self-tapping owing to a modification to the design of the leading threads. Usually two or more screws are required for functioning, although one screw has been suggested for some applications if sufficient inter-

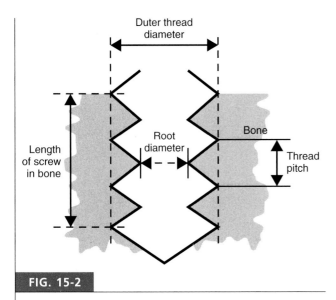

FIG. 15-2

Screw parameters. For screw pull-out the bone must shear along the outer diameter (*dotted line*).

fragment approximation can be achieved to create adequate friction between the bone surfaces for stability. The quality of bone also determines screw-holding ability; cortical bone is approximately ten times stronger than cancellous bone. The thickness of the cortex and the degree of osteopenia (bone density) are thus critical for fixation strength and influence the number of screws required for adequate stability. Using screws in a bicortical manner appreciably increases the strength of fixation.

Anatomical constraints limit the number or size of screws that can be applied in a given region. As a result, screws are often combined with plates to achieve adequate stability and increased strength of fixation. The optimal site for a single plate application is on the side of the bone subjected to tension; usually two plates are applied to achieve better fixation stability (Fig. 15-4). Owing to anatomical constraints such as soft tissue thickness, sometimes thinner plates are used (such as for forearm fracture stabilization), but these plates possess sufficient stiffness (function of the width of the plate times its thickness cubed) to prevent undesired fracture motion as a result of bending loads (Fig. 15-5).

Screws should be inserted with a torque driver and the tightness of all screws rechecked; if this is not done, one screw may bear most of the load and possibly fail. Some plates use a specially designed screw hole slot, countersunk to accommodate the

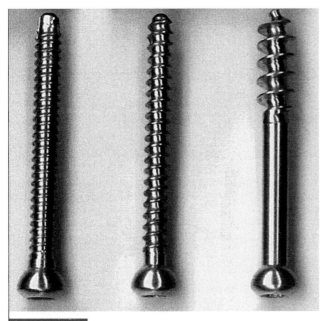

FIG. 15-3

Types of bone screws. Left to right: cortical, cancellous, and cancellous lag.

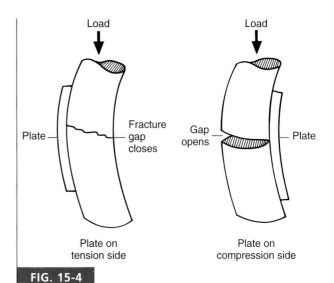

FIG. 15-4

Effect of plate placement. A plate located on the compression side causes the fracture to gap when loaded.

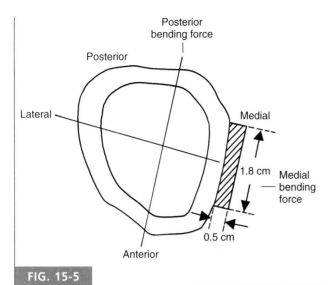

FIG. 15-5

Effect of loading direction on plate stiffness. The rigidity of the plate is EI, where E is the modulus of the plate material and I is the moment of inertia of the plate. $I = bh^3/12$ (I_1 = posterior bending; I_2 = medial bending; $I_1 = 0.5 \times 1.8^3/12 = 0.243$; $I_2 = 1.8 \times 0.5^3/12 = 0.01875$), where b is the base dimension and h is its height. Thus, the plate is 13 times more rigid in posterior bending than in medial bending.

screw head, whose center is offset with respect to the screw head to obtain interfragmentary compression as the screw is tightened. An alternative method to achieve compression is to pre-bend the plate before application so that when the attachment screws are tightened, the bone fragments are approximated as the plate straightens. Some new plate designs use threaded holes to engage the screw so that bicortical screw insertion is not as essential for maximum fixation stability.

Plates can also be used to span gaps created by severe fractures or tumor surgery and are frequently used with bone grafts for this application. Unless the graft is exactly sized, the plate will bear the entire load across the defect. The bending moment on the plate-screw fixation linearly increases with defect size and thus the plate requires adequate stabilization, particularly at the more highly loaded, proximal end where at least three screws are needed. Multiple-holed plates enable selection of the best osseous sites for screw purchase and should permit anchoring of the graft by at least two additional screws.

The major surgical considerations for the use of plates are the requirements of a large exposure for their insertion and the possibility of compromising periosteal blood supply by the exposure or plate insertion (some plate designs have inferior feet or ridges to minimize this possibility). There is also interest in polymeric plates that would be more flexible to achieve a greater degree of micromotion at the fracture that could be advantageous to bone healing and minimize stress shielding.

Hip fracture devices can be internal or external in their application; the most common external device is a side plate affixed to the femur supporting an internal, sliding lag screw through the neck across the fracture.

The relationship of biomechanical forces borne by the device and borne by the bone (load bearing, load sharing) influences fracture healing and device survival. An important factor is the ability of the device to slide to consolidate the fracture during healing. Internal devices for fixation are usually intramedullary nails (IM) and in comparison with external devices are subject to less loading force because of their location being closer to the neutral bending axis of the bone (Fig. 15-6). Their size is critical because their bending and torsional stiffness are proportional to the diameter to the fourth power. This is why one large nail provides more rigid fixation than does multiple smaller rods. Size, amount of curvature, and amount of reaming are also important because the stability of the fixation relies on load transfer to the bone; often, distal and

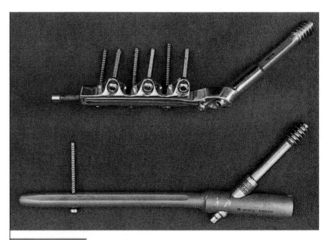

FIG. 15-6

Typical intermedullary and extramedullary devices. *Top,* Medoff sliding plate; *bottom,* intermedullary hip screw.

proximal screws inserted through the bone and nail are used to increase torsional stability (Fig. 15-7). Bending of the nail as a result of insertion in a curved medullary cavity can make insertion of the distal screws difficult.

External fixation devices are also used for fracture stabilization; multiple transcutaneous pins are inserted into the bone and stabilized with an external bar(s) or ring(s). Factors that influence mechanical stability and rigidity of these constructs are the number, diameter, orientation, and length of these pins and their relation with respect to the fracture; however, these factors are subject to surgical considerations for frame application. Large, short pins located close to the fracture provide the most rigid fixation (Fig. 15-8).

Spinal implants used for deformity correction or fracture fixation consist of various combinations of rods, wires, plates, and screws. The junctions between these components are often the site of failure, such as fatigue or fretting as a result of cyclic loading. A specific problem is that the size and the loca-

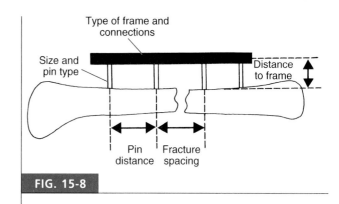

FIG. 15-8

Typical external fixator showing the variable that influences fixation stability.

tion of appropriate sites for device attachment to the spine are limited. This is important because these devices are subject to appreciable forces during flexion and extension of the neck, and torso and fixation failure can occur.

Summary

1 The optimal frequency of waveform and the total number of cycles of bone healing are under investigation. Rigid and semirigid (micromotion) devices can result in bone healing. Gross motion, instability, and inadequate blood supply may lead to nonunion.

2 Factors determining optimal fixations for specific fracture applications are:

    a. Mechanical considerations, such as the types and magnitude of forces to which the fixation will be subjected and expected cycle history
    b. Bone quality and strength
    c. Surgical and anatomical considerations
    d. The energy involved in the original injury and the amount of soft tissue damage.

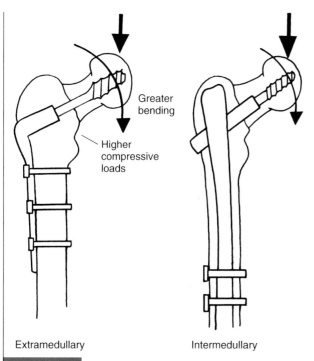

FIG. 15-7

The extramedullary device is less rigid and when loaded has greater deflection, creating higher medial stresses in the femur.

SUGGESTED READING

Burstein, A.H. & Wright, T.M. (1994). *Fundamentals of Orthopaedic Biomechanics*. Baltimore: Williams & Wilkins.
Cochran, G.V.B. (1982). *A Primer of Orthopaedic Biomechanics*. London: Churchill Livingstone.
Dycheyne, P., & Hastings, G.W. (Eds.) (1984). *Functional Behavior of Orthopaedic Biomaterials*. Boca Raton, FL: CRC Press.

Frankel, V.H. (1998). Results of prescription of pulse ultrasound therapy in fracture management. In Z. Szabo, J. Lewis, G. Fantini, & R. Savalgi (Eds.), *Surgical Technology International VII. International Developments in Surgery and Surgical Research.* San Francisco: Universal Medical Press, Inc. Surgical Technology International.

Fung, Y.C. (1981). *Biomechanics: Mechanical Properties of Living Tissues.* New York: Springer-Verlag.

Ghista, D.N. (Ed.) (1981). *Biomechanics of Medical Devices.* New York: Dekker.

Gozna, E.R., Harrington, I.J., & Evans, D.C. (1982). *Biomechanics of Musculoskeletal Injury.* Baltimore: Williams & Wilkins.

Kasser, J.M. (Ed.) (1995). *Orthopaedic Knowledge Update 5.* Rosemont, IL: AAOS.

Mow, V.C. & Hayes, W.C. (Eds.) (1991). *Basic Orthopaedic Biomechanics.* New York: Raven Press.

Özkaya, N. & Nordin, M. (1998). *Fundamentals of Biomechanics* (2nd ed.). New York: Springer-Verlag.

Pauwels, F. (1976). *Biomechanics of the Normal and Diseased Hip.* Berlin: Springer-Verlag.

Radin, E.L. (Ed.) (1992). *Practical Biomechanics for the Orthopedic Surgeon.* New York: Churchill Livingstone.

Sarmiento, A., McKellop, H.A., Llinas, A., et al. (1996). Effect of loading and fracture motions on diaphyseal tibial fractures. *J Orthop Res, 14*(1), 80–84.

Simon, S.R. (1994). *Orthopedic Basic Science.* Rosemont, IL: AAOS.

Spivak, J.M., Di Cesare, P.E., Feldman, D.S., et al. (Eds.) (1999). *Orthopaedics—A Study Guide.* New York: McGraw-Hill.

Tencer, A.F. & Johnson, K.D. (1994). *Biomechanics in Orthopedic Trauma.* London: M. Dunitz..

Uhthoff, H.K. (Ed.) (1980). *Current Concepts of Internal Fixation of Fractures.* Berlin: Springer-Verlag.

Valenta, J. (Ed.) (1993). *Biomechanics.* Amsterdam: Elsevier.

White, A.A. & Panjabi, M.M. (Eds.) (1990). *Clinical Biomechanics of the Spine.* Philadelphia: Lippincott.

Wolff, J. (1986). *Das Gesetz der Transformation der Knochen* [The law of bone remodeling]. P. Maquet & R. Fulong (Trans.). Berlin: Springer-Verlag. (Original work published in 1892).

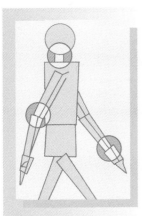

CHAPTER 16

Biomechanics of Arthroplasty

Debra E. Hurwitz, Thomas P. Andriacchi, Gunnar B.J. Andersson

Introduction

As designs for total joint replacements evolve, there is an increasing need to improve the understanding of the biomechanics of these joints. For instance, reducing loads on a total joint replacement during daily activities and designing implants to withstand these loads will both increase the likelihood of normal joint function and lower the probability of implant failure. As implants are put into younger and more active patients, the loads placed on the implants are often several times greater, thereby increasing the likelihood of mechanical failure. Mechanical problems associated with total joint replacements include issues related to wear of the bearing surface, mechanical failure of the implant, loosening of the implant from the bone, and dislocation of the implant at the articulating surfaces. Important biomechanical information addressing each of these issues has been obtained from in vitro cadaver testing, model simulation of the joint motions and loads, and in vivo studies of human locomotion.

The overall goals of joint replacement are to provide long-term restoration of function and pain relief. Several mechanical challenges must be met to achieve these goals. For example, the control of joint motion and stability in total knee replacements is achieved through an intricate biomechanical interaction between the shapes of the replaced surfaces and the remaining ligaments and muscles.

To meet one design objective, compromises with respect to another design objective must often be made. For example, the femoral stem of cementless total hip replacements requires initial rotatory stability for bony ingrowth into the porous material to occur. The rotational stability of early cementless total hip replacements was insufficient and was increased by designing implants with greater medullary canal fill. However, implants with increased medullary canal fill were stiffer because of their larger size and were thus associated with greater stress shielding.

Forces acting at the hip or knee joint are dependent on the external forces acting on the limb and the internal forces primarily generated by muscle contraction. Joint forces have been measured with implanted transducers or estimated using inverse dynamics and analytical methods (Tables 16-1 and 16-2). By measuring the external ground reaction forces, approximating the limb segment inertial properties, and locating the three-dimensional position of the joint centers during dynamic activities, the intersegmental hip forces and external moments can be obtained using inverse dynamics. Even with simplifications to the anatomy, solving for the muscle and contact forces at the hip and knee remains an indeterminate problem. Thus, a unique solution for individual muscle forces is not possible without further assumptions or simplifications.

In general, two approaches have been used to solve the indeterminate problem. The first is a "re-

TABLE 16-1

Hip and Knee Contact Forces Measured In Vivo in Patients With Instrumented Implants

Activity	Typical Peak Force (Body Weights)	Number of Patients	Time Since Surgery (Months)	Reference
Hip Force				
Walking normal to fast speeds	2.7–3.6	2	1–2	Kotzar et al., 1991
Stair climbing	2.6			
Walking slow speed (crutches)	2.6	1	1	Davy et al., 1988
Ascending stairs	2.6			
Walking	2.7–4.3	2	8–33	Bergmann et al., 1993, 1995
Ascending stairs	3.4–5.5			
Descending stairs	3.9–5.1			
Walking	1.8–3.3	2	6	Rydell, 1966
Walking slow speed	2.7	1	15	English & Kilvington, 1979
Knee Contact Force				
Walking normal to fast speeds	2.3–2.5	1	12	Taylor et al., 1997

TABLE 16-2

Analytical Methods of Estimating Peak Hip and Knee Contact Force

Activity	Magnitude (BW)	Method	Reference
Hip Force			
Walking	4.8	Reduction method	Paul, 1976
Stair ascending	7.2	Reduction method	Paul, 1976
Stair descending	7.1		
Walking slow with cane	2.2	Optimization-maximize	Brand & Crowninshield, 1980
Walking slow without cane	3.4	endurance	
Walking	5.0		Crowninshield et al., 1978
Stair climbing	7.4		
Chair rising	3.3		
Walking	5.5	Quasi static-minimize muscle forces	Seireg & Arvikar, 1975
Knee Force			
Walking	3.2	Reduction method	Harrington, 1983
Walking	4	Reduction method	Morrison, 1970
Walking	3	Optimization	Schipplein & Andriacchi, 1991
Walking	7	Optimization	Seireg & Arvikar, 1975

duction" method that groups muscles into functional units, thereby reducing the indeterminate problem to a determinate one. The second approach uses optimization methods in which the force is distributed among the muscles in such a manner that some physical parameter such as minimum muscle stress, maximum muscle endurance, or minimum joint reaction force is optimized (Brand, Pedersen, & Friederich, 1986; Crowninshield & Brand, 1981; Crowninshield et al., 1978; Seireg & Arvikar, 1975). However, function in patients with total joint replacements may not be normal and may be influenced less by minimizing energy than by other factors such as pain or implant stability. One alternative to optimization methods is to generate a range of muscle forces able to maintain mechanical equilibrium at the joint. Rather than obtain a single value for the contact or muscle force, this parametric approach determines a range of agonist muscle force distributions needed to balance the external moment and a selected level of antagonistic activity (Foucher et al., 1997; Hurwitz, D. E., 1994. Functional Biomechanics of the Hip As Related to Total Hip Replacements. Unpublished doctoral dissertation. University of Illinois at Chicago).

Forces at the Hip Joint

The peak resultant forces during gait measured with strain-gauged prostheses have ranged from 1.8 to 4.36 times body weights (Table 16-1). Bergmann et al. (1993) have conducted the most extensive in vivo studies on forces during daily activities (Fig. 16-1) and have shown that the peak loads and torsional moments increase with walking speed. In general, the force at the hip joint reached an initial peak in early stance and a second peak in late stance. Many of the failure mechanisms in total joint replacements are affected not only by load magnitude but also by the cyclic nature of the loads. Thus, in evaluating cyclic fatigue, one must consider two cycles of load variation for each step.

Independent measurements at different institutions seem to indicate that stems with similar features experience similar peak forces. In many instances, differences between the measured forces can be attributed to variations in the hip position during gait (Noble, Helmke, & Paul, 1993). Analytical models generally predict higher contact forces than those measured by in vivo instrumented total hip replacements. This may be the result of employing anatomical simplifications, using inadequate optimization cri-

A

Activities: Walking, Jogging, Stairs, Stumbling

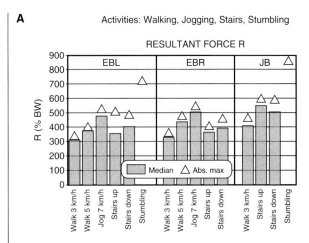

B

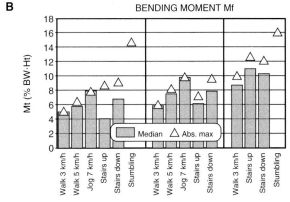

C

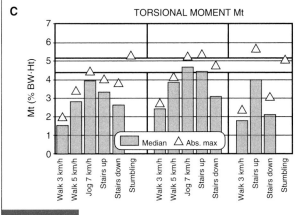

FIG. 16-1

Joint loading during different activities for two patients, EB (EBL: left hip and EBR: right hip) and JB. The median load values (column height) and absolute maxima (triangle) are given. The resultant force is in the top graph (**A**) the bending moment in the frontal plane is in the middle graph (**B**) and the torsional moment in the transverse plane is in the bottom graph (**C**). The *gray bar* indicates the fixation strength of cementless implants (14). *Reprinted with permission from Bergmann G., Graichen, F., & Rohlmann, A. (1995). Is staircase walking a risk for the fixation of hip implants?* J Biomechanics, 28(5), 535–553.

teria to determine the agonistic and antagonistic muscle activity, and assuming normal function. Identifying how patients with total hip replacements alter their function during gait could improve analytical predictions of joint force. In vivo force measurements have often been obtained during the early postoperative period when patients may still have compromised function.

Rotational Moments About the Implant

Out-of-plane loads may be detrimental to both initial and long-term implant stability, especially in uncemented stems (Berzins, Sumner, & Andriacchi, 1993; Phillips, Nguyen, & Munro, 1991). Excessive bone-implant motion prevents bone ingrowth into porous coatings and may lead to failure of the biological fixation (Pilliar, Lee, & Maniatopoulus, 1986). The largest torsional moments measured in vivo during activities of daily living (Bergmann, Graichen, & Rohlmann, 1995) reach the average experimental strength of implant fixation (33.1 Nm) as determined from in vitro tests (Phillips, Nguyen, & Munro, 1991) (Fig. 16-1). In vitro testing of prostheses implanted in human femurs indicate that the amount of initial bone-implant motion is sensitive to the off-axis loading that frequently occurs during stair climbing and rising from a chair (Fig. 16-2) (Berzins, Sumner, & Andriacchi, 1993). Furthermore, resultant proximal translations were twice as high with a straight stem as with a curved stem at load angles encountered during these activities (Berzins, Sumner, & Andriacchi, 1993).

Walking with a decreased hip range of motion during daily activities may minimize the out-of-plane force components (anterior-posterior). Thus, decreased sagittal plane motion during walking often reported in patients with total hip replacements (Hurwitz, Chertack, & Andriacchi, 1992; Murray, Brewer, & Zuege, 1972; Stauffer, Smidt, & Wadsworth, 1974; White, Yack, & Lesswing, 1992) may be beneficial for implant stability by reducing the rotational moments about the implant stem. Dynamic hip range of motion during gait in patients with uncemented total hip replacements has been related to the metaphyseal fill of the femoral stem (Hurwitz et al., 1992). It was concluded that a reduction in the dynamic range of hip motion was an adaptive response to decrease torsional micromo-

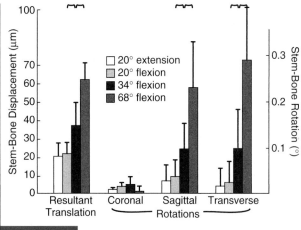

FIG. 16-2

Distal motions as a function of flexion angle (mean and standard deviation) There were significant differences between 20 and 34° and between 34 and 68° for the resultant translation and the transverse rotation, but for the sagittal rotation only the difference between the 20 and 34° was significant. *Reprinted with permission from Berzins, A., Sumner, D.R., Andriacchi, T.P., et al. (1993). Stem curvature and load angle influence the initial relative bone implant motion of cementless femoral stems. J Orthop Res, 11(5), 758–769.*

tion produced by out-of-plane loads when the hip reaches greater ranges of flexion.

Reconstructed Joint Geometry

Alterations in joint anatomy impact on hip biomechanics by altering the contact area, the contact force, and the strength and moment-generating capacity of the muscles. The effect of variations in acetabular position, anteversion angle, head-neck angle, neck length, and joint center location on the muscles' capacity (moment-generating capacity) and the resultant hip force have all been mathematically modeled (Delp & Maloney, 1993; Doehring et al., 1996; Johnston, Brand, & Crowninshield, 1979). These analyses assume that alterations in joint and femoral geometry do not alter the manner in which subjects perform the activities.

The mechanical ability of the abductors is affected by head-neck angle, neck length, and joint center position, all of which are frequently altered during a total hip replacement. A decreased head-neck angle (varus hip) increases the mechanical ad-

vantage of the abductors (Fig. 16-3) (Delp, Komattu, & Wixson, 1994). Joint contact forces therefore should be minimized with small head-neck angles (Johnston, Brand, & Crowninshield, 1979). Decreased head-neck angles also improve joint stability through increased congruence by turning the femoral head deeper into the acetabulum. Moving the greater trochanter laterally also increases the mechanical advantage of the abductors. Clinically, increased abductor/adductor strength has been associated with increased neck length and a more distal greater trochanter position (Hurwitz & Andriacchi, 1997).

Neck angle and neck length have an impact not only on the abductor muscle force and resultant hip force but also on the bending moments in the proximal femur. A varus hip or an increased neck length increases bending moments in the proximal femur by increasing the moment arm of the forces transmitted along the shaft of the femur. Prostheses must be designed to resist these bending moments. Decreasing the neck length or increasing the head-neck angle (valgus) will decrease the bending moments in the stem; however, these alterations compromise the abductor function and increase the joint reaction force (Case Study 16-1). The abductors are important during the single-legged stance phase of gait because their contraction pulls the rim of the pelvis toward the greater trochanter and prevents the contralateral side of

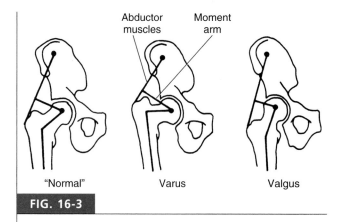

FIG. 16-3

The abductor mechanism changes with head-neck angle or neck length. A valgus neck angle decreases the moment arm, whereas a varus neck angle or an increased neck length increases the moment arm. *Reprinted with permission from Hurwitz D.E. & Andriacchi, T.P. (1998). Biomechanics of the hip. In J. Callaghan, A. Rosenberg, & H. Rubash (Eds.), The Adult Hip (pp. 75–86). New York: Raven Press.*

CASE STUDY 16-1

Cemented Total Hip Replacement

A 65-year-old woman, with chronic pain caused by osteoarthrosis in the hip. Severe cartilage degeneration and reactive periarticular bony changes leading to loss of congruency had been affecting her hip function and daily activities such as gait. After a careful documentation of the patient's history, physical examination, and radiographic information, a total cemented total hip replacement is performed (Fig. cs16-1-1).

The picture shows the stage of the total hip arthroplasty after surgery. The head-neck angle is in valgus. This valgus position will decrease bending moments in the stem prosthesis but will increase the joint reaction force as a result of reduction in the mechanical advantage of the abductor muscles (lever arm shortens [c]). The figure is marked with the line of action of the abductor muscles (A), the line of gravity (white line), the line of the lever arm (b) from the center of rotation to the line of gravity, and the line of action of the reaction force at the estimated point of contact of the femoral head and the acetabular unit (J). In addition, the line of gravity (white line) is depicted with the line of action of gravity force (W).

The picture was made during a single-leg position, in which the line of gravity moves toward the hip, decreasing the abductor moment arm relative to the body weight. Thus, the patient adapts her gait and posture to decrease the demand on the abductor muscles by leaning over her leg and thereby limping a little.

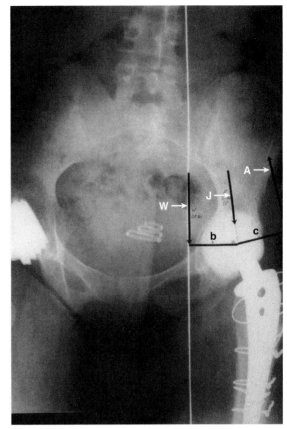

Case Study Figure 16-1-1.

the pelvis from dropping as a result of the weight of the swinging leg and upper body. If changes in the neck angle, neck length, and joint center position decrease the abductor moment arm relative to the body weight and no compensation in function occurs, then an increase in the resultant force would be expected. Subjects may, however, adapt their gait to lessen the demand on these muscles when the moment-generating capacity of the abductors is compromised.

Alterations in hip center location have a large effect on the moment-generating capacity of the muscles and the resultant hip force (Doehring et al., 1996; Johnston, Brand, & Crowninshield, 1979). Predicted joint forces are minimized when the joint center is moved medial, inferior, and anterior (Fig. 16-4). This position maximizes the moment-generating capacity of the abductors and brings the hip center closer to the line of action of the foot floor reaction force, thus decreasing the external moment that needs to be balanced by muscle forces (Doehring et al., 1996; Johnston, Brand, & Crowninshield, 1979).

Although the models can predict hip joint center positions that minimize the resultant force, these positions may not be practical for the acetabular component. Pathological conditions strongly influence the potential locations of the hip center. For instance, osteoarthritis frequently results in the femoral head being displaced laterally, superiorly, and posteriorly.

Large joint forces are analytically predicted for hip centers that are located superior, lateral, and posterior as compared with the original location (Johnston, Brand, & Crowninshield, 1979). High joint forces were obtained with superior lateral hip centers in an experimental set-up in which a loading fixture simulated the hip abductors, adductors, and extensors during single-legged stance and stair climbing (Gore et al., 1977). Superior displacements of the hip center reduce the moment-generating capacity of the abductors, adductors, flexors, and extensors as a result of alterations in muscle lengths and moment arms (Doehring et al., 1996). Increasing the neck length or advancing the greater

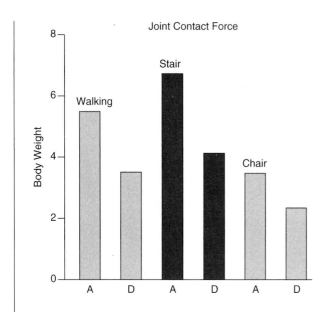

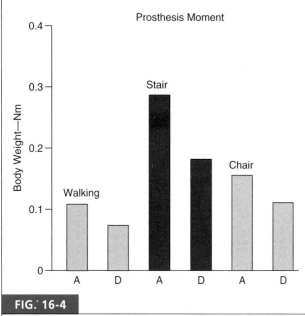

FIG. 16-4

Peak contact forces at the hip and peak moments about the neck-stem junction of the prosthesis during level walking, stair climbing, and rising from a chair under the following conditions: A = normal location of the hip center and D = hip center 20 mm medial, 20 mm inferior, and 10 mm anterior. Peak forces were based on an optimization approach that minimized muscle stresses. *Reprinted with permission from Johnston, R.C., Brand, R.A., & Crowninshield, R.D. (1979). Reconstruction of the hip.* J Bone Joint Surg, *61A(5), 646.*

trochanter partially compensates for these losses in muscle moment-generating capacities (Delp, Komattu, & Wixson, 1994).

In general, the analytical and experimental results on the effect of joint geometry on hip joint forces are consistent with clinical patient studies. Clinical studies have associated inferior functional outcomes with superior placement of the joint center (Box & Noble, 1993) and have associated decreases in abductor strength and loss of passive hip flexion motion with superior placements of the joint centers unless compensated with an increased neck length (Hurwitz & Andriacchi, 1997). Higher femoral loosening rates have been associated with joint centers placed superior and lateral as opposed to those placed in an anatomical position (Yoder et al., 1988), while higher volumetric polyethylene wear is associated with decreased femoral offsets and decreased abductor moment arms (Robinson et al., unpublished data. The effefct of implant position in polyethylene wear in total hip arthroplasty).

Stem Position Within the Femoral Canal

Both clinical experience and biomechanical stress analyses suggest that a valgus stem position provides better results than does a varus position (Andriacchi et al., 1976; Collis & Oregon, 1977; Galante, Rostoker, & Doyle, 1975). Finite element models indicate that varus stems sustain greater peak stresses than those in valgus or neutral for the same loading conditions (Andriacchi et al., 1976). Subjects with a Mueller-cemented stem in a varus position walk with more abnormalities than those with a valgus stem despite the fact that subjects in both groups had an excellent clinical outcome (Hodge, Andriacchi, & Galante, 1991). The gait abnormalities in the varus group may be suggestive of a biomechanical adaptation to either micromotion or abnormal stress patterns present in varus stems.

Periprosthetic Bone Loss

Periprosthetic bone loss associated with uncemented femoral stems has been well documented (Bryan et al., 1994; Engh & Bobyn, 1988; Engh et al., 1992), and concerns have been raised with regards to the long-term clinical implications of this phenomenon. Osteolysis, stress shielding, and generalized limb unloading all may play a role in periprosthetic bone loss. Wear debris has been implicated in osteolysis and implant failure (Amstutz et al., 1992). Wear particles from the polyethylene and other implant materials are found in the joint fluid and adjacent tissues. Even small amounts of wear can generate large numbers of polyethylene particles that are as small as or smaller than a micrometer. These wear particles result in a foreign-body reaction with increased macrophage activity and intercellular secretion of mediators that stimulate osteoclasts and result in periprosthetic bone loss (Jasty et al., 1993; Willert & Buchhorn, 1993). Not unexpectedly, undersized or unstable components have a higher incidence of osteolytic lesions than do those with stable fixation (Noble, 1995).

Stress shielding results from a decrease in the stress distribution in the femoral bone as a result of the presence of the implant stem that has a greater or equivalent mechanical stiffness as compared with the femur. Changes in the loading environment result in bone remodeling. Once bone ingrowth occurs in the cementless prosthesis, load transfer can occur through these areas of bony attachment. However, bone remodeling does not result in the restoration of normal cortical strain levels (Engh et al., 1992). The fit of the prosthesis within the femoral canal (Jasty et al., 1994), as well as the material properties (stiffness) of the stem (Cheal, Spector, & Hayes, 1992; Weinans, Huiskes, & Grootenboer, 1992), affects the amount of stress-shielding (Fig. 16-5).

Bone loss also can result from limb disuse (Goethgen et al., 1991). Postoperative subjects with total hip replacements continue to walk asymmetrically, with decreased forces on the operated side as compared with the contralateral side (Bryan et al., 1996; Long et al., 1993). Tibial bone loss is unaffected by implant characteristics and most likely results from generalized limb disuse associated with asymmetries in joint loading conditions. A 16% decrease in proximal tibial bone mineral content has been demonstrated in subjects with long-term total hip replacements, and this decrease has been related to an asymmetry in the peak vertical intersegmental knee force during gait (Bryan et al., 1996). Preoperative gait mechanics of patients with hip osteoarthritis have been shown to be correlated with the bone mineral density of the proximal femur (Fig. 16-6) (Hurwitz et al., 1997). The greater the bone loss preoperatively, the less stiff the femur and the more that likely stress shielding and associated bone resorption will occur postoperatively (Engh &

Bobyn, 1988; Engh et al., 1992). Autopsy studies have also shown that the lower the bone mineral density or content of the contralateral femur, the greater the reduction in periprosthetic bone on the affected side, which further implies that preoperative bone mineral density influences the extent of postoperative bone loss (Engh et al., 1992; Maloney et al., 1996).

Forces at the Knee Joint

The knee joint depends primarily on soft tissues for stability while sustaining large joint reaction forces at the tibiofemoral and patellofemoral articulations. The peak forces during walking predicted by the analytical models (Morrison, 1970; Schipplein & Andriacchi, 1991; Seireg & Arvikar, 1975) varied from 3 to 7 body weights and are similar to those measured in vivo (2.3 to 2.5 body weights) in a single patient with a distal femoral replacement and rotating knee hinge (Taylor et al., 1997) (Tables 16-1 and 16-2). The magnitude and cyclic nature of the compressive force in the tibiofemoral joint are important considerations in the design of a total knee replacement. General characteristics of the predicted forces at the knee joint show three peaks

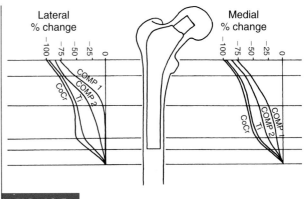

FIG. 16-5

Percent change in the strain energy density within the medial and lateral regions of the medial and lateral cortex from a three-dimensional finite element model. The greatest reduction in strain energy density was found for the femur with the stiffest implant (CoCr). The femur with the most flexible implant (Composite 1) had the smallest reduction in strain energy density (*Comp1* and *Comp2*, composite materials; *Cocr*, cobalt chromium; *Ti*, titanium) (*Personal communication, R.N. Natarajan*).

during stance phase. Thus, failure as a result of cyclic fatigue of both interfaces and implant materials is an important consideration in total knee replacement designs (Ducheyne, Kagan, & Lacey, 1978; Kagan, 1977; Landy & Walker, 1988). In addition, the portion of the tibial plateau that is loaded varies with knee flexion angle (Fig. 16-7). In many designs of total knee replacements, a large contact area only occurs for a limited portion of the knee range of motion with a much smaller contact area occurring at other flexion angles. The smaller the contact area, the larger the contact stresses.

One consideration in the factors producing wear on the tibiofemoral articulation is the tractive

rolling of the femur on the tibia as the knee flexes. A two-dimensional model using input from gait analysis has demonstrated the presence and location of tractive forces on the tibial surface (Wimmer & Andriacchi, 1997). The model shows that a reversal of the tractive force occurred at the posterior end of the contact region, suggesting that the effect of tractive forces should be considered in the evaluation of damage mechanisms. Different types of gait can cause different tractive forces on the tibial surface. Thus, one of the important variables in the consideration of factors leading to polyethylene damage may be a variation in the tractive force associated with the gait of a particular patient.

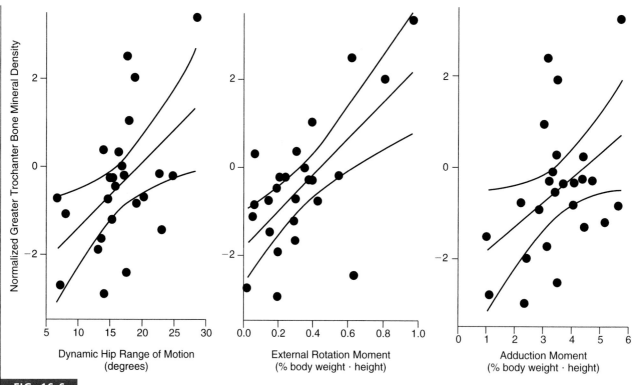

FIG. 16-6

The hip range of motion and external adduction and external rotation moments were significant predictors of the normalized bone mineral density of the greater trochanter in the patients with hip osteoarthritis. The abductors are the primary structures responsible for balancing the adduction moment. Because the abductors insert on the greater trochanter, a reduced adduction moment may reflect reduced forces in this region and may result in bone loss. Similarly, the anterior fibers of the gluteus medius and minimus are recognized as primary internal rotators. Thus, the decreased external rotation moment in early stance may also be reflective of decreased abductor muscle forces. *Modified with permission from Hurwitz, D.E., Foucher, K.C., Sumner, D.R., et al. (1998). Hip motion and moments during gait relate directly to proximal femoral bone mineral density in patients with osteoarthritis. J Biomechanics 31(10), 919–925.*

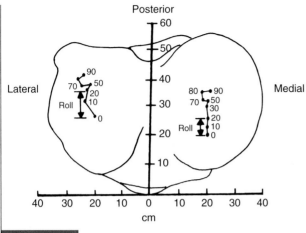

FIG. 16-7

The tibial-femoral contact moves posteriorly with knee flexion. The contact on the lateral side moves posteriorly much more during flexion (0–20°) than does the medial side because the lateral femoral condyle is rolling on a larger radius than is the medial femoral condyle. Beyond 20°, sliding motion begins on both condyles. *Reprinted with permission from Andriacchi, T.P., Stanwyck, T.S., & Galante, J.O. (1986). Knee biomechanics and total knee replacement. Arthroplasty, 1(3), 211–219.*

Medial-Lateral Load Distribution

One of the major problems limiting the use of total knee replacement in the 1970s was tibial component loosening (Bargren, Blaha, & Freeman, 1983; Ducheyne, Kagan, & Lacey, 1978; Hsieh & Walker, 1972; Kagan, 1977). Tibial component loosening was related to the load imbalance between the medial and lateral surface of the tibia that often occurs during walking and other activities. The early designs of the all-polyethylene tibial component were not sufficient to sustain this load imbalance. During walking, approximately 70% of the load across the knee joint is normally sustained by the medial compartment of the knee (Morrison, 1970; Schipplein & Andriacchi, 1991; Harrington, 1983). The adduction moment is a major determinate of the load distribution between the medial and lateral plateaus (Schipplein & Andriacchi, 1991) (Fig. 16-8). In fact, among normal subjects, the adduction moment is a significant predictor of the bone distribution

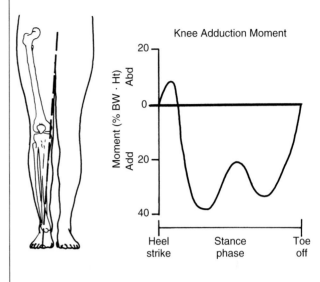

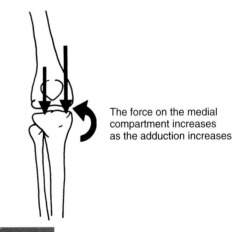

FIG. 16-8

An illustration of the adduction moment during walking and the resultant greater load across the medial compartment of the knee compared with the lateral compartment. *Reprinted with permission from Andriacchi, T.P. (1993). Functional analysis of pre- and post-knee surgery: Total knee arthroplasty and ACL reconstruction. J Biomechanics Eng, 115, 575–581.*

between the proximal medial and lateral tibia (Hurwitz et al., 1997).

The load asymmetry at the knee resulting from the adduction moment during gait provides a strong rationale for maintaining proper limb align-

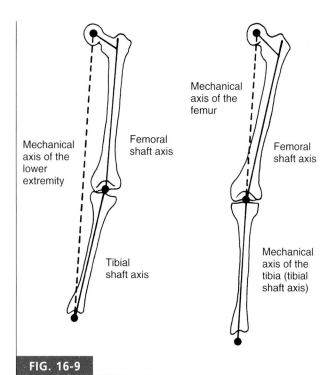

FIG. 16-9

Left, In a lower extremity with varus deformity, the mechanical axis passes medial to the knee. *Right,* When alignment is normal, the mechanical axis of the femur is in line with the mechanical axis of the tibia (tibial shaft axis). The *line* represented by the mechanical axes of the femur and the tibia is coincident with the mechanical axis of the lower extremity in this situation. *Reprinted with permission from Krachow, K.A. (1995). Surgical principles in total knee arthroplasty: Alignment, deformity, approaches and bone cuts. In J.J. Callagan, D.A. Dennis, W.G. Paprosky, et al. (Eds.), Orthopaedic Knowledge Update: Hip and Knee Reconstruction (pp. 269–276). Rosemont, IL: AAOS.*

ment following total knee replacement and uni-compartmental arthroplasty (Fig. 16-9) (Bargren, Blaha, & Freeman, 1983; Brugioni, Andriacchi, & Galante, 1990; Weinstein, Andriacchi, & Galante, 1986). Knees with a varus alignment are more likely to have a substantial load imbalance that creates stresses that could eventually lead to tibial component loosening (Case Study 16-2). Increased wear has been demonstrated in the medial compartment of knees initially in varus preoperatively and in the lateral compartment for those in valgus preoperatively (Wasielewski et al., 1994). To address problems associated with this load imbal-

Knee Arthroplasty

A 70-year-old man suffering from disabling left knee pain as a result of a severe genu varus and progressive left knee joint degeneration. The abnormal load resulting from the genu varus deformity creates a load imbalance characterized by a decrease in contact area at the lateral left tibia plateau and an increase of the contact stresses at the medial tibia plateau resulting in progressive wear in the medial tibiofemoral compartment. (Fig. cs16-2-1).

The patient has an impairment and is unable to walk more than half a mile. He wishes to maintain his active lifestyle. A first trial of conservative treatment was unsuccessful. A careful examination ensures the presence of a functional extensor mechanism. Moreover, complete imaging studies confirm the severe articular surface degeneration. The decision of knee arthroplasty was made to avoid a more severe joint degeneration and improve patient's lifestyle.

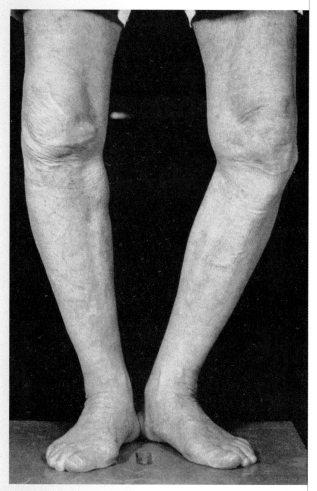

Case Study Figure 16-2-1.

ance, tibial component designs were modified to have a metal backing of the polyethylene articulating surface, and surgical instrumentation was modified to allow for proper alignment of the mechanical axis.

Patellofemoral Joint and Loads

As the incidence of tibial component loosening substantially decreased in the early 1980s, patellofemoral problems began to emerge as a primary issue in total knee replacement (Rorabeck et al., 1995; Rosenberg et al., 1988). The magnitude of the retropatellar force as well as the contact area on the retropatellar surface varies with knee flexion angle (Ahmed, Burke, & Hyder, 1987; Huberti & Hayes, 1984). Loads between two and three body weights have been reported at the patellofemoral joint for various activities of daily living. It was shown that for walking, the loads are relatively low but because the knee flexes beyond approximately 40° during activities such as stair climbing, the loads can reach levels of several body weights. The high magnitude of these forces poses a great risk to the mechanical integrity of the implant as well as the implant's fixation to bone.

The external knee flexion moment as measured with gait analysis is reflective of net quadriceps muscle activity. Alterations in the external flexion moment during stair climbing have been related to both the curvature of the patellar flange (Andriacchi & Hurwitz, 1997) and the height of the patella (Martel et al., 1990). Two groups of patients with different total knee replacement designs that differed primarily in the anterior curvature of the patellar flange in the region of the femoral trochlea were evaluated while climbing stairs. Both groups were selected on the basis of a good clinical outcome. One design group (nonanatomical trochlea) had a smaller radius on the patellar flange that caused the patella to articulate more anteriorly and distally than the second design (anatomical trochlea) that had a larger radius in this region. The second design more closely replicated the femoral trochlear anatomy. The group with the design that placed the patella more anteriorly had a slight buckling (increased flexion) of the knee in late stance (Fig. 16-10). There was also an increase in the moment at the knee sustained by the quadriceps in late stance concurrent with

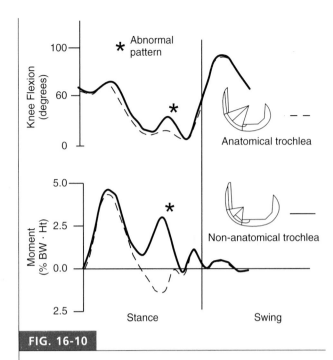

FIG. 16-10

(Top) The moment tending to flex the knee during stair climbing demonstrated differences in stair climbing function between the patients with nonanatomical femoral trochlea and anatomical femoral trochlea designs. *Reprinted with permission from Andriacchi, T.P., Yoder, D., Conley, A., et al. (1997). Patellofemoral design influences function following total knee arthroplasty. J Arthroplasty, 12(3), 243–249.* ***(Bottom)*** Patients with the nonanatomical femoral trochlea had increased knee flexion in late stance phase (shown by *). The increased knee flexion was balanced by an increase in the flexion moment (balanced by net quadriceps contraction) during late stance phase. *Reprinted with permission from Andriacchi, T.P. & Hurwitz, D.E. (1997). Gait biomechanics and total knee arthroplasty. Am J Knee Surg, 10(4), 255–260.*

the increase in knee flexion. Patients in the other group did not have these abnormal characteristics. In the design of a total knee replacement, the replication of an anatomical curvature of the femoral trochlea requires more bone resection of the distal anterior femur than does a nonanatomical curvature. Thus, many designs compromise between the restoration of normal anatomy and a more extensive resection of the distal femur. These results suggest that replication of normal patellofemoral anatomy is important because it will have a significant effect on both function and patellar loading.

Joint Line Height

In some instances, the joint line is elevated following total knee replacement, which results in an inferior movement of the position of the retropatellar contact on the femur. Elevated joint lines, which affect patella function and patella subluxation, have been correlated with wear patterns (Wasielewski et al., 1994), decreased longevity of the patellar component (Rosenberg et al., 1988), decreased clinical outcome (Junnosuke et al., 1993), and decreased range of motion (Ritter, Faris, & Keating, 1988). The height of the patella with respect to the joint line has been associated with significant changes in the flexion moment of the knee during stair climbing (Fig. 16-11). When the patellar position was changed 15 mm inferior to its normal position, more than 50% reduction in the flexion moment during stair climbing was noted (Martell et al., 1990).

Posterior Cruciate Ligament

Differing opinions exist with regards to the benefits of retaining, substituting for, or removing the posterior cruciate ligament (Andriacchi & Galante, 1988; Li et al., 1995; Rorabeck et al., 1993), with no definitive answers with regard to which design results in better wear rates, clinical outcome, or range of motion. Some studies indicate no substantial differences in loosening or radiolucent lines (Ranawat et al., 1993; Stern & Insall, 1992; Wright & Bartel, 1986) or range of motion (Hirsch, Lotke, & Morrison, 1994) between the different designs. In fact, the preoperative range of motion may have a greater influence on the postoperative range of motion than any influence attributable to design differences (Harvey et al., 1993; Maloney & Schurman, 1992). The decision of whether to retain or remove the posterior cruciate ligament imposes design criteria on the amount of constraint that the articulating surfaces need to provide.

Retention of the posterior cruciate ligament requires that the joint line be accurately reproduced for the kinematics to remain normal. Otherwise, the knee kinematics can be altered and loads across the joint may even be increased. Limited knee flexion (Ritter, Faris, & Keating, 1988) and posterior polyethylene wear (Swany & Scott, 1993) have both been associated with posterior cruciate ligaments that are too tight and result in posterior tracking of the femur on the tibia. Posterior cruciate-retaining designs generally have an unconstrained but conforming tibial

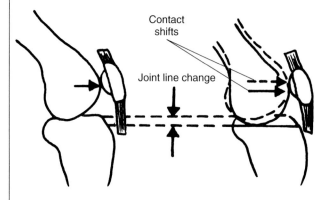

Interaction Between Tibiofemoral Joint Line Position and Patellofemoral Mechanics

Contact shifts

Joint line change

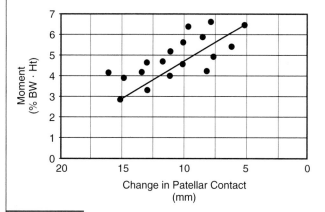

Stair Climbing Knee Flexion Moment and Joint Line Change

Moment (% BW · Ht) vs. Change in Patellar Contact (mm)

FIG. 16-11

The position of the retropatellar contact is related to the location of the joint line. Typically, in total knee replacement the joint line is shifted superiorly, causing a downward movement of the location of the retropatellar contact at any flexion angle. The retropatellar position is related to the flexion moment during stair climbing.
Reprinted with permission from Andriacchi, T.P. (1993). Functional analysis of pre and post-knee surgery: Total knee arthroplasty and ACL reconstruction. J Biomechanics Eng, 115, 575–581.

component to increase the contact area and minimize the stresses and resulting polyethylene wear. As discussed earlier, the lateral side of the knee can be unweighted during the stance phase of gait and can result in the knee being in a varus position. The flat articular surfaces frequently used with posterior cruciate-retaining designs permit large contact areas but can result in edge loading and high stresses if the implant is tilted.

Removal of the posterior cruciate ligament necessitates that posterior stability now results from increased tibial-femoral constraint. In the absence of a posterior cruciate ligament, the posteriorly directed shear force is instead sustained by the interfaces of the articulating surfaces (Andriacchi & Galante, 1988). Although more constrained designs are inherently more stable, they may limit the passive range of motion by restricting the amount of rollback needed to achieve deep knee flexion (Fig. 16-12). Substituting designs are also more constraining with a cam mechanism used to maintain the posterior position of the femur relative to the tibia.

Variations in the knee kinematics and moments during stair climbing suggest that posterior cruciate-retaining patients have more normal function while ascending stairs than do patients with knees in which the posterior cruciate ligament is removed (Dorr et al., 1988; Kelman et al., 1989). Patients with cruciate-sacrificing knee replacements had a tendency to reduce the moment sustained by the quadriceps by leaning forward during the portion of the support phase of ascending stairs when the quadriceps moment would reach a peak value (Fig. 16-13) (Andriacchi, Galante, & Fermier, 1982). This finding was also consistent with a study in which electromyographic activity was measured during

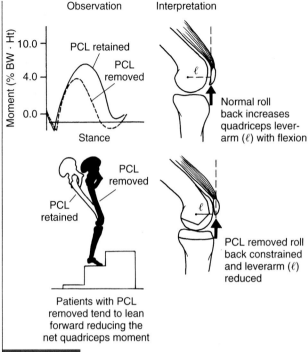

Stair Climbing in Patients Following Total Knee Replacement

FIG. 16-13

Patients with designs that remove or substitute for the posterior cruciate ligament tend to reduce the knee flexion moment and thus the resulting demand on the quadriceps. The mechanism they use for the adaptation is a forward lean of the torso. The biomechanical explanation for the adaptation seen in these patients can be related to the normal posterior movement of the tibiofemoral contact with flexion, which is reduced when the posterior cruciate ligament is removed and constraint is added to the articular surface. *Reprinted with permission from Andriacchi, T.P. (1993). Functional analysis of pre- and post-knee surgery: Total knee arthroplasty and ACL Reconstruction. J Biomechanics Eng, 115, 575–581.*

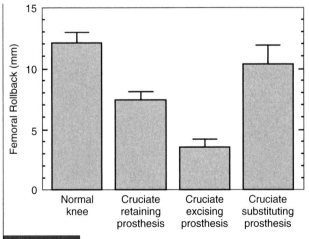

FIG. 16-12

Femoral rollback as a function of prosthesis type during stair descent at 90° of knee flexion. *Reprinted with permission from Mahoney, O.M., Noble, P.C., Rhoads, D.D., et al. (1994). Posterior cruciate function following total knee arthroplasty. A biomechanical study. J Arthroplasty, 9(6), 569–78.*

stair climbing (Dorr et al., 1988). In that study, patients with posterior cruciate ligament-sacrificing designs required increased use of the soleus muscle while stair climbing. The increased soleus activity was suggestive of a forward lean in the patients with posterior cruciate ligament-sacrificing designs similar to that described in other studies (Andriacchi, Galante, & Fermier, 1982). In a more recent study by Wilson et al. (1996), patients with posterior cruciate ligament-sacrificing designs were compared with normal subjects while walking and stair climbing. Although the study did not report a statistical difference, there was a 25% reduction in the peak

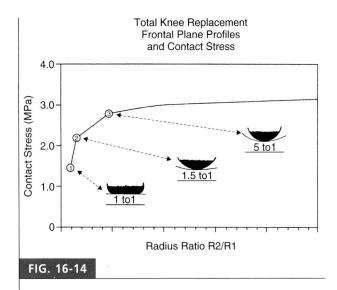

Total Knee Replacement
Frontal Plane Profiles
and Contact Stress

FIG. 16-14

The predicted contact stress increases as the conformity decreases. *Modified with permission from Andriacchi, T.P. & Natarajan, R.N. (1993). Conformity and polyethylene damage in total knee replacement (Internal Communication 97–5110–206 3MZ). Zimmer, Inc.*

flexion moment during stair climbing between normal subjects and patients following total knee replacement. The lack of a statistically significant difference in that study may have been associated with the small sample size of the test population.

The functional differences between the posterior cruciate ligament-retaining and sacrificing designs were associated with the normal posterior movement of the femur on the tibia (rollback) with flexion. This finding has been explained by the dynamic interaction between the posterior cruciate ligament and tibiofemoral rollback with flexion. The lever arm of the quadriceps (Andriacchi, Stanwyck, & Galante, 1986) normally increases with knee flexion. The functional adaptations seen among patients with cruciate-sacrificing designs were likely associated with the need to compensate for the lack of normal femoral rollback in knees in which the cruciate ligament is removed. Thus, rollback must occur in the early phases of flexion to have an appropriate quadriceps lever arm to sustain normal stair climbing.

Conformity

The degree of conformity between the femoral component and the tibial component depends on the ratio of the radii of the two components. As the radius of the tibial component increases relative to that of the femoral component, the conformity decreases and the contact stress between the two components increases (Fig. 16-14). Conformity is frequently used to characterize the articulation between a dished tibial surface and a rounded femoral component, but it can also be used to describe the articulation between a flat tibial surface and a flat femoral component. A flat geometry has a conformity of one and does not constrain the rotational or translational movement as required with a posterior cruciate-retaining design. A dished geometry achieves conformity and constraint as needed for the posterior cruciate ligament-sacrificing designs. To maintain the sagittal plane kinematics, the femoral component must have a smaller posterior radius and a larger distal radius. Thus, it is not possible to achieve conformity in the sagittal plane in both flexion and extension (Fig. 16-15).

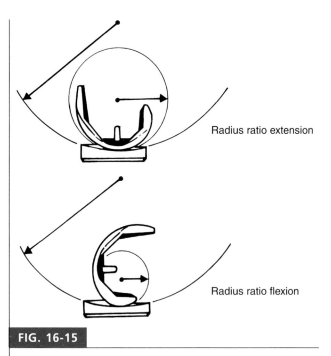

Radius ratio extension

Radius ratio flexion

FIG. 16-15

The radius of the femoral component varies with knee flexion angle. Thus, in the sagittal plane it is not possible to achieve optimal conformity in both flexion and extension. *Reprinted with permission from Andriacchi, T.P. & Natarajan, R.N. (1993). Conformity and polyethylene damage in total knee replacement (Internal Communication 97–5110–206 3MZ). Zimmer, Inc.*

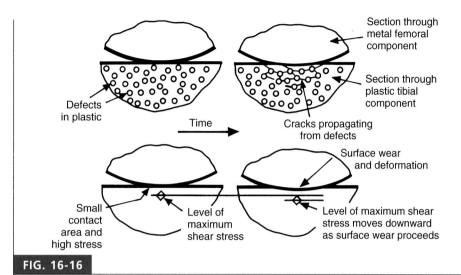

FIG. 16-16

A model of delamination wear in polyethylene with intergranular defects. The lower diagram explains a possible reason why delamination does not occur if there are no defects in the material. *Reprinted with permission from Walker, P.S. & Blunn, G.W. (1997). Keynote Lecture II: Modern design of total knee replacement. In S. Niwa, X. Yoshino, M. Kurosaka, K. Shino, S. Yamamoto (Eds.),* Reconstruction of the Knee Joint *(pp. 129–142). Tokyo: Springer-Verlag.*

Constraint

In general, proper soft tissue balance is necessary for a satisfactory outcome. In the presence of complex bony deformities such as a severe valgus deformity, satisfactory stability is often unobtainable and constraint must be provided by the implant design. Historically, a hinged prosthesis, which provides maximum constraint, was advocated for those patients with severe valgus deformities. Hinged prostheses, however, have been associated with a poor clinical outcome (Bargar, Cracchiolo, & Amstutz, 1980; Hui & Fitzgerald, 1980; Rand, Chao, & Stauffer, 1987). A more contemporary alternative to the hinged prosthesis is a highly constrained but unlinked total knee replacement (constrained condylar knee). This design eliminates the need for ligament balancing by providing medial lateral stability through a rectangular polyethylene tibial post. This highly constrained design has provided adequate outcome for elderly low-demand patients with severe valgus deformities (Bullek, Scuderi, & Insall, 1996).

Polyethylene

Polyethylene damage has been closely related to its thickness (Collier et al., 1991; Wright & Bartel, 1986), the material properties, the presence of third-body particles (cement), and areas of high contact stress (Bargren, Blaha, & Freeman, 1983). Defects in the polyethylene serve as sites for crack initiation and propagation (Fig. 16-16). Increasing the polyethylene thickness to at least 8 to 10 mm will reduce contact stresses and should decrease the amount of wear (Collier et al., 1991). Metal backing was initially introduced to more evenly distribute the load to the underlying cancellous bone of the proximal tibia. However, overall component thickness needed to be increased following the introduction of metal backing so that an adequate polyethylene thickness was maintained. The multivariate nature of the causes of polyethylene damage makes it difficult to draw definitive conclusions on failure mechanisms from retrieval studies. Moreover, the diverse nature of the contact stress distribution (compressive, tensile, and shear) may result in different damage modes. Deformation, pitting, cracking, and abrasion are all examples of polyethylene damage modes.

Anterior Cruciate Ligament

During total knee replacement, the anterior cruciate ligament is either already absent or usually removed. In the case when only one compartment of the knee requires replacement (unicompartmental knee arthroplasty), both cruciate ligaments are frequently retained. Gait studies of total knee replacement patients (Andriacchi, Galante, & Fermier, 1982; Chao, Laughman, & Stauffer, 1980; Kelman et al., 1989; Simon et al., 1983) show that normal function is not achieved in the majority of the patients despite improvements in stride lengths and knee motion and clinical status. Numerous subsequent studies demonstrated differences in the flexion-extension moment during level walking. These variations in the flexion-extension moments at the knee could not be related to any specific design but instead suggested the possibility that loss of joint proprioception or the functionality of the anterior cruciate ligament may have been a factor (Weinstein, Andriacchi, & Galante, 1986). The removal of the anterior cruciate ligament was common to all total knee replacement designs and may be one of the factors that limit a patient's recovery of total normal function. Similar patterns of abnormal flexion-extension moments (Berchuck et al., 1990) have been reported in patients following injury to the anterior cruciate ligament.

Summary

1 The effect of forces on the stability of a total joint replacement depends not only on its magnitude but also on its orientation and point of application.

2 Magnitude, orientation, and point of application of the loads at joints influence the stresses, bending moments, and rotational moments of the implant, and are critical for the implant stability and longevity.

3 Understanding the dynamic loads during daily activities provides critical information for addressing clinical problems such as mechanical loosening of implants, amount of wear, bone resorption, and the choice of rehabilitation and surgical protocols.

4 The evolution of total joint replacement has been aided by information generated from biomechanical studies.

REFERENCES

Ahmed, A.M., Burke, D.L., & Hyder, A. (1987). Force analysis of the patellar mechanism. *J Orthop Res, 5,* 69.

Amstutz, H.C., Campbell, P., Kossovsky, N., et al. (1992). Mechanism and clinical significance of wear debris-induced osteolysis. *CORR, 276,* 7–18.

Andriacchi, T.P. (1993). Functional analysis of pre- and post-knee surgery: Total knee arthroplasty and ACL reconstruction. *J Biomechanics Eng, 115,* 575–581.

Andriacchi, T.P. & Galante, J.O. (1988). Retention of the posterior cruciate ligament in total knee arthroplasty. *J Arthroplasty,* S13–19.

Andriacchi, T.P., Galante, J.O., Belytschko, T.B., et al. (1976). A stress analysis of femoral stem in total hip prostheses. *J Bone Joint Surg, 58A*(5),618–624.

Andriacchi, T.P., Galante, J.O., & Fermier, R.W. (1982). The influence of total knee replacement design on walking and stair-climbing. *J Bone Joint Surg, 64A,* 1328.

Andriacchi, T.P. & Hurwitz, D.E. (1997). Gait biomechanics and total knee arthroplasty. *Am J Knee Surg, 10*(4), 255–260.

Andriacchi, T.P. & Natarajan, R.N. (1993). Conformity and polyethylene damage in total knee replacement (Internal Communication 97–5110–206 3MZ). Zimmer, Inc.

Andriacchi, T.P., Stanwyck, T.S., & Galante, J.O. (1986). Knee biomechanics and total knee replacement. *Arthroplasty, 1*(3),211–219.

Andriacchi, T.P., Yoder, D., Conley, A., et al. (1997). Patellofemoral design influences function following total knee arthroplasty. *J Arthroplasty, 12*(3), 243–249.

Bargar, W.L., Cracchiolo, A., & Amstutz, H.C. (1980). Results with constrained total knee prosthesis in treating severely disabled patients and patients with failed total knee replacement. *J Bone Joint Surg, 62A,* 504–512.

Bargren, J.H., Blaha, J.D., & Freeman, M.A.R. (1983). Alignment in total knee arthroplasty. Correlated and clinical observations. *Clin Orthop, 173,* 178.

Berchuck, M., Andriacchi, T.P., Bach, B.R. Jr., et al. (1990). Gait adaptations by patients who have a deficient ACL. *J Bone Joint Surg, 72A,* 871–877.

Bergmann, G., Graichen, F., & Rohlmann, A. (1993). Hip joint loading during walking and running measured in two patients. *J Biomechanics, 26*(8), 969–990.

Bergmann, G., Graichen, F., & Rohlmann, A. (1995). Is staircase walking a risk for the fixation of hip implants? *J Biomechanics, 28*(5), 535–553.

Berzins, A., Sumner, D.R., & Andriacchi, T.P. (1993). Stem curvature and load angle influence the initial relative bone-implant motion of cementless femoral stems. *J Orthop Res, 11*(5), 758–769.

Berzins, A., Sumner, D.R., Andriacchi, T.P., et al. (1993). Stem curvature and load angle influence the initial relative bone implant motion of cementless femoral stems. *J Orthop Res, 11*(5), 758–769.

Box, G. & Noble, P.C. (1993). The position of the joint center and the functional outcome of total hip replacement. *ORS Trans, 18,* 525.

Brand, R.A. & Crowninshield, R.D. (1980). The effect of cane use on hip contact force. *CORR, 147,* 181–184.

Brand, R.A., Pedersen, D.R., & Friederich, J.A. (1986). The sensitivity of muscle force predictions to changes in physiologic cross-sectional area. *J Biomechanics, 19*(8), 589–596.

Brugioni, D.J., Andriacchi, T.P., & Galante, J.O. (1990). A functional and radiographic analysis of the total condylar knee arthroplasty. *J Arthroplasty, 5*(2),173–180.

Bryan, J.M., Sumner, D.R., Hurwitz, D.E., et al. (1996). A possible confounding effect of altered load history on the assessment of periprosthetic bone loss ten years following successful cementless total hip arthroplasty: Assessment by dual energy x-ray absorptiometry and gait analysis. *J Orthop Res, 14*(5), 762–768.

Bryan, J.M., Tompkins, G., Sumner, D.R., et al. (1994). Quantifying proximal femoral bone loss following cementless total hip arthroplasty using dual energy x-ray absorptiometry. *Trans ORS, 19*, 580.

Bullek, D.D., Scuderi, G.R., & Insall J.N. (1996). The constrained condylar knee prosthesis: An alternative for the valgus knee in the elderly. In J.N. Insall, N.W. Scott, & G.R. Scuderi (Eds.), *Current Concepts in Primary and Revision Total Knee Arthroplasty* (pp. 85–89). Philadelphia: Lippincott-Raven Press, Ltd.

Chao, E.Y., Laughman, R.K., & Stauffer, R.N. (1980). Biomechanical gait evaluation of pre- and postoperative total knee replacement patients. *Arch Orthop Trauma Surg, 97*, 309.

Cheal, E.J., Spector, M., & Hayes, W.C. (1992). Role of loads and prosthesis material properties on the mechanics of the proximal femur after total hip arthroplasty. *J Orthop Res, 10*(4), 5–22.

Collier, J.P., Mayor, M.B., McNamara, J.L., et al. (1991). Analysis of the failure of 122 polyethylene inserts from uncemented tibial knee components. *Clin Orthop, 273*, 232–242.

Collis, D.K. & Oregon, E. (1977). Femoral stem failure in total hip replacement. *J Bone Joint Surg, 59A*(8), 1033–1041.

Crowninshield, R.D. & Brand, R.A. (1981). A physiologically based criterion of muscle force prediction in locomotion. *J Biomechanics, 14*(11), 793–801.

Crowninshield, R.D., Johnston, R.C., Andrew, J.G., et al. (1978). A biomechanical investigation of the human hip. *J Biomechanics, 11*, 75–85.

Davy, D.T., Kotzar, G.M., Brown, R.H., et al. (1988). Telemetric force measurements across the hip after total hip arthroplasty. *J Bone Joint Surg, 70A*(1), 45–50.

Delp, S.L., Komattu, A.V., & Wixson, R.L. (1994). Superior displacement of the hip in total joint replacement: Effects of prosthetic neck length, neck-stem angle, and anteversion angle on the moment-generating capacity of the muscles. *J Orthop Res, 12*, 860–869.

Delp, S.L. & Maloney, W. (1993). Effects of hip center location on the moment-generating capacity of the muscles. *J Biomechanics, 26*(4,5), 485–499.

Doehring, T.C., Rubash, H.E., Shelly, F.J., et al. (1996). The effect of superior and superolateral relocations of the hip center on hip joint forces: An experimental and analytical analysis. *J Arthroplasty, Sept 11*(6), 693–703.

Dorr, L.D., Ochsner, J.L., Gronley, J., et al. (1988). Functional comparison of posterior cruciate-retained versus cruciate-sacrificed total knee arthroplasty. *Clin Orthop, 236*, 36.

Ducheyne, P., Kagan, A., & Lacey, J.A. (1978). Failure of total knee arthroplasty due to loosening and deformation of the tibial component. *J Bone Joint Surg, 60A*, 384.

Engh, C.A. & Bobyn, J.D. (1988). The influence of stem size and extent of porous coating on femoral bone resorption after primary cementless hip arthroplasty. *CORR, 231*, 7–28.

Engh, C.A., McGovern, T.F., Bobyn, J.D., et al. (1992). A quantitative evaluation of periprosthetic bone remodeling after cementless total hip arthroplasty. *J Bone Joint Surg, 74A*, 1009–1020.

Engh, C.A., O'Connor, D., Jasty, M., et al. (1992). Quantification of implant micromotion, strain shielding and bone resorption with porous-coated anatomical medullary locking femoral prostheses. *CORR, 285*, 13–29.

English, T.A. & Kilvington, M. (1979). In vivo records of hip loads using a femoral implant with telemetric output (a preliminary report). *J Biomed Eng, 1*(2),111–15.

Foucher, K.C., Hurwitz, D.E., Andriacchi, T.P., et al. (1997). Reductions in hip contact forces due to gait adaptations in preoperative total hip replacement patients persist even if antagonistic muscle activity is increased. *21st Annual Meeting of American Society of Biomechanics*, 192–193.

Galante, J.O., Rostoker, W., & Doyle, J.M. (1975). Failed femoral stem in total hip prostheses. A report of six cases. *J Bone Joint Surg, 57A*(2), 230–236.

Goethgen, C.B., Sumner, D.R., Platz, C., et al. (1991). Changes in tibial bone mass after primary cementless and revision cementless total hip arthroplasty in canine models. *J Orthop Res, 9*, 820–827.

Gore, D.R., Murray, M.P., Gardner, G.M., et al. (1977). Roentgenographic measurements after Muller total hip replacement. *J Bone Joint Surg, 59A*(7), 948–953.

Harrington, I.J. (1983). Static and dynamic loading patterns in knee joints with deformities. *J Bone Joint Surg, 65A*, 247–259.

Harvey, I.A., Barry, K., Kirby, S.P., et al. (1993). Factors affecting the range of movement of total knee arthroplasty. *J Bone Joint Surg, 75B*(6), 950–955.

Hirsch, H.S., Lotke, P.A., & Morrison, L.D. (1994). The posterior cruciate ligament in total knee surgery: Save, sacrifice, or substitute? *CORR, 309*, 64–68.

Hodge, W.A., Andriacchi, T.P., & Galante, J.O. (1991). A relationship between stem orientation and function following total hip arthroplasty. *J Arthroplasty, 6*(3), 229–235.

Hsieh, H. & Walker, P.S. (1972). Stabilizing mechanisms of the loaded and unloaded knee joint. *J Bone Joint Surg, 58A*, 87–93.

Huberti, H.H. & Hayes, W.C. (1984). Patellofemoral contact pressures. *J Bone Joint Surg, 66A*, 715–724.

Hui, F.C. & Fitzgerald, R.H. (1980). Hinged total knee arthroplasty. *J Bone Joint Surg, 62A*, 513–519.

Hurwitz, D.E. & Andriacchi, T.P. (1997). Biomechanics of the hip. In J. Callaghan, A. Rosenberg, & H. Rubash (Eds.), *The Adult Hip* (pp. 75–89). New York: Raven Press, Ltd.

Hurwitz, D.E., Chertack, C.C., & Andriacchi, T.P. (1992). How gait changes in preoperative and postoperative patients with total hip replacements. *Proceedings of NACOB II, The Second North American Congress on Biomechanics*, 313–314.

Hurwitz, D.E., Foucher, K.C., Sumner, D.R., et al. (1998). Hip motion and moments during gait relate directly to proximal femur bone mineral density in patients with hip osteoarthritis. *J Biomechanics, 31*(10), 919–925.

Hurwitz, D.E., Guyton, J.A., Andriacchi, T.P., et al. (1992). How canal fill in uncemented total hip replacements affects the biomechanics of gait. *38th Annual Meeting of the Orthopaedic Research Society, 17*(1), 281.

Hurwitz, D.E., Sumner, D.R., Andriacchi, T.P., et al. (1998). Dynamic knee loads during gait predict proximal tibial bone distribution. *J Biomechanics, 31*(5),423–30.

Jasty, M., Bragon, C., Lee, K., et al. (1993). Wear of polyethylene in total joint arthroplasty. In B.F. Morrey (Ed.), *Biological Material and Mechanical Considerations of Joint Replacement* (pp. 103–117). New York: Raven Press Ltd.

Jasty, M., O'Connor, D.O., Henshaw, R.M., et al. (1994). Fit of the uncemented femoral component and the use of cement influence the strain transfer to the femoral cortex. *J Orthop Res, 12*, 648–656.

Johnston, R.C., Brand, R.A., & Crowninshield, R.D. (1979). Reconstruction of the hip. *J Bone Joint Surg, 61A*(5), 639–652.

Junnosuke, R., Saito, S., Yamamoto, K., et al. (1993). Factors influencing the postoperative range of motion in total knee arthroplasty. *Bull Hosp Joint Dis, 53*(3),35–40.

Kagan, A. (1977). Mechanical causes of loosening in knee joint replacements. *J Biomechanics, 10*, 387.

Kelman, G.J., Biden, E.N., & Phil, et al. (1989). Gait laboratory analysis of a posterior cruciate-sparing total knee arthroplasty in stair ascent and descent. *Clin Orthop, 248*, 21.

Kotzar, G.M., Davy, D.T., Goldberg, V.M., et al. (1991). Telemeterized in vivo hip joint force data. A report on two patients after total hip surgery. *J Orthop Res, 9*, 621–633.

Krachow, K.A. (1995). Surgical principles in total knee arthroplasty: Alignment, deformity, approaches and bone cuts. In J.J. Callagan, D.A. Dennis, W.G. Paprosky, & A.G. Rosenberg (Eds.), *Orthopaedic Knowledge Update Hip and Knee Reconstruction* (pp. 269–276). Rosemont, IL: AAOS.

Landy, M.M. & Walker, P.S. (1988). Wear of ultra-high-molecular weight polyethylene components of 90 retrieved knee prostheses. *J Arthroplasty (Suppl)*, 73–85.

Li, E., Ritter, M., Moilanen, T., et al. (1995). Point-counterpoint total knee arthroplasty. *J Arthroplasty, 10*(4), 560–570.

Long, W.T., Dorr, L.D., Healy, B., et al. (1993). Functional recovery of noncemented total hip arthroplasty. *CORR, 288*, 73–77.

Mahoney, O.M., Noble, P.C., Rhoads, D.D., et al. (1994). Posterior cruciate function following total knee arthroplasty. A biomechanical study. *J Arthroplasty, 9*(6), 569–578.

Maloney, W.J. & Schurman, D.J. (1992). The effects of implant design on range of motion after total knee arthroplasty. Total condylar versus posterior stabilized total condylar designs. *CORR, 278*, 147–152.

Maloney, W.J,, Sychterz, C., Bragdon, C., et al. (1996). The Otto Aufranc Award. Skeletal response to well fixed femoral components inserted with and without cement. *Clin Orthop, Dec*(333), 15–26.

Martell, J.M., Andriacchi, T.P., Rosenberg, A.G., et al. (1990). The relationship between changes in patellar height and function following total knee replacement. Transcript of the *36th Annual Meeting of the Orthopaedic Research Society, 15*(1),169.

Morrison, J.B. (1970). The mechanics of the knee joint in relation to normal walking. *J Biomechanics, 3*, 51–61.

Murray, M.P., Brewer, B.J., & Zuege, R.C. (1972). Kinesiologic measurements of functional performance before and after McKee-Farrar total hip replacement. *J Bone Joint Surg, 54A*(2), 237–256.

Noble, P.C. (1995). The design of cementless femoral prostheses. In J.J. Gallaghan, D.A. Dennis, & A.G. Rosenberg (Eds.), *Orthopaedic Knowledge Update: Hip and Knee Reconstruction* (pp. 127–138). Rosemont, IL: AAOS.

Noble, P.C., Helmke, H.W., & Paul, J.P. (1993). Femoral position critically affects the interpretation of intra-vital hip force data. *Trans ORS, 18*(2), 443.

Paul, J.P. (1976). Approaches to design: Force actions transmitted by joints in the human body. *Proc Res Soc London, 192*, 163–72.

Phillips, T.W., Nguyen, L.T., & Munro, S.D. (1991). Loosening of cementless femoral stems: A biomechanical analysis of immediate fixation with loading vertical, femur horizontal. *J Biomechanics, 24*(1), 37–48.

Pilliar, R.M., Lee, J.M., & Maniatopoulus, C. (1986). Observations on the effect of movement on bone ingrowth into porous-surfaced implants. *Clin Orthop, 208*, 108–113.

Ranawat, C.S., Flynn, W.F., Saddler, S., et al. (1993). Long-term results of the total condylar knee arthroplasty. *Clin Orthop, 286*, 94–102.

Rand, J.A., Chao, E.Y.S., & Stauffer, R.W. (1987). Kinematic rotating hinge knee arthroplasty. *J Bone Joint Surg 69A*, 489–497.

Ritter, M.A., Faris, P.M., & Keating, E.M. (1988). Posterior cruciate ligament balancing during total knee arthroplasty. *J Arthroplasty, 3*, 323.

Rorabeck, C.H., Bourne, R.B., Lewis, P.L., et al. (1993). The Miller/Galante knee prosthesis for the treatment of osteoarthrosis: A comparison of the results of partial fixation with cement and fixation without any cement. *J Bone Joint Surg, 75*, 402.

Rorabeck, C.H., Dorr, L.D., Hofmann, A.A., et al. (1995). Controversial issues in knee arthroplasty. *Orthop Crossfire, 18*(9), 905–914.

Rosenberg, A.G., Andriacchi, T.P., Barden, R., et al. (1988). Patellar component failure in cementless total knee arthroplasty. *Clin Orthop, 236*, 106.

Rydell, N.W. (1966). Forces acting on the femoral head-prosthesis: A study on strain gauge supplied prostheses in living persons. *Acta Orthop Scand (Suppl)*, 88, 37.

Schipplein, O.D. & Andriacchi, T. (1991). Interaction between active and passive knee stabilizers during level walking. *J Orthop Res, 9*, 113–119.

Seireg, A. & Arvikar, R.J. (1975). The prediction of muscular load sharing and joint forces in the lower extremities during walking. *J Biomechanics, 8*, 89–102.

Simon, S.R., Trieshmann, H.W., Burdett, R.G., et al. (1983). Quantitative gait analysis after total knee arthroplasty for monarticular degenerative arthritis. *J Bone Joint Surg, 65*, 605.

Stauffer, R.N., Smidt, G.L., Wadsworth, J.B. (1974). Clinical and biomechanical analysis of gait following Charnley total hip replacement. *CORR, 99*, 70–77.

Stern, S.H. & Insall, J.H. (1992). Posterior stabilized prosthesis results after follow-up of nine to twelve years. *J Bone Joint Surg, 74A*, 980.

Swany, M.R. & Scott, R.D. (1993). Posterior polyethylene wear in posterior cruciate ligament retaining total knee arthroplasty. *J Arthroplasty, 8*, 439–446.

Taylor, S.J., Walker, P.S., Cannon, P.J., et al. (1997). The forces in the distal femur and knee during different activities measured by telemetry. *Transactions of the 43rd Annual ORS Meeting*, 259.

Walker, P.S. & Blunn, G.W. (1997). Keynote Lecture II: Modern design of total knee replacement. In S. Niwa, X. Yoshino, M. Kurosaka, K. Shino, S. Yamamoto (Eds.), *Reconstruction of the Knee Joint* (pp. 129–142). Tokyo: Springer-Verlag.

Wasielewski, R.C., Galante, J.O., Leighty, R.M., et al. (1994). Wear patterns on retrieved polyethylene tibial inserts and their relationship to technical considerations during total knee arthroplasty. *CORR, 299*, 31–43.

Weinans, H., Huiskes, R., & Grootenboer, H.J. (1992). Effects of material properties of femoral hip components on bone remodeling. *J Orthop Res, 10*, 845–53.

Weinstein, J.N., Andriacchi, T.P., & Galante, J.O. (1986). Factors influencing walking and stairclimbing following unicompartmental knee arthroplasty. *J Arthroplasty, 1*(2), 109–115.

White, S.C., Yack, H.J., & Lesswing, A.L. (1992). Pre- and post surgical gait of a total hip replacement patient. *Trans 7th Annual East Coast Gait Conference 1992;* Session 11, Richmond Virginia.

Willert, H. & Buchhorn, G.H. (1993). Particle disease due to wear of ultrahigh molecular weight polyethylene. Findings from retrieval studies. Wear of polyethylene in total joint arthroplasty. In B.F. Morrey (Ed), *Biological Material and Mechanical Considerations of Joint Replacement* (pp. 87–102). New York: Raven Press Ltd.

Wilson, S.A., McCann, P.D., Gotlin, R.S., et al. (1996). Comprehensive gait analysis in posterior-stabilized knee arthroplasty. *J Arthroplasty, 11*(4),359–367.

Wimmer, M.A. & Andriacchi, T.P. (1997). Tractive forces during rolling motion of the knee: Implications for wear in total knee replacement. *J Biomechanics, 30*(2),131–37.

Wright, T.M. & Bartel, D.L. (1986). The problem of surface damage in polyethylene total knee components. *Clin Orthop, 205*, 67–74.

Yoder, S.A., Brand, R.A., Pedersen, D.R., et al. (1988). Total hip acetabular component position affects component loosening rates. *CORR, 228*, 79–87.

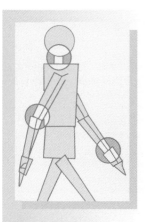

CHAPTER 17

Engineering Approaches to Standing, Sitting, and Lying

Chris J. Snijders

Biomechanics of Standing

Muscles extending from the neck to the ankle are continually active to prevent collapse of the skeleton. In view of this function, these muscles are known as postural muscles. Obviously, these muscles are comparatively strong and do not tire easily. In skeletal musculature, postural and phasic muscles—also known as slow and fast muscles—are present (see Chapter 6). The morphological differences are particularly marked in the muscles of birds, but in humans this distinction is less evident because of the mixed composition of muscles. It is assumed that the force proportion of postural to phasic muscles is 3:2. Exercise, especially participation in high-level sports or athletic training, can change this proportion to even 5:1. Selective training of postural (red) muscles is advantageous because these muscles are stronger and deliver more work than do phasic (white) muscles. The neurologist and muscle physiologist Vladimir Janda (1980) pointed to the following relationship between postural and phasic muscles in agonist and antagonist action:

1. Postural muscles tend to spontaneous functional or even anatomical shortening. This manifests itself in a higher muscle tonus.
2. Postural muscles have an inhibiting effect on their phasic partners (inhibition of an antagonist muscle by the agonist).
3. With insufficient variety in muscle use, postural muscles can be activated disproportionately, which leads to inhibition and weakening of phasic muscles (pseudoparesis). This process can lead to an imbalance between groups of muscles, resulting in poor posture with loss of mobility and increase of joint load.

Figure 17-1*A* illustrates the distal crossed syndrome according to Janda (1980), which involves shortened back extensor and hip flexor muscles versus weakened abdominal and buttock muscles. Anterior pelvic tilt and hyperlordosis are the result, which also manifests in walking with insufficient hip extension (normal is 5 to 10°). A similar imbalance is the crossed proximal syndrome with shortened pectoralis major, cervical trapezius, levator scapulae, and, less pronounced, the sternocleidomastoid muscles versus the weakened fixator muscles of the scapulae (rhomboideus, distal and medial parts of the trapezius, and the serratus anterior muscles) and the deep flexor muscles of

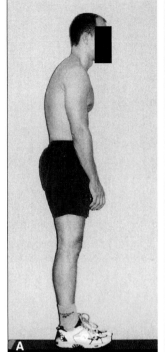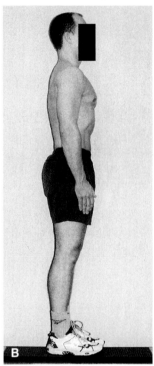

FIG. 17-1

A, Illustration of poor posture. **B,** Illustration of good posture.

the neck. This manifests itself in postural deterioration with the head placed forward, the shoulder blades raised and abducted, the upper part of the cervical spine overextended, and the shoulders moved forward. Figure 17-1*B* illustrates the result of strengthening of phasic muscles and stretching of postural muscles allowing for posterior tilt of the pelvis, backward movement of the shoulders, and elevation of the head by moving the chin in the direction of the ears.

The unconstrained standing posture is often studied because of the typical individual characteristics. One of these characteristics is the location of the mass center of gravity (Fig. 17-2*A*, F_g, F_v). The point of application of the resultant force on the feet (F_v) can be measured with the aid of a force plate (Fig. 17-2*B*) and is called the center of pressure (COP). A triangular plate with force transducers under the three corners can measure the position of the COP as shown in Figure 17-2, *C & D* (Moll van Charante, Snijders, & Mulder, 1991; Snijders & Verduin, 1973). The amount of sway around a mean equilibrium position reflects the

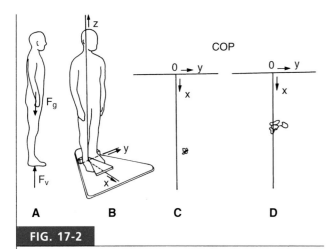

FIG. 17-2

A, The resultant force between ground and feet (F_v) equals body weight (F_g). **B,** F_v position (center of pressure path, COP) can be measured with a force plate with force transducers under the corners depicting in a three-dimensional force system (x, y, z). The person recorded in **C** rests more on the left leg but has less sway than the person in **D** in x and y directions.

condition of neuromuscular control. Consumption of alcohol or certain medicines causes greater swaying. Marksmen, conversely, stand significantly more stable. Most force plates have a rectangular design with four force transducers under the corners. Such construction, however, has the disadvantage of static overdetermination. Because standing is not a pure static equilibrium as a result of accelerations and decelerations of body mass during swaying, the COP does not represent the exact position of the mass center of gravity of the body. Recordings show that the COP is always located in front of the ankle axis at the site of the os navicularis. Therefore, in standing, calf muscles are always active (Fig. 17-3, *A & B*). Figure 17-3, *C & D* presents the location of forces in relation to foot geometry taken from different literature sources (Snijders, 1991).

Standing in shoes in general means standing on uneven ground because a heel of elastic rubber has a certain height for shock absorption and because at the ball of the foot, the sole must be thin to give good flexibility. It is better to look at the inclination of the foot, not at the height of the heel, because the inclination determines the degree to which a person loads the forefoot. With any given heel height, the inclination of the foot depends on the length of the foot. With a certain heel height, the angle of incli-

nation of the smaller foot is greater than that of the larger foot. In practice, however, it is often the smallest women who wear the highest heels. In Figure 17-4, the angle is 40°. Recommended angles are 10 to 14°, which translates to heel heights of 3 to 4 cm maximum.

In Figure 17-5*A*, a chock is placed under a plaster cast around the lower leg and foot. This position of the chock causes discomfort because it is placed in front of the ankle joint and causes a counterclockwise moment, $M = F_v.a$. The foot and cast can be regarded as a single entity, so equilibrium is obtained with a clockwise moment from force F_b exerted by the tibia on the cast. A moment about the ankle joint in the opposite direction occurs when the foot hits the ground with force F at heel strike (Fig. 17-5). The heel of a shoe produces a lever arm with respect to the ankle joint (Fig. 17-5*C*) that is consid-

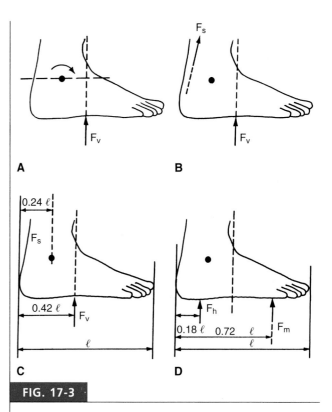

FIG. 17-3

A, The foot-ground reaction force (F_v) is always in front of the ankle axis (*black circle*). **B,** Therefore, the calf muscles (F_s) have to be constantly active. **C,** Mean values of lever arms for calf muscles and foot ground reaction forces in relation to foot length (ℓ). The data is derived from different sources. **D,** Lever arms for resultant forces on the heel (F_h) and the forefoot (F_m) in relation to foot length (ℓ).

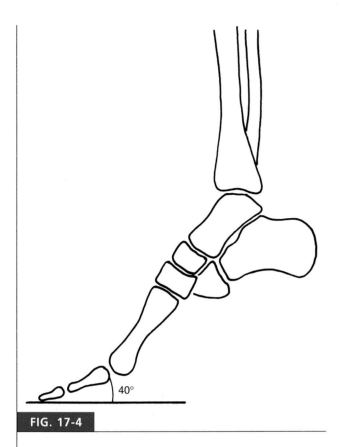

FIG. 17-4

Diagram of a foot in a high-heeled shoe with a "plateau sole." The angle of inclination of the foot is 40°.

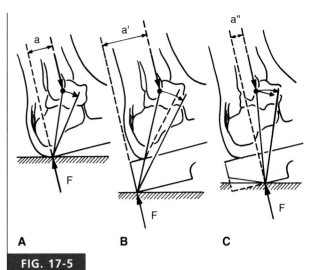

FIG. 17-5

A, Heel strike produces a moment on the foot, which claps on the ground. **B,** A heel on a shoe increases this moment of the foot and the movement of the ankle. **C,** Cutting off the back edge of the heel reduces the downward moment on the foot and produces a more horizontal movement of the ankle. (F = ground reaction force at heel strike; a, a', a" = leverarm force F.)

erably larger than with a bare foot (Fig. 17-5*B*). This moment claps the forefoot down on the ground, which can be reduced by cutting off the back edge of the heel (Fig. 17-5*D*). The latter produces a more horizontal movement of the ankle. This provision is relevant for normal, sport, and orthopaedic shoes.

Excessive mobility or play is characteristic of an unstable joint, as compared with that of the healthy joint. In the following, instability refers to a susceptibility to tilting or falling as a result of interfering forces. In the top view of the foot (Fig. 17-6), one can identify three points where great forces are possible. Hence, both in the lateral and frontal view of the foot, two points of support are found at a distance from one another. In the posterior view, however, only one point of support at the heel exists. In this unstable situation, the heel must get stability from the ball if the ankle fails. A stable positioning of the foot in a shoe means little if the shoe itself is unstable in relation to the ground because of a stiletto heel or a curved sole.

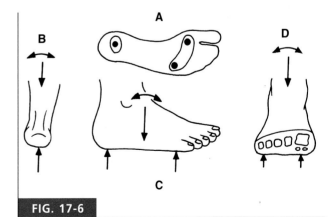

FIG. 17-6

With three points of support in the top view (**A**) both in the lateral (**C**) and the frontal view (**D**) of the foot, two points of support are found at a distance from each other. Such stable situations are not found in the dorsal (**B**) view with only one point of support at the heel.

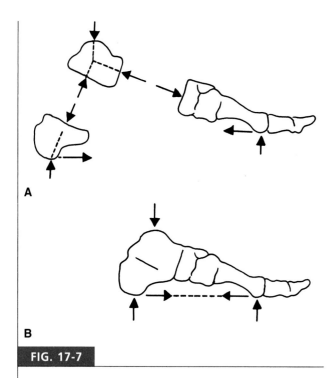

FIG. 17-7

A, The arch of the foot compared with a Roman arch. **B,** Flat joint surfaces in an arch experience compression while shear is avoided.

Free-Body Diagram in Stooped Postures

The mass center of gravity of the total body lies vertically above the feet. Some joint axes are indicated on the skin. Z = center of gravity; F_g = upper body weight force; F_v = body mass reaction force; F_s = back muscle force; F_{rg} = reaction force of the weight force; F_{rs} = reaction force of the back muscle force; a = leverarm of upper body weight; b = leverarm of back muscle force.

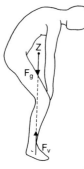

Calculation Box Figure 17-1-1.

Case A. The large ratio between lever arms a and b causes large muscle forces in the lower back. As an approximation, F_g is 500 N in a person with a body height of 180 cm and a body weight of 770 N. With a = 27 cm and b = 5 cm, the back muscle force can be calculated: $F_s = a/b.F_g = 27/5 \times 500 = 2700$ N .

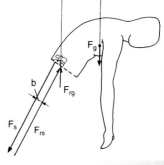

Calculation Box Figure 17-1-2.

Case B. In the next case, the lever arm a is 11 cm, which results in back muscle force $F_s = a/b.F_g = 11/5 \times 500 = 1100$ N. This reduction of 60% of muscular force illustrates that keeping the trunk more upright has dramatic influence on (static) work load, with the lever arm a as the most important factor. Thus, a more upright posture reduces muscle and disc load considerably.

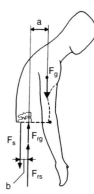

Calculation Box Figure 17-1-3.

Body weight is carried by the arch of the foot, which resembles the form of a Roman arch (Fig. 17-7*A*). The arch mechanism relies on the firm connection between the two ends. In the foot, this function is ascribed to the plantar aponeurosis. Schematic free-body diagrams of parts of the foot (Fig. 17-7*B*) show the interesting feature of an arch: the joint reaction forces in the hind foot are perpendicular to the flat joint surfaces. Thus, shear loading that would tend to dislocate predominantly flat joints is avoided (Snijders et al., 1993).

Stooped postures often occur because of the role of the eyes in combination with the work of the hands. This raises large muscle forces in the lower back as a result of the large ratio of the lever arm (a) of upper body weight (F_g) and the lever arm (b) of back muscle force (F_s). A cross-section at the level of L5–S1 shows that the mass center of gravity of the body part above this cross-section is situated at the armpits (Calculation Box 17-1, Case A). The equilibrium of forces in the vertical direction shows that the weight force (F_g) equals its reaction force in the spine (F_{rg}). It is assumed that this reaction force acts in the middle of the intervertebral disc (the axis of

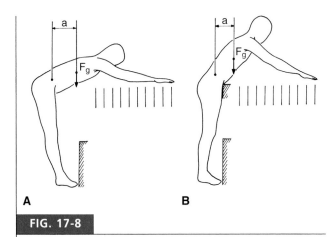

FIG. 17-8

A, An obstacle prevents the feet from advancing any further, leading to a forced posture. **B,** Same reach distance, but a more comfortable position, thanks to suitable support of the pelvis. The lever arm **a** is reduced by 30%, and the arms and eyes are in a better position. (F_g = center of gravity upper body; a = lever arm center of rotation spine to F_g.)

this joint). F_g and F_{rg} form a clockwise moment with $M = F_g.a$. The equilibrium of moments comes from the couple formed by back muscle force F_s and its reaction force F_{rs} on the disc. The total force on the disc is the (vectorial) sum of F_{rs} and F_{rg}. The equilibrium of moments yields: $F_g.a = F_s.b$. So, the total muscle force $Fs = a/b.F_g$.

REACHING

Conditions like those shown in Figure 17-8A occur at work when the person reaches as far as possible to a distant object while the feet cannot be placed any further forward, either because of the design of the machine involved or because the toes touch a tank with liquid. The provision of a support for the pelvis as shown in Figure 17-8B allows for the same reach but with greatly improved posture. This measure reduces the lever arm by approximately 30% and the arms and eyes are in a much more suitable position. In the workplace, people often seek support for the pelvis or upper legs by using the edge of a table or bench.

BIOMECHANICS OF THE PELVIS

With reference to Figure 17-8, the largest forces always act in the longitudinal direction of the spine. The position of the intervertebral discs is optimal because they are perpendicular to the longitudinal orientation of the spine. However, the sacroiliac (SI) joint surfaces are parallel to the largest forces and are not protected against dislocation by the closed form of a ball and socket joint. Thus, the SI joints are vulnerable to shearing because of their predominant flat surfaces, which are almost parallel to the plane of maximal load (Fig. 17-9). In a biomechanical model, Snijders et al. (1993) made the assumption that in addition to strong ligament support, muscle forces are always required for compression of the SI

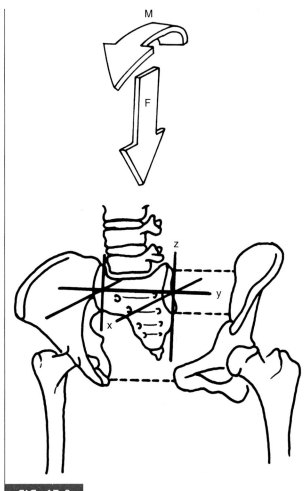

FIG. 17-9.

Schematic drawing illustrating that the sacroiliac joint is vulnerable to shear when loaded in the sagittal plane (moment M/Force F). Integrity of the joint relies on ligament support; joint compression by muscle force can raise friction and prevent shear.

joints to raise friction, which resists shearing. This so-called self-bracing is also expected in sitting with reference to ligament creep by the load of upper body weight.

FLAT VERSUS BALL AND SOCKET JOINT

The different joints in the human body have a wide variety of often highly irregular forms. By comparing a ball and socket joint (or cylindrical joint) with completely flat joint surfaces, some main principles of load transfer can be identified. If a transverse force is applied to the bones in Figure 17-10A, shearing must occur to produce stress in ligaments, which stops the movement. The bones are no longer in line. A ball and socket joint (Fig. 17-10B) is better protected against transverse forces. When a flat joint is loaded with a bending moment (Fig. 17-10C), the joint reaction force can shift to the edge of the joint surface and can produce with ligament or muscle force F_ℓ a couple with moment $M = F_\ell.2r$. When a ball and socket joint is loaded with a moment (Fig. 17-10D), the joint reaction force cannot shift to the edge of the joint surface. Here, F_n and F_ℓ form a couple with moment $M = F_\ell.r$. This shows that a flat joint can transfer a "factor two" larger bending moment than a spherical or cylindrical joint at the hip joints. In Figure 17-10, C & D, the joint reaction force is perpendicular to the tangent to the joint surfaces at the bone contact point. This holds when friction can be neglected. At the spherical hip joint the problem of a lesser moment of force has

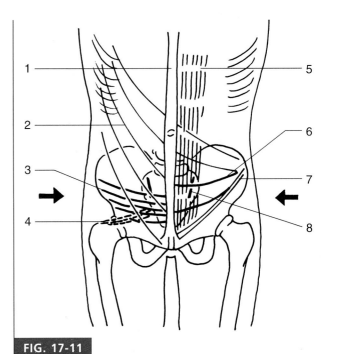

FIG. 17-11

Transversely oriented muscle forces that cross the sacroiliac (SI) joints can press the sacrum in between the hip bones. Such forces caudal to the SI joints may contribute to the mechanism of the pelvic arch by opposing lateral movement of the hip bones. (1) linea alba, (2) external oblique abdominal, (3) transverse abdominal, (4) piriformis, (5) rectus abdominis, (6) internal oblique abdominal, (7) ilioinguinal ligament, and (8) SI joint.

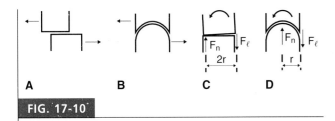

FIG. 17-10

A, Forces near and in the plane of a flat joint result in shearing before this movement is stopped by ligaments. **B,** A ball and socket joint is well protected against shear. **C,** Because of the greater lever arm, a pure bending moment can be better transferred by a flat joint than by a ball and socket joint (**D**) (F_n delineates joint reaction force, F_ℓ is the ligament or muscle force, r represents the lever arms).

been removed by means of the trochanter major, which enlarges the lever arm of muscles considerably. From this comparison, it can be concluded that SI joints are vulnerable to shear but can transfer large bending moments and compression (Snijders et al., 1993).

Muscle forces that cross the SI joint surfaces can produce compression, in combination with forces in ligaments and fascia. This protective system requires the concerted action of muscles in the back, pelvis, and legs. Some muscles with the appropriate transverse direction are indicated in Figure 17-11. SI joint stability can also be ascribed to the mechanism of the pelvic arch, which relies on the protection against lateral movement of the hip bones. Figure 17-12 compares the arch of the foot and the arch of the pelvis. The effect of a pelvic belt distal to the SI joints also can be seen (Snijders et al., 1993). The pelvic arch receives bi-

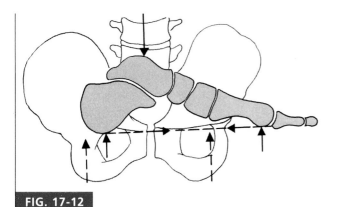

FIG. 17-12

Analogy between the arch of the pelvis and the arch of the foot. This shows analogy between the load on the sacroiliac joint and the load on a tarsal joint. The (horizontal) line of action of a pelvic belt distal to the sacroiliac joints is also seen. *Reprinted with permission from Snijders, C.J., Vleeming, A., & Stoeckart, R. (1993). Transfer of lumbosacral load to iliac bones and legs. Part I: Biomechanics of self-bracing of the sacroiliac joints and its significance for treatment and exercise.* Clin Biomechanics, 8, *285–294.*

lateral support from the hip joints. When one sits on the ischial tuberosities, the supportive forces are below the SI joints and the mechanism of the arch is absent.

Sitting

It is possible to predict whether a chair is comfortable or not, independent of the size of the person. Evaluation of design criteria on the basis of biomechanical aspects demonstrates the poor design of much furniture. Body posture is highly influenced by the form of a chair. A good sitting posture is characterized by minimal muscle effort, which is produced with proper support by arm rests, back rest, seat, and foot rest. Nonetheless, the first law of good seating is the ability to change posture regularly (Case Study 17-1).

ARM RESTS

The importance of arm rests is often underestimated. Arm rests unload the shoulder girdle, which is a loose construction hanging on the spine by means of ligaments and muscles. The weight of the arms is 10% of body weight, which is considerable. In chairs without arm rests, the arms are placed on the table, crossed before the chest, or laid in the lap. In cars, arm rests are often absent or too low. Drivers tend to turn to the side of the door and put their arm on the edge of the window. The other arm rests on the lap or is put on the back rest of the passenger seat. Because of the weight of the arms, the driving wheel is often held at the lower side. A proper arm rest must be placed below the mass centers of upper and lower arm. A support at the wrist is therefore useless. In cockpit seats, arm rests are adjustable in height but only by turning about an axis adjusted to the back rest. This construction is a logical error because in a high position the arm rest only supports the wrist and leaves air below the elbow of the tall pilot.

CASE STUDY 17-1

Postural Problems at VDT Workstations

A female computer operator works at a VDT workstation that includes a corner computer desk fixed at a certain height, an office chair without adjustable features, CPU, monitor, keyboard, and mouse. The VDT operator complains about pain in the right shoulder, wrist, and low back region. The work setup necessitates excessive arm extension that puts an increased load on the shoulder joint and mechanical pressure on the elbow and forearm, affecting underlying soft tissues of the arm. The unsupported sitting posture shown in the figure below creates increased disc pressure, particularly in the lumbar spine.

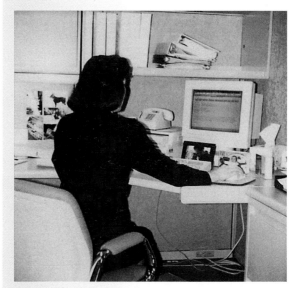

Case Study Figure 17-1-1.

BACK REST

The back rest provides stability for the vertically erected trunk, analogous to Figure 17-8B. However, in prolonged sitting, the prevention of a lumbar kyphosis seems to be the most important function of the back rest. The significance of a lumbar support can be illustrated with the so-called click-clack phenomenon (Fig. 17-13) (Snijders, 1970, On the form of the human thoraco-lumbar spine and some aspects of its mechanical behavior. Thesis, Eindhover). This can be experienced when one sits upright on the edge of a straight chair. Slow forward translation of the trunk increases lumbar lordosis, whereas slow backward translation moves the center of gravity above the ischial tuberosities into an unstable posi-

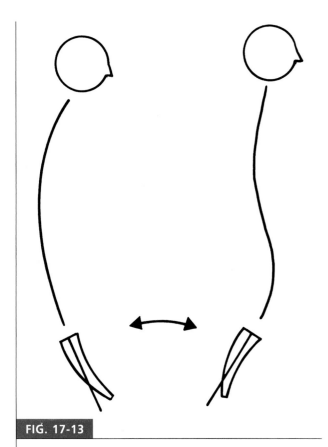

FIG. 17-13

The lumbopelvic click-clack phenomenon. Lumbar lordosis is the result of a mass center of gravity of the trunk at the ventral side of the ischial tuberosities (*right*). The mass center of gravity of the trunk dorsal to the ischial tuberosities forces the lumbar spine into kyphosis (*left*). The latter can be prevented by the exertion of lumbar support on the upper side of the pelvis and the lumbar spine.

tion. Further translation results in backward tilt of the pelvis and lumbar kyphosis. The reader can easily perform this test. The function of a lumbar support is to exert a firm force on the upper side of the pelvis and the lumbar area to prevent tilting of the spine into kyphosis. This support should not reach higher than the lower edge of the scapulae. The thoracic spine is stiff enough (ribs) and a higher back rest pushes the shoulder blades forward, which "overrules" the lumbar support and hinders the shoulders to stretch and to turn to the left and the right. The absence of a back rest, like sitting on a crutch, always leads to a C-form of the spine.

SEAT

The weight of the trunk, head, and (part of) the arms is almost completely carried by the ischial tuberosities. This leads to a simple representation of the static equilibrium of the upper body in sitting. The aim of Figure 17-14 is to illustrate that a horizontal seat always raises friction at the ischial tuberosities, that friction can be completely eliminated by means of a moderate seat angle, and that the angle between seat and back rest is optimal between 90 and 95°, which is met by the classical rocking chair (Snijders, 1988). In Figure 17-14B, a free-body diagram of the trunk is given, with a cross-section at the upper legs and support forces at the seat and the back rest. The mass center of gravity of this part of the body is near the armpits. The line of action of the gravitational force (F_g) and the back rest (F_b) intersects at point S. The resultant force exerted by the seat on the ischial tuberosities (F_t) must also intersect at point S for static equilibrium. The magnitude of the three forces is found by the composition of the triangle of forces. It can be concluded from the direction of F_t that a back rest force always raises a horizontal force component (F_h) at the ischial tuberosities. The consequence is friction on the skin and underlying tissues that causes discomfort.

From Figure 17-14C, it can be seen that with a slightly inclined seat surface at the ischial tuberosities, the resultant seat force (F_t) stands nearly perpendicular to the surface. There is a reduced force component in the shear direction. When the back rest is tilted further, the seat angle must follow because F_t becomes more inclined. In Figure 17-15, the relation between back rest angle and seat angle is given for the condition that friction is absent (Goossens & Snijders, 1995). This relation was found with a biomechanical model of

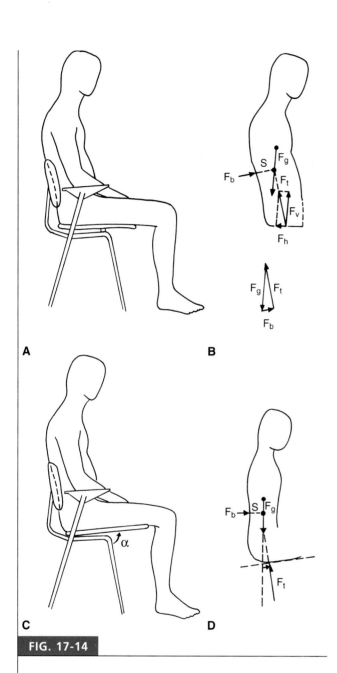

FIG. 17-14

A, Sitting with maximal support. **B,** Free-body diagram of the trunk. Back rest force (F_b) and upper body weight force (F_g) intersect in the point S. The resultant seat force at the ischial tuberosities (F_t) must intersect in S as well, and therefore inclines backward. The horizontal component (F_h) must come from friction acting on skin and underlying tissues. **C–D,** By tilting the seat slightly backwards (α), the resultant seat force (F_t) becomes nearly perpendicular to the seat surface and friction on the ischial tuberosities is significantly reduced.

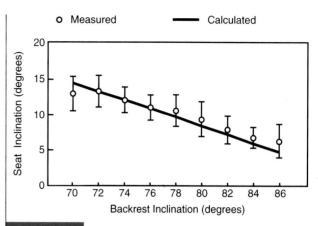

FIG. 17-15

Relation between back rest angle and seat angle. No friction exists at the ischial tuberosities. The *solid line* is from a model calculation. The *vertical bars* represent measurements (n = 10), including tall and small persons.

the total body divided in five links and was verified by measurements on 10 healthy subjects with different body height. Back rest inclination is larger in auditoriums, cars, and easy chairs at home. This facilitates a horizontal direction of looking and has the advantage that the back rest contributes in carrying the trunk. Head rests cannot carry the head when they are positioned too far forward. Figure 17-16A illustrates that the head rest can only give

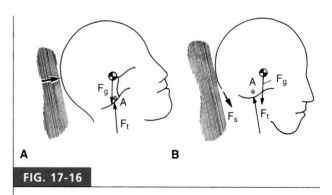

FIG. 17-16

A, The mass center of gravity (represented by a circle and gravitational force F_g) is behind the atlanto-occipital joint axis A (F_t represents the joint reaction force). With support of a head rest, no muscle forces are needed for equilibrium of the head ($F_g = F_t$). **B,** The head rest is positioned too far forward and is useless. Muscle force F_s remains needed for equilibrium and F_t increases.

support when the mass center of gravity of the head is dorsal to the axis of the atlanto-occipital joint (A). In Figure 17-16B, the head rest hinders movement because the head cannot be tilted backward. This design error can be recognized in trains and buses in which people nod or rest with the head sideways.

CHAIR AND TABLE

A chair is important for a good posture, but when tasks such as reading and writing are involved, the height and inclination of the desk or table play a dominating role. Despite good chairs, postures with the back bent, sagging, or twisted can be observed. Problems arise when such extreme postures are maintained for long periods of time. In the relaxed posture according to Figure 17-17A the direction of vision with the head upright is given (dotted line). However, reading with the trunk upright requires a sharp bend in the cervical spine, which cannot be sustained for a long time. Furthermore, in this position the reading distance is larger than 25 to 35 cm (the height of the table must coincide with approximately the level of the elbows). Consequently, children and adults always bend forward with a curved spine over the table (Fig. 17-17B) and urgings to sit up straight are useless.

In the past, inclined desks were common. The fixed angle was approximately 12° because at a higher angle, paper will slip downward on paper be-

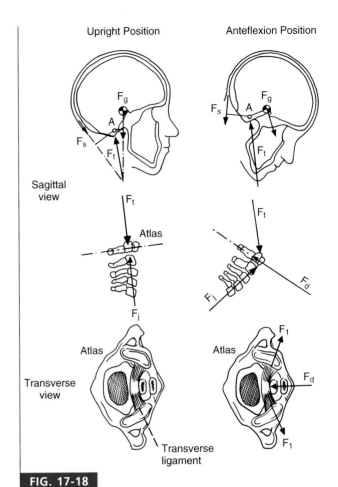

FIG. 17-18

Anteflexion of the head leads to a larger lever arm of the weight force (F_g) with respect to the atlanto-occipital joint axis (A) than in the upright position. For equilibrium, greater neck muscle forces (F_s) are needed. Forward inclination also raises tension in the ligamentum transversum atlantis (F_1) to transmit the force from the dens (F_d), which is directed transversely to the cervical spine. This force follows from the equilibrium of the atlas, with joint reaction forces F_t and F_j.

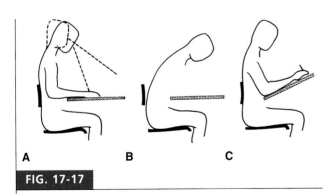

FIG. 17-17

A, Reading while sitting upright demands, forced by the eyes, a bend in the cervical spine. Moreover, the reading distance is too large. **B,** Therefore, the back is bent. **C,** A proper height and a small inclination of the desk (up to 12°) brings the page to the eyes, instead of the reverse.

neath it (Snijders et al., 1990). A steeper angle also is inappropriate for arm support. Anteflexion of the head leads to increased neck muscle force with almost a factor of three. Furthermore, ligaments such as the ligamentum transversum atlantis (Fig. 17-18) are loaded considerably in anteflexion, while this load is almost absent in the upright position (Snijders et al.,1991).

In a forward-bent position of the trunk and head, considerable muscle forces are needed. A pro-

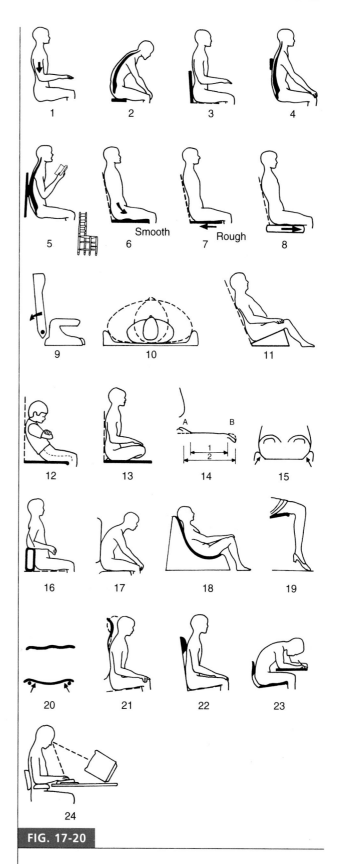

FIG. 17-19

The vicious circle of pain.

longed, continuous contraction (above approximately 20% of voluntary maximal contraction) causes a lack of oxygen, accumulation of sour metabolites, and intracellular shortage of potassium. Pain is the result, which can lead to muscle spasm, which closes a vicious circle (Fig. 17-19). Prolonged isometric contractions can even cause an inflammation process with fibrosing; the result is a passive shortening of the respective muscle. Entering this vicious circle is also ascribed to cold and stress. Attempts to cut this circle are analgesia, muscle relaxation, and improvement of circulation by massage and heat radiation. These efforts involve the treatment of symptoms, while the improvement of the work posture addresses the origin of the muscle spasm. Some biomechanical problems in sitting are illustrated in Figure 17-20.

1. The absence of an arm rest loads the loose shoulder girdle, which hangs from the spine with ligaments and muscles.
2. Sitting without a back rest always leads to a C-form of the spine.
3. A back rest must leave space for the buttocks. With a straight back rest starting from the seat, no proper support can be given to the upper side of the pelvis and the lumbar spine. A support that is too high does not provide force on the lumbar area and a C-form of the spine is the result.
4. If the back rest is too high (as it is in some folding chairs), it gives no support to the lumbar area and the back bends in a C-form.

FIG. 17-20

Examples of poor chair design leading to poor posture.

5. A vertical, straight, and high back rest also promotes lumbar kyphosis.

6. On a horizontal slippery seat, the bottom slides forward and the body sags in the chair because the friction force (F_b in Fig. 17-14A) is absent.

7. On a rough horizontal seat, the friction force (F_b in Fig. 17-14B) causes discomfort; people avoid back support and adopt a posture as in Fig. 17-17B.

8. When sitting on a horizontal cushion like on a lounge chair, the cushion is moved by the horizontal force component at the ischial tuberosities (reaction force of F_b in Fig. 17-14B) and moves into the room.

9. Further tilting of the back rest must be coupled to the same increase of seat inclination. In airplanes, however, seats remain almost horizontal.

10. Broad persons are jammed by lateral supports. In common cars, such pronounced lateral supports are useless because curves are not taken with more than 30 m/s² (0.3 g centripetal acceleration). A back rest with a uniform moderate curvature fits everybody and provides sufficient lateral support.

11. Elderly people do not appreciate a low or deep sinking seat.

12. The length of the seat in a chair for adults is too large for children.

13. The lengths of seats in easy chairs or lounge chairs are often too large for adults.

14. Although the length of this seat (2) seems to be sufficient, the effective seat length (1) is far too small because of a useless elevation at the dorsal side and a too large radius at the foreside. A radius of approximately 30 to 50 mm is sufficient.

15. Pronounced lateral supports on seats have no use, also common in cars. Broad people experience painful jamming on the thighs.

16. A back support that is too low cannot give stability to the trunk (analogous to Fig. 17-8B).

17. Arm rests are even more important in easy chairs than in straight chairs because the arms cannot rest on a table.

18. Easy chairs exist with a pronounced C-form.

19. A seat that is too high causes pressure on the thighs, which promotes "sleeping legs."

20. Seats must be straight in the anteroposterior direction. The curvature in the lateral direction should remain moderate. Forms

molded to the individual anatomy should be restricted to the severely handicapped.

21. A head rest that is placed too far forward hinders upright sitting.

22. Tall people experience hindrance from a head rest that pushes against the shoulder (analogous to 5).

23. When reading and writing at a horizontal desk, adults and children always show flexion of the thoracolumbar spine. This forward bending is independent of the chair.

24. Neck and shoulder complaints are reported with visual display units. When it is not necessary to look at the keyboard all the time, the optimal height of the screen is approximately at eye level (Snijders et al., 1991; Wall et al., 1992).

LEG-CROSSING

The majority of people cross their legs often when sitting, alternating left over right and right over left (Fig. 17-21). There may be many reasons to do this, but in the literature there is no scientific proof about the benefit or demerit of leg-crossing. One ex-

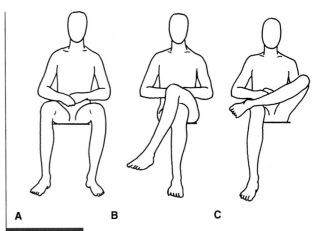

FIG. 17-21

Even in sitting with the support of back rest and arm rests, the internal oblique abdominal muscles are significantly more active as compared with when supine. Crossing the legs (upper legs crossed or ankle on knee) lowers this activity. Therefore, leg-crossing is assumed to be functional and should be allowed for in work places (except car seats and cockpit seats).

ception is the observation that leg-crossing (upper legs crossed or ankle on knee) may result in less activity of the internal oblique abdominal muscles that have the same orientation as the transverse abdominal muscles (Fig. 17-11) (Snijders et al., 1995). By crossing the legs, an alternative and less fatiguing means is found for self-bracing of the SI joints.

Lying

A bed is a body support surface on which prolonged and complete rest must be found. It is a combination of a mattress, a mattress carrier, and a bed frame or bedstead. However, in many countries it is customary to sleep on a spread-out mat on the floor. Three types of mattresses can be distinguished: polyether, foam rubber, and internally sprung. There are several kinds of mattress carriers, like the wire-spiral mat, the hardboard bottom, lathes that can tilt, the box spring, and a carrier simply made of planks with distances of approximately 7 cm. Many combinations of mattress and mattress carrier are possible, but not every combination is appropriate. A good bed should (1) adapt to body curvatures, (2) remain flat, (3) have a pleasant spring action, (4) have good ventilation, and (5) not be too warm or too cold. Aspects 1 to 3 concern body support that evenly spreads the pressure on protruding (bony) parts, gives a straight spine when lying on the side, and gives a natural S-shape to the spine in the supine posture. Lying on a horizontal surface is special because each body part receives separate support with minimal pressure on skin, and underlying tissues and joints can be kept in a relaxed position. The result must be that for static equilibrium, muscle action is superfluous.

For separate support of the head, a pillow is needed. The thickness of the pillow is related to the curvature of the spine: the more curved (especially in older people), the thicker the pillow (Fig. 17-22). If the pillow is too thin, the head must be tilted backward. A pillow that is too thick is inconvenient because it causes a bend in the cervical spine. This bend can also occur when the pillow is hard, with the shape of a coconut resulting in a concentrated force on the head at the side of the crown. Pillows must be pliable to also support the neck.

A bed that is too hard results in restless change of posture to unload areas with disturbed blood flow. Normally, people change posture 20 times per night. One can imagine that large pressure occurs with thin people. But this may also hold for heavy people because with an increase of volume, the weight increases with the third power (m³) but the support surface only with the second power of length (m²).

The most unconstrained form of the lumbar spine is found when the angle between the trunk and femur is 135° (Keegan, 1953). Furthermore, the muscle running from the lumbar spine to the femur (m. psoas major, part of the m. iliopsoas) can be shortened, which raises tension in this muscle and causes a hollow back in supine posture. This can be improved by exorotation of the legs and, if this is insufficient, by lying on the side. When lying on the side, the spine should not bend laterally, resembling the scoliotic form. This occurs in persons with pronounced waists and little give of the mattress in the

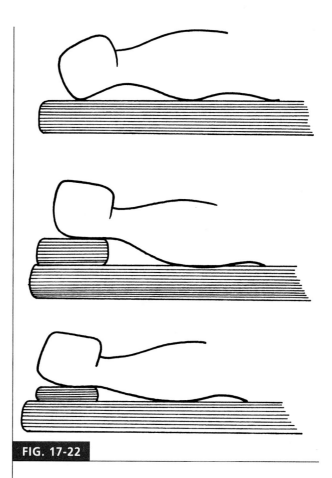

FIG. 17-22

Pillows must be pliable to also support the neck. The thickness of the pillow is related to the curvature of the spine because hyperextension or a sharp bend of the cervical spine should be avoided.

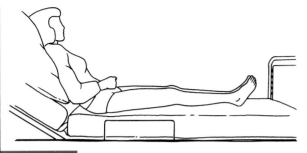

FIG. 17-23

Sitting in bed results in shear on the coccyx (here, approximately 100 N). This is analogous to the horizontal seat of Figure 17-14.

region of the shoulder and the hip. Therefore, the criterion of conformity has been introduced. This is the sinking of two square plates of 20 × 20 cm at a distance of 60 cm, each loaded with 20 kg (a shoulder and a hip), measured in relation to a point on the mattress in the middle between the plates. The greater the depth to which the plates sink, the greater the conformity. In a comparative study, a level difference of more than 3.5 cm was judged as good, a difference of 2.5 to 3.5 cm as reasonable, and of less than 2.5 cm as moderate (Het Bed, 1979).

SITTING IN BED

Sitting in bed is common, especially in hospitals in which the head portion can be raised upward. With a horizontal mattress, the same biomechanical model holds as in Figure 17-14. Sitting in bed on a horizontal mattress (Fig. 17-23) gives rise to shear forces (in the order of magnitude of 100 N) on the skin and underlying tissues of the bottom. As a consequence, the pelvis moves little by little on the mattress, the night dress creeps upward, and the underwear pulls tight in the crotch (Snijders, 1988). Taller people have the advantage that they can come to a stop with the feet against the board at the foot end. Figure 17-23 shows that lumbar support is absent, which causes lumbar kyphosis and the pelvis to rest on the os coccyx instead of on the ischial tuberosities. The combination of pressure and shear is a provocation of decubitus skin ulcerations (Case Study 17-2).

Decubitus Skin Ulcerations

A 90-year-old man, with a pelvic fracture and cognitive limitations. In his second week of hospitalization, the patient is spending 100% of his time in bed. Prolonged pressure and shear stresses in the skin linearly affect the oxygen saturation of the tissue and thus the nutrition of it. In association with the natural aging of the collagen tissue and the slower metabolism associated with advanced age, the inactivity increases the likelihood of developing a decubitus ulcer.

DECUBITUS

It is assumed that prolonged pressure (without shear) of 35 to 40 mm Hg (4.6–5.3 kPa) can be tolerated. Shear decreases the tolerable pressure considerably (Fig. 17-24). Oxygen saturation was measured without (upper curve) and with (lower curve) a shear stress of 3.1 kPa (Goossens, Zegers, Hoek van Dijke, & Snijders, 1994). This diagram shows a dramatic decrease of saturation in the case of additional shear force. Therefore, sitting in bed is a provocation of decubitus skin ulcerations, which can be solved by tilting the mattress in ac-

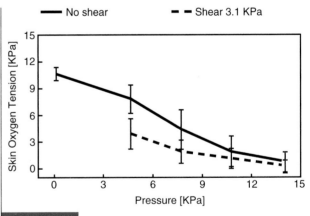

FIG. 17-24

Oxygen saturation in subcutaneous tissue under pressure (*upper curve*) decreases dramatically by adding 3.1 kPa shear stress (*lower curve*). *Reprinted with permission from Goossens, R.H.M., Zegers, R., Hoek van Dijke, G.A., et al. (1994). Influence of shear on skin oxygen tension. J Clin Physiol, 14, 111–118.*

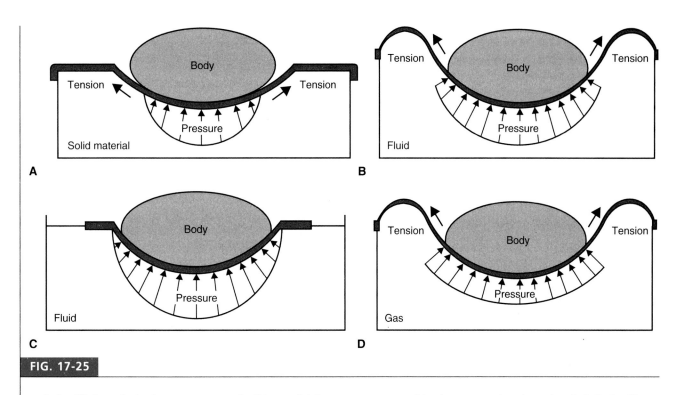

FIG. 17-25

A, Equilibrium of a body on a mattress of solid material. Restricted support surface. **B,** Fluid mattress with an elastic envelope. The highest pressure is at the deepest point. **C,** Fluid mattress with a loose cover; less shear than in **B. D,** Equilibrium of the body on gas. A favorable, uniform pressure distribution over almost the maximal available supporting surface.

cordance with Figure 17-14*C*. This folding principle is now applied in hospital beds and in beds for home care.

The medium for antidecubitus mattresses can be divided in four groups: solid material, fluid, gas, and a combination of these media. Solid materials are foam, sheepskin, woolen blankets, etc. Deep impression of the material results in a larger force (Fig. 17-25*A*). The ideal material should have a horizontal (isotonic) and adjustable spring characteristic. For fluid, a good envelope is needed (Fig. 17-25*B*). Tensile forces in this envelope contribute to body support, but raise shear stresses. The supported surface is large but still the largest stresses are at the deepest point. Gas allows for the application of equal pressure along a large surface (Fig. 17-25*D*). Chambers are necessary to follow the contour of the body. Combinations of the foregoing are the "air-fluidized" beds, hammocks, etc. For home situations, gas support is preferred, with an adjustable spring characteristic to accommodate body weight. In all cases, the largest body surface is involved in support when the body sinks deep in the mattress (Holscher et al., 1994).

Summary

1 Any deviation from the anatomical posture generates increased tension in soft tissue and increased loading on the skeletal structures.

2 The design of human tools should include knowledge of biomechanics and its effect on humans.

3 Use and adaptation of supports, including arm rests, back rests, and adjustable desks or beds, will help to decrease the load on musculoskeletal structures.

4 The most important factor to reducing load on the lumbar spine during lifting is to keep the load close to the body. For engineering purposes, the goal is to reduce the lever arm of the object.

REFERENCES

Goossens, R.H.M. & Snijders, C.J. (1995). Design criteria for the reduction of shear forces in beds and seats. *J Biomechanics*, 28(2),225–230.

Goossens, R.H.M., Zegers, R., Hoek van Dijke, G.A., et al. (1994). Influence of shear on skin oxygen tension. *J Clin Physiol*, 14, 111–118.

Het Bed. *Instituut voor Huishoudtechnisch Advies (IVHA) van de Nederlandse Vereniging van Huisvrouwen. Testreport* (in Dutch). Gravenhage: 1979.

Holscher, T.G., Goossens, R.H.M., Snijders, C.J., et al. (1994). A new low-cost anti-decubitus mattress for home care: Requirements and development. *J Rehab Sci*, 7(2),53–58.

Janda, V. (1980). *Muskelfunktionsdiagnostik. Verlag für Medizin Dr. Ewald Fischer*. Leuven, Acco Verlag; Heidelberg.

Keegan, J. (1953). Alterations of the lumbar curve related to posture and seating. *J Bone Joint Surgery, 35*, 589–603.

Moll van Charante, A.W., Snijders, C.J., & Mulder, P.G.H. (1991). Posture control and the risk of industrial accident: A stabilographic investigation in a naval shipyard. *Ann Occup Hygiene, 35*(5),505–515.

Snijders, C.J. (1988). Biomechanical analysis of seated posture. *ICAART 88: International Conference of the Association for the Advancement of Rehabilitation Technology.* Montreal, 472–473.

Snijders, C.J. (1991). Biomechanics of foot gear, hallux valgus and splay foot. In M.H. Jahss (Ed), *The Foot and its Disorders* (2nd ed.). Philadelphia: W.B. Saunders.

Snijders, C.J., Aghina, J.C.F.M., Riel, M.P.J.M., et al. (1990). Reading and inclined surfaces. *Lancet, 335*(8692), 802.

Snijders, C.J., Hoek van Dijke, G.A., & Roosch, E.R. (1991). A biomechanical model for the analysis of the cervical spine in static postures. *J Biomechanics, 24*(9),783–792.

Snijders, C.J., Slagter, A.H.E., Strik, R., et al. (1995). Why leg-crossing? The influence of common postures on abdominal muscle activity. *Spine, 20*(18),1989–1993.

Snijders, C.J. & Verduin, M. (1973). Stabilograph, an accurate instrument for sciences interested in postural equilibrium. *Agressologie, 14C*, 1520.

Snijders, C.J., Vleeming, A., & Stoeckart, R. (1993). Transfer of lumbosacral load to iliac bones and legs. Part I: Biomechanics of self-bracing of the sacroiliac joints and its significance for treatment and exercise. *Clin Biomechanics, 8*, 285–294.

Wall, M., de Riel, M.P.J.M., van Aghina, J.C.F.M., et al. (1992). Improving the sitting posture of CAD/CAM workers by increasing VDU monitor working height. *Ergonomics, 35*(4), 427–436.

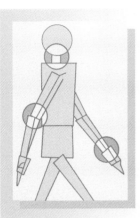

CHAPTER 18

Biomechanics of Gait

Ann E. Barr, Sherry I. Backus

Introduction

Bipedal locomotion, or gait, is a functional task requiring complex interactions and coordination among most of the major joints of the body, particularly of the lower extremity. This fundamental task has been the subject of study by scientists for several centuries, both with respect to description of typical body movements and of pathological conditions and therapeutic interventions. Gait analysis and training in one form or another is a staple of physical therapy and rehabilitation medicine practice. As technological advances become both more sophisticated and affordable, detailed biomechanical analyses of gait increasingly can be performed in a clinical setting. This means that the biomechanics of gait need to be more broadly understood by both clinicians and researchers. In the paragraphs that follow, the anatomical characteristics of the major joints of the lower limb and trunk will be summarized and their behavior during level walking in healthy adults will be described. More detailed anatomy of the relevant joints and tissues can be found in other chapters of this book.

Anatomical Considerations

HIP

During gait, motion about the coxofemoral, or hip, joint is triaxial: flexion-extension occurs about a mediolateral axis; adduction-abduction occurs about an anteroposterior axis; and internal-external rotation occurs about a longitudinal axis. Although flexion-extension movements are of the highest amplitude, motions in the other two planes are substantial and consistent both within and between individuals. In addition, impairments in all three movement planes can cause problematic deviations of the typical gait pattern at the hip and other joints.

KNEE

In the case of the knee, three degrees of freedom of angular rotation are also possible during gait. The primary motion is knee flexion-extension about a mediolateral axis. Knee internal-external rotation and adduction-abduction (varus-valgus) may also occur, but with less consistency and amplitude among healthy individuals owing to soft tissue and bony constraints to these motions.

ANKLE AND FOOT

Ankle motion is restricted by the morphological constraints of the talocrural joint, which permits only plantarflexion (extension) and dorsiflexion (flexion). Although frequently modeled in gait analysis as a rigid segment, the foot is required to act as both a semirigid structure (as a spring during weight transfer and a lever arm during push-off) and a rigid structure that permits adequate stability to support body weight.

The movements of the ankle, subtalar, tarsal, metatarsal, and phalangeal joints contribute to the smooth progression of the body's center of mass through space. There are constant adjustments in these joints in response to the characteristics of the supporting terrain and to the actions of the muscles that cross them, which provides a smooth interaction between the body and the wide variety of supporting surfaces encountered when walking. The loss of normal motion or muscular function at these joints has a direct effect not only on the foot and ankle but also on the remainder of the joints of the lower extremity.

UPPER BODY

The pelvis and thorax may be considered separately or, as in many studies in the literature, as a rigid unit comprised of the head, arms, and trunk (pelvis + thorax), or HAT, segment. The upper limbs and head have not received as much attention as the trunk and lower limbs in the literature. Studies that do exist indicate that shoulder motions occur primarily as flexion-extension and internal-external rotation at the glenohumeral joints. Elbow flexion-extension and forearm pronation-supination occur. Cervical spine motion is primarily in flexion-extension and rotation to stabilize visual gaze or facilitate the vestibulo-ocular reflex as the body is propelled through the environment.

Methods of Gait Analysis

The information presented in this chapter is summarized from the scientific and clinical literature in which various laboratory methods have been used to measure gait characteristics, including stride analysis, angular kinematic analysis, force plate and foot pressure analysis, and electromyographic (EMG) analysis. In stride analysis, the temporal sequence of stance and swing are quantified using either simple tools, such as a stopwatch and ink and paper, or electromechanical instruments, such as pressure-sensitive switches imbedded in shoe inserts or applied to the bottom of the foot. Stride analysis data are used to calculate basic time-distance variables, which will be described in detail.

Angular kinematic analysis uses electrogoniometry, accelerometry, and optoelectronic techniques. Electrogoniometers are available in uniaxial and multiaxial configurations and are attached directly to the body segments on either side of the joint or joints of interest for the direct measurement of angular displacement. Accelerometers are attached to the body segments of interest for the direct measurement of segmental acceleration from which segmental velocities and displacements are then derived. Optoelectronic techniques involve the use of video cameras to capture images of an individual walking. Such systems usually include the use of reference markers, which are attached to the subject, to estimate the location of joint axes and to assist in digitization. Such camera systems require careful calibration to locate anatomical markers and are often permanently installed in a "gait laboratory." Force plate and foot pressure analysis techniques involve the recording of information at the foot-floor interface during the stance phase of gait. Force plates measure the resultant ground reaction force beneath the foot and the location of its point of application in the plane of the supporting surface. Pressure plates or insoles measure the load distribution beneath the foot during stance. Force and pressure plates are often combined with angular kinematic methods for the calculation of kinetic variables, such as joint moments.

EMG is used to record muscle activation during walking. Both surface and intramuscular sensing techniques are used in gait analysis. EMG is typically combined with stride or angular kinematic analysis to provide information about phasic muscle activation patterns. EMG helps to explain the motor performance underlying the kinematic and kinetic characteristics of gait.

Gait Cycle

Bipedal locomotion is a cyclic activity consisting of two phases for each limb, stance and swing. Gait is more or less symmetrical with regard to angular motions of the major joints, muscle activation pat-

terns, and load bearing of the lower extremities and, as a result, is efficient in translating the body's center of mass in the overall direction of locomotion. A full gait cycle is defined by the occurrence of a sequential stance phase and swing phase by one limb, or a stride (Figs. 18-1 and 18-2). The limits of a stride can be demarcated by the occurrence of a specific gait event (e.g., initial contact) on one limb to the next occurrence of that same event on the ipsilateral limb.

Stance phase occupies 60% of the stride and consists of two periods of double limb support (initial and terminal), when the contralateral foot is in contact with the ground, and an intermediate period of single limb support, when the contralateral limb is engaged in swing phase. Stance can be decomposed into six events or periods. Initial contact or heel contact is defined as the instant the foot makes contact with the floor. Loading response is an interval during which the sole of the foot comes into con-

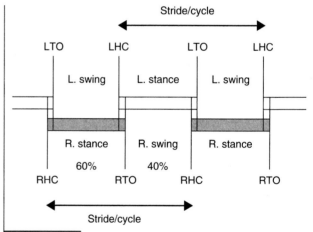

FIG. 18-1

Schematic diagram of the temporal sequence of the gait cycle or stride showing complete right (*shaded bars*) and left strides. *HC,* heel/initial contact; *TO,* toe off, *R,* right; *L,* left. The areas of overlap between HC and TO represent periods of double limb support, which coincide with the occurrence of pre-swing on the trailing limb and loading response on the leading limb. In the case of the right stride, initial double limb support (lasting ~10% of the stride) occurs from RHC to LTO, and terminal double limb support (lasting ~10% of the stride) occurs from LHC to RTO. *Reprinted with permission from Barr, A.E. (1998). Gait analysis. In J. Spivak & J. Zuckerman (Eds.),* Orthopaedics—A Comprehensive Study Guide. *New York: McGraw-Hill.*

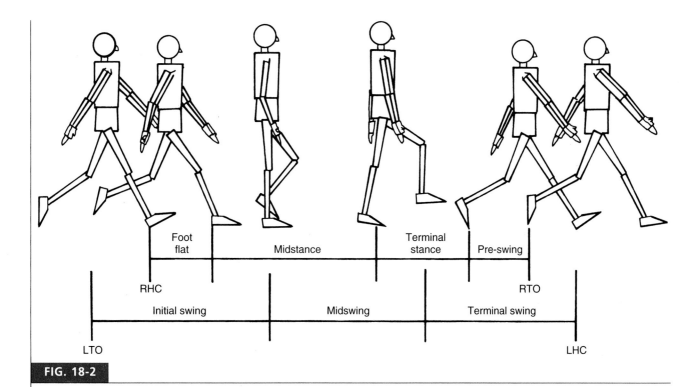

FIG. 18-2

Schematic diagram of the spatial sequence of the gait cycle or stride showing stance phase on the right and swing phase on the left. *HC,* heel/initial contact; *TO,* toe off, *R,* right; *L,* left. Stance phase is demarcated by two events, HC and TO, and broken into four periods, loading response (foot flat) (from ~0 to 10% of the stride), midstance (from ~10 to 30% of the stride), terminal stance (from ~30 to 50% of the stride), and pre-swing (from ~50 to 60 % of the stride).

Swing phase is demarcated by two events, TO and HC, and broken into three periods, initial swing (from ~60 to 70% of the stride), mid-swing (from ~70 to 85% of the stride), and terminal swing (from ~85 to 100% of the stride). *Reprinted with permission from Barr, A.E. (1998). Gait analysis. In J. Spivak & J. Zuckerman (Eds.),* Orthopaedics—A Comprehensive Study Guide. *New York: McGraw-Hill.*

tact with the floor and the weight of the body is accepted onto the supporting limb. The loading response period coincides with the end of initial double limb support at approximately 10 to 12% of the stride. Midstance is the period during which the tibia rotates over the stationary foot in the direction of locomotion. The beginning of midstance coincides with single limb support and lasts from approximately 10 to 30% of the stride. Terminal stance is the period during which the weight of the body is transferred from the hind and midfoot regions onto the forefoot. It occurs from 30 to 50% of the stride and coincides with the beginning of terminal double limb support. Pre-swing occurs simultaneously with terminal double limb support and lasts from approximately 50 to 60% of the

stride. During pre-swing, weight is transferred onto the contralateral limb in preparation for swing phase. The end of pre-swing corresponds to toe off at which moment the foot breaks contact with the floor, thereby demarcating the beginning of swing phase.

Swing phase occupies 40% of the gait cycle and is decomposed into three periods. Initial swing lasts from approximately 60 to 73% of the stride (approximately one third of swing phase), from toe off until the swinging foot is opposite the stance foot. Mid-swing ends when the tibia of the swinging limb is vertically oriented and lasts from 73 to 87% of the stride. Terminal swing lasts from 87 to 100% of the stride and ends at the moment of initial contact.

TABLE 18-1	
Ranges of Normal Values for Time-Distance Parameters of Adult Gait at Free Walking Velocity	
Stride or cycle time	1.0 to 1.2 m/sec[a]
Stride or cycle length	1.2 to 1.9 m[b]
Step length	0.56 to 1.1 m[a]
Step width	7.7 to 9.6 cm[a]
Cadence	90 to 140 steps/minute[b]
Velocity	0.9 to 1.8 m/sec[b]

Reprinted with permission from Barr, A.E. (1998). Gait analysis. In J. Spivak & J. Zuckerman, (eds.), Orthopedics: A Comprehensive Study Guide. New York: McGraw-Hill.

[a]*Values adapted from multiple sources as summarized in Craik, R.L. & Oatis, C.A. (1995). Gait Analysis: Theory and Application. St. Louis: Mosby.*

[b]*Values adapted from Whittle, M.W. (1991). Gait Analysis: An Introduction. Oxford: Butterworth-Heinemann.*

Time-Distance Variables

Time-distance variables are derived from the temporal and spatial occurrence of the stance and swing phases. Normal values of these quantities are provided in Table 18-1.

Stride time refers to the time it takes to perform a single stride. Stride length refers to the distance covered by a stride in the direction of locomotion. Step is defined as the occurrence of an event on one foot until the next occurrence of that same event on the opposite foot. It is most commonly delineated by sequential contralateral initial contact. Laterality is determined by the swinging limb; for example, right step is delineated by left initial contact to the subsequent right initial contact. Step length refers to the distance covered by a step in the direction of locomotion. Step width refers to the distance covered by a step perpendicular to the direction of locomotion as measured from the points of contact on

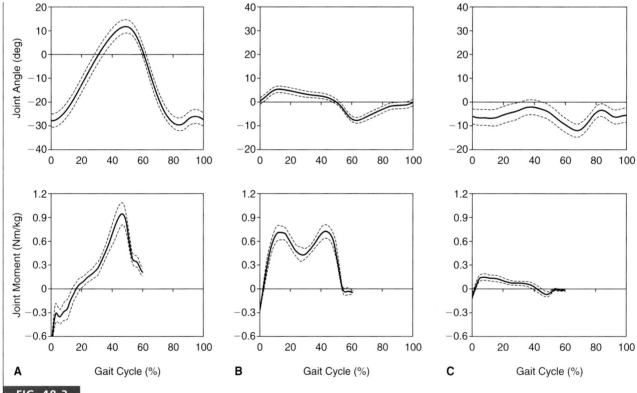

A Gait Cycle (%) **B** Gait Cycle (%) **C** Gait Cycle (%)

FIG. 18-3

Angular displacements and moments of the hip during level walking at freely chosen velocity among normal subjects (25 males, 4 females; 15 to 35 years of age). *Solid lines* indicate mean values (ordinate) over the course of a single stride (abscissa). *Dashed lines* indicate 90% bootstrap confidence intervals. **A** (*top*), Hip flexion (<0) and extension (>0) position; **A** (*bottom*), Hip extensor (<0) and flexor (>0) moment; **B** (*top*), Hip abduction (<0) and adduction (>0) position; **B** (*bottom*), Hip adductor (<0) and abductor (>0) moment; **C** (*top*), Hip external rotation (<0) and internal rotation (>0) position; **C** (*bottom*), Hip internal rotator (<0) and external rotator (>0) moment.

the heels. Two sequential steps comprise a stride. Although step variables may differ from right to left within an individual, stride variables will remain constant regardless of whether stride is delineated by right or left initial contacts, because stride consists of the sums of right and left steps.

Cadence is a measure of step frequency that is defined as the number of steps taken per unit time and is usually expressed in steps per minute. Velocity is defined as the distance covered in the direction of locomotion per unit time and is usually expressed in meters per second.

Angular Kinematics

This discussion will focus on joint angular displacements about the motion axes of the major lower limb and axial segments during level walking. Figures 18-3 through 18-7 show examples of angular displacements at these motion segments over the course of the stride in a healthy adult population (Calculation Box 18-1).

HIP

At initial contact, the hip is flexed approximately 30° (Fig. 18-3A, top). Throughout terminal stance phase, the hip extends until it reaches approximately 10° of extension. During pre-swing and throughout the majority of swing phase, the hip flexes to approximately 35°, and then begins to extend just prior to the next initial contact as the lower limb is extended for placement of the foot on the ground.

The hip is neutral with respect to adduction-abduction at initial contact (Fig. 18-3B, top). By the end of initial double limb support or early midstance, the hip achieves its maximum adduction position of approximately 5°. Throughout the remainder of stance, the hip abducts to approximately 10° at toe off, then steadily adducts throughout swing in preparation for the next initial contact.

Hip rotational motions are more variable across individuals during gait (Fig. 18-3C, top). At initial contact, the hip is externally rotated approximately 5° and remains so throughout loading response and early midstance. It begins to internally rotate to within 2° of neutral rotation by the middle of terminal stance, then reverses direction and externally rotates, as the heel begins to rise, to its peak of 15° of external rotation during initial swing. As the limb swings past the opposite stance leg during mid-

swing, its hip internally rotates to within 3° of neutral, then it oscillates between 3 and 5° of external rotation during terminal swing. Except for perhaps a brief period during the middle of terminal swing, the hip never achieves an internally rotated position during gait.

CALCULATION BOX 18-1

Bootstrap Method for the Statistical Calculation of Confidence Intervals

The bootstrap method for the calculation of confidence intervals is an iterative technique whereby a population of gait data time history curves (e.g., joint angular displacement or joint moment with respect to percent of the gait cycle) is sampled with replacement. This sampling is known as a bootstrap iteration.

Each curve in the population of interest is first analyzed using a Fourier series representation, and a mean curve for the entire population is constructed by averaging the Fourier coefficients. Then, for each bootstrap iteration, a sample of curves, equal in number to the population of curves from which the sample is taken, is randomly selected with replacement and a multiplier is calculated for that iteration, b, using the following formula:

$$M[b] = \max_{0 \le t_j \le t_{max}} \frac{|\bar{F}(t_j)_{af} - \bar{F}(t_j)_{bs}|}{\sigma(t_j)_{bs}}$$

where $\bar{F}(t_j)_{af}$ is the mean of all curves at point t_j of the gait cycle, $\bar{F}(t_j)_{bs}$ is the mean of the bootstrap sample at the same point of the gait cycle, and $\sigma(t_j)_{bs}$ is the standard deviation of the bootstrap sample at the same point of the gait cycle (Lenhoff, et al., 1996; and personal communication).

After the final bootstrap iteration, the multipliers, M[b], are sorted by magnitude and an M value is selected corresponding to the desired confidence limit at each point in time. For example, if a 90% confidence interval is desired, the value for M is selected such that it is larger than 90% of the remaining M values at a given point in the gait cycle. The standard deviation of the population mean is then multiplied by the appropriate M value at each point in time of the gait cycle to obtain the confidence interval envelope.

The stability of the confidence intervals obtained by the bootstrap method increases as the population size increases and as the number of bootstrap iterations increases. The curves depicted in Figures 18-3 through 18-5 were analyzed using the bootstrap method. For more specific computational details, see Lenhoff et al. (1996).

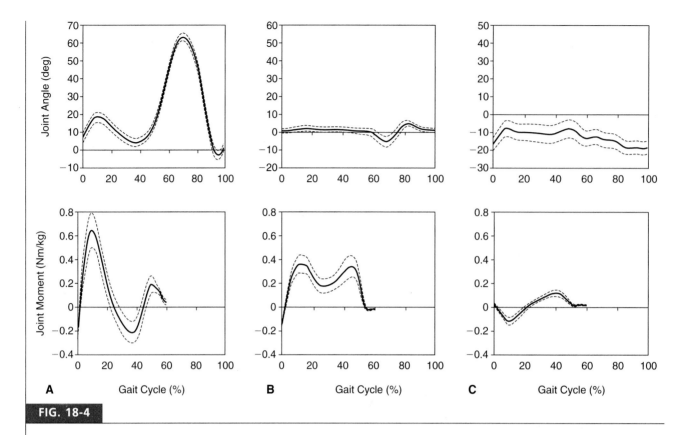

FIG. 18-4

Angular displacements and moments of the knee during level walking at freely chosen velocity among normal subjects (25 males, 4 females; 15 to 35 years of age). *Solid lines* indicate mean values (ordinate) over the course of a single stride (abscissa). *Dashed lines* indicate 90% bootstrap confidence intervals. **A** (*top*), Knee extension (<0) and flexion (>0) position; **A** (*bottom*), Flexor (<0) and extensor (>0) moment; **B** (*top*), Knee abduction (<0) and adduction (>0) position; **B** (*bottom*), Knee adductor (<0) and abductor (>0) moment; **C** (*top*), Knee external rotation (<0) and internal rotation (>0) position; **C** (*bottom*), Knee internal rotator (<0) and external rotator (>0) moment.

KNEE

At initial contact, the knee is almost fully extended, then it gradually flexes to its support phase peak flexion of approximately 20° during the early portion of midstance (Fig. 18-4*A*, top). During the latter portion of midstance, it again extends almost fully, and then flexes to approximately 40° during preswing. Immediately following toe off, the knee continues to flex to its peak flexion of 60 to 70° at midswing, then extends again in preparation for the next initial contact.

In the adduction-abduction plane of motion, the knee is quite stable during stance phase because of the presence of bony and ligamentous constraints in the relatively extended knee position. Individual skeletal alignment plays a major role in adduction-abduction movements at the knee. In the normal sample presented in Figure 18-4*B* (top), which is predominantly males (25 males/29 subjects), the knee remains in a slightly adducted (varus) position throughout stance but fluctuates only within 2 to 3° of neutral. During pre-swing and initial swing, as weight is shifted onto the opposite limb, the knee may abduct (move into valgus) as much as 10°, but it then regains its adducted position by terminal swing.

Internal and external rotation about the knee during gait, as in the case of adduction-abduction, is determined primarily by bony and ligamentous mechanisms and is variable across individuals. In addition, the placement of reference markers during optoelectronic gait analysis may introduce specific offsets into angular calculations. For example, in the data presented in Figure 18-4, there was an external rotation offset as a result of placement of the ankle markers on the medial and lateral malleoli. Such technical differences may result in slight discrepancies between the absolute value of joint angular position at the knee as reported by different laboratories, although the relative displacement range and overall patterns of motion should be similar.

In the normal sample of predominantly males (25 males/29 subjects) depicted in Figure 18-4*C* (top), the knee is maintained in an externally rotated position throughout stance and fluctuates between 10 and 20°. Rotational motions about the knee are strongly coupled with flexion-extension motions. A comparison of Figure 18-4, *A–C* (top) illustrates that during periods when the knee is flexing, it also internally rotates; whereas during periods when the knee is extending, it also externally rotates. This coupling is related to the bony morphology of the femoral condyles and tibial plateaus as well as the displacements induced in this articulation by, especially, the anterior and posterior cruciate ligaments.

ANKLE AND FOOT

Talocrural Joint

At initial contact, the ankle joint is neutral or slightly plantarflexed 3 to 5° (Fig. 18-5, top). From initial contact to loading response, the ankle plantarflexes (i.e., extends) to a maximum of 7° as the foot is lowered to the supporting surface. Throughout midstance, the ankle dorsiflexes (i.e., flexes) to a maximum of 15° as the lower leg rotates anteriorly and medially over the supporting foot. During terminal stance and pre-swing, the ankle plantarflexes to approximately 15° as body weight is transferred onto the contralateral limb. Immediately following toe off, the ankle rapidly dorsiflexes to the neutral position to attain toe clearance and then may plantarflex slightly during terminal swing in preparation for initial contact.

Subtalar Joint

The subtalar joint rotates in both stance and swing (Fig. 18-6, bottom), but it is the motion during stance that influences the weight-bearing alignment of the entire lower extremity. Like the ankle joint, the arc of motion at the subtalar joint is small compared with the knee and the hip, but it is the motion present at this joint that permits the foot to adapt to a variety of surfaces. The subtalar joint functions as a mitered hinge during gait to transmit internal and external rotation from the tibia to rotations (eversion and inversion) about the foot. The subtalar joint also transmits inversion and eversion from the foot to external and internal rotation about the tibia.

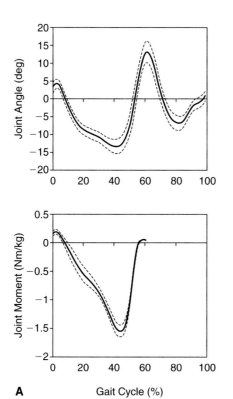

FIG. 18-5

Angular displacements and moments of the ankle during level walking at freely chosen velocity among normal subjects (25 males, 4 females; 15 to 35 years of age). *Solid lines* indicate mean values (ordinate) over the course of a single stride (abscissa). *Dashed lines* indicate 90% bootstrap confidence intervals. *Top,* ankle dorsiflexion (flexion) (<0) and plantarflexion (extension) (>0) position; *bottom,* ankle plantarflexor (extensor) (<0) and dorsiflexor (flexor) (>0) moment.

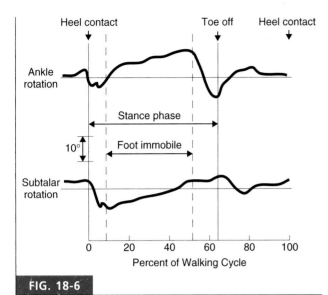

FIG. 18-6

Ankle and subtalar rotations during normal walking in a single subject. Reprinted with permission from Wright, D.G., Desai, S.M., & Henderson, W.H. (1964). Action of the subtalar and ankle-joint complex during the stance phase of walking. *J Bone Joint Surg, 46A(2),* 361–382.

During loading response, the subtalar joint begins everting until peak eversion is reached by early midstance (Fig. 18-6, bottom). Peak eversion averages 4 to 6°. This rapid eversion is followed by gradual inversion, with peak inversion achieved by preswing. The foot drifts back to neutral during swing followed by minimal inversion during the last 20% of the stride.

Subtalar eversion is one of the mechanisms for shock absorption as body weight is transferred onto the supporting foot during loading response and early midstance. Subtalar eversion is a normal passive response to initial contact with the heel. Because the body of the calcaneus is lateral to the longitudinal axis of the tibia at initial contact, as load is applied to the talus, eversion occurs at the subtalar joint. Eversion of the subtalar joint unlocks the midtarsal joint to produce a relatively flexible forefoot.

When the body's center of mass is translated more laterally as stance progresses, the calcaneal support of the talus is decreased and the calcaneus inverts. This is coupled with internal tibial rotation resulting from the shape of the ankle joint. Subtalar inversion helps to bring about stability of the foot during single limb stance (Box 18-1).

Midtarsal joint

Motion about the transverse axis of the midtarsal joint affects the longitudinal arch of the foot. Following forefoot contact during loading response, the longitudinal arch flattens during single limb support. The restoration of the arch occurs with heel rise.

Midtarsal extension is another of the mechanisms for shock absorption as body weight is lowered onto the stance limb during loading response and early midstance. This motion, which accompanies forefoot contact at the onset of midstance, occurs after subtalar eversion.

Finally, the interaction between the subtalar joint and the midtarsal joint is such that if motion at the subtalar joint is limited, then motion at the midtarsal joint will be limited. Similarly, when motion at the talonavicular joint is prevented, almost no motion is permitted at the subtalar joint.

BOX 18-1 *Joint Compensation: In- and Out-Toeing*

There is an important inter-relationship between the motion at the ankle joint and the subtalar joint during gait that permits compensation between the joints. If this compensatory mechanism fails, there is increased stress in these joints and possibly an increased incidence of secondary degenerative arthritis. For example, the degree of in-toeing (internal rotation at the ankle joint) and out-toeing (external rotation at the ankle) affects the amount of motion required at the subtalar joint. In the case of an individual with excessive out-toeing, the range of motion required at the ankle joint is decreased, and at the subtalar joint, the motion required is increased. This occurs because the greatest motion will always occur about the axis that is closest to perpendicular to the plane of progression. With out-toeing, the ankle joint axis is even less perpendicular to the plane of progression than normal. The subtalar joint axis becomes oriented more perpendicular to the plane of progression, and subsequently undergoes a larger angular excursion. The reverse occurs with increased in-toeing; the ankle joint axis becomes more perpendicular to the plane of progression and the range of motion required at the ankle joint is increased. At the subtalar joint, the motion required is then decreased. One of the compensations seen clinically for the loss of ankle range of motion is increased out-toeing, so that the motion required for walking can occur at the subtalar joint.

Forefoot and Interphalangeal Joints

At initial contact, the toes are off the ground with the metatarsophalangeal joints in 25° of extension. The toes then flex to neutral after forefoot contact at the end of loading response. A neutral position is maintained throughout midstance. During terminal stance, as the heel rises, the metatarsophalangeal joints (collectively known as the metatarsal break) extend to approximately 21° while the toes remain in contact with the ground and the hind foot lifts up into the air. This metatarsophalangeal extension places tension on the plantar aponeurosis, which in turn exerts a passive hind foot (calcaneal) inversion force. Tightening of the plantar aponeurosis also results in supination of the foot and accentuation, or heightening, of the longitudinal arch of the foot. The subsequent stiffening of the intertarsal joints from the calcaneus to the metatarsal break imparts rigidity to the entire foot and facilitates push-off.

A maximum of 58° of toe extension is reached during pre-swing. During swing, the toes flex slightly but remain in extension. Finally, there is a minimal increase in toe extension in preparation for initial contact. Little or no flexion occurs at the metatarsophalangeal joint during walking, although some may be present during athletic activities.

Little or no motion occurs at the interphalangeal joints during gait with the exception that during pre-swing, slight flexion is occasionally noted.

TRUNK AND PELVIS

At initial contact, the pelvis is tilted anteriorly approximately 7° (Fig. 18-7A, bottom), rotated for-

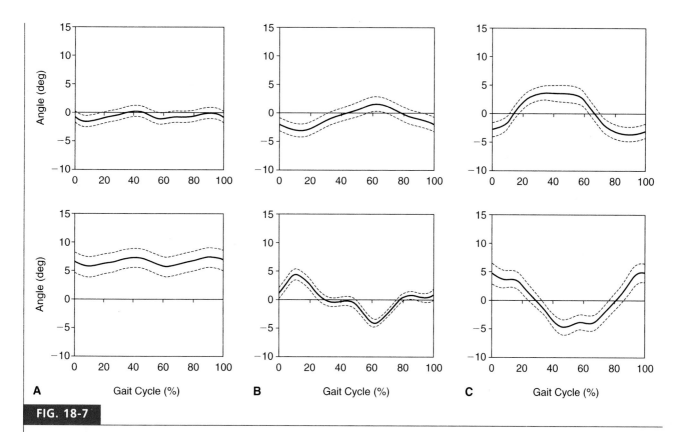

FIG. 18-7

Angular rotation of the trunk and pelvis during level walking at freely chosen velocity among normal subjects (25 males, 4 females; 15 to 35 years of age). *Solid lines* indicate mean values (ordinate) over the course of a single stride (abscissa). *Dashed lines* indicate 90% bootstrap confidence intervals. **A** (*top*), Trunk posterior (< 0) and anterior (>0) lean; **A** (*bottom*), Pelvis posterior (<0) and anterior (>0) tilt; **B** (*top*), Trunk downward (< 0) and upward (>0) tilt with respect to the stance limb; **B** (*bottom*), Pelvis downward (<0) and upward (>0) tilt with respect to the stance limb; **C** (*top*), Trunk backward (< 0) and forward (>0) rotation with respect to the stance limb; **C** (*bottom*), Pelvis backward (<0) and forward (>0) rotation with respect to the stance limb.

ward approximately 5° (Fig. 18-7C, bottom), and is level from right to left. During the loading response, the pelvis tilts upward on the stance limb side to a maximum of 5°, then it regains neutral tilt at the next initial contact of the swinging limb (Fig. 18-7B, bottom). During stance phase, the pelvis rotates backward on the stance limb side and tilts anteriorly (bottom of Fig. 18-7 C & B, respectively). The total excursion for anteroposterior tilt is approximately 5°; for lateral tilting, approximately 10°; and for forward and backward rotation, approximately 10°.

Trunk motion during gait is opposite in direction, or out of phase, to the motions of the pelvis (Fig. 18-7, A–C, top). For example, at initial contact, the trunk is rotated backward approximately 3° while the pelvis is rotated forward approximately 5°. The amplitudes of the angular displacements of the trunk segment as reflected in the movement of the shoulder girdle are only slightly attenuated in comparison with the pelvic movements, as can be easily appreciated by comparing the top (trunk) to bottom (pelvis) plots in Figure 18-7.

CENTER OF MASS

The body's center of mass remains located within the pelvis anterior to the sacrum throughout the gait cycle. It undergoes sinusoidal displacements in all three planes with peak to peak excursions of approximately

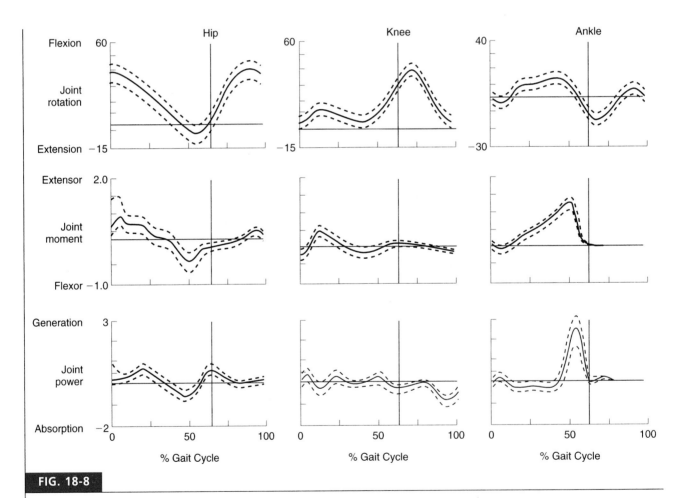

FIG. 18-8

Joint power profiles in watts/kg of body weight (bottom row) of the hip (left column), knee (middle column), and ankle (right column) for flexion-extension motions (top row) during level walking. The middle row shows the joint moments in Nm/kg body weight. Joint motions are in degrees. *Reprinted with permission from Gage, J.R. (1991).* Gait Analysis in Cerebral Palsy *(p. 31). London: Mac Keith Press.*

3 cm in the vertical direction, 4 cm in the lateral direction, and 2 cm in the anteroposterior direction.

Segmental Kinetics

In gait analysis, the human body is modeled as a mechanical system of anatomical segments linked together by the joints. Kinetic computations in gait analysis make use of angular kinematic and force data.

JOINT MOMENTS

A moment is defined as the vector cross-product of a force vector and the perpendicular distance of the joint center from the line of action of that force vector. Moments are frequently expressed in Nm per kg of body weight in gait analysis (i.e., normalized to body weight). The effect of moments is to cause a tendency for joint rotation. In this discussion, the term moment will refer to the internal moment generated about the joint in question. A knee extensor moment, for example, refers to the internal moment of force that tends to rotate the knee joint in the direction of extension and occurs when the line of action of the tibiofemoral reaction force vector passes posteriorly to the axis of knee flexion-extension (i.e., when the external moment tends to cause knee flexion). Activation by the knee extensors is required to counterbalance the tendency for knee flexion caused by the external flexion moment. Internal moments are assumed to be generated by the muscles, soft tissues, and joint contact forces acting on the joint and are inferred from inverse dynamics calculations of external moments. As such, the internal moment is an expression of the net effect of internal active and passive structures and is strictly accurate in the case where a muscle group is contracting unopposed by antagonist activation. At certain periods during normal gait and for longer periods during gait in many pathological conditions, agonist-antagonist coactivation may be present. In such cases, reported values for net internal moments will underestimate the actual muscular forces occurring. However, this terminology is prevalent in the literature and useful for the calculation of other kinetic variables. Plots of the internal moments occurring about the hip, knee, and ankle joints during level walking in healthy adults are depicted in Figures 18-3 through 18-5 and 18-8.

Hip

At initial contact, there is an extensor moment about the hip that fluctuates at first, then stabilizes at approximately 5 Nm/kg (Fig. 18-3A, bottom). This extensor moment persists through early midstance and then reverses to a flexor moment in the latter third of midstance. For the remainder of stance, there is a hip flexor moment that peaks at approximately 1 Nm/kg near the end of terminal stance.

Although the hip moment about the anteroposterior axis is adductor at initial contact (Fig. 18-3B, bottom), it rapidly reverses to an abductor moment of approximately 0.7 Nm/kg during loading response. As the opposite limb swings near the midline of the body during midstance, the stance limb hip abductor moment decreases to approximately 0.4 Nm/kg, but it once again increases to 0.7 Nm/kg during terminal stance (Box 18-2).

BOX 18-2 | *Gait Deviations*

Loss of hip abductor strength or pain of the coxofemoral joint as a result of arthritic degeneration results in profound gait deviations. One possible pathological gait pattern is Trendelenburg gait, which results from the failure of the hip abductors to produce a sufficient abductor moment during loading response and terminal stance. This pattern is easily observed as a lateral drop of the pelvis on the side opposite the weakness during stance on the weak side. Another way of describing this pattern is excessive adduction of the weak hip during stance phase.

Another pathological gait pattern seen with abductor weakness or coxofemoral pain is the lateral lurch. In this pattern, the trunk is displaced toward the affected stance limb during loading response, where it remains throughout terminal stance. This is observed as excessive lateral displacement of the trunk toward the affected side. The result of this gait deviation is to reduce the required hip abductor moment by displacing the body's center of mass closer to the hip adduction-abduction rotation axis.

Both of these gait deviations effectively reduce compression across the coxofemoral joint by reducing contraction force of the hip abductors, thereby alleviating joint pain. The Trendelenburg pattern is a simple mechanical result of hip abductor weakness. The lateral lurch is a compensation for hip abductor weakness.

By the end of loading response, the peak hip external rotator moment of approximately 0.18 Nm/kg is achieved (Fig. 18-3C, bottom). The external rotator moment gradually decreases until the middle of terminal stance. Throughout the remainder of terminal stance and pre-swing, a slight hip internal rotator moment occurs.

Knee

At initial contact, there is a small knee flexor moment (Fig. 18-4A, bottom). During early midstance, an extensor moment peak of approximately 0.6 Nm/kg occurs. During terminal stance, a second low amplitude extensor moment of 0.2 Nm/kg occurs (Case Study 18-1).

As was the case with adduction-abduction about the knee, knee adduction-abduction moments are controlled primarily through bone and soft tissue constraints. Therefore, the terminology for these moments at the knee refers to passive restraints, not to muscular control.

An abductor moment persists about the knee throughout stance with two peaks of approximately 0.4 Nm/kg during loading response and ter-

---

CASE STUDY 18-1

Gait Adaptations in an Individual With Anterior Cruciate Ligament Deficiency

Some individuals with anterior cruciate ligament (ACL) deficiency demonstrate a "quadriceps avoidance" gait pattern associated with reduction of the stance phase knee extensor moment by as much as 140% (Andriacchi & Birac, 1993). The angular motion and moment data plotted below show just such a clinical example.

The subject of this analysis was a 60-year-old male who had sustained a partial tear of the right ACL approximately 10 years prior to the gait analysis. The injury was not surgically repaired. The subject had minor complaints of functional deficits, primarily on descending stairs.

The flexion-extension motion plot (average of three trials) of the affected right knee shows a flattening and a reduction of the support phase peak knee flexion. The knee is main-

tained in 10 to 15° of flexion throughout midstance. Associated with this motion adaptation is a marked decrease of the knee extensor moment during the early stance phase (see corresponding right knee moment plot).

This adaptation is hypothesized to prevent unrestrained anterior translation of the tibia by the patellar tendon through reduction in quadriceps activation. EMG analysis of the quadriceps muscles in studies of ACL deficiency is consistent with this hypothesis. This effective behavioral mechanism to reduce mechanical instability of the knee seems to be subconscious on the part of injured subjects. However, it may be possible to train individuals to use this adaptation in a conservative management program for ACL injury (Andriacchi, 1993).

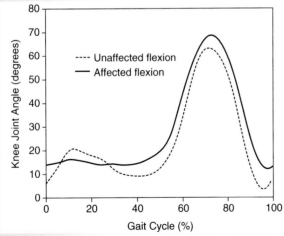
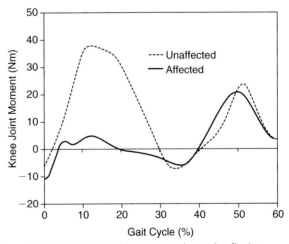

Case Study Figure 18-1-1. Effect of anterior cruciate ligament injury on knee motion and moments about the flexion-extension axis. Data were obtained during three trials of walking at freely chosen velocity and averaged. The figure (left) shows the difference between the ACL-deficient knee (affected) and unaffected knee flexion angles. The figure (right) shows the corresponding knee moments with values greater than zero representing knee extensor moments and values less than zero representing knee flexor moments.

minal stance (Fig. 18-4*B*, bottom). During midstance, the knee abductor moment decreases to approximately 0.2 Nm/kg. In individuals who achieve abduction (valgus) positions of the knee, the moment profile may be shifted toward adductor moments, and midstance adductor moments may occur.

A knee internal rotator moment peak of 0.18 Nm/kg occurs at the transition between loading response and midstance. The knee rotation moment then reverses direction during the latter portion of midstance, reaching an external rotator moment peak of approximately 0.15 Nm/kg during terminal stance.

Ankle

Immediately after initial contact, there is a slight dorsiflexor (i.e., flexor) moment of approximately 0.2 Nm/kg about the ankle that rapidly reverses to a plantarflexor (i.e., extensor) moment for the remainder of stance (Fig. 18-5, bottom). The plantarflexor moment peak is approximately 1.6 Nm/kg at 45% of the stride, or the latter portion of terminal stance.

JOINT POWER

Joint power is defined as the product of joint angular velocity and the corresponding internal moment at a given point in time and is expressed in watts/kg of body weight. It fluctuates continuously throughout the gait cycle and can be either negative or positive in value. Joint power indicates the generation or absorption of mechanical energy by muscle groups and other soft tissues. Profiles for joint power about the flexion-extension axes during level walking in healthy adults are depicted in Figure 18-8.

Hip

From initial contact through early midstance, the concentrically contracting hip extensors generate power to a peak of approximately 1 watt/kg (Fig. 18-8, bottom left). From midstance to terminal stance, power absorption by the eccentrically contracting hip flexors controls the backward acceleration of the thigh segment until approximately 50% of the stride. From pre-swing to mid-swing, power generation by the concentrically contracting hip flexors acts to pull off the swinging limb.

Knee

During loading response, power absorption by the eccentrically contracting quadriceps controls knee flexion (Fig. 18-8, bottom-middle). During early midstance, power generation by the concentrically contracting quadriceps extends the knee while the contralateral limb is engaged in swing. During pre-swing, power absorption by the eccentrically contracting quadriceps controls knee flexion while the stance limb unloads in preparation for swing and the transfer of body weight onto the contralateral limb. During terminal swing, power absorption by the eccentrically contracting hamstrings controls the forward acceleration of the swinging thigh, leg, and foot segments.

Ankle

During midstance, power absorption by the eccentrically contracting plantarflexors controls the tibia as it rotates over the stationary foot (Fig. 18-8, bottom right). During pre-swing, a high-magnitude power generation peak of 2 to 3 watts/kg by the concentrically contracting plantarflexors represents approximately two thirds of the total energy generated during walking and is believed to contribute significantly to propulsion in gait.

WORK AND ENERGY TRANSFER

Work is defined as the integral of power with respect to time and is expressed in Joules/kg of body weight. Work is an estimate of the flow of mechanical energy from one body segment to another and is used to determine overall mechanical energy efficiency during gait. When work is positive in value, the internal moment and joint angular velocity are acting in the same direction, a concentric muscle contraction is indicated, and mechanical energy is being generated. When work is negative in value, the internal moment and joint angular velocity are acting in opposite directions, an eccentric contraction is indicated, and mechanical energy is being absorbed. During periods of energy generation, the muscle is working on the limbs to produce movement. During periods of energy absorption, the limbs are working on the muscles, which must then contract to resist the tendency for muscle elongation.

Muscular Control

Muscle activation patterns are also cyclic during gait (Figs. 18-9 through 18-11). Muscle contraction type varies between the eccentric control of joint angular accelerations, such as in hamstrings activation during terminal swing, and the concentric initiation of movement, such as in tibialis anterior activation in pre-swing. In normal individuals, agonist-antagonist coactivation is of relatively short duration and occurs during periods of kinematic transition (e.g., terminal swing to initial contact). The presence of prolonged or out-of-phase agonist-antagonist coactivation during gait in individuals with pathology may indicate skeletal instability as well as motor control deficiencies.

HIP

During early stance phase, the hip extensors act concentrically while the hip abductors stabilize the lateral aspect of the coxofemoral joint (Fig. 18-9). The lower fibers of the gluteus maximus show increasing activation intensity from initial contact to the middle of loading response that tapers off by the end loading response. The upper fibers of the gluteus maximus and the gluteus medius (and probably the gluteus minimus) increase activation intensity through loading response and taper off by the end of midstance. The posterior fibers of the tensor fascia lata are moderately activated at the onset of loading response while the anterior fibers become activated later and persist into terminal stance.

During pre-swing and initial to mid-swing, the hip flexors act to advance the limb, particularly when walking velocity is changing. The adductor longus is activated earliest in terminal stance and persists the longest to early mid-swing. The rectus femoris is the second hip flexor activated during pre-swing and remains activated a short time into early initial swing. The iliacus, sartorius, and gracilis have short periods of activation predominantly during initial swing.

The hip adductors are activated during transitions between stance and swing, as are the hamstring muscle group. This activation pattern can be interpreted as the dynamic control of the swinging

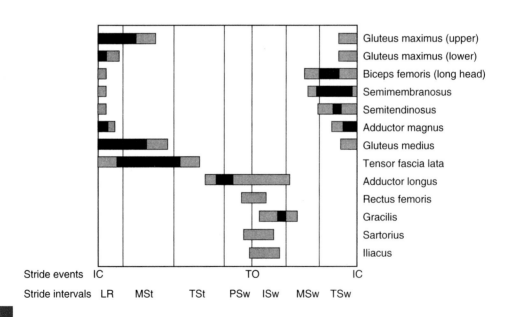

FIG. 18-9

Phasic pattern of electromyographic (EMG) activity of the muscles of the hip during level walking in healthy adults. Gray regions represent activation below 20% of maximum voluntary contraction. Black regions represent activation above 20% of maximum voluntary contraction. *IC*, initial contact; *TO*, toe off; *LR*, loading response; *MSt*, midstance; *TSt*, terminal stance; *PSw*, pre-swing; *ISw*, initial swing; *MSw*, midswing; and *TSw*, terminal swing. *Adapted with permission from Perry, J. (1992). Gait Analysis: Normal and Pathological Function. Thorofare, NJ: SLACK Incorporated.*

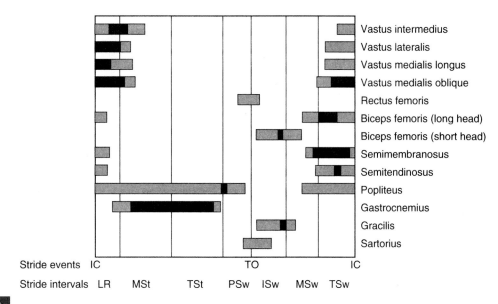

| Stride events | IC | | | TO | | | IC |
| Stride intervals | LR | MSt | TSt | PSw | ISw | MSw | TSw |

FIG. 18-10

Phasic pattern of electromyographic (EMG) activity of the muscles of the knee during level walking in healthy adults. Gray regions represent activation below 20% of maximum voluntary contraction. Black regions represent activation above 20% of maximum voluntary contraction. *IC,* initial con-

tact; *TO,* toe off; *LR,* loading response; *MSt,* midstance; *TSt,* terminal stance; *PSw,* pre-swing; *ISw,* initial swing; *MSw,* mid-swing; and *TSw,* terminal swing. *Adapted with permission from Perry, J. (1992). Gait Analysis: Normal and Pathological Function. Thorofare, NJ: SLACK.*

limb that is tending to flex and abduct at the hip. The function of the muscles during such periods is to control the acceleration of the rotating joints to ensure the precise placement of the foot on the support surface in anticipation of the upcoming stance phase. This explains the hamstrings and adductor magnus activity during terminal swing.

KNEE

During stance phase, the quadriceps muscle group (vasti) is relied on to control the tendency for knee flexion collapse with weight acceptance and single limb support (Fig. 18-10). This muscle group is activated during terminal swing and then acts eccentrically during weight acceptance as the knee rotates from the fully extended position at initial contact to its peak support phase flexion of approximately 20° during loading response. Thereafter, the quadriceps act concentrically to extend the knee through early midstance as the body's center of mass is raised vertically over the supporting limb and the anterior orientation of the ground reaction force vector precludes the need for further muscular control of knee flexion.

Most of the hamstrings muscles are activated in late mid-swing or terminal swing. Their function at the knee is probably to control the angular acceleration into knee extension. This is consistent with their presumed action at the hip, or the control of hip flexion in preparation for the upcoming stance phase. The short head of the biceps femoris is activated earlier than are the other hamstrings muscles in early mid-swing and probably assists in flexing the knee for foot clearance.

The gracilis and sartorius muscles also may contribute to swing phase knee flexion when they are activated during late pre-swing, initial swing, and early mid-swing. However, these muscles may very well be acting as primary hip flexors during this period.

ANKLE AND FOOT
Talocrural Joint

From EMG studies on the muscles that cross the ankle, the dorsiflexor muscles are shown to be firing concentrically during swing to allow for foot clearance and eccentrically during loading response to control the placement of the foot by ankle plantarflexion (Fig. 18-11). The plantarflexors are consistently firing eccentrically during stance to control

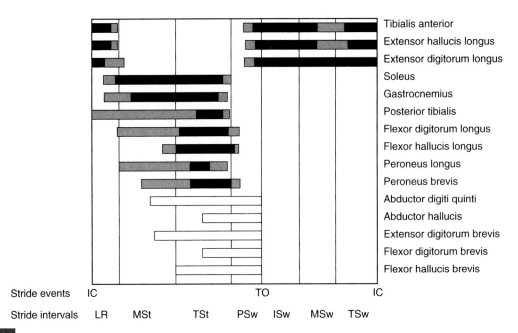

| Stride events | IC | | | TO | | | IC |
| Stride intervals | LR | MSt | TSt | PSw | ISw | MSw | TSw |

FIG. 18-11

Phasic pattern of electromyographic (EMG) activity of the muscles of the ankle and foot during level walking in healthy adults. Gray regions represent activation below 20% of maximum voluntary contraction. Black regions represent activation above 20% of maximum voluntary contraction. *White bars* for the intrinsic muscles of the foot indicate phasic data only for which relative intensity as a percent of maximum voluntary contraction is not shown. *IC,* initial contact; *TO,* toe off; *LR,* loading response; *MSt,* midstance; *TSt,* terminal stance; *PSw,* pre-swing; *ISw,* initial swing; *MSw,* mid-swing; and *TSw,* terminal swing. *Adapted with permission from Perry, J. (1992).* Gait Analysis: Normal and Pathological Function. *Thorofare, NJ: SLACK Incorporated.*

the advancement of the tibia over the foot, to stabilize the knee, and concentrically to assist push-off.

The onset of muscle activity in the dorsiflexors begins just prior to foot-off during pre-swing. Winter and Yak (1987) reported that these muscles remain active throughout swing and loading response with peak electrical activity seen in the first 15% of the gait cycle during weight acceptance, when they must assist in controlling the fall of the center of mass (Fig. 18-11). They are virtually silent during mid- and terminal stance (Box 18-3).

The soleus and the medial head of the gastrocnemius begin activation at approximately 10% of the gait cycle, as single limb support begins (Fig. 18-11). They continue firing throughout the stance phase until pre-swing, when single limb support ends and the opposite foot makes contact with the ground. The lateral head of the gastrocnemius may not begin activation until midstance. During midstance, the plantarflexors eccentrically contract to restrain forward motion of the tibia. During terminal stance, as the heel begins to rise, the gastrocnemius contin-

BOX 18-3 Timing Effects on Gait Patterns

The peak electrical activity of the dorsiflexors corresponds to a high demand on the pretibial muscles as body weight is transferred onto the supporting foot. These muscles fire eccentrically to decelerate the rate of ankle plantarflexion. If there is inappropriate timing or insufficient force of contraction in the pretibial muscles, a drop-foot or foot-slap gait pattern may be present. In addition, restrained ankle plantarflexion provides some shock absorption during the loading response. During swing, the tibialis anterior and the toe extensors function to dorsiflex the foot for toe clearance. Loss of normal function in the pretibial muscle during swing frequently results in increased knee and hip flexion, or a steppage gait pattern.

ues to contract to begin active ankle plantarflexion. During this phase, they provide a stable tibia over which the femur may advance. Peak electrical activity is seen at 50% of the gait cycle.

Although both the soleus and gastrocnemius muscles share a common insertion, the role of the soleus is somewhat different from that of the gastrocnemius because of the soleus' origin on the tibia. The soleus, as a one-joint muscle, provides a direct link between the tibia and the calcaneus and is thought to be the dominant decelerating plantarflexion force. The gastrocnemius, as a two-joint muscle, plays a direct role in knee flexion during midstance (Fig. 18-10).

The remaining five posterior muscles are smaller in size and as perimalleolar muscles lie closer to the ankle joint (Fig. 18-11). These five muscles are tibialis posterior, flexor hallucis longus, flexor digitorum longus, peroneus longus, and peroneus brevis. These muscles play a greater role at the subtalar joint and the foot than at the ankle but still create a plantarflexion force at the ankle joint.

The tibialis posterior begins firing at initial contact and remains active through single limb stance until opposite initial contact. The flexor digitorum longus begins firing next at opposite toe off and also continues until opposite initial contact. The flexor hallucis longus is active from 25% of the gait cycle into pre-swing. Peroneus brevis and longus activity begins early in stance and continues into terminal stance or pre-swing. Note that the activity in these muscles is subject to considerable variation across individuals.

The posterior calf muscles function as a group and cease functioning by 50% of the gait cycle when opposite initial contact has occurred. The continuation of plantarflexion past this point probably serves to balance the body because the opposite foot has already accepted the body's weight. In a small group of healthy adults, Sutherland et al. (1980) used a nerve block to the tibial nerve to further describe the role of the ankle plantarflexors, particularly the gastrocnemius and soleus during gait. They concluded that these muscles did not serve as a propulsion mechanism during pre-swing. Instead, they concluded that these muscles should be thought of as maintaining forward progression, step length, and gait symmetry. If the plantarflexors do not function normally, an increase in ankle dorsiflexion is seen with a shortened step by the swinging limb. In addition, the swinging limb strikes the ground prematurely as a result of the lack of restraint of the tibial movement of the stance limb.

In summary, during the first arc of plantarflexion following initial contact, the dorsiflexors are firing eccentrically to decelerate the rate of plantarflexion and footfall onto the ground. During the first arc of dorsiflexion, the plantarflexors are firing eccentrically to control the rate of dorsiflexion and tibial progression over the stationary foot. During the second arc of plantarflexion, just prior to weight transfer onto the opposite limb, the plantarflexors are firing to maintain walking velocity and step length. Finally, during the last arc of motion, dorsiflexion during swing, the dorsiflexors are firing concentrically to allow foot clearance.

Subtalar Joint

As the foot makes contact with the floor, subtalar eversion occurs as a shock-absorbing mechanism. The inverters fire to decelerate this eversion (Fig. 18-11). The tibialis anterior acts to restrain the subtalar joint during loading response. With its greatest activity seen during loading response, the tibialis anterior is quiet by midstance.

Although the activation patterns of the tibialis posterior have been reported with various patterns of activity by different investigators, there is agreement that it is a stance phase muscle. It becomes active during loading response and remains active throughout stance until early pre-swing. Perry (1992) proposed that the activation during loading response provides early subtalar control. In addition, the variability of activity in this muscle may be indicative of its function as a reserve force to supplement insufficient varus control by the ankle muscles.

Soleus activity is seen during midstance with progressively increasing activity in terminal stance. Despite its major function as an ankle plantarflexor, this muscle also has considerable inversion leverage, especially as a result of its large cross-sectional area. By pre-swing there is a rapid decline in activity, and the muscle remains quiet during swing. The long toe flexors are the last inverters to be activated. The flexor digitorum longus and the flexor hallucis longus begin activation during midstance and cease firing during pre-swing.

The muscles that are responsible for eversion at the subtalar joint are the extensor digitorum longus, peroneus tertius, peroneus longus, and peroneus brevis. The first two lie anterior to the subtalar joint axis, while the last two lie posterior to the subtalar joint axis. The extensor digitorum longus is active during loading response and quiet with the onset of midstance. Little information is available about the firing of the peroneus tertius, but Perry (1992) reports similar timing as the extensor digitorum longus.

The peroneus longus and brevis initiate activity during forefoot loading and demonstrate their peak activity during terminal stance. Both the timing and intensity of the EMG signals in the peroneus brevis and longus are closely coordinated. Activity in these muscles ceases by the middle of pre-swing. The peroneus longus has peak electrical activity at 50% of the gait cycle during push-off.

Midtarsal Joint

The midtarsal joint is supported primarily by the tibialis posterior. Because the activity of the long toe flexors and the lateral plantar intrinsic muscles begins before the toes flex, these muscles may well contribute to the support of the midtarsal joint.

Forefoot and Interphalangeal Joints

The flexor digitorum longus and the flexor hallucis longus begin activation during midstance and cease firing during pre-swing. These muscles stabilize the metatarsophalangeal joints and add toe support to supplement forefoot support. The intrinsic muscles of the forefoot and interphalangeal joints include the abductor hallucis, adductor hallucis, flexor digitorum brevis, flexor hallucis brevis, and abductor digiti quinti. These muscles become active at approximately 20 to 30% of the walking cycle and cease when the foot leaves the ground. These muscles aid in the stabilization of the longitudinal arch and of the toes at the metatarsophalangeal joint.

Although the kinematics, kinetics, and muscular control of the major joints have been presented separately, they are functionally inter-related during gait. The musculoskeletal system must undergo highly integrated, precisely coordinated actions in both timing and amplitude for efficient locomotion to occur. This requires not only an intact musculoskeletal system, or physical plant, but also a functioning nervous system, or controller. The nervous system must be able to instantaneously assess pertinent aspects of the external and internal environments to act or respond appropriately to a variety of functional contexts. Motion limitations or other pathology of any participating joint will have a subsequent effect on all other participating joints. It is the complex integration of anatomy, biomechanics, and muscular control that permits normal walking.

Summary

1 Motion about the hip joint during gait occurs in all three planes: flexion-extension, adduction-abduction, and internal-external rotation. Flexion-extension is the primary motion occurring about the knee joint during gait, although varus-valgus and rotational motions are present to a lesser extent.

2 Because of its bony morphology, the talocrural joint undergoes only plantarflexion and dorsiflexion during gait. Subtalar, midtarsal, and phalangeal motion further assist in providing adaptation to the support surface as well as rigidity for propulsion.

3 The upper body, including the pelvis and trunk, undergoes sinusoidal displacements in all three cardinal planes. The trunk and pelvis rotate in opposite directions while the head usually remains stable. The swinging of the arms involves shoulder flexion-extension and rotation, elbow flexion-extension, and forearm pronation-supination.

4 The gait cycle, or stride, is defined as the occurrence of an event on one lower limb until the next occurrence of the same event on the same lower limb. It is most typically demarcated by sequential ipsilateral initial contact. Stance phase occupies 60% of the stride and is divided into six events or periods: initial contact, loading response, midstance, terminal stance, pre-swing, and toe off. Swing phase occupies 40% of the stride and is divided into periods: initial swing, mid-swing, and terminal swing.

5 Internal joint moments indicate the net moment of force generated by muscles, bones, and passive soft tissues that counteract the tendency for joint rotation caused by gravity.

6 Joint power is the product of joint angular velocity and the corresponding internal moment at a given point in time. It indicates the generation or absorption of mechanical energy by muscle groups and other soft tissues.

7 Coactivation of agonist-antagonist muscle groups usually occurs during periods of kinematic transition when a joint may be reversing the direction of rotation.

8 Motion limitations or disorders of motor control affecting any of the lower limb segments will potentially alter the patterns of movement and motor control at all other joints during gait.

REFERENCES

Andriacchi, T.P. & Birac, D. (1993). Functional testing in the anterior cruciate ligament-deficient knee. *Clin Orthop Rel Res, 288*(March), 40–47.

Barr, A.E. (1998). Gait analysis. In J. Spivak & J. Zuckerman (Eds.), *Orthopaedics—A Comprehensive Study Guide.* New York: McGraw-Hill.

Craik, R.L. & Oatis, C.A. (1995). *Gait Analysis: Theory and Application.* St. Louis: Mosby.

Gage, J.R. (1991). *Gait Analysis in Cerebral Palsy.* London: Mac Keith Press.

Lenhoff, M.W., Santner, T.J., Otis, J.C., et al. (1996). Bootstrap simultaneous prediction and confidence intervals for gait data. *Gait Post, 4*(2), 172.

Perry, J. (1992). *Gait Analysis: Normal and Pathological Function.* Thorofare, NJ: SLACK Incorporated.

Sutherland, D.H., Cooper, L., & Daniel, D. (1980). The role of the ankle plantarflexors in normal walking. *J Bone Joint Surg, 62A*(3), 354–363.

Whittle, M.W. (1991). *Gait Analysis: An Introduction.* Oxford: Butterworth-Heinemann.

Winter, D.A. & Yak, H.J. (1987). EMG profiles during normal human walking: Stride-to-stride and inter-subject variability. *Electronencephalogr Clin Neurophysiol, 67,* 402–411.

Wright, D.G., Desai, S.M., & Henderson, W.H. (1964). Action of the subtalar and ankle-joint complex during the stance phase of walking. *J Bone Joint Surg, 46A*(2), 361–382.

Index

Page numbers in *italics* denote figures; those followed by a *t* denote tables.